VOLUME ONE HUNDRED AND SEVENTY ONE

ADVANCES IN IMMUNOLOGY

Microglial Advances in Neurodegenerative Diseases

ASSOCIATE EDITORS

Fritz Melchers†

University of Basel, Basel, Switzerland

Chen Dong

Shanghai Jiaotong University School of Medicine,
Tsinghua University School of Medicine

Hao Wu

Boston Children's Hospital, Harvard Medical School

† Deceased

VOLUME ONE HUNDRED AND SEVENTY ONE

ADVANCES IN IMMUNOLOGY

Microglial Advances in Neurodegenerative Diseases

Edited by

SUBASHCHANDRABOSE CHINNATHAMBI

Department of Neurochemistry, National Institute of Mental Health and Neuro Sciences Hospital (NIMHANS), Institute of National Importance, Bangalore, Karnataka, India

ELSEVIER

ACADEMIC PRESS
An imprint of Elsevier

Academic Press is an imprint of Elsevier
125 London Wall, London, EC2Y 5AS, United Kingdom
50 Hampshire Street, 5th Floor, Cambridge, MA 02139, United States

First edition 2026

ISBN: 978-0-443-47054-7
ISSN: 0065-2776

For information on all Academic Press publications
visit our website at https://www.elsevier.com/books-and-journals

Publisher: Zoe Kruze
Acquisitions Editor: Leticia Lima
Editorial Project Manager: Palash Sharma
Production Project Manager: James Selvam
Cover Designer: Muthukumaran Thangaraj

Typeset by MPS Limited, India

Contents

Contributors

Yukti
Department of Biochemistry, University of Delhi South Campus, Dhaula Kuan, New Delhi, India

Anusree Adityan
Department of Neurochemistry, National Institute of Mental Health and Neuro Sciences Hospital (NIMHANS), Institute of National Importance, Bangalore, Karnataka, India

Lucas H.M. Alfredo
Research Laboratory in bionanomaterials, LPbio, Department of Chemistry, Federal University of Viçosa, Viçosa, MG; National Institute of Science and Technology of Bioanalytics-Lauro Kubota (INCTBio-LK), Campinas, SP, Brazil

Vaishnavi Ananathanarayana
Department of Neurochemistry, National Institute of Mental Health and Neuro Sciences Hospital (NIMHANS), Institute of National Importance, Bangalore, Karnataka, India

Wesley C.P. Aquino
Research Laboratory in bionanomaterials, LPbio, Department of Chemistry, Federal University of Viçosa, Viçosa, MG; National Institute of Science and Technology of Bioanalytics-Lauro Kubota (INCTBio-LK), Campinas, SP, Brazil

Zabin Bagewadi
Department of Biotechnology, KLE Technological University, Vidyanagar, Hubballi, Karnataka, India

Neha P. Bochageri
School of Chemical Engineering, The University of Adelaide, Adelaide, South Australia, Australia

Anastasia Bougea
Department of Neurology, Medical School National and Kapodistrian University of Athens, Athens, Greece

Madhura Chandrashekar
Department of Neurochemistry, National Institute of Mental Health and Neuro Sciences Hospital (NIMHANS), Institute of National Importance, Bangalore, Karnataka, India

Hariharakrishnan Chidamabram
Department of Neurochemistry, National Institute of Mental Health and Neuro Sciences Hospital (NIMHANS), Institute of National Importance, Bangalore, Karnataka, India

Subashchandrabose Chinnathambi
Department of Neurochemistry, National Institute of Mental Health and Neuro Sciences Hospital (NIMHANS), Institute of National Importance, Bangalore, Karnataka, India

Venkata Chaitanya Chirumamilla
The Zickler Family Prenatal Pediatrics Institute, Children's National Hospital, Washington, DC, United States

Indrani Datta
Department of Biophysics, National Institute of Mental Health and Neurosciences, Institute of National Importance, Bengaluru, Karnataka, India

Jemmyson R. de Jesus
Research Laboratory in bionanomaterials, LPbio, Department of Chemistry, Federal University of Viçosa, Viçosa, MG; National Institute of Science and Technology of Bioanalytics-Lauro Kubota (INCTBio-LK), Campinas, SP, Brazil

Joshua De Leon
Department of Foundations of Medicine, NYU Grossman Long Island School of Medicine, Mineola, NY, United States

Manuel Debasa-Mouce
NeuroAging Group (NEURAL), Clinical Neurosciences Research Laboratory (LINC), Health Research Institute of Santiago de Compostela (IDIS), Santiago de Compostela, Spain

Ateendra Kumar Dubey
Department of Biochemistry, University of Delhi South Campus, Dhaula Kuan, New Delhi, India

Shelly Gulkarov
Department of Medicine, NYU Grossman Long Island School of Medicine, Mineola, NY, United States

Claudia Z. Han
Department of Pathology and Immunology; Brain Immunology and Glia (BIG) Center, Washington University in St. Louis School of Medicine, St. Louis, MO, United States

Hao Huang
Department of Medicine, University Medical Center Hamburg-Eppendorf (UKE), Hamburg, Germany; Institute of Neuroimmunology and Multiple Sclerosis, University Medical Center Hamburg-Eppendorf (UKE), Hamburg, Germany

Gouri H. Illanad
Department of Biotechnology, KLE Technological University, Vidyanagar, Hubballi, Karnataka, India

Hem Chandra Jha
Mehta Family School of Biosciences and Biomedical Engineering, Indian Institute of Technology, Indore, Madhya Pradesh, India

Sushmita Jha
Department of Bioscience and Bioengineering, Indian Institute of Technology, Jodhpur, India

Himanshi Jindal
Mehta Family School of Biosciences and Biomedical Engineering, Indian Institute of Technology, Indore, Madhya Pradesh, India

Rachel J. Johnston
Department of Pathology and Immunology; Brain Immunology and Glia (BIG) Center, Washington University in St. Louis School of Medicine, St. Louis, MO, United States

Deena Krishnan
Department of Human Genetics and Molecular Biology, Bharathiar University, Coimbatore, Tamil Nadu, India

Yangchen Li
Department of Pathology and Immunology; Brain Immunology and Glia (BIG) Center, Washington University in St. Louis School of Medicine, St. Louis, MO, United States

Elvira Mass
Developmental Biology of the Immune System, Life and Medical Sciences (LIMES) Institute, University of Bonn, Bonn, Germany

Amit Mishra
Cellular and Molecular Neurobiology Unit, Indian Institute of Technology Jodhpur, Jodhpur, Rajasthan, India

Srija Mukherjee
Mehta Family School of Biosciences and Biomedical Engineering, Indian Institute of Technology, Indore, Madhya Pradesh, India

Ashitha Siddappa Niranjana Murthy
Department of Psychiatry, National Institute of Mental Health, and Neuroscience (NIMHANS), Centre for Brain and Mind, Bengaluru, India

Muthuraman Muthuraman
Department of Neurology, University Hospital Würzburg, Würzburg; Institute of Computer Science, University Augsburg, Augsburg, Germany

Alberto Ouro
NeuroAging Group (NEURAL), Clinical Neurosciences Research Laboratory (LINC), Health Research Institute of Santiago de Compostela (IDIS), Santiago de Compostela; de Investigación Biomédica en Red en Enfermedades Neurodegenerativas (CIBERNED), Instituto de Salud Carlos III, Madrid, Spain

Nicole A. Pagán Torres
Department of Pathology and Immunology; Brain Immunology and Glia (BIG) Center, Washington University in St. Louis School of Medicine, St. Louis, MO, United States

Marcos V.S. Pereira
Research Laboratory in bionanomaterials, LPbio, Department of Chemistry, Federal University of Viçosa, Viçosa, MG; National Institute of Science and Technology of Bioanalytics-Lauro Kubota (INCTBio-LK), Campinas, SP, Brazil

Vijay Kumar Prajapati
Department of Biochemistry, University of Delhi South Campus, Dhaula Kuan, New Delhi, India

Allison B. Reiss
Department of Foundations of Medicine; Department of Medicine, NYU Grossman Long Island School of Medicine, Mineola, NY, United States

Iare S. Ribeiro
Research Laboratory in bionanomaterials, LPbio, Department of Chemistry, Federal University of Viçosa, Viçosa, MG; National Institute of Science and Technology of Bioanalytics-Lauro Kubota (INCTBio-LK), Campinas, SP, Brazil

Dibyam Debasish Sahu
Department of Biophysics, National Institute of Mental Health and Neurosciences, Institute of National Importance, Bengaluru, Karnataka, India

Vaishali Saini
Mehta Family School of Biosciences and Biomedical Engineering, Indian Institute of Technology, Indore, Madhya Pradesh, India

Murugan Sevanan
Division of Biotechnology, Karunya Institute of Technology and Sciences (Deemed to be University), Coimbatore, Tamil Nadu, India

Lipika Sha
Department of Bioscience and Bioengineering, Indian Institute of Technology, Jodhpur, India

Anushka Sharma
Department of Biochemistry, University of Delhi South Campus, Dhaula Kuan, New Delhi, India

Sanyukta Sharma
Department of Biochemistry, University of Delhi South Campus, Dhaula Kuan, New Delhi, India

R. Sivasamy
Department of Human Genetics and Molecular Biology, Bharathiar University, Coimbatore, Tamil Nadu, India

Swathi Suresh
Department of Neurochemistry, National Institute of Mental Health and Neuro Sciences Hospital (NIMHANS), Institute of National Importance, Bangalore, Karnataka, India

Riddhi Upadhyay
Division of Biotechnology, Karunya Institute of Technology and Sciences (Deemed to be University), Coimbatore, Tamil Nadu, India

Gowshika Velmurugan
Department of Neurochemistry, National Institute of Mental Health and Neuro Sciences Hospital (NIMHANS), Institute of National Importance, Bangalore, Karnataka, India

Varsha Vishnu
Department of Psychiatry, National Institute of Mental Health, and Neuroscience (NIMHANS), Centre for Brain and Mind, Bengaluru, India

Biju Viswanath
Department of Psychiatry, National Institute of Mental Health, and Neuroscience (NIMHANS), Centre for Brain and Mind, Bengaluru, India

Chaitali Vora
Mehta Family School of Biosciences and Biomedical Engineering, Indian Institute of Technology, Indore, Madhya Pradesh, India

CHAPTER ONE

Alzheimer's disease: Extracellular Tau internalization in neuro-glial axis and its propagation mechanisms

Subashchandrabose Chinnathambi[a,*], Swathi Suresh[a], Gowshika Velmurugan[a], and Amit Mishra[b]

[a]Department of Neurochemistry, National Institute of Mental Health and Neuro Sciences Hospital (NIMHANS), Institute of National Importance, Bangalore, Karnataka, India
[b]Cellular and Molecular Neurobiology Unit, Indian Institute of Technology Jodhpur, Jodhpur, Rajasthan, India
*Corresponding author. e-mail address: subashneuro@nimhans.ac.in

Contents

Advances in Immunology, Volume 171
ISSN 0065-2776, https://doi.org/10.1016/bs.ai.2025.11.004

Abstract

Tau is a protein associated with microtubules that is essential to the central nervous system's extracellular and intracellular functions. Aberrant post-translational changes cause Tau to dissociate from microtubules in pathological circumstances like Tauopathies and also in AD (AD). The free Tau can diffuse into the extracellular space, contributing to neurofibrillary tangles formation and paired helical filaments. Moreover, pathogenic Tau can spread in a prion-like manner from diseased neurons to healthy ones exacerbating Tau pathology. By stimulating the NLRP3 inflammasome and other pathways, extracellular Tau has an impact on microglia. This, in turn, triggers inflammatory responses and leads to neuroinflammation. Astrocytes, the predominant brain cells, absorb extracellular Tau and undergo morphological and functional changes that result in the production of neurotoxic compounds, which ultimately cause neurodegeneration. The uptake of Tau by astrocytes results in a proinflammatory phenotype and cellular senescence, which intensify neuroinflammatory processes and oxidative stress and accelerate the advancement of neurodegenerative illnesses.

Abbreviations

AD	AD.
ApoE	Apo lipoprotein E.
CB2	Cannabinoid receptor type2.
cGAS	cyclic GMP-AMP synthase.
CME	Clathrin-mediated endocytosis.
CNS	Central nervous system.
CX3CL1	C motif chemokine ligand1.
CX3CR1	C-C chemokine receptor 1.
DAMP	Damage associated molecular pattern.
DSBS	Double-stranded DNA breaks.
ERF	Extracellular signal regulated kinase feedback.
GPCR	G protein coupled receptor.
GSDMD	Gasdermin D.
HMGB1	High mobility group box 1.
HSPG	Heparan sulfate proteoglycan.
IL	Interleukin.
IRAK	Interleukin 1 receptor associated kinase.
icTau	intracellular Tau.
IRF7	Interferon regulatory factor 7.
IRF7	Interferon regulatory factor 7.
JAK	Janus kinase.
LDLR	Low density lipoprotein receptor.
LRP1	Low-density lipoprotein receptor-related protein.
M1 receptor	Muscarinic 1 receptor.

M3 receptor	Muscarinic 3 receptor.
MAPK	Mitogen activated protein kinase.
MyD88	Myeloid differentiation primary response88.
MT	Microtubule.
NFkB	Nuclear factor kappa light chain enhancer of activated b cells.
NFT	Neurofibrillary tangles.
NLRP3	NOD like receptor family pyrin domain containing 3.
p38	Protein 38.
PAMP	Pattern associated molecular pattern.
PFF	Pre formed fibrils.
PHF	Paired helical filaments.
PQBP1	Polyglutamine binding protein 1.
PRRs	Pattern recognition receptors.
RAF	Rapidly accelerated fibrosarcoma.
RAGE	Receptor for advanced glycation end products.
RAS	Rat sarcoma protein.
SASP	Senescence-associated secretory phenotype.
STAT	Signal transducers and activators of transcription.
STING	Stimulator of interferon genes.
TGFβ	Transforming growth factor β.
TLR4	Toll like receptor 4.
TNTs	Tunneling nanotube dependent endocytosis.
TRAF6	TNF receptor associated factor 6.
TREM2	Triggering receptor expressed on myeloid cells 2.
Tyk2	Tyrosine kinase 2.
xcTau	Extracellular Tau.
xcTauOs	Extracellular Tau oligomers;.

1. Introduction

Tau is a protein associated with microtubules which stabilizes neuronal microtubules and thereby stimulates the development of axons. Tau is a highly soluble, naturally unfolded protein with minimal aggregation propensity (Chinnathambi et al., 2025b; Chinnathambi, 2025; Gorantla et al., 2019; Jeganathan et al., 2012; Nanjundaiah et al., 2021; Shkumatov et al., 2011; Wang & Mandelkow, 2016). They are widely dispersed throughout the neurons of central nervous system (CNS) and are mainly responsible stability of microtubules in axons (Balmik & Chinnathambi, 2022a; Gorantla et al., 2017a; Michalicova et al., 2020; Vijay Nalini et al., 2019). The intracellular trafficking and microtubule stability are regulated by Tau proteins, which are part of the intracellular matrix (Qureshi et al., 2025; Zhao et al., 2021). Tau has an important physiological role in regulating microtubule polymerization and suppressing MT dynamics. Dysregulation of the microtubule complex and Tau results in Tau detachment, loss of MT stability, and disintegration, which ultimately disrupts MT-dependent transport and impairs cellular viability and polarity maintenance (Brunello et al., 2020). Tau monomers can aggregate to form higher order fibrils and oligomers (Kent et al., 2020). Tau is phosphorylated and hyperphosphorylated under pathological conditions and this leads to the formation self-aggregates which results in pathogenic conformations in neurodegenerative diseases, termed Tauopathies (Amir Mishan et al., 2019; Qureshi et al., 2025). Tau misfolding and aggregation are major hallmark of AD pathology (Chinnathambi & Dubey, 2024; Granholm & Hamlett, 2024). Pathogenic Tau can spread in prion-like fashion, from diseased neurons to healthy neurons (Sonawane & Chinnathambi, 2018), which serve as seeds for template misfolding and aggregation (Zhu et al., 2022). The phosphorylation state of Tau, which is markedly elevated in AD and other Tauopathies, affects the activity of Tau (Balmik et al., 2019; Hanger et al., 2014). Aberrant post-translational processes (Sonawane et al., 2022), such as hyperphosphorylation, truncation, deamination, and methylation (Balmik & Chinnathambi, 2021), etc., may alter Tau under pathological circumstances (Avila et al., 2004), and cause structural alterations, aggregation, NFT development, and synaptic dysfunction in AD (Wu et al., 2021). All These changes may cause Tau to separate from MTs and build up in a free form. When neurons deteriorate, this free Tau might diffuse freely into the extracellular space (Gomez-Ramos et al., 2006) and also these alterations result in Tau protein aggregation and the development of neurofibrillary tangles (NFT) and paired helical filaments (PHF), which are typical signs and symptoms of Tauopathies, including AD. PHFs and NFTs build up and cause apoptosis, neuronal loss, and impairment of physiological activities. This leads to cognitive impairment and, in the advanced stages of the disease, death (Sinsky et al., 2021). The soluble dimers and oligomers that are assembled using the pathogenic Tau protein as a template eventually clump together to produce insoluble paired helical filaments (PHFs) and NFTs (Chu et al., 2024).

2. Pathophysiology of Tau

2.1 Tau and microtubule

Tau is microtubule associated protein which is a known component of neuronal cytoskeleton. The cytoskeleton mainly consists of three principles types of filaments: microtubules, actin filaments and intermediate filaments

(Hohmann & Dehghani, 2019). Microtubules are present throughout all cell types and these are long cytoskeletal filaments. These are made up of heterodimers of αβ tubulin (Dubey & Chinnathambi, 2021) which forms a hollow cylinder comprising 13 protofilaments (Cleary & Hancock, 2021). Microtubules are essential for the regulation of many cellular processes including cell division, morphology of cell, and intracellular transport of organelles (Tabeshmehr & Eftekharpour, 2023). It is distributed throughout the brain under physiological circumstances and also binds to microtubules directly and dynamically controls their shape and function (Medina & Avila, 2020). Tau is a microtubule associated protein (MAP) in neuron that inhibits microtubule dynamics while promoting assembly and bundling of microtubule. Abnormal Tau is involved in neurodegenerative illnesses, including Parkinson's disease (PD) and AD (AD), where Tau forms insoluble aggregates which leads to neurotoxicity (Venkatramani & Panda, 2019). Tau involves in axonal microtubule formation and also in its stabilization (Weingarten et al., 1975). Tau – microtubule complex is altered by hyperphosphorylation of Tau or dysregulation due to genetic mutation which results in Tau detachment and this condition cause disassembly and instability of microtubules and disruption of axonal transport (Garcia & Cleveland, 2001).

2.2 Tau interaction with other cytoskeleton protein

Tau and other microtubule associated proteins, such as MAP2, bind to filamentous actin in addition to microtubules, causing actin filaments to bundle and cross-link (Cabrales Fontela et al., 2017) and it also regulates actin microtubule interaction (Balmik & Chinnathambi, 2022b). Tau regulates actin stability by its direct interaction and also it influence synaptic plasticity (Biswas & Kalil, 2018). This interaction with filamentous actin plays an important role in postsynaptic reorganizations and dendritic spine formation (Cabrales Fontela et al., 2017). The connections between actin and microtubules in the neuronal growth cones are mediated by Tau proteins. Development of neurons depends on the growth cone's morphological alterations, which are facilitated by Tau-mediated cytoskeletal connections. Due to the arrangement of microtubules and actin filaments, Tau preferentially accumulates in the distal ends of axons during axonal development Also in growth cone the disruption of actin structures affects Tau localization within the growth cones (Mohan & John, 2015). Actin filament over stabilization can potentially cause Tau mediated neurotoxicity by disrupting cytoskeleton (Tabeshmehr & Eftekharpour, 2023) and Tau also interacts with intermediate filaments (Mohan & John, 2015) and the intermediate filament system collapses as a result of microtubule disruption (Ebneth et al., 1998). The primary components of neurofibrillary lesions in most adult-onset dementias are the neuron-specific cytoskeletal proteins Tau and neurofilament, which are abundant in axons, controlled by many of the same protein kinases, and interact physically. These two proteins have identical function in learning and memory, long-term synaptic potentiation, axonal transport, the microtubule stability and functions in axons, and also scaffolding of organelles (Yuan & Nixon, 2023).

2.3 Crosstalk between Tau physiology and pathology

Tau monomers and filaments aggregate to generate Tau intermediates, which are soluble in physiological fluids. The production of NFTs is aided by hyperphosphorylation (Gerson et al., 2016). Tau proteins that are hyperphosphorylated irregularly cause an increase in microtubule depolymerisation, which results in insoluble cytoplasmic Tau oligomers from Tau monomers that eventually combine into protomers and then the formation of paired helical filaments takes place by twisting of two protomers around one another. These filaments then aggregate and eventually forms neurofibrillary tangles (NFTs) (Gorantla et al., 2020; Mamun et al., 2020). Neurofibrillary tangles are neuropathological hallmarks of AD (Granholm & Hamlett, 2024). Phosphorylation and dephosphorylation are out of equilibrium in pathological condition which leads to increased abnormal phosphorylation (Köpke et al., 1993). Tau hyperphosphorylation causes its dissociation from microtubules and also disrupts the function of microtubules and microtubule stability (Qiang et al., 2018; Sonawane et al., 2020). Soluble Tau oligomer formed Tau monomers in the process of aggregation are primary drivers of toxicity and also neurofibrillary tangles (NFTs) are toxic species due to their presence in brain Tau pathology (Hill et al., 2020). These consequences were linked to aberrant neurotransmission, intracellular calcium mobilization, synapse loss, neuronal death, and long-term abnormalities in neurite outgrowth (Usenovic et al., 2015). The most prevalent post translational modification of Tau is phosphorylation (Balmik et al., 2019), and dynamic modulation of this process is essential for modifying Tau function (Neddens et al., 2018). Phosphorylated Tau affects the stability of microtubules and it further develops Tau monomers into Tau oligomers (Chinnathambi & Das, 2023). Tau aggregates further form Tau fibrils and finally, it leads to the formation of neurofibrillary tangles (Granholm & Hamlett, 2024). Tau is phosphorylated disproportionately at specific points in AD (Chidambaram & Chinnathambi, 2020) and other Tauopathies, which probably contributes to its toxicity (Guha et al., 2020). Abnormal Tau causes destabilization of microtubules, disruption of axonal transport, and also it dysregulates synaptic plasticity in pathological conditions (Vacchi et al., 2020). Under physiological condition the main role of Tau is stabilizing the microtubule (Gorantla et al., 2017b) and also preventing MTs from depolymerizing by reducing tubulin dissociation at both MT ends (Barbier et al., 2019). Tau also plays a role in regulation of axonal transport (Vacchi et al., 2020). Tau as a synaptic protein accelerates synaptic plasticity in physiological conditions (Robbins et al., 2021). Under pathological condition Tau abnormally phosphorylates and forms aggregation into filamentous inclusions which are referred to as neurofibrillary tangles (Pooler et al., 2013), and post translational modification give rise to abnormal phosphorylation of Tau (Chinnathambi & Rangappa, 2025; Sonawane & Chinnathambi, 2020).

3. Tau propagation from diseased neurons to healthy neurons

3.1 Tau and neurodegeneration in AD

AD is a prominent form of age-related dementia (Gorantla et al., 2019), and around 25 million people are affected worldwide. The presence of two main categories of pathological brain abnormalities characterizes AD pathologically: (1) Amyloid beta (Aβ) accumulates extracellularly which leads to plaque formation and cerebral amyloid angiopathy. (2) Tau protein aggregates intercellularly which results in the formation of neurofibrillary tangles (NFTs) and neuropil threads (Balmik et al., 2022; Xia et al., 2020). Neurofibrillary tangles (NFTs) cause death of neuron as well as loss of synapse which results in cognitive death. This happens due to hyperphosphorylation of Tau protein in NFTs (Hardy & Selkoe, 2002). Both NFTs or Aβ deposits exhibits the direct neurotoxic effect and indirectly propagate chronic inflammation and which is responsible for neurodegeneration in AD (Kapoor & Chinnathambi, 2023b). The pathophysiology of AD develops in the hippocampus and expands as the disease proceeds. As the illness progresses, the hippocampus becomes less effective in helping the brain maintain normal functions (Sonawane et al., 2022). Besides extracellular amyloid-beta (Aβ) plaques (Sonawane et al., 2021), phosphorylated Tau (P-Tau), and intracellular neurofibrillary tangles (NFTs), AD is characterized by a variety of cellular alterations, including deregulation of microRNAs, imbalance in hormones, defective mitophagy and degeneration of synapse (Morton et al., 2021). Tau accumulates in each neuron independently, but it may also aggregate in an extrinsic regulation way in which Tau aggregates (Dubey et al., 2022) are transferred from one cell to another (Yamada, 2017). Tau aggregation ultimately leads to neurodegeneration by decreasing the level of soluble functional Tau, sequestering other cell components, or impairing axonal transport (Gao et al., 2018; Vijay Nalini et al., 2019). Tau oligomers partake in Tau spreading which favors its assembly via the nucleation process, whereas Tau monomers induce neurodegeneration and apoptosis of cells (Sebastian-Serrano et al., 2018). Disruption of Tau homeostasis can also cause neurodegeneration. Two factors that can contribute to Tau-mediate neurodegeneration are the toxic function produced by Tau abnormalities and also the detrimental impacts of loss of normal Tau function (Gendron & Petrucelli, 2009). A pathological disease that predominantly affects neurons is referred to as neurodegeneration (Przedborski et al., 2003). Neurodegeneration is caused by two different but related disease characteristics, which is a common neuropathological background: (i) deposits of aberrant proteins within the cell bodies of brain tissue, either extracellularly or as neuronal or glial; and (ii) general mechanisms of programmed cell death, such as apoptotic cell death and autophagocytosis (Matej et al., 2019). AD (AD) is a complicated neurodegenerative disorder and also is defined by neuronal death and neuronal dysfunction (Moya-Alvarado et al., 2016). Parkinson's disease, amyotrophic lateral sclerosis, prion disease, Huntington's disease and motor neuron disease are other neurodegeneration disease apart from AD. Neurodegeneration can be caused by dysregulation of the neuronal network, and synapses, and also the accumulation of physiologically modified protein variations in brain (Lamptey et al., 2022) (Fig. 1).

3.2 Extracellular Tau internalization in neurons

The release and transsynaptic transport of pathogenic Tau may be regulated by presynaptic neuronal activity (Sokolow et al., 2015). Pathological Tau which is secreted in extracellular space can be internalized into neighbour cells like neurons and glial cells (Chinnathambi et al., 2025a). Either at the somatodendritic compartment or axonal terminal, the internalization of Tau can take place. Tau proteins are transferred anterogradely or retrogradely after internalization (Zhao et al., 2021). Through different cellular mechanism, the various Tau species will be internalized i.e. monomeric Tau and small oligomeric

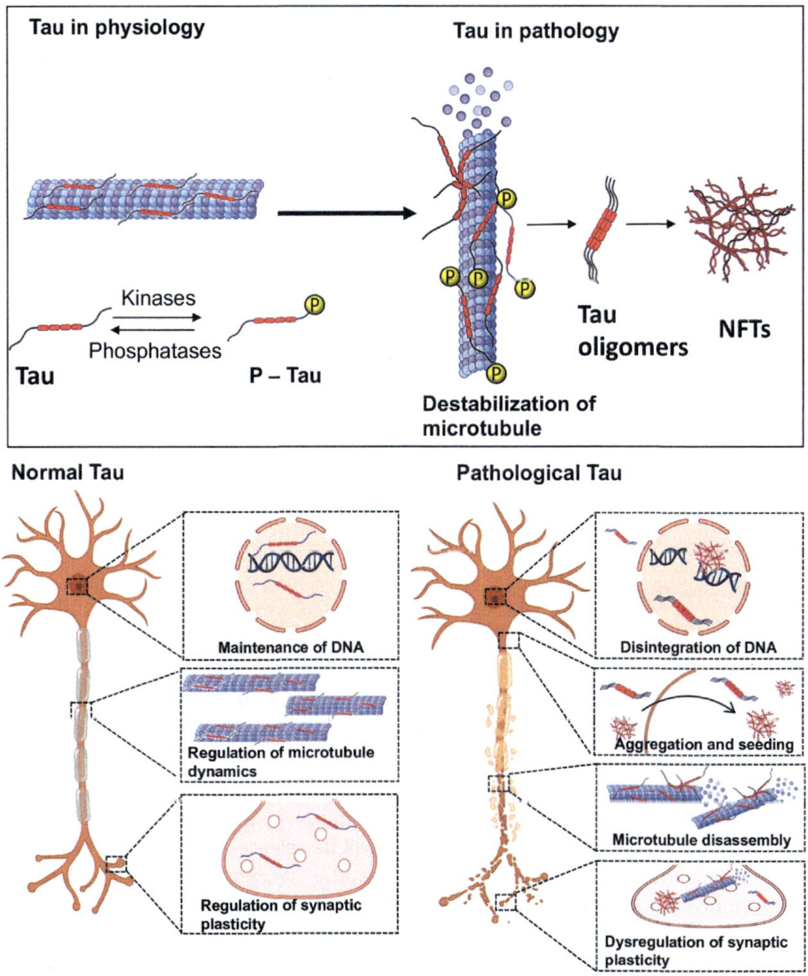

Fig. 1 Pathophysiology of Tau. In the physiological state Tau protein plays different role according to its localization in neurons. In axon Tau maintain microtubule stability and also regulates axonal transport, in dendrite Tau regulates synaptic plasticity. In pathological state, the normal Tau undergoes hyperphosphorylation and it get detaches from microtubule which forms Tau fibrils, eventually forms the NFTs. Tau cause disruption of axonal transport and also dysregulates synaptic plasticity in pathological condition leading to neurodegeneration.

Tau are internalized by macropinocytosis and the Tau aggregates are internalized by dynamin dependent endocytosis (Brunello et al., 2020; Chidambaram & Chinnathambi, 2025; Chinnathambi et al., 2025a). From (Fig. 2) extracellular Tau (xcTau) is present in a various vesicle, including

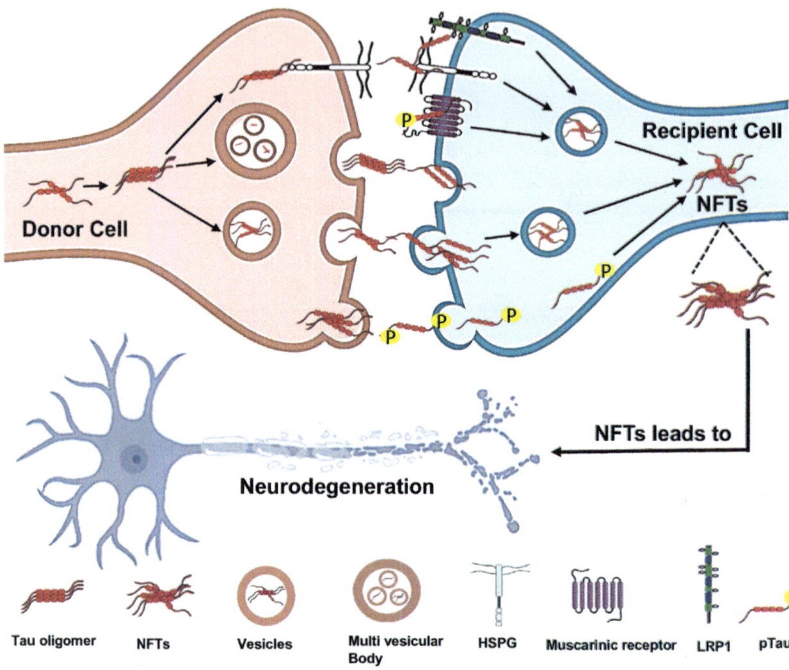

Fig. 2 Tau propagation from diseases neuron to healthy neuron. Tau propagates in a prion like manner from diseased neurons to healthy neurons. Tau is a microtubule associated protein, aggregates into pathological forms within neurons in neurodegenerative diseases. These aggregations are released into extracellular space, Tau present in extracellular space contributes in progressive spread. In the above figure, diseased neurons containing aggregated Tau will be released into extracellular space and these are internalized by neighboring healthy neurons. After internalized Tau species induce the misfolding and aggregation of normal Tau protein in the recipient neurons, leading to Tau pathology propagation. Extracellular Tau transfer contributes to the spread of Tau pathology through interactions with cell surface receptors such as LRP1 and as well as regulation by muscarinic receptors.

exosomes and ectosomes, as well as free protein. Tau aggregates enter the extracellular space, and nearby cells like neurons and glial cells can internalize them through endocytic, pinocytic, and phagocytic processes (Brunello et al., 2020). xcTau aggregates can also be taken up by neurons, which function as seeds to cause the formation of Tau protein aggregates. Neurons release Tau species, including monomers, oligomers, and aggregates, through exosomes. Exosomes aid in the development of Tau pathology since they help in the trans-synaptic transmission of Tau between neurons. (Wang et al., 2017). xcTau is taken up by the recipient cells, where it seeds soluble Tau to propagate

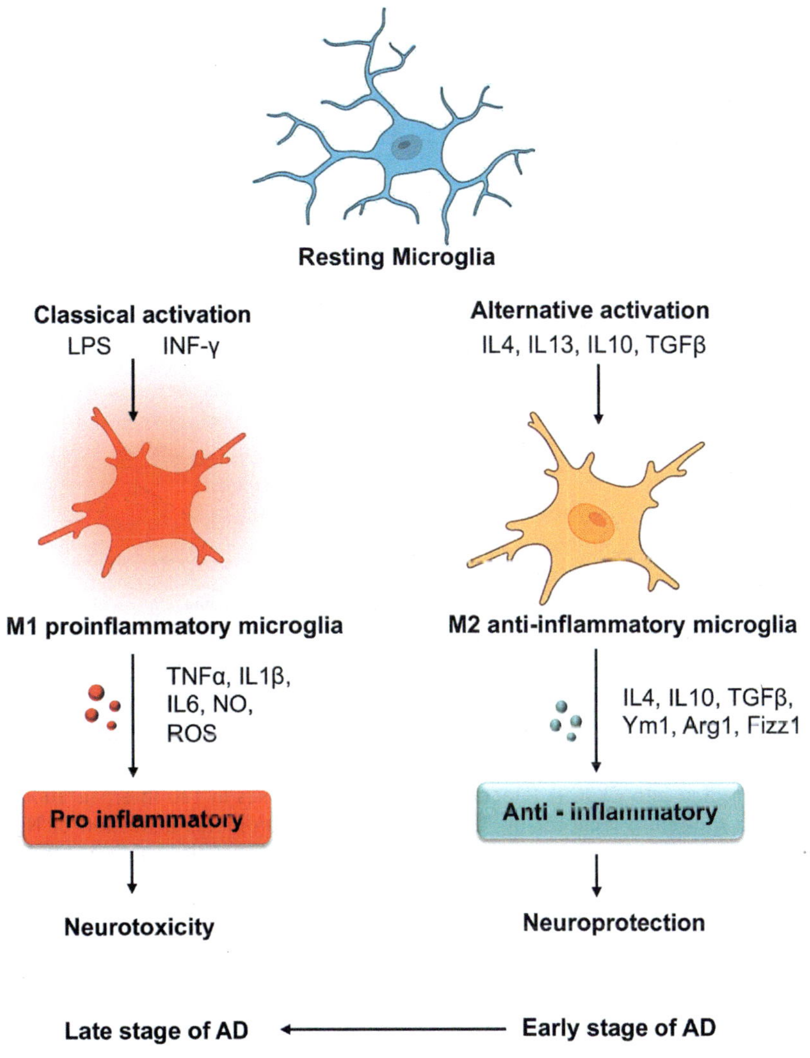

Fig. 3 Activation of microglia. Diagrammatic representation of the microglia's polarization and phenotypic change. In a normal state, microglia are stationary. Different phenotypes can be acquired by resting microglia through a variety of stimulus. M2 microglia exhibit an anti-inflammatory phenotype, whereas M1 microglia generally exhibit a pro-inflammatory phenotype.

the Tau disease by trans-cellular propagation (Yamada, 2017). In the neurotoxic impact generated by Tau the plasma membrane receptors have been identified as M1 and M3. The internalization of xcTau can be mediated by the activation of muscarinic M1 receptors, which are subject to agonist-induced

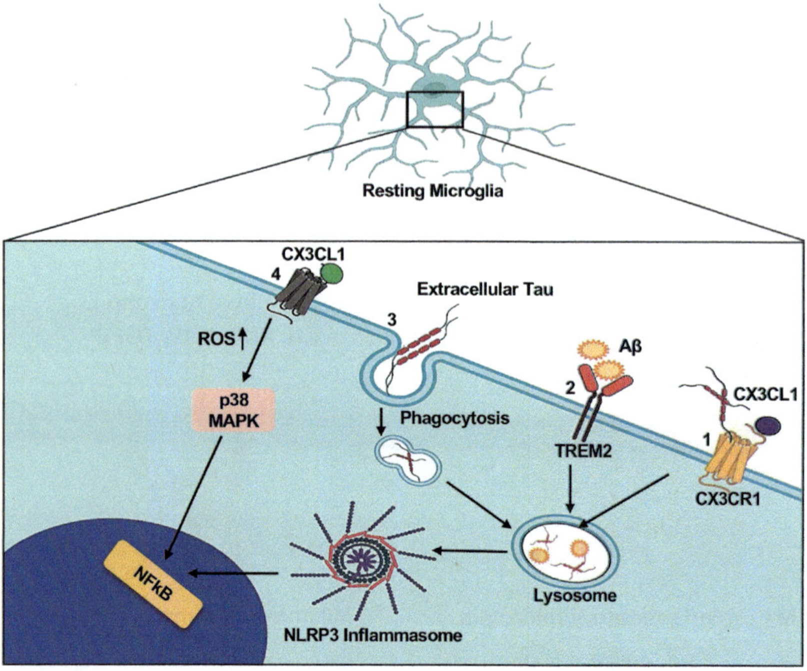

Fig. 4 Extracellular Tau internalization and its role in microglia. Diagram depicting the interaction between Tau pathology and neuroinflammation which contributes in development of AD pathology. Extracellular Tau competes with CX3CL1 for its binding into CX3CR1 (Fractalkine receptor) partakes in Tau internalization, Aβ binds to triggering receptor on TREM2. Tau and Aβ promotes activation of NLRP3 inflammasome which further triggers production of proinflammatory cytokines. CX3CL1 involved in regulation of microglial activation and phagocytosis. Tau and Aβ promote activation of p38 MAPK and NFkB, also these triggers the production of ROS. NFkB regulates proinflammatory cytokines production.

receptor internalization, this is known as sequestration. This process involves the protein extracellular dephosphorylated Tau. The neurotoxicity caused by xcTau implies that this protein must be in its dephosphorylated form to act as an agonist for the muscarinic receptor (Sebastian-Serrano et al., 2018). Dysfunction of M1 receptors contributes to several clinical alterations seen in AD, including neuroinflammation, neurofibrillary tangles, and parenchymal and cerebrovascular amyloid accumulation (Wysocka et al., 2020). The internalization of Tau present in extracellular space occurs by phagocytosis, clathrin – and dynamin-mediated endocytosis, and receptor- or heparan sulfate proteoglycan (HSPG)-mediated endocytosis (Perea et al., 2020). LRP1 is an endocytic receptor that binds and breaks down monomeric Tau forms, causing them to be degraded, and facilitates the seeding of pathogenic Tau forms (Cooper et al., 2021). Tau protein dissemination is controlled by low-density lipoprotein receptor-related protein 1 (LRP1) (Chen et al., 2022a). xcTau plays significant roles in signaling functions that lead to the neurodegenerative processes in Alzheimer's and also related Tauopathies (Chinnathambi et al., 2024; Medina & Avila, 2014) (Figs. 3 and 4).

4. Extracellular Tau internalization and its role in microglia

4.1 Classical Activation of Microglia

The four phases of activation of microglia are as follows: M1 is the most similar to the traditional (pro-inflammatory) activation stage, whereas M2a, M2b, and M2c are the alternate activation stages (Bell-Temin et al., 2015). M1 type activation in microglia produce neurotoxicity and inflammation by the production of inflammatory mediators, whereas M2 type activation in microglia produces neuroprotectivity and anti-inflammatory mediators (Guo et al., 2022). Classical activation—M1 type: pro-inflammatory activation following tissue damage results in the synthesis of TNFα, IL1β, superoxides, nitric oxide, ROS, and proteases (Das & Chinnathambi, 2019). Interleukin 1α (IL-1α) significantly stimulated both ERK activation and NF-κB (Miyazaki et al., 2000). From (Fig. 5) interleukin 6 (IL 6) stimulates the synthesis of pro-inflammatory cytokines produced from microglia and increases the proliferation of microglial cells (Recasens et al., 2021). Alternate activation—M2 type: following sufficient inflammatory response, tissue healing, and extracellular matrix reconstitution—related to the release of IL4, IL13, IL10, and TGFβ—are necessary (Das & Chinnathambi, 2019). The JAK-STAT signalling pathway is triggered by the IL-10 receptor. Particularly, IL-10 causes the activation of Stat3 and affects the activation of Tyk2, which is connected to the IL-10 receptor b chain, and Jak1, which is connected to the IL-10 receptor a chain (Riley et al., 1999). Through the JAK/STAT6 pathway, IL-4 may partially facilitate the polarization of M2 microglia and macrophages (He et al., 2020). Proinflammatory cytokine release is controlled by the transcription pathway of nuclear factor kappa B (NF-κB) (Lappas et al., 2002). The NLRP3 inflammasome, NFkB in microglia, and caspase-1 can all be activated. On the one hand, activated caspase-1 cleaves GSDMD, generating an N-terminal structural domain and causing a cell membrane perforation that leads to pyroptosis. Conversely, cleaved IL-1β and IL-18 precursors by active caspase-1

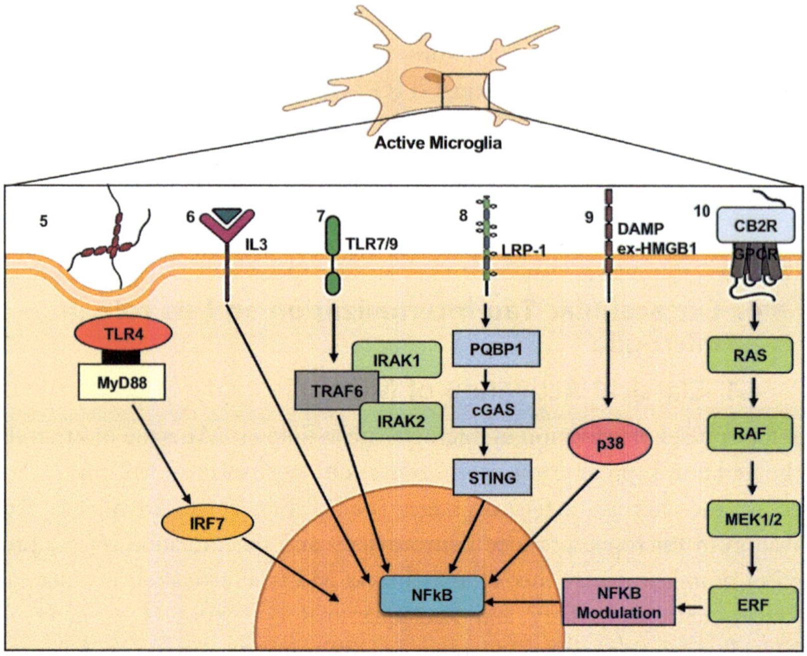

Fig. 5 Toll like receptor (TLR4) signals through adaptor protein MyD88 / IRF7 which leads to activation of central inflammatory mediators NFkB. Pathogen recognition receptor – Toll like receptor (TLR4) signals through adaptor protein MyD88 / IRF7 which leads to activation of central inflammatory mediators NFkB. IL3 signaling influence the activation state and function of microglia in response to extracellular Tau. Due to stress cell condition PAMP/DAMP activates and this leads to activation of TLR7/TLR9. TLR7/9 activates TNF receptor-associated factor 6 (TRAF6), IRAK1, and IRAK4 and influence activation of NFkB. DAMP is represented by the protein HMGB1. HMGB1 stimulates the production of proinflammatory cytokines via promoting the phosphorylation of MAPK p38 and the activation of NF-κB. Extracellular monomeric Tau is taken up by microglia via surface receptors; LRP1 this activates PQBP1, cGAS, STING causing NF-κB activation in microglia.

increase extracellular levels of IL-1β and IL-18 and intensify neuroinflammatory reactions. Neuroinflammation triggers pyroptosis in microglia, which results in the ongoing advancement of the disease, and it also encourages the synthesis of several pathological indicators of neurological disorder (Wu et al., 2022).

4.2 Extracellular Tau internalization in microglia

Macrophages in the brain called microglia are responsible for preserving the central nervous system (CNS) homeostasis (Das & Chinnathambi, 2019;

Das & Chinnathambi, 2020; Perea et al., 2020). Microglia originate from hematopoietic cells and these are sustained through the recruitment of blood-borne monocytes (Cartier et al., 2014) and also it is tissue-resident macrophages (Chinnathambi et al., 2023). Microglial cells regulate the physiological phagocytosis of synapses or synaptic fragments which is a process known as trogocytosis and synaptic pruning, which regulates the growth, maturity, and plasticity of neuronal ensembles (Verkhratsky et al., 2021). Microglia activation is induced by Tau pathology (Desale & Chinnathambi, 2020), indicating a vicious loop between active microglia and Tau pathology (Wang & Xie, 2022). Activated microglia release toxic products and pro-inflammatory substances that can harm neurons (Kim et al., 2023) and also results in a persistent state of neuroinflammation. Microglia contribute to phagocytosis (Desale & Chinnathambi, 2021), neurodegeneration, and inflammation in AD. They have a complex involvement in the disease (Miao et al., 2023). One of the main characteristics of neuroinflammation in AD is the buildup of activated microglia surrounding damaged regions (Cai et al., 2022). Tau can be released to extracellular space through various mechanisms like micro vesicle shedding, exosomes release, secretory lysosomes, and direct transfer from the cytoplasm across the plasma membrane (Wang et al., 2017). Tau is actively discharged into the extracellular area in addition to being in the cytoplasm of neurons (Yamada, 2017). The Tau released from dying cells was the source of xcTau, whereas the extracellular tangles arised from the intracellular Tau (icTau) aggregates that pre-existed in the dead cells (Sebastian-Serrano et al., 2018). xcTau released by Tau-pathological neurons and Tau filament propagation from diseased neurons can have an impact on microglia (Vogels et al., 2019). Through endocytic, pinocytic, and phagocytic processes, Tau aggregates in the extracellular space will be internalized by nearby cells, including glial and neuronal cells (Brunello et al., 2020; Chinnathambi et al., 2025a) and also due to its interactions with certain cell receptors, secreted extracellular will be toxic to surrounding cells (Zhang et al., 2021). xcTau that has aggregated penetrates cells and transfers a misfolded condition to icTau (Frost et al., 2009). Neuronal death can lead to the accumulation of Tau in the extracellular space. Consequently, the xcTau would spread and lead to the death of the cell (Gomez-Ramos et al., 2006). xcTau leads to the development of AD and is harmful to nearby cells (Vogels et al., 2019). xcTau causes activated microglia to engulf stressed neurons in a primary phagocytic response (Pampuscenko et al., 2020).

4.3 Phagocytosis of Tau in microglia

Microglia can internalize the xcTau which is toxicity inducing component by phagocytosis or pinocytosis or through secretion of chemokines and interferons (Chidambaram et al., 2024a, 2024b; Kapoor & Chinnathambi, 2023a). Bulk phagocytosis occurs in microglia due to its activation which further cause the engulfment of synapses and this in turn causes loss of synaptic connection and neuronal death (Das & Chinnathambi, 2019). From (Fig. 3) Through a microglial receptor called fractalkine C-X3-C motif chemokine receptor (CX3CR1), extracellular hyperphosphorylated Tau is internalized and phagocytosed by reactive microglia. Phagocytosis impairment in turn contributes to abnormal build-up of Tau and Aβ proteins (Chinnathambi et al., 2024; Kapoor & Chinnathambi, 2023a). In the AD brain, fractalkine production is downregulated indicating Tau competition with its receptor CX3CR1. The chemokine receptor CX3CR1 directly binds to Tau and facilitates its internalization allowing microglia to phagocytose and internalize xcTau species (Chidambaram & Chinnathambi, 2020; Chidambaram et al., 2020). Lack of CX3CR1 facilitates the phagocytosis of Aβ rather than Tau (Perea et al., 2020), and also microglia's phagocytosis of Tau and amyloid-beta (Aβ) is enhanced by TLR4 activation (Zhou et al., 2020).

Inflammatory bursts and memory loss are caused due to phagocytosis of synapses. Extracellular oligomers Tau activates microglia which further results in an increase of inflammation and phagocytosis matrix depositions (Chinnathambi & Chidambaram, 2024; Das & Chinnathambi, 2020; Desale et al., 2024). In some pathological circumstances, the decoupling of microglia's phagocytosis and activation capabilities might hasten the process of neurodegeneration. An inflammatory response can be triggered or exacerbated by the dysregulation of microglial phagocytosis processes, which can hinder the removal of debris and lead to brain disorders like AD (Chidambaram et al., 2022; Das & Chinnathambi, 2021; Perea et al., 2020).

4.4 Activation of NLRP3 inflammasome by Aβ and Tau

An essential channel for communication between neurons and microglia is the CX3CL1/CX3CR1 axis (Bolós et al., 2017). Chemokine receptor CX3CR1 is primarily expressed on microglia, where it binds to fractalkine (CX3CL1) ligand, which is expressed in neurons in both a membrane-bound state and soluble, therefore keeping the microglia in an inactive state (Chidambaram et al., 2020). CX3CL1 is the only chemokine that is expressed more in the central nervous system than in peripheral nervous system (Pawelec et al., 2020). In extracellular space Tau competes with CX3CL1, the native ligand of CX3CR1, for binding to this receptor involved in Tau internalization (Bolós et al., 2017). Triggering receptor expressed on myeloid cells 2 (TREM2) is mostly expressed in CNS microglia and has a role in CNS microglia migration, survival, proliferation, and phagocytosis (Li et al., 2023b). Transmembrane receptor TREM2 is expressed nearly exclusively in the microglia of the central nervous system. In the preclinical stage of AD, TREM2 and ApoE 4 may have synergistic effects (Li et al., 2023c). TREM2 binds to apolipoprotein like APOE and hence promotes the absorption of amyloid-beta by microglia (Lyu et al., 2023). Aβ binds directly to TREM2 (Zhao et al., 2018), both Tau and Aβ contribute to the activation of NLRP3 inflammasome by causing lysosomal damage (Jung et al., 2022). Phagocytosis is caused by activated microglia i.e. through various surface receptors, microglia detect pathogenic Tau species and initiate phagocytosis (Chen & Yu, 2023). The activation of the NLR family pyrin domain-containing protein 3 (NLRP3) inflammasome causes Tau hyperphosphorylation and aggregation by modifying Tau phosphatases and kinases (Ising et al., 2019). Specifically, the NOD-, LRR-, and pyrin domain-containing 3 (NLRP3) inflammasome is important for the development and progression of Aβ-plaque formation and Tau-induced pathologies (Hanslik & Ulland, 2020). The dimeric transcription factor NF-κB controls the expression of genes linked to apoptosis, oxidative stress, and inflammation, among other stress-related responses (Guo et al., 2013b). The NFKB pathway produces the pro-inflammatory cytokines and these are stimulated by soluble CX3CL1 activating the microglia-specific receptor CX3CR1, which phosphorylates p38MAPK kinase (Qin et al., 2020), p38MAPK plays a vital role in inflammation (Hanslik & Ulland, 2020).

4.5 NFkB activation by various receptors

From (Fig. 4) a nonspecific molecular pattern on patho-proteins is identified by microglial PRRs, including Toll-like receptor 4, as a death signal. (TLR4), which eventually causes the activation of the major inflammatory mediator NfκB by signaling through the adaptor protein MyD88/IRF7 (Das & Chinnathambi, 2019). IL-3 mediates the Tau pathology and is associated with sTREM2 (Desale & Chinnathambi, 2020; Wang et al., 2022). The release of chemokines or inflammatory cytokines and the attraction of immune cells are encouraged by the activation of DAMP-sensing receptors, which results in an inflammatory response (Ma et al., 2024). Through their pattern recognition receptors (PRRs), microglia identify pathogen-associated and damage-associated molecular patterns (DAMPs and PAMPs, respectively), which are indicators of pathogenic insult (Bivona et al., 2023). Activation of TLR7/TLR9 results in the formation of a Myddosome complex, which is made up of MyD88, IRAK1, and IRAK4, and then recruits TNF receptor-associated factor 6 (TRAF6), which is activated one after the other (Suthers & Sarantopoulos, 2017). A classic DAMP is represented by the protein high mobility group box 1 (HMGB1) (Mueller, 2012). HMGB1 stimulates the production of proinflammatory cytokines by promoting the phosphorylation of MAPK p38 and the activation of NF-kappaB via RAGE (Qin et al., 2009). On NF- B activation, DAMP-induced signaling (by RAGE or TREM-1) converges with PAMP-mediated signaling (Mueller, 2012). Extracellular monomeric Tau is taken up by microglia in parallel via surface receptors; LRP1/polyglutamine binding protein 1 (PQBP1)/cyclic GMP-AMP synthase (cGAS)/Stimulator of interferon genes (STING) causes nuclear factor NF-κB activation in microglia, which in turn causes neuronal death (Chen & Yu, 2023). Microglial GPCR–CB2, an endogenous cannabinoid receptor that is more highly expressed on immune cells, senses the xcTau protein load. In the brain of AD, CB2 is seen to encircle Tau deposits and amyloid plaques (Das & Chinnathambi, 2019). The RAF/MEK/ERK cascade is one of the downstream signaling pathways that are triggered by Ras activation (Moriuchi et al., 2020) GPCR induces the NF-κB activation (Ye, 2001).

5. Extracellular Tau internalization and its role in astrocyte

5.1 Internalization of extracellular Tau in astrocyte

The most prevalent type of neural cell in the brain is astrocyte. They are essential to the glymphatic system, blood-brain barrier, synapse, and neuronal function (Reid et al., 2020). Astrocytes act as fundamental players in the pathogenic process which leads to neuronal injury and also these are implicated in several central nervous system illnesses (Ferrer, 2018). Astrocytes absorb Tau fibrils from extracellular space and also Tau can be absorbed from dystrophic neurites, synapses, or dead neurons by phagocytosis (Eltom et al., 2024). Hyperphosphorylated Tau from damaged and deteriorating neurons is taken up by astrocytes (De Calignon et al., 2012).

Tau can be internalized as monomers, truncated preformed Tau fibrils (PFF), or aggregates (Fleeman & Proctor, 2021) by astrocytes. Internalization of Tau mechanisms includes phagocytosis, lipid raft dependent endocytosis, tunneling nanotube dependent endocytosis (TNTs), macropinocytosis, and Clathrin-mediated endocytosis (CME) (Chinnathambi et al., 2025a; Zhao et al., 2021). Astrocytes aid in the breakdown of Tau filaments by infiltrating extracellular "ghost" tangles (Zilka et al., 2012). From (Fig. 6) extracellular Tau oligomers (xcTauOs) are extensively internalized by astrocytes, and their intracellular buildup modifies neuro/gliotransmitter processing, impairing synaptic function. Tau oligomers

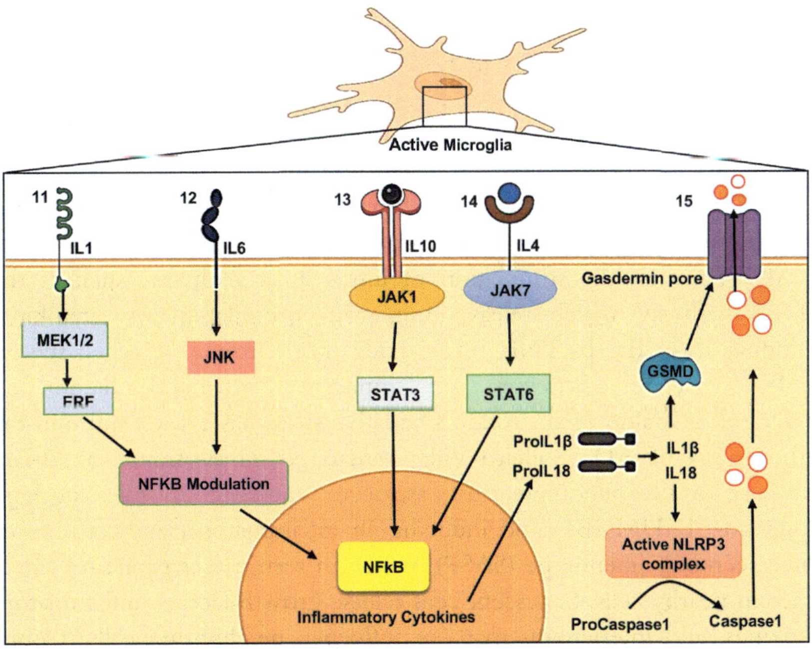

Fig. 6 Activation of NLRP3 inflammasome. Microglia can be activated in different ways i.e., Classical activation – M1 activation and Alternative activation – M2 activation. Interleukin 1α (IL-1α) and significantly stimulated both ERK activation and NF-κB and Interleukin-6 (IL-6) stimulates the synthesis of pro-inflammatory cytokines produced from microglia. IL1 and IL6 are M1 activation upon encountering Extracellular Tau it activates NFkB. IL10 and IL4 are M2 activation, IL10 activates JAK1/STAT3 which activates NFkB and IL4 activates JAK7/STAT6 which further induces the activation of NFkB to release proinflammatory cytokines. Proinflammatory cytokine release is regulated by the transcription pathway of nuclear factor kappa B (NFkB) and activated caspase-1 cleaves GSDMD. Proinflammatory cytokines are released outside the microglia by Gasdermin pore which further intensify neuroinflammatory reactions.

internalize through heparan sulfate proteoglycans (HSPGs) (Puliatti et al., 2023). LRP1 is a large member of the LDLR family, and it is well known that LDL receptors cooperate with HSPGs (Rauch et al., 2020). In reactive astrocytes, LRP1 is highly expressed (Mckee et al., 2022). Astrocytic Tau internalization modifies morphology and functionality of astrocytes (Fleeman & Proctor, 2021). Astrocytes are stimulated by high Tau levels and this lead to the production of neurotoxic substances that leads to neurodegeneration (Wang & Ye, 2021) (Fig. 7).

5.2 Astrocytic response to extracellular Tau uptake

The accumulation of Tau fibrils induces chronic inflammation and neurotoxic phenotype in astrocytes (Eltom et al., 2024). Tau propagated transcellularly to astrocytes which triggers cellular senescence/senescence associated secretory phenotype [SASP] (Olson et al., 2019). Cellular senescence refers to a group of conditions in which cells cease to divide and subsequently display several cellular and molecular alterations (Han et al., 2020). Dysregulated astrocytic regulation increases oxidative stress and cytotoxicity, which causes the formation of Aβ plaques and also aggregates in AD. Through the stimulation of intracellular pathways such as the NF-κB pathway which releases numerous proinflammatory cytokines including IL-6, IL-1β, TNF, nitric oxide (NO), reactive oxygen species (ROS), reactive astrocytes are implicated in neuroinflammation (Rodríguez-Giraldo et al., 2022). Oxidative stress has a key feature in the pathogenesis of AD (Solleiro-Villavicencio & Rivas-Arancibia, 2018). Exposure to Tau oligomers causes astrocyte senescence by releasing high group box 1 (HMGB1) and inducing an inflammatory senescence-associated secretory phenotype (SASP), which in turn causes paracrine senescence in nearby cells. Senescent cells release growth factors, inflammatory cytokines, and interleukins that can influence neighboring cells (Coppe et al., 2010). xcTau can induce the SASP (Gaikwad et al., 2021). Senescent cells produce the Senescence-associated secretory phenotype (SASP) factors and can induce senescence in normal cells it also increases chronic inflammation (Li et al., 2023a). Damage-associated molecular pattern molecules (DAMPs), which is HMGB1 actively secrete and passively release outside the cells, influencing immunological responses and inflammation (Chen et al., 2022b). Intra neuronal Tau accumulation gradually causes oxidative stress in astrocytes (Batenburg et al., 2022). Reactive oxygen species (ROS) are produced excessively under oxidative stress, which leads to mitochondrial dysfunction (Guo et al., 2013a).

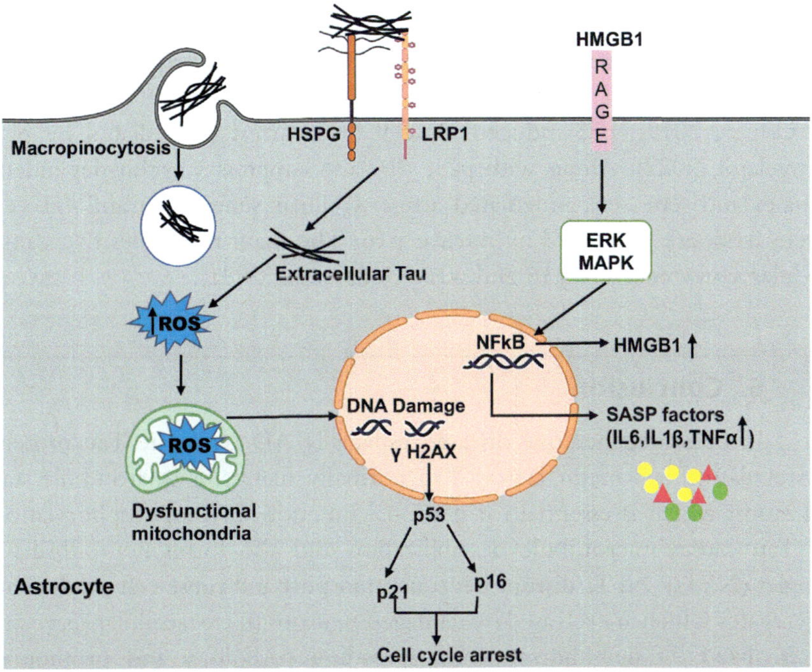

Fig. 7 Extracellular Tau internalization and role in astrocyte. Hyperphosphorylated Tau is internalized by astrocyte from injured and degenerating neuron. Pre formed Tau fibril, taken up by astrocytes through micropinocytosis and through a non heparan sulfate proteoglycan (HSPG) mediated mechanism the Tau monomers are internalized into astrocyte. TauO exposure induce HMGB1 release, HMGB1 activates rage and on surface of target cells, TLR4 promotes the expression of [IL1β, IL16, and TNFα]. LRP1 [Low density lipoprotein related protein1] is a master regulator of Tau internalization by neurons, also in reactive astrocyte, LRP1 is highly expressed which is mainly in AD. Pathological TauO triggers astrocyte senescence and contributes inflammation, tissue deteriotion through SASP. Extracellular HMGB1 serves as vital inflammatory SASP component initiates and spread of cellular senescence. Extracellular Tau increases oxidative stress and this leads to mitochondrial dysfunction, DNA damage. γ-H2AX [Histone 2A family member] is cellular senescence marker, also this is double stranded DNA breaks sensitive marker. Expression of p21 is up regulated by p53, p21 supress cyclin D dependent kinase CDK2 activity and initiates cell cycle arrest and p16 blocks cell cycle entry to S phase.

Mitochondrial dysfunction and nuclear DNA damage are caused by the accumulation of ROS (Zhao et al., 2022). Histone γ-H2AX [replacement histone] is phosphorylated at serine-139, which is located at the C-terminal of the H2AX histone. It is a typical indicator of senescence in cells. The most sensitive indicator of double-stranded DNA breaks (DSBs) is histone γ-H2AX (Bernadotte et al., 2016). p53 is activated by cellular stresses, including DNA damage (Lowe, 1999). p53 increases the expression of p21, due to cellular stress, such as oxidative stress or damage of DNA (Shamloo & Usluer, 2019). p53-induced G_1 cell cycle arrest is mediated by p21 (Engeland, 2022). Along with p21, p16 also suppresses cyclin-dependent kinases and senescence-mediated arrest. Cellular senescence and G1 cell cycle arrest are promoted by nuclear p16. The main molecules that cause cellular senescence are p16 and p21 (Ueda et al., 2021).

6. Conclusion

In neurodegenerative diseases, especially AD (AD) the Tau protein dysregulation is a major factor. Tau normally maintains microtubule stabilization which is essential for neuronal function. Hyperphosphorylation of Tau causes microtubule destabilization and also forms neurofibrillary tangles (NFTs). NFTs disrupt neuronal transport and cause cell death. Tau aggregates which are released by damaged neurons to extracellular space are internalized by neighboring cells, spreading pathology and promoting neurodegeneration. Microglia internalize xcTau in response to Tau pathology, which exacerbates the condition through inflammation. The NLRP3 inflammasome and NFkB are triggered by activation of microglial receptors which contributes to neuroinflammation. xcTau uptake alters the astrocyte morphology and function. Astrocytic response to Tau uptake triggers cellular senescence and the secretion of proinflammatory cytokines, causing neuroinflammation. Understanding these mechanisms highlights the potential therapeutic target to mitigate neurodegenerative in AD.

Acknowledgements

We are grateful to Chinnathambi's lab members for their scientific discussions, helpful suggestions and critical reading of the manuscript. We also greatly acknowledge internal support from the Department of Neurochemistry, National Institute of Mental Health and Neuro Sciences (NIMHANS), Institute of National Importance, Bangalore.

Competing interest

The authors declare no competing interests.

Funding

This project is supported by National Institute of Mental Health and Neuro Sciences (NIMHANS), Institute of National Importance, Bangalore.

Ethical approval and consent to participate

Not applicable.

Author contributions

SBC, SS, GV and AM conducted the literature survey, analyzed the data and wrote the manuscript. SBC conceived, designed, supervised, initial draft, review editing and wrote the paper. All authors read and approved the final paper.

Data availability

All the data have been included in the manuscript.

Consent for publication

Not applicable.

References

Amir Mishan, M., Rezaei Kanavi, M., Shahpasand, K., & Ahmadieh, H. (2019). Pathogenic Tau protein species: Promising therapeutic targets for ocular neurodegenerative diseases. *Journal of Ophthalmic and Vision Research, 14*, 491–505.

Avila, J., Lucas, J. J., Perez, M., & Hernandez, F. (2004). Role of tau protein in both physiological and pathological conditions. *Physiological Reviews, 84*, 361–384.

Balmik, A. A., & Chinnathambi, S. (2021). Methylation as a key regulator of Tau aggregation and neuronal health in Alzheimer's disease. *Cell Communication and Signaling: CCS, 19*, 51.

Balmik, A. A., & Chinnathambi, S. (2022a). Inter-relationship of histone deacetylase-6 with Tau-cytoskeletal organization and remodeling. *European Journal of Cell Biology, 101*, 151202.

Balmik, A. A., & Chinnathambi, S. (2022b). Inter relationship of histone deacetylase 6 with Tau-cytoskeletal organization and remodeling. *European Journal of Cell Biology, 101*, 151202.

Balmik, A. A., Das, R., Sonawane, S. K., & Chinnathambi, S. (2022). Aggregation species of amyloid-β and Tau oligomers in Alzheimer's disease: Role in therapeutics and diagnostics. In T. Govindaraju (Ed.). *Alzheimer's disease: Recent findings in pathophysiology, diagnostic and therapeutic modalities*. The Royal Society of Chemistry.

Balmik, A. A., Sonawane, S. K., & Chinnathambi, S. (2019). Modulation of Actin network and Tau phosphorylation by HDAC6 ZnF UBP domain. *bioRxiv*702571.

Barbier, P., Zejneli, O., Martinho, M., Lasorsa, A., Belle, V., Smet-Nocca, C., ... Landrieu, I. (2019). Role of Tau as a microtubule-associated protein: Structural and functional aspects. *Frontiers in Aging Neuroscience, 11*.

Batenburg, K. L., Kasri, N. N., Heine, V. M., & Scheper, W. (2022). Intraneuronal tau aggregation induces the integrated stress response in astrocytes. *Journal of Molecular Cell Biology, 14*.

Bell-Temin, H., Culver-Cochran, A. E., Chaput, D., Carlson, C. M., Kuehl, M., Burkhardt, B. R., ... Jr (2015). Novel molecular insights into classical and alternative activation states of microglia as revealed by stable isotope labeling by amino acids in cell culture (SILAC)-based proteomics. *Molecular & Cellular Proteomics: MCP, 14*, 3173–3184.

Bernadotte, A., Mikhelson, V. M., & Spivak, I. M. (2016). Markers of cellular senescence. Telomere shortening as a marker of cellular senescence. *Aging (Albany NY), 8*, 3–11.

Biswas, S., & Kalil, K. (2018). The microtubule-associated protein tau mediates the organization of microtubules and their dynamic exploration of actin-rich lamellipodia and filopodia of cortical growth cones. *The Journal of Neuroscience, 38*, 291–307.

Bivona, G., Iemmolo, M., Agnello, L., Lo Sasso, B., Gambino, C. M., Giglio, R. V., ... Ciaccio, M. (2023). Microglial activation and priming in Alzheimer's disease: State of the art and future perspectives. *International Journal of Molecular Sciences, 24*.

Bolós, M., Llorens-Martín, M., Perea, J. R., Jurado-Arjona, J., Rábano, A., Hernández, F., & Avila, J. (2017). Absence of CX3CR1 impairs the internalization of Tau by microglia. *Molecular Neurodegeneration, 12*, 59.

Brunello, C. A., Merezhko, M., Uronen, R. L., & Huttunen, H. J. (2020). Mechanisms of secretion and spreading of pathological tau protein. *Cellular and Molecular Life Sciences: CMLS, 77*, 1721–1744.

Cabrales Fontela, Y., Kadavath, H., Biernat, J., Riedel, D., Mandelkow, E., & Zweckstetter, M. (2017). Multivalent cross-linking of actin filaments and microtubules through the microtubule-associated protein Tau. *Nature Communications, 8*, 1981.

Cai, Y., Liu, J., Wang, B., Sun, M., & Yang, H. (2022). Microglia in the neuroinflammatory pathogenesis of Alzheimer's disease and related therapeutic targets. *Frontiers in Immunology, 13*, 856376.

Cartier, N., Lewis, C.-A., Zhang, R., & Rossi, F. M. V. (2014). The role of microglia in human disease: Therapeutic tool or target? *Acta Neuropathologica, 128*, 363–380.

Chen, K., Martens, Y. A., Meneses, A., Ryu, D. H., Lu, W., Raulin, A. C., ... Zhao, N. (2022a). LRP1 is a neuronal receptor for α-synuclein uptake and spread. *Molecular Neurodegeneration, 17*, 57.

Chen, R., Kang, R., & Tang, D. (2022b). The mechanism of HMGB1 secretion and release. *Experimental & Molecular Medicine, 54*, 91–102.

Chen, Y., & Yu, Y. (2023). Tau and neuroinflammation in Alzheimer's disease: Interplay mechanisms and clinical translation. *Journal of Neuroinflammation, 20*, 165.

Chidambaram, H., & Chinnathambi, S. (2020). G-Protein coupled receptors and tau-different roles in Alzheimer's disease. *Neuroscience, 438*, 198–214.

Chidambaram, H., & Chinnathambi, S. (2025). LC3-associated endocytosis facilitates extracellular Tau aggregate internalization and degradation in microglia. *Brain Network Disorders*.

Chidambaram, H., Das, R., & Chinnathambi, S. (2020). Interaction of Tau with the chemokine receptor, CX3CR1 and its effect on microglial activation, migration and proliferation. *Cell BioSciences, 10*, 109.

Chidambaram, H., Das, R., & Chinnathambi, S. (2022). G-protein coupled purinergic P2Y12 receptor interacts and internalizes Tau(RD)-mediated by membrane-associated actin cytoskeleton remodeling in microglia. *European Journal of Cell Biology, 101*, 151201.

Chidambaram, H., Desale, S. E., & Chinnathambi, S. (2024a). Purinergic receptor P2Y12-mediated Tau internalization in microglia. *Methods in Molecular Biology, 2754*, 457–470.

Chidambaram, H., Desale, S. E., Qureshi, T., & Chinnathambi, S. (2024b). Microglial uptake of extracellular Tau by actin-mediated phagocytosis. *Methods in Molecular Biology, 2761*, 231–243.

Chinnathambi, S. (2025). Histone deacetylase's regulates Tau function in Alzheimer's disease. *Advances in Protein Chemistry and Structural Biology, 143*, 339–361.

Chinnathambi, S., & Chidambaram, H. (2024). G-protein coupled receptors regulates Tauopathy in neurodegeneration. *Advances in Protein Chemistry and Structural Biology, 141*, 467–493.

Chinnathambi, S., & Das, R. (2023). Microglia degrade Tau oligomers deposit via purinergic P2Y12-associated podosome and filopodia formation and induce chemotaxis. *Cell BioSciences, 13*, 95.

Chinnathambi, S., Das, R., & Desale, S. E. (2023). Tau aggregates improve the purinergic receptor P2Y12-associated podosome rearrangements in microglial cells. *Biochimica et Biophysica Acta (BBA) - Molecular Cell Research, 1870*, 119477.

Chinnathambi, S., & Dubey, T. (2024). Photo-excited dyes: Emerging technique against Tau protein aggregation. *Methods in Molecular Biology, 2754*, 105–116.

Chinnathambi, S., & Rangappa, N. (2025). *SUMO inhibits Tau aggregation in Alzheimer's disease. Advances in protein chemistry and structural biology*. Academic Press.

Chinnathambi, S., Rangappa, N., & Chandrashekar, M. (2025a). Chapter One - Internalization of extracellular Tau oligomers in Alzheimer's disease. In G. S. Makowski (Ed.). *Advances in clinical chemistry*. Elsevier.

Chinnathambi, S., Velmurugan, G., Ananthanaraya, V., Chandrashekar, M., & Rangappa, N. (2024). *G-protein coupled receptors (GPCRs) interacts with Tau protein in Alzheimer's disease. Advances in protein chemistry and structural biology*. Academic Press.

Chinnathambi, S., Velmurugan, G., Suresh, S., Adithyan, A., & Chandrashekar, M. (2025b). Nuclear Tau accumulation in Alzheimer's disease. *Advances in Protein Chemistry and Structural Biology, 143*, 323–337.

Chu, D., Yang, X., Wang, J., Zhou, Y., Gu, J.-H., Miao, J., ... Liu, F. (2024). Tau truncation in the pathogenesis of Alzheimer's disease: A narrative review. *Neural Regeneration Research, 19*, 1221–1232.

Cleary, J. M., & Hancock, W. O. (2021). Molecular mechanisms underlying microtubule growth dynamics. *Current Biology, 31*, R560–R573.

Cooper, J. M., Lathuiliere, A., Migliorini, M., Arai, A. L., Wani, M. M., Dujardin, S., ... Strickland, D. K. (2021). Regulation of tau internalization, degradation, and seeding by LRP1 reveals multiple pathways for tau catabolism. *The Journal of Biological Chemistry, 296*, 100715.

Coppe, J. P., Desprez, P. Y., Krtolica, A., & Campisi, J. (2010). The senescence-associated secretory phenotype: The dark side of tumor suppression. *Annual Review of Pathology, 5*, 99–118.

Das, R., & Chinnathambi, S. (2019). Microglial priming of antigen presentation and adaptive stimulation in Alzheimer's disease. *Cellular and Molecular Life Sciences: CMLS, 76*, 3681–3694.

Das, R., & Chinnathambi, S. (2020). Actin-mediated microglial chemotaxis via G-protein coupled purinergic receptor in Alzheimer's disease. *Neuroscience, 448*, 325–336.

Das, R., & Chinnathambi, S. (2021). Microglial remodeling of actin network by Tau oligomers, via G protein-coupled purinergic receptor, P2Y12R-driven chemotaxis. *Traffic (Copenhagen, Denmark), 22*, 153–170.

De Calignon, A., Polydoro, M., Suarez-Calvet, M., William, C., Adamowicz, D. H., Kopeikina, K. J., ... Hyman, B. T. (2012). Propagation of tau pathology in a model of early Alzheimer's disease. *Neuron, 73*, 685–697.

Desale, S. E., Chidambaram, H., & Chinnathambi, S. (2024). α-Linolenic acid induces microglial activation and extracellular Tau internalization. *Methods in Molecular Biology, 2754*, 471–481.

Desale, S. E., & Chinnathambi, S. (2020). Role of dietary fatty acids in microglial polarization in Alzheimer's disease. *Journal of Neuroinflammation, 17*, 93.

Desale, S. E., & Chinnathambi, S. (2021). Phosphoinositides signaling modulates microglial actin remodeling and phagocytosis in Alzheimer's disease. *Cell Communication and Signaling: CCS, 19*, 28.

Dubey, T., & Chinnathambi, S. (2021). Photodynamic sensitizers modulate cytoskeleton structural dynamics in neuronal cells. *Cytoskeleton, 78*, 232–248.

Dubey, T., Sonawane, S., Mannava, C., Nangia, A., Chandrashekar, M., & Chinnathambi, S. (2022). The inhibitory effect of Curcumin-Artemisinin co-amorphous on Tau aggregation and Tau phosphorylation. *Colloids and Surfaces B: Biointerfaces, 221*, 112970.

Ebneth, A., Godemann, R., Stamer, K., Illenberger, S., Trinczek, B., Mandelkow, E.-M., & Mandelkow, E. (1998). Overexpression of Tau protein inhibits kinesin-dependent trafficking of vesicles, mitochondria, and endoplasmic reticulum: Implications for Alzheimer's disease. *Journal of Cell Biology, 143*, 777–794.

Eltom, K., Mothes, T., Libard, S., Ingelsson, M., & Erlandsson, A. (2024). Astrocytic accumulation of tau fibrils isolated from Alzheimer's disease brains induces inflammation, cell-to-cell propagation and neuronal impairment. *Acta Neuropathologica Communications, 12*, 34.

Engeland, K. (2022). Cell cycle regulation: p53-p21-RB signaling. *Cell Death & Differentiation, 29*, 946–960.

Ferrer, I. (2018). Astrogliopathy in Tauopathies. *Neuroglia, 1*, 126–150.

Fleeman, R. M., & Proctor, E. A. (2021). Astrocytic propagation of tau in the context of Alzheimer's disease. *Frontiers in Cellular Neuroscience, 15*, 645233.

Frost, B., Jacks, R. L., & Diamond, M. I. (2009). Propagation of Tau misfolding from the outside to the inside of a cell*. *Journal of Biological Chemistry, 284*, 12845–12852.

Gaikwad, S., Puangmalai, N., Bittar, A., Montalbano, M., Garcia, S., Mcallen, S., ... Kayed, R. (2021). Tau oligomer induced HMGB1 release contributes to cellular senescence and neuropathology linked to Alzheimer's disease and frontotemporal dementia. *Cell Reports, 36*, 109419.

Gao, Y. L., Wang, N., Sun, F. R., Cao, X. P., Zhang, W., & Yu, J. T. (2018). Tau in neurodegenerative disease. *Annals of Translational Medicine, 6*, 175.

Garcia, M. L., & Cleveland, D. W. (2001). Going new places using an old MAP: Tau, microtubules and human neurodegenerative disease. *Current Opinion in Cell Biology, 13*, 41–48.

Gendron, T. F., & Petrucelli, L. (2009). The role of tau in neurodegeneration. *Molecular Neurodegeneration, 4*, 13.

Gerson, J. E., Mudher, A., & Kayed, R. (2016). Potential mechanisms and implications for the formation of tau oligomeric strains. *Critical Reviews in Biochemistry and Molecular Biology, 51*, 482–496.

Gomez-Ramos, A., Diaz-Hernandez, M., Cuadros, R., Hernandez, F., & Avila, J. (2006). Extracellular tau is toxic to neuronal cells. *FEBS Letters, 580*, 4842–4850.

Gorantla, N. V., Das, R., Chidambaram, H., Dubey, T., Mulani, F. A., Thulasiram, H. V., & Chinnathambi, S. (2020). Basic limonoid modulates chaperone-mediated proteostasis and dissolve Tau fibrils. *Scientific Reports, 10*, 4023.

Gorantla, N. V., Das, R., Mulani, F. A., Thulasiram, H. V., & Chinnathambi, S. (2019). Neem derivatives inhibits Tau aggregation. *Journal of Alzheimer's Disease & Reports, 3*, 169–178.

Gorantla, N. V., Khandelwal, P., Poddar, P., & Chinnathambi, S. (2017a). Global conformation of Tau protein mapped by Raman spectroscopy. *Methods in Molecular Biology, 1523*, 21–31.

Gorantla, N. V., Shkumatov, A. V., & Chinnathambi, S. (2017b). Conformational dynamics of intracellular Tau protein revealed by CD and SAXS. In C. Smet-Nocca (Ed.). *Tau protein: Methods and protocols*. New York, NY: Springer New York.

Granholm, A.-C., & Hamlett, E. D. (2024). The role of Tau pathology in Alzheimer's disease and down syndrome. *Journal of Clinical Medicine, 13*, 1338.

Guha, S., Johnson, G. V. W., & Nehrke, K. (2020). The crosstalk between pathological Tau phosphorylation and mitochondrial dysfunction as a key to understanding and treating Alzheimer's disease. *Molecular Neurobiology, 57*, 5103–5120.

Guo, C., Sun, L., Chen, X., & Zhang, D. (2013a). Oxidative stress, mitochondrial damage and neurodegenerative diseases. *Neural Regeneration Research, 8*, 2003–2014.

Guo, R.-M., Xu, W.-M., Lin, J.-C., Mo, L.-Q., Hua, X.-X., Chen, P.-X., ... Feng, J.-Q. (2013b). Activation of the p38 MAPK/NF-κB pathway contributes to doxorubicin-induced inflammation and cytotoxicity in H9c2 cardiac cells. *Molecular Medicine Reports, 8*, 603–608.

Guo, S., Wang, H., & Yin, Y. (2022). Microglia polarization from M1 to M2 in neurodegenerative diseases. *Frontiers in Aging Neuroscience, 14*, 815347.

Han, X., Zhang, T., Liu, H., Mi, Y., & Gou, X. (2020). Astrocyte senescence and Alzheimer's disease: A review. *Frontiers in Aging Neuroscience, 12*, 148.

Hanger, D. P., Lau, D. H., Phillips, E. C., Bondulich, M. K., Guo, T., Woodward, B. W., ... Noble, W. (2014). Intracellular and extracellular roles for tau in neurodegenerative disease. *Journal of Alzheimer's Disease: JAD, 40*(1), S37–S45.

Hanslik, K. L., & Ulland, T. K. (2020). The role of microglia and the Nlrp3 inflammasome in Alzheimer's disease. *Frontiers in Neurology, 11*, 570711.

Hardy, J., & Selkoe, D. J. (2002). The amyloid hypothesis of Alzheimer's disease: Progress and problems on the road to therapeutics. *Science (New York, N. Y.), 297*, 353 356.

He, Y., Gao, Y., Zhang, Q., Zhou, G., Cao, F., & Yao, S. (2020). IL-4 Switches microglia/macrophage M1/M2 polarization and alleviates neurological damage by modulating the JAK1/STAT6 pathway following ICH. *Neuroscience, 437*, 161–171.

Hill, E., Wall, M. J., Moffat, K. G., & Karikari, T. K. (2020). Understanding the pathophysiological actions of Tau oligomers: A critical review of current electrophysiological approaches. *Frontiers in Molecular Neuroscience, 13*.

Hohmann, T., & Dehghani, F. (2019). The cytoskeleton-A complex interacting meshwork. *Cells, 8*.

Ising, C., Venegas, C., Zhang, S., Scheiblich, H., Schmidt, S. V., Vieira-Saecker, A., ... Heneka, M. T. (2019). NLRP3 inflammasome activation drives tau pathology. *Nature, 575*, 669–673.

Jeganathan, S., Chinnathambi, S., Mandelkow, E. M., & Mandelkow, E. (2012). Conformations of microtubule-associated protein Tau mapped by fluorescence resonance energy transfer. *Methods in Molecular Biology, 849*, 85–99.

Jung, E. S., Suh, K., Han, J., Kim, H., Kang, H. S., Choi, W. S., & Mook-Jung, I. (2022). Amyloid-beta activates NLRP3 inflammasomes by affecting microglial immunometabolism through the Syk-AMPK pathway. *Aging Cell, 21*, e13623.

Kapoor, M., & Chinnathambi, S. (2023a). TGF-β1 signalling in Alzheimer's pathology and cytoskeletal reorganization: A specialized Tau perspective. *Journal of Neuroinflammation, 20*, 72.

Kapoor, M., & Chinnathambi, S. (2023b). TGF-β1 signalling in Alzheimer's pathology and cytoskeletal reorganization: A specialized Tau perspective. *Journal of Neuroinflammation, 20*, 72.

Kent, S. A., Spires-Jones, T. L., & Durrant, C. S. (2020). The physiological roles of tau and Aβ: Implications for Alzheimer's disease pathology and therapeutics. *Acta Neuropathologica, 140*, 417–447.

Kim, S., Sharma, C., Jung, U. J., & Kim, S. R. (2023). Pathophysiological role of microglial activation induced by blood-borne proteins in Alzheimer's disease. *Biomedicines, 11*, 1383.

Köpke, E., Tung, Y. C., Shaikh, S., Alonso, A. C., Iqbal, K., & Grundke-Iqbal, I. (1993). Microtubule-associated protein tau. Abnormal phosphorylation of a non-paired helical filament pool in Alzheimer disease. *Journal of Biological Chemistry, 268*, 24374–24384.

Lamptey, R. N. L., Chaulagain, B., Trivedi, R., Gothwal, A., Layek, B., & Singh, J. (2022). A review of the common neurodegenerative disorders: Current therapeutic approaches and the potential role of nanotherapeutics. *International Journal of Molecular Sciences, 23*.

Lappas, M., Permezel, M., Georgiou, H. M., & Rice, G. E. (2002). Nuclear factor kappa B regulation of proinflammatory cytokines in human gestational tissues in vitro. *Biology of Reproduction, 67*, 668–673.

Li, X., Li, C., Zhang, W., Wang, Y., Qian, P., & Huang, H. (2023a). Inflammation and aging: Signaling pathways and intervention therapies. *Signal Transduction and Targeted Therapy, 8*, 239.

Li, Y., Xu, H., Wang, H., Yang, K., Luan, J., & Wang, S. (2023b). TREM2: Potential therapeutic targeting of microglia for Alzheimer's disease. *Biomedicine & Pharmacotherapy = Biomedecine & Pharmacotherapie, 165*, 115218.

Li, Y., Xu, H., Wang, H., Yang, K., Luan, J., & Wang, S. (2023c). TREM2: Potential therapeutic targeting of microglia for Alzheimer's disease. *Biomedicine & Pharmacotherapy, 165*, 115218.

Lowe, S. W. (1999). Activation of p53 by oncogenes. *Endocrine-Related Cancer, 6*, 45–48.

Lyu, S., Lan, Z., & Li, C. (2023). The triggering receptor expressed on myeloid cells 2-apolipoprotein· E signaling pathway in diseases. *Chinese Medical Journal (Engl), 136*, 1291–1299.

Ma, M., Jiang, W., & Zhou, R. (2024). DAMPs and DAMP-sensing receptors in inflammation and diseases. *Immunity, 57*, 752–771.

Mamun, A. A., Uddin, M. S., Mathew, B., & Ashraf, G. M. (2020). Toxic tau: Structural origins of tau aggregation in Alzheimer's disease. *Neural Regeneration Research, 15*, 1417–1420.

Matej, R., Tesar, A., & Rusina, R. (2019). Alzheimer's disease and other neurodegenerative dementias in comorbidity: A clinical and neuropathological overview. *Clinical Biochemistry, 73*, 26–31.

Mckee, C. A., Lee, J., Cai, Y., Saito, T., Saido, T., & Musiek, E. S. (2022). Astrocytes deficient in circadian clock gene Bmal1 show enhanced activation responses to amyloid-beta pathology without changing plaque burden. *Scientific Reports, 12*, 1796.

Medina, M., & Avila, J. (2014). The role of extracellular Tau in the spreading of neurofibrillary pathology. *Frontiers in Cellular Neuroscience, 8*.

Medina, M., & Avila, J. (2020). Editorial: Untangling the role of Tau in physiology and pathology. *Frontiers in Aging Neuroscience, 12*, 146.

Miao, J., Ma, H., Yang, Y., Liao, Y., Lin, C., Zheng, J., ... Lan, J. (2023). Microglia in Alzheimer's disease: Pathogenesis, mechanisms, and therapeutic potentials. *Frontiers in Aging Neuroscience, 15*, 1201982.

Michalicova, A., Majerova, P., & Kovac, A. (2020). Tau protein and its role in blood–brain barrier dysfunction. *Frontiers in Molecular Neuroscience, 13*.

Miyazaki, T., Katagiri, H., Kanegae, Y., Takayanagi, H., Sawada, Y., Yamamoto, A., ... Tanaka, S. (2000). Reciprocal role of ERK and NF-kappaB pathways in survival and activation of osteoclasts. *The Journal of Cell Biology, 148*, 333–342.

Mohan, R., & John, A. (2015). Microtubule-associated proteins as direct crosslinkers of actin filaments and microtubules. *IUBMB Life, 67*, 395–403.

Moriuchi, Y., Iwagawa, T., Tsuhako, A., Koso, H., Fujita, Y., & Watanabe, S. (2020). RasV12 expression in microglia initiates retinal inflammation and induces photoreceptor degeneration. *Investigative Ophthalmology & Visual Science, 61*, 34.

Morton, H., Kshirsagar, S., Orlov, E., Bunquin, L. E., Sawant, N., Boleng, L., ... Reddy, P. H. (2021). Defective mitophagy and synaptic degeneration in Alzheimer's disease: Focus on aging, mitochondria and synapse. *Free Radical Biology & Medicine, 172*, 652–667.

Moya-Alvarado, G., Gershoni-Emek, N., Perlson, E., & Bronfman, F. C. (2016). Neurodegeneration and Alzheimer's disease (AD). What can proteomics tell us about the Alzheimer's brain? *Molecular & Cellular Proteomics: MCP, 15*, 409–425.

Mueller, C. (2012). Danger-associated molecular patterns and inflammatory bowel disease: Is there a connection? *Digestive Diseases (Basel, Switzerland), 30*(3), 40–46.

Nanjundaiah, S., Chidambaram, H., Chandrashekar, M., & Chinnathambi, S. (2021). Role of microglia in regulating cholesterol and Tau pathology in Alzheimer's disease. *Cellular and Molecular Neurobiology, 41*, 651–668.

Neddens, J., Temmel, M., Flunkert, S., Kerschbaumer, B., Hoeller, C., Loeffler, T., ... Hutter-Paier, B. (2018). Phosphorylation of different tau sites during progression of Alzheimer's disease. *Acta Neuropathologica Communications, 6*, 52.

Olson, A., Hussong, S. A., Kayed, R., & Galvan, V. (2019). Tau-induced astrocyte senescence: A novel mechanism for neuronal dysfunction in Alzheimer's disease. *Innovation in Aging, 3*, S91.

Pampuscenko, K., Morkuniene, R., Sneideris, T., Smirnovas, V., Budvytyte, R., Valincius, G., ... Borutaite, V. (2020). Extracellular tau induces microglial phagocytosis of living neurons in cell cultures. *Journal of Neurochemistry, 154*, 316–329.

Pawelec, P., Ziemka-Nalecz, M., Sypecka, J., & Zalewska, T. (2020). The impact of the CX3CL1/CX3CR1 axis in neurological disorders. *Cells, 9*.

Perea, J. R., Bolos, M., & Avila, J. (2020). Microglia in Alzheimer's disease in the context of Tau pathology. *Biomolecules, 10*.

Pooler, A. M., Polydoro, M., Wegmann, S., Nicholls, S. B., Spires-Jones, T. L., & Hyman, B. T. (2013). Propagation of tau pathology in Alzheimer's disease: Identification of novel therapeutic targets. *Alzheimer's Research & Therapy, 5*, 49.

Przedborski, S., Vila, M., & Jackson-Lewis, V. (2003). Neurodegeneration: What is it and where are we? *The Journal of Clinical Investigation, 111*, 3–10.

Puliatti, G., Li Puma, D. D., Aceto, G., Lazzarino, G., Acquarone, E., Mangione, R., ... Grassi, C. (2023). Intracellular accumulation of tau oligomers in astrocytes and their synaptotoxic action rely on amyloid precursor protein intracellular domain-dependent expression of glypican-4. *Progress in Neurobiology, 227*, 102482.

Qiang, L., Sun, X., Austin, T. O., Muralidharan, H., Jean, D. C., Liu, M., ... Baas, P. W. (2018). Tau does not stabilize axonal microtubules but rather enables them to have long labile domains. *Current Biology: CB, 28*, 2181–2189 e4.

Qin, B., Li, Y., Liu, X., Gong, D., & Zheng, W. (2020). Notch activation enhances microglial CX3CR1/P38 MAPK pathway in rats model of vincristine-induced peripheral neuropathy. *Neuroscience Letters, 715*, 134624.

Qin, Y. H., Dai, S. M., Tang, G. S., Zhang, J., Ren, D., Wang, Z. W., & Shen, Q. (2009). HMGB1 enhances the proinflammatory activity of lipopolysaccharide by promoting the phosphorylation of MAPK p38 through receptor for advanced glycation end products. *Journal of Immunology, 183*, 6244–6250.

Qureshi, T., Chandrashekar, M., Ananthanarayana, V., Kumarappan, M., Rangappa, N., Velmurugan, G., & Chinnathambi, S. (2025). Chapter Fourteen - Nuclear podosomes regulates cellular migration in Tau and Alzheimer's disease. In R. Donev (Ed.). *Advances in protein chemistry and structural biology*. Academic Press.

Rauch, J. N., Luna, G., Guzman, E., Audouard, M., Challis, C., Sibih, Y. E., ... Kosik, K. S. (2020). LRP1 is a master regulator of tau uptake and spread. *Nature, 580*, 381–385.

Recasens, M., Almolda, B., Pérez-Clausell, J., Campbell, I. L., González, B., & Castellano, B. (2021). Chronic exposure to IL-6 induces a desensitized phenotype of the microglia. *Journal of Neuroinflammation, 18*, 31.

Reid, M. J., Beltran-Lobo, P., Johnson, L., Perez-Nievas, B. G., & Noble, W. (2020). Astrocytes in Tauopathies. *Frontiers in Neurology, 11*, 572850.

Riley, J. K., Takeda, K., Akira, S., & Schreiber, R. D. (1999). Interleukin-10 receptor signaling through the JAK-STAT pathway. Requirement for two distinct receptor-derived signals for anti-inflammatory action. *The Journal of Biological Chemistry, 274*, 16513–16521.

Robbins, M., Clayton, E., & Kaminski Schierle, G. S. (2021). Synaptic tau: A pathological or physiological phenomenon? *Acta Neuropathologica Communications, 9*, 149.

Rodríguez-Giraldo, M., González-Reyes, R. E., Ramírez-Guerrero, S., Bonilla-Trilleras, C. E., Guardo-Maya, S., & Nava-Mesa, M. O. (2022). Astrocytes as a therapeutic target in Alzheimer's disease–comprehensive review and recent developments. *International Journal of Molecular Sciences, 23*, 13630.

Sebastian-Serrano, A., De Diego-Garcia, L., & Diaz-Hernandez, M. (2018). The neurotoxic role of extracellular Tau protein. *International Journal of Molecular Sciences, 19*.

Shamloo, B., & Usluer, S. (2019). p21 in Cancer research. *Cancers (Basel), 11.*

Shkumatov, A. V., Chinnathambi, S., Mandelkow, E., & Svergun, D. I. (2011). Structural memory of natively unfolded tau protein detected by small-angle X-ray scattering. *Proteins, 79*, 2122–2131.

Sinsky, J., Pichlerova, K., & Hanes, J. (2021). Tau protein interaction partners and their roles in Alzheimer's disease and other tauopathies. *International Journal of Molecular Sciences, 22.*

Sokolow, S., Henkins, K. M., Bilousova, T., Gonzalez, B., Vinters, H. V., Miller, C. A., ... Gylys, K. H. (2015). Pre-synaptic C-terminal truncated tau is released from cortical synapses in Alzheimer's disease. *Journal of Neurochemistry, 133*, 368–379.

Solleiro-Villavicencio, H., & Rivas-Arancibia, S. (2018). Effect of chronic oxidative stress on neuroinflammatory response mediated by CD4(+)T cells in neurodegenerative diseases. *Frontiers in Cellular Neuroscience, 12*, 114.

Sonawane, S. K., Chidambaram, H., Boral, D., Gorantla, N. V., Balmik, A. A., Dangi, A., ... Chinnathambi, S. (2020). EGCG impedes human Tau aggregation and interacts with Tau. *Scientific Reports, 10*, 12579.

Sonawane, S. K., & Chinnathambi, S. (2018). Prion-Like propagation of post-translationally modified Tau in Alzheimer's disease: A hypothesis. *Journal of Molecular Neuroscience, 65*, 480–490.

Sonawane, S. K., & Chinnathambi, S. (2020). A green tea polyphenol epigallocatechin-3-gallate modulates Tau post-translational modifications and cytoskeletal network. *bioRxiv* 2020.03.22.002014.

Sonawane, S. K., Dubey, T., Balmik, A. A., Das, R., & Chinnathambi, S. (2022). Alzheimer's disease pathology: A Tau perspective. In T. Govindaraju (Ed.). *Alzheimer's disease: Recent findings in pathophysiology, diagnostic and therapeutic modalities*. The Royal Society of Chemistry.

Sonawane, S. K., Uversky, V. N., & Chinnathambi, S. (2021). Baicalein inhibits heparin-induced Tau aggregation by initializing non-toxic Tau oligomer formation. *Cell Communication and Signaling: CCS, 19*, 16.

Suthers, A. N., & Sarantopoulos, S. (2017). TLR7/TLR9- and B cell receptor-signaling crosstalk: Promotion of potentially dangerous B cells. *Frontiers in Immunology, 8*, 775.

Tabeshmehr, P., & Eftekharpour, E. (2023). Tau; One protein, so many diseases. *Biology, 12*, 244.

Ueda, S., Tominaga, T., Ochi, A., Sakurai, A., Nishimura, K., Shibata, E., ... Nagai, K. (2021). TGF-β1 is involved in senescence-related pathways in glomerular endothelial cells via p16 translocation and p21 induction. *Scientific Reports, 11*, 21643.

Usenovic, M., Niroomand, S., Drolet, R. E., Yao, L., Gaspar, R. C., Hatcher, N. G., ... Parmentier-Batteur, S. (2015). Internalized Tau oligomers cause neurodegeneration by inducing accumulation of pathogenic Tau in human neurons derived from induced pluripotent stem cells. *The Journal of Neuroscience, 35*, 14234–14250.

Vacchi, E., Kaelin-Lang, A., & Melli, G. (2020). Tau and alpha synuclein synergistic effect in neurodegenerative diseases: When the periphery is the core. *International Journal of Molecular Sciences,* 21.

Venkatramani, A., & Panda, D. (2019). Regulation of neuronal microtubule dynamics by tau: Implications for tauopathies. *International Journal of Biological Macromolecules, 133*, 473–483.

Verkhratsky, A., Sun, D., & Tanaka, J. (2021). Snapshot of microglial physiological functions. *Neurochemistry International, 144*, 104960.

Vijay Nalini, G., Das, R., Balaraman, E., & Chinnathambi, S. (2019). Transition metal nickel prevents Tau aggregation in Alzheimer's disease. *International Journal of Biological Macromolecules, 156.*

Vogels, T., Murgoci, A.-N., & Hromádka, T. (2019). Intersection of pathological tau and microglia at the synapse. *Acta Neuropathologica Communications, 7*, 109.

Wang, P., & Ye, Y. (2021). Filamentous recombinant human Tau activates primary astrocytes via an integrin receptor complex. *Nature Communications, 12*, 95.

Wang, Q., & Xie, C. (2022). Microglia activation linking amyloid-β drive tau spatial propagation in Alzheimer's disease. *Frontiers in Neuroscience, 16.*

Wang, Y., Balaji, V., Kaniyappan, S., Krüger, L., Irsen, S., Tepper, K., ... Mandelkow, E.-M. (2017). The release and trans-synaptic transmission of Tau via exosomes. *Molecular Neurodegeneration, 12*, 5.

Wang, Y., & Mandelkow, E. (2016). Tau in physiology and pathology. *Nature Reviews. Neuroscience, 17*, 22–35.

Wang, Z. B., Ma, Y. H., Sun, Y., Tan, L., Wang, H. F., Yu, J. T., & Alzheimer's Disease Neuroimaging, I. (2022). Interleukin-3 is associated with sTREM2 and mediates the correlation between amyloid-beta and tau pathology in Alzheimer's disease. *Journal of Neuroinflammation, 19*, 316.

Weingarten, M. D., Lockwood, A. H., Hwo, S. Y., & Kirschner, M. W. (1975). A protein factor essential for microtubule assembly. *Proceedings of the National Academy of Sciences of the United States of America, 72*, 1858–1862.

Wu, M., Zhang, M., Yin, X., Chen, K., Hu, Z., Zhou, Q., ... Liu, D. (2021). The role of pathological tau in synaptic dysfunction in Alzheimer's diseases. *Translational Neurodegeneration, 10*, 45.

Wu, X., Wan, T., Gao, X., Fu, M., Duan, Y., Shen, X., & Guo, W. (2022). Microglia pyroptosis: A candidate target for neurological diseases treatment. *Frontiers in Neuroscience, 16*, 922331.

Wysocka, A., Palasz, E., Steczkowska, M., & Niewiadomska, G. (2020). Dangerous liaisons: Tau interaction with muscarinic receptors. *Current Alzheimer Research, 17*, 224–237.

Xia, Y., Prokop, S., Gorion, K. M., Kim, J. D., Sorrentino, Z. A., Bell, B. M., ... Giasson, B. I. (2020). Tau Ser208 phosphorylation promotes aggregation and reveals neuropathologic diversity in Alzheimer's disease and other tauopathies. *Acta Neuropathologica Communications, 8*, 88.

Yamada, K. (2017). Extracellular Tau and its potential role in the propagation of Tau pathology. *Frontiers in Neuroscience, 11*, 667.

Ye, R. D. (2001). Regulation of nuclear factor kappaB activation by G-protein-coupled receptors. *Journal of Leukocyte Biology, 70*, 839–848.

Yuan, A., & Nixon, R. A. (2023). Posttranscriptional regulation of neurofilament proteins and tau in health and disease. *Brain Research Bulletin, 192*, 115–127.

Zhang, H., Cao, Y., Ma, L., Wei, Y., & Li, H. (2021). Possible mechanisms of Tau spread and toxicity in Alzheimer's disease. *Frontiers in Cell and Developmental Biology, 9.*

Zhao, J., Wu, H., & Tang, X. Q. (2021). Tau internalization: A complex step in tau propagation. *Ageing Research Reviews, 67*, 101272.

Zhao, X., Chen, B., Wu, L., & Zhao, G. (2022). Role of mitochondria in nuclear DNA damage response. *Genome Instability & Disease, 3*, 285–294.

Zhao, Y., Wu, X., Li, X., Jiang, L. L., Gui, X., Liu, Y., ... Xu, H. (2018). TREM2 Is a receptor for beta-amyloid that mediates microglial function. *Neuron, 97*, 1023–1031 e7.

Zhou, Y., Chen, Y., Xu, C., Zhang, H., & Lin, C. (2020). TLR4 Targeting as a promising therapeutic strategy for Alzheimer disease treatment. *Frontiers in Neuroscience, 14.*

Zhu, Y., Gandy, L., Zhang, F., Liu, J., Wang, C., Blair, L. J., ... Wang, L. (2022). Heparan sulfate proteoglycans in Tauopathy. *Biomolecules, 12.*

Zilka, N., Kazmerova, Z., Jadhav, S., Neradil, P., Madari, A., Obetkova, D., ... Novak, M. (2012). Who fans the flames of Alzheimer's disease brains? Misfolded tau on the crossroad of neurodegenerative and inflammatory pathways. *Journal of Neuroinflammation, 9*, 47.

CHAPTER TWO

Brain macrophages in neurodegeneration

Rachel J. Johnston[a,b], Nicole A. Pagán Torres[a,b], Yangchen Li[a,b], and Claudia Z. Han[a,b,*]
[a]Department of Pathology and Immunology, Washington University in St. Louis School of Medicine, St. Louis, MO, United States
[b]Brain Immunology and Glia (BIG) Center, Washington University in St. Louis School of Medicine, St. Louis, MO, United States
*Corresponding author. e-mail address: claudiah@wustl.edu

Contents

Abstract

Brain macrophages are not uniform responders to neurodegeneration, but anatomically specialized populations whose functions depend on niche, developmental history, and regulatory state. The goal of this chapter is to discuss how parenchymal

Advances in Immunology, Volume 171
ISSN 0065-2776, https://doi.org/10.1016/bs.ai.2026.06.005

microglia and brain border associated macrophages as components of a distributed macrophage network that operates across the central nervous system. Microglia are embedded within the parenchyma and are central to surveillance, synaptic remodeling, myelin maintenance and tissue repair, whereas BAMs occupy vascular, meningeal, and choroid plexus interfaces where they regulate barrier function, immune surveillance, fluid dynamics and solute clearance. Across disease settings, these populations repeatedly converge and diverge on pathological programs, including inflammatory activation, lysosomal stress, lipid handling and maladaptive crosstalk with neighboring cells. Future studies on how these populations are alike and different and development of technology to allow precise targeting of these populations will be essential towards enhancing macrophage protection of the brain.

1. Introduction

The central nervous system (CNS) contains a specialized network of resident macrophages that occupy anatomically and functionally distinct niches. These include microglia, which reside within the parenchyma, and border-associated macrophages (BAMs), which populate CNS interfaces such as the meninges, perivascular spaces, and choroid plexus (Rustenhoven & Kipnis, 2022; Brioschi, Han & Colonna, 2025; Penati et al., 2025). Although both populations belong to the CNS macrophage compartment, they differ in developmental origin, anatomical localization, transcriptional identity, turnover dynamics, and physiological roles in neurodegeneration.

2. Microglia: Historical debate and embryonic origin

The origin of microglia has been contested for decades. Pio del Río-Hortega hypothesized that microglia had a mesodermal, likely meningeal origin (Penfield, 1932). This idea was overshadowed for decades by the notion that microglia, like other glial cells, were of neuro-ectodermal origin. Subsequent electron microscopy and immunohistochemistry studies showed that microglia demonstrate morphological features similar to those of macrophages, lending new weight to del Rio-Hortega's hypothesis (Murabe & Sano, 1982). This was further supported by immunohistochemical analysis showing microglial expression of macrophage markers, including F4/80, Fc receptor, and CD11b in mice (Perry et al., 1985). Genetic evidence later demonstrated that PU.1, a transcription factor required for myeloid lineage development, is necessary for microglial development (McKercher et al., 1996). Together, these studies shifted the field decisively toward a myeloid origin for microglia, but their specific embryonic origin and developmental timeline remained unclear.

Early descriptive studies showed that amoeboid microglia appear in the rodent neuroepithelium during embryogenesis and express monocytic markers (Wang et al., 1996). In humans, microglia-like cells were observed as early as gestational week (GW) 4.5 (Hutchins et al., 1990; Menassa & Gomez-Nicola, 2018). Progressive colonization of the spinal cord occurs around GW9, with a major wave of microglial influx and distribution around GW16, and broadly ramified microglia distributed throughout the brain by GW22 (Rezaie & Male, 1999). Together, these studies suggested that microglia are derived from hematopoietic precursors prior to the onset of bone marrow hematopoiesis.

During embryogenesis, hematopoiesis proceeds in overlapping waves that arise from the extraembryonic yolk sac (YS), intraembryonic hematopoietic sites, and later the fetal liver (Tavian & Peault, 2005). In mice, the first, or primitive, wave of hematopoiesis begins in the YS around E7.5 and generates the earliest erythroid and myeloid cells (Moore & Metcalf, 1970; McGrath et al., 2003). At E8.5, hematopoietic progenitors arise first within the para-aortic splanchnopleure and then in the aorta, gonads, and mesonephros (AGM) region, which gives rise to definitive hematopoiesis (Medvinsky et al., 1993). At around E10.5, both YS- and AGM-derived progenitors begin to colonize the fetal liver, becomes as the major hematopoietic origin after day E11.5 and generates multiple hematopoietic lineages, including monocytes (Naito et al., 1990; Kumaravelu et al., 2002). These overlapping waves of hematopoiesis contributed to long-standing uncertainty about the timing and source of microglial emergence.

Fate-mapping experiments in mice later clarified the embryonic origin of microglia. Microglia arise from erythro-myeloid progenitor cells (EMPs), which emerge from the YS between E7.5 and E8.5, with no contribution from the fetal liver or bone marrow (Ginhoux et al., 2010; Ginhoux et al., 2013; Ginhoux & Guilliams, 2016; Thion et al., 2018; Silvin et al., 2023). Notably, EMPs produce macrophages in a MYB-independent process and without an intermediate stage (Hoeffel et al., 2015). Rather, EMPs differentiate into macrophages through a transcription factor program reliant on PU.1, RUNX1, and IRF8 (Kierdorf, Erny, et al., 2013; Mass et al., 2016, 2023; Kierdorf et al., 2019). After the establishment of the embryonic circulatory system, microglial progenitors emerge from the YS and infiltrate the brain between E9.5 and E10.5 (Ginhoux et al., 2010; Thion, Ginhoux & Garel, 2018). As the blood-brain barrier (BBB) matures around E13.5, later entry of circulating immune cells into the brain parenchyma becomes increasingly restricted (Profaci et al., 2020), Fig. 1.

Evidence from human development supports a similar transition from primitive yolk sac macrophages to nascent microglia within the developing head. Using single-cell transcriptomics, At Carnegie stage (CS) 11, CD45+ hematopoietic cells are detectable in the yolk sac, with a smaller population already present in the developing head; these have been

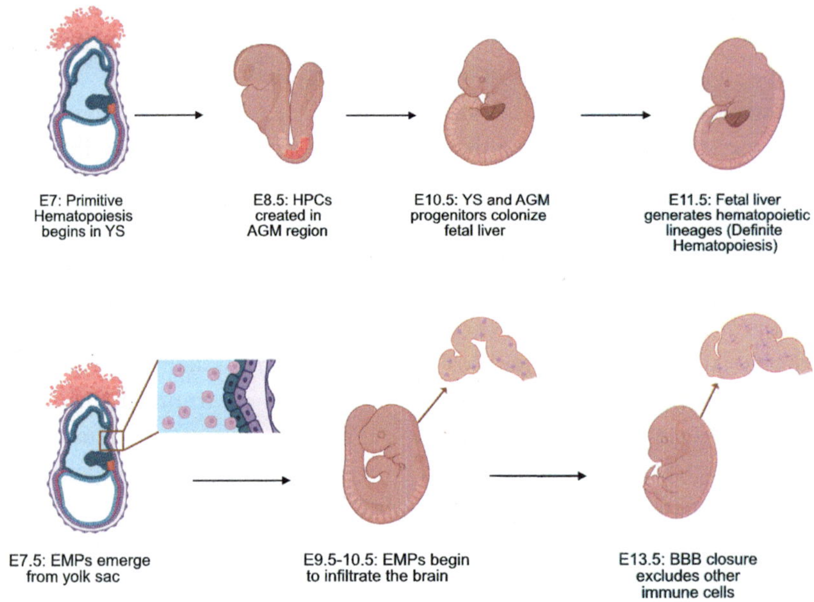

Fig. 1 Waves of hematopoiesis and staged microglia development during embryogenesis. (top) Schematic depicting sequential waves of hematopoiesis across embryonic development. Primitive hematopoiesis begins in the yolk sac around E7.0-E8.5, generating early erythroid cells and erythromyeloid progenitors. Definitive hematopoiesis emerges in the aorta-gonad-mesonephros (AGM) region beginning around E8.5-E10.5, producing hematopoietic stem cells that subsequently migrate to and expand within the fetal liver beginning around E10.5-E11.5, where hematopoiesis becomes the dominant source of circulating progenitors. (bottom) Schematic illustrating the developmental progression of microglia from yolk sac–derived progenitors across embryonic timepoints. Erythromyeloid progenitors generated in the yolk sac between E7.5-E8.5 give rise to macrophage precursors that migrate into the developing brain beginning around E9.5-E10.5. Following brain colonization, microglia undergo proliferation and maturation, progressing through early developmental stages toward mature microglial states characterized by increasing cellular complexity and acquisition of homeostatic microglial identity.

proposed to represent yolk sac-derived primitive macrophages that give rise to microglial precursors following migration into the CNS (Bian et al., 2020). Between CS11 and CS23, head macrophage populations undergo a transcriptional transition marked by declining inflammatory regulators, including *IRF7* and *STAT1*, and increasing expression of factors associated with acquisition of a microglial identity, such as *BHLHE41*, *NR4A1*, and *SALL1* (Bian et al., 2020). These findings place the emergence of human microglia at the transition between early hematopoietic migration and tissue-specific reprogramming within the developing CNS.

2.1 Microglia: Developmental maturation and persistence

Microglia undergo a stepwise maturation program after entering the CNS, with marked changes in transcriptional state, chromatin landscape, morphology, and long-term maintenance. Mouse microglia profiled across developmental timepoints found that early microglia express genes associated with cell cycle progression and differentiation, including *Mcm5* and *Dab2* (Matcovitch-Natan et al., 2016). Early microglia also retained substantial similarity to yolk sac macrophages despite occupying a distinct tissue environment, supporting the idea that newly seeded microglia initially preserve aspects of an earlier developmental program. At these early stages, microglia were enriched for gene ontology categories related to neurogenesis, neural migration, and cytokine secretion, consistent with their involvement in neural development and circuit refinement. Genes such as *Csf1* and *Cxcr2,* which have been linked to neuronal development, peaked shortly before birth and declined in adulthood, whereas genes including *Cd14* and *Pmepa1* were more prominent in adult microglia (Matcovitch-Natan et al., 2016). Importantly, these transcriptional transitions were accompanied by stage-specific changes in chromatin accessibility and enhancer activity, indicating that developmental progression is coupled to remodeling of the underlying regulatory landscape.

Consistent with rodent studies, human fetal microglia are present in the brain early and undergo further regional dispersal as development proceeds. Shortly after neural tube closure, at approximately GW4.5, IBA1+ microglia are detected in the leptomeninges, ventricular edge, and choroid plexus, from which they infiltrate the telencephalon and diencephalon (Kracht et al., 2020). By GW12, many microglia already display ramified processes resembling those of adult cells, indicating that morphological differentiation begins early in fetal life. Additionally, fetal microglia acquire core homeostatic features early in development, including expression of canonical microglial genes such as *CSF1R*, *CX3CR1*, *P2RY12*, *P2RY13*, and *TMEM119* as development proceeds (Kracht et al., 2020).

Mechanistically, the transition from fetal to postnatal human microglia is accompanied by extensive remodeling of both the transcriptome and enhancer landscape, establishing development stage-specific gene regulatory networks rather than a simple linear progression toward an adult endpoint (Han et al., 2023). Fetal microglia were enriched for programs related to cell cycle, ATP metabolism, phagocytosis, lysosomal function, adhesion, and motility, whereas postnatal microglia preferentially expressed genes involved in cytokine signaling, antigen processing and presentation, and immune priming (Han et al., 2023). Within fetal life itself, second-trimester microglia upregulated genes linked to immune regulation and phagocytosis, including *AHR*, *NR4A2*, *TIMD4*, and *CLEC7A*, indicating that substantial maturation occurs during gestation (Han et al., 2023). As seen in mice, (Matcovitch-Natan et al., 2016), these stage-specific states were associated with distinct regulatory programs, with fetal microglia preferentially engaging MiTF-TFE family members, MAF, and MEF2-centered networks and postnatal microglia preferentially engaging IRF, STAT, KLF, and SMAD-centered networks (Han et al., 2023). Single-cell chromatin and transcriptomic analyses likewise identified both shared and stage-biased microglial substates, including lysosomal, proliferative, immune-modulatory, interferon-responsive, and phagocytic populations, indicating that heterogeneity is a built-in feature of microglial development rather than a deviation from a single resting state (Han et al., 2023).

In adulthood, homeostatic microglia are defined by a core molecular signature that includes P2RY12, TMEM119, SIGLECH, GPR34, and SALL1. SALL1 is particularly important within this program because it acts as a microglia-selective transcriptional regulator that maintains the homeostatic state and distinguishes microglia from peripheral and BAMs. Loss of *Sall1* in microglia results in downregulation of their homeostatic identity, adoption of a more activated morphology, and upregulation of genes associated with inflammation and aging (Buttgereit et al., 2016; Fixsen et al., 2023). These findings indicate that SALL1 is not simply a marker of mature microglia, but an active repressor of alternative macrophage states and a key stabilizer of microglial identity. This signature, identified through independent transcriptomic and proteomic studies, is maintained in a cell-autonomous manner by TGFβ1 signaling through SMAD4 (Butovsky et al., 2014; Brioschi et al., 2023; Fixsen et al., 2023) and is progressively lost as microglia transition into disease-associated states. Establishing this baseline identity is essential for interpreting how microglia change in neurodegeneration.

Once established in the parenchyma, microglia are maintained largely through self-renewal rather than continual replacement by circulating monocytes, distinguishing them from many other tissue-resident macrophage populations. Fate-mapping studies in mice showed that microglia renew slowly under homeostatic conditions, with approximately 2 % of the population turning over at a given time and the overall population renewed on the order of months, while total microglial density remains relatively stable across the lifespan (Hashimoto et al., 2013; Yona et al., 2013). Importantly, this renewal was not uniform across the CNS, but varied according to local microenvironment, indicating that regional niche signals continue to shape microglial maintenance long after developmental colonization is complete (Tay et al., 2017).

2.2 Homeostatic functions of microglia

The developmental programs that establish microglial identity also position these cells to perform a wide range of homeostatic functions in the mature CNS. As long-lived, self-renewing macrophages of the parenchyma, microglia continuously survey the local environment, remove cellular and molecular debris, shape neural circuit structure, and support tissue integrity through interactions with neurons, synapses, oligodendrocytes, and other glial populations. By sensing changes in the local microenvironment and calibrating their responses accordingly, microglia preserve cellular integrity, maintain normal neuronal activity, and help prevent the accumulation of damage that could compromise circuit function. Microglial homeostatic functions can be divided into several major categories, including surveillance and phagocytosis, synaptic remodeling, trophic support for neuronal survival, and regulation of oligodendrocyte lineage cells and myelin. These categories are presented separately for clarity, but in vivo they are mechanistically and temporally intertwined. As a result, some concepts introduced above in the context of development reappear below as specific examples of ongoing homeostatic function. Rather than reflecting redundancy in microglial biology, this overlap underscores the extent to which microglia use a shared set of core behaviors to support multiple aspects of CNS homeostasis.

2.2.1 Surveillance, phagocytosis and synaptic remodeling

A core homeostatic function of microglia is continuous surveillance of the parenchyma coupled to phagocytic clearance. Under resting conditions, microglial processes are highly dynamic and repeatedly sample the surrounding tissue, allowing microglia to detect local perturbations and respond rapidly to changes in the microenvironment. Ultrastructural analyses have identified cellular inclusions in both microglial soma and primary processes (Wake et al., 2009; Tremblay, Lowery & Majewska, 2010), indicating that phagocytic activity occurs across multiple cellular compartments rather than being confined to the cell body.

These surveillance behaviors extend to direct interactions with synaptic structures. Microglial processes form transient contacts with synapses, often accompanied by local process enlargement or bulb formation, and these contacts have been observed across multiple spine and synapse classes, whereas interactions with dendritic shafts were not detected (Wake et al., 2009). Consistent with this, most microglial profiles are associated with at least one synapse-related element, including pre- and postsynaptic structures as well as perisynaptic astrocytic processes (Tremblay, Lowery & Majewska, 2010).

During development, these interactions contribute to active synaptic remodeling through a molecularly defined pathway. Complement proteins C1q and C3 localize to subsets of synapses in the developing visual system and mediate their elimination, establishing that the classical complement cascade, long considered an innate immune mechanism, is repurposed in the brain to tag synapses for pruning (Stevens et al., 2007). Microglia mediate this pruning by phagocytosing C3-tagged inputs via complement receptor 3 (CR3). In the retinogeniculate system, microglia preferentially engulf less-active presynaptic retinal ganglion cell inputs during the peak period of pruning, and mice lacking C3 or CR3 show lasting deficits in eye-specific segregation, demonstrating that complement-dependent microglial pruning is required for proper circuit refinement, not merely passive debris removal (Schafer et al., 2012). This developmental pruning pathway is directly relevant to neurodegeneration, because the same C1q–C3 microglia axis is aberrantly reactivated in Alzheimer's disease models, where it drives early synapse loss before overt plaque deposition (Hong et al., 2016).

Synaptic remodeling by microglia is also shaped by instructive signals from neighboring glial cells. Astrocyte-derived IL-33 promotes microglial engulfment of excitatory synaptic material during postnatal circuit maturation, indicating that glial crosstalk helps direct where and when microglia prune synapses (Vainchtein et al., 2018). In addition to direct engulfment of synaptic elements, microglia can remodel the extracellular environment around synapses. Neuronal IL-33 promotes microglial uptake of extracellular matrix components in the hippocampus, and disruption of this pathway leads to matrix accumulation at synapses, impaired synaptic plasticity, and defective memory consolidation, showing that microglia regulate circuit function not only by removing synaptic material but also by shaping the perisynaptic matrix (Nguyen et al., 2020). Recent work further indicates that developmental microglial remodeling is not limited to synaptic pruning alone. A type I interferon-responsive microglial state emerges during cortical development and participates in engulfment of whole neurons during periods of tissue remodeling, indicating that distinct microglial states can specialize in different forms of developmental clearance and circuit refinement (Escoubas et al., 2024).

Taken together, these studies show that microglial remodeling of neural circuits operates through multiple, partially overlapping mechanisms, including complement-dependent pruning, cytokine-directed engulfment, extracellular matrix remodeling, and state-specific forms of developmental clearance. By shaping synapse number, circuit refinement, and activity-dependent plasticity, these processes have lasting consequences for sensory processing, learning, memory, and behavior. These functions also connect naturally to broader developmental roles of microglia beyond synaptic remodeling alone, including support of neuronal survival, gliogenesis, and tissue maturation.

2.2.2 Support of neuronal and glial development

Because microglia enter the CNS early, they are positioned to influence multiple aspects of neural development that remain foundational for later homeostasis. Beyond their roles in synaptic remodeling, microglia interact extensively with neural progenitors, neurons, and glia during development and help shape the cellular environment in which later homeostatic functions are carried out (Li & Barres, 2018).

Microglia support selected neuronal populations during defined developmental windows. For instance, attenuating microglial activity with minocycline during a specific postnatal window increased apoptosis of cortical layer V neurons (Ueno et al., 2013). Importantly, treated microglia remained capable of engulfment, indicating that the phenotype was not due solely to impaired clearance of dying cells. The same study identified microglia-derived IGF-1 as a trophic factor contributing to neuronal survival, supporting the idea that microglia provide active trophic support in addition to their better-known phagocytic roles (Ueno et al., 2013). This trophic function is not restricted to early development. In the mature brain, microglia are required for learning-dependent synapse formation, and microglial BDNF is a key mediator of this effect. Selective removal of BDNF from microglia largely recapitulated the learning deficits seen after microglial depletion, reduced motor learning-dependent spine formation, and decreased neuronal TrkB phosphorylation, extending the concept of microglial trophic support into adult circuit plasticity (Parkhurst et al., 2013). More recent work further showed that microglial BDNF contributes to development of experience-dependent social behaviors and medial prefrontal cortex maturation during a juvenile critical period, indicating that trophic support by microglia continues to shape circuit refinement beyond the earliest postnatal stages (Komori et al., 2024).

Microglia have likewise been implicated in shaping glial development. *In vitro*, both astrocytes and microglia support oligodendrocyte lineage survival and differentiation, although astrocytes provide stronger long-term support, indicating that microglial effects are important but not exclusive (Pang et al., 2013). In the developing hypothalamus, embryonic microglia influence gliogenesis, and altered expression of cytokines including *Ccl2* and *Cxcl10* has been linked to changes in progenitor proliferation and lineage output (Marsters et al., 2020). More generally, astrocyte-microglia crosstalk is a broader feature of CNS development and homeostasis (Matejuk & Ransohoff, 2020). Consistent with this, depletion of microglia during embryonic cortical development reduced precursor proliferation and astrogenesis, indicating that microglia contribute to shaping glial as well as neuronal outcomes during development (Antony et al., 2011).

2.2.3 Regulation of oligodendrocytes and myelin

Among the developmental interactions between microglia and glia, the relationship with the oligodendrocyte lineage is especially important because it links early gliogenesis to later myelin formation and maintenance. Microglia support oligodendrocyte-lineage cells and contribute to myelin homeostasis across development and adulthood. A transient population of amoeboid microglia is present in early postnatal white matter, such as the corpus callosum. Depletion of microglia during this period reduces oligodendrocyte progenitor cell numbers, indicating that microglia help sustain the oligodendrocyte precursor cells (OPC) pool during active myelinogenesis (Hagemeyer et al., 2017). Short-term depletion in the adult brain also decreased OPC abundance without immediately affecting mature oligodendrocytes or myelin proteins, supporting an ongoing role in oligodendrocyte lineage maintenance (Hagemeyer et al., 2017). Microglia can also influence OPC proliferation through defined signaling pathways; for example, microglial neuropilin-1 promotes OPC proliferation by activating PDGFRα signaling in trans during development and demyelination (Sherafat et al., 2021).

Recent work refined this model by showing that microglia are critical for regulating myelin growth and preserving myelin integrity over time. In a microglia-deficient model, oligodendrocyte differentiation and initial axon wrapping were largely preserved, but later myelin growth became dysregulated, producing overly thick sheaths, expansion of the innermost myelin membrane, and abnormal myelin protrusions extending away from the axon (McNamara et al., 2023). These abnormalities became more consequential with age, progressing to patchy demyelination and cognitive deficits in adulthood (McNamara et al., 2023), indicating that microglia are require for long-term maintenance of myelin health.

Taken together, these studies establish microglia as a developmentally distinct, self-renewing macrophage population whose identity and functional range are shaped by yolk sac origin, early CNS colonization, and progressive tissue-specific reprogramming. From embryonic development through adulthood, microglia carry out a broad set of homeostatic functions that preserve CNS structure and circuit function. Many of these activities depend on maintenance of a defined homeostatic molecular program, and disruption of that program is increasingly understood to drive, rather than simply reflect, neurodegeneration. Defining how microglial homeostasis is established, maintained, and lost is therefore central to understanding their role in CNS disease. The second major CNS macrophage compartment, the border-associated macrophages, shares a partially overlapping developmental origin with microglia but occupies distinct anatomical niches, maintains a separate transcriptional identity, and performs complementary functions at CNS interfaces.

3. Border-associated macrophages (BAMs): Historical view, ontogeny, and molecular distinction from microglia

BAMs comprise the macrophage populations that reside at CNS interfaces rather than within the parenchyma itself (Fig. 2, Table 1). Historically, these cells were thought to derive from circulating blood monocytes and to be rapidly replaced by bone marrow-derived cells, based largely on irradiation bone marrow chimera studies. That model was later revised because irradiation disrupts CNS barriers and induces local inflammatory cues that artificially enhance leukocyte entry, thereby confounding conclusions about normal BAM turnover and origin (Hickey & Kimura, 1988; Hickey, Vass & Lassmann, 1992; Kierdorf, Katzmarski, et al., 2013; Kierdorf et al., 2019). Subsequent fate-mapping and single-cell

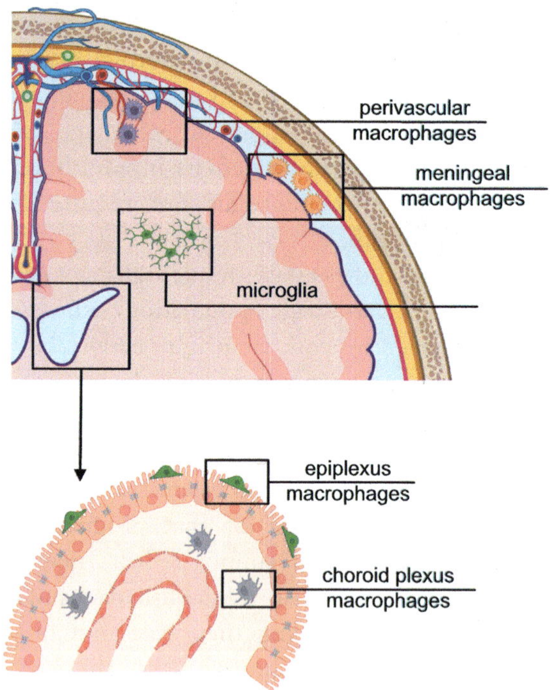

Fig. 2 Schematic illustrating the distribution of BAM subsets within the CNS border regions, including the meninges and choroid plexus, and microglia within the brain parenchyma. Distinct BAM populations occupy dural, subdural, perivascular, and choroid plexus compartments.

Table 1 Table summarizing major central nervous system macrophage populations, including microglia and multiple BAM subtypes. Key features compared across cell types include developmental origin, representative marker expression, and transcriptional characteristics, highlighting distinctions among macrophage populations at central nervous system interfaces.

Cell type	Origin	Cell markers	Transcriptional profile	
Microglia	Embryonic yolk sac	SALL1,P2RY12, TMEM119,SIGLEC-H	*Tmem119, Siglech, Slc2a5,P2ry12, Sparc, Fcrls, Sall1,Hexb, Trem2*	
Subdural meningeal BAM	Yolk sac, fetal liver	CD206,CD38,CD169, CD163,CD36,LYVE1	*Lyve1, P2rx7,Ccr1, Egfl7*	*Mrc1, Cd163,Cd169, Cd36,Apoe, Ms4a7,Ms4a6c, Stab1,Lyz2, Pf4, Cbr2,Tgfbi*
Perivascular BAM	Mostly yolk sac		*Lyve*1	
Dural meningeal BAM	Yolk sac, fetal liver			
Choroid Plexus BAM	Yolk sac, fetal liver		*Ccnd2, Ttr, Lilra5*	
Epiplexus Kolmer BAM	Mostly yolksac		Significantly similar to microglia	

Source: Adapted from (Penati et al., 2025).

studies showed that BAMs, like microglia, are largely embryonically derived, but differ from microglia in developmental trajectory, anatomical niche, transcriptional identity, and maintenance dynamics (Goldmann et al., 2016; Van Hove et al., 2019; Utz et al., 2020). This divergence is evident already during development: BAM-lineage cells are associated with a CD206/MRC1-positive program and later acquisition of markers such as LYVE1, whereas microglial-lineage cells progressively acquire SALL1 and other genes linked to parenchymal microglial identity (Utz et al., 2020). Rather than behaving as a single monocyte-replaced compartment, BAMs comprise a heterogeneous family of interface macrophages whose origin and turnover vary by location (Goldmann et al., 2016; Van Hove et al., 2019). This is especially evident in the distinction between relatively long-lived leptomeningeal and many perivascular populations and the more dynamic dural and stromal choroid plexus compartments. Together, these findings establish BAMs as a distinct CNS macrophage system specialized for vascular, meningeal, and ventricular interfaces rather than as peripheral macrophages transiently visiting the brain (Brioschi et al., 2023; Brioschi, Han & Colonna, 2025; Penati et al., 2025).

3.1 BAM subtype organization and developmental features

BAMs are commonly grouped into perivascular, meningeal, dural, stromal choroid plexus, and epiplexus macrophages, although nomenclature varies across studies. These populations occupy distinct interface niches and should not be treated as a single homogeneous compartment.

3.1.1 Perivascular macrophages

Perivascular macrophages (PVMs) reside within the Virchow-Robin spaces between endothelial and glial basement membranes and are found predominantly along arteries and arterioles, with a smaller population also associated with venous vessels (Masuda et al., 2022). They were historically identified by strong expression of CD206/MRC1 (Galea et al., 2005). Current models suggest that PVMs are predominantly yolk-sac derived, but mature canonical PVM identity is acquired indirectly rather than fixed as an early embryonic endpoint. Yolk-sac-derived progenitors first populate meningeal compartments prenatally, and a canonical CD206-positive, LYVE1-positive, P2RY12-negative PVM population is then specified postnatally from perinatal meningeal macrophages as the perivascular space develops (Van Hove et al., 2019; Utz et al., 2020; Masuda et al., 2022).

This postnatal establishment requires integrin-mediated signaling through Talin-1 and the presence of arterial vascular smooth muscle cells (Masuda et al., 2022). Under homeostatic conditions, PVMs are maintained largely through local renewal with limited monocyte replenishment. At least two functionally distinct PVM states have been described, distinguished by LYVE1 and MHC II expression: LYVE1-positive PVMs are enriched along arteries and arterioles and are associated with homeostatic surveillance functions, whereas MHC II-positive PVMs are enriched along veins and venules and show stronger immune-interaction and antigen-presentation programs (Mrdjen et al., 2018; Drieu et al., 2022). Ongoing PVM identity is further shaped by niche-dependent signals, including IL-34, and by c-MAF-associated transcriptional programs (Moura Silva et al., 2021; Van Hove et al., 2025). Transcriptionally, PVMs share broad myeloid programs with microglia but remain a distinct embryo-derived BAM population characterized by expression of genes such as *Mrc1* and *Cd36* and by relatively high CD45 levels (Goldmann et al., 2016; Mrdjen et al., 2018; Brioschi et al., 2023). During neuroinflammation, these resident CNS myeloid populations continue to follow distinct trajectories rather than collapsing into a single macrophage state (Jordão et al., 2019).

3.1.2 Meningeal macrophages

Meningeal BAMs occupy the leptomeningeal and subdural compartments, where they reside alongside fibroblast-like stromal cells and meningeal vasculature. Relative to dural and choroid plexus macrophages, leptomeningeal macrophages are often described as comparatively homogeneous, though more recent single-cell studies have begun to identify transcriptional heterogeneity within this population as well (Van Hove et al., 2019; Mildenberger, Stifter & Greter, 2022). Homeostatic meningeal BAMs express LYVE1 but not SALL1, distinguishing them from microglia, and they remain largely distinct from CCR2-dependent monocyte populations under steady-state conditions (Mrdjen et al., 2018; Van Hove et al., 2019). Like other CNS macrophages, their development depends on PU.1, and their numbers are reduced in *Irf8*-deficient mice, indicating shared but subtype-specific myeloid transcription factor requirements (Goldmann et al., 2016). Meningeal BAMs are largely embryonically derived and relatively long-lived, although fate-mapping studies indicate that a small fraction of the leptomeningeal population can be replaced by circulating monocytes over time (Goldmann et al., 2016; Utz et al., 2020).

3.1.3 Dural macrophages

Dural macrophages are particularly heterogeneous and differ from leptomeningeal macrophages in phenotype, turnover, and functional specialization. At least two major populations have been identified: an *Mrc1*-high, *Folr2*-positive, *Mgl2*-positive subset that is largely embryo-derived and comparatively long-lived, and a more MHC II-high, *Mrc1*-low subset that expands after birth and is more extensively replenished by monocyte-derived cells (Van Hove et al., 2019; Amann et al., 2024; Dalmau Gasull et al., 2024). These populations broadly parallel the TIMD4/LYVE1/FOLR2-positive long-lived macrophage subsets and the more MHC II-high monocyte-replenished subsets described across multiple tissues (Dick et al., 2022). In adulthood, monocyte-derived cells contribute to replenishment of both dural populations, with higher replacement rates in the MHC II-high subset, although a proportion of dural macrophages retains embryonic origin throughout life (Van Hove et al., 2019; Amann et al., 2024). A major refinement to this model came from the demonstration that skull bone marrow supplies the dura with monocytes through direct vascular channels, establishing the skull as a local myeloid reservoir for the adjacent meninges under homeostatic conditions (Herisson et al., 2018; Cugurra et al., 2021). This anatomical arrangement helps explain why the dura is a particularly dynamic immune niche at the CNS border, integrating vascular, lymphatic, and local marrow-derived immune inputs (Cugurra et al., 2021). More recent work has further resolved dural macrophage heterogeneity by identifying extrasinusoidal macrophages as a distinct subset, reinforcing the view that the dura is not a uniform meningeal compartment but an especially diverse and immunologically active BAM niche (Amann et al., 2024).

3.1.4 Stromal choroid plexus macrophages

Stromal choroid plexus macrophages occupy the blood-CSF interface within the stroma of the choroid plexus, distinct from the epiplexus macrophages that reside on the ventricular-facing epithelial surface (Goldmann et al., 2016). They are prenatally established primarily from YS progenitors, but unlike leptomeningeal and perivascular BAMs, they are substantially replaced by circulating monocytes after birth, making the choroid plexus stroma one of the CNS macrophage compartments with the highest monocyte replenishment rates under homeostatic conditions (Goldmann et al., 2016; Bastos et al., 2025). This high turnover likely reflects the unique vascular permeability of the choroid plexus stroma. Development of this population is notably less dependent on IRF8 than meningeal BAMs, and unlike microglia is not impaired by MYB deficiency, emphasizing the subtype-specific nature of BAM developmental requirements (Goldmann et al., 2016). The choroid plexus macrophage compartment is substantially more heterogeneous than earlier models suggested. Three biologically distinct choroid plexus macrophage subsets have been identified, distinguished by differential expression of CD163, MHC II, and CD9 (Dani et al., 2021; Du et al., 2026). These subsets arise from separate hematopoietic waves, occupy distinct anatomical niches within the choroid plexus, and differ in their dependence on CSF1 and IL-34 for survival (Du et al., 2026). TGFβ signaling is required to maintain their tissue-specific identities, and corresponding populations are also present in the human choroid plexus.

3.1.5 Epiplexus (Kolmer) macrophages

Epiplexus, or Kolmer, macrophages lie on the ventricular-facing epithelial surface of the choroid plexus and remain among the least well-characterized BAM populations because they are difficult to isolate and identify histologically (Ling, Kaur & Lu, 1998; Mundt, Greter & Becher, 2022). Recent single-cell and spatial work have confirmed their identity as a distinct choroid plexus macrophage subset, marked by CD9 expression and localized to the apical side of the epithelial layer, distinguishing them anatomically and molecularly from the stromal CD163+ and MHC II+ macrophage populations (Du et al., 2026). Current evidence suggests that epiplexus macrophages are embryo derived and likely yolk-sac derived, although the extent of any fetal liver contribution has not been rigorously excluded by negative fate-mapping approaches (Otero & Antonson, 2025). They express a mixed transcriptional program that includes BAM-associated genes such as *Lyz2* and *Apoe*, together with genes more typically associated with microglia or disease-associated microglial states, including *Trem2*, *Hexb*, *Tmem119*, *P2ry12*, *Sparc*, and *Sall1* (Li et al., 2019; Van Hove et al., 2019). Independent *P2ry12*-CreER studies have corroborated P2RY12 expression in a subset of IBA1+ choroid plexus cells at the epithelial surface, consistent with epiplexus identity (McKinsey et al., 2020). This mixed signature places epiplexus macrophages in a distinctive position within the broader CNS macrophage landscape. Epiplexus macrophages are ideally situated for CSF surveillance because their location on te ventricular-facing epithelial surface places them in direct contact with CSF (Ling, Kaur & Lu, 1998). Classic ultrastructural studies further indicate that epiplexus macrophages possess phagocytic and lysosomal features, supporting the view that they can participate in immune monitoring at the blood-CSF interface.

3.2 Homeostatic functions of BAMs

Whereas microglia are specialized for parenchymal homeostasis, BAMs are specialized for homeostatic functions at CNS interfaces. Their anatomical position at blood vessel walls, meningeal surfaces, and the choroid plexus places them at sites of molecular exchange, barrier regulation, waste handling, and communication between the CNS and peripheral compartments. BAMs are therefore best viewed not as redundant microglia outside the parenchyma, but as interface-adapted macrophages with niche-specific homeostatic tasks.

3.2.1 Vascular and barrier-associated support

Perivascular macrophages contribute to the vascular microenvironment through ongoing interactions with endothelial and perivascular cells. *In vitro*, co-culture of brain endothelial cells with blood-derived macrophages, used as a proxy for perivascular macrophages, increases trans-endothelial electrical resistance through a cAMP-independent mechanism, suggesting that macrophage-derived signals can strengthen endothelial barrier properties (Zenker et al., 2003). In circumventricular organs such as the area postrema, where vessels are fenestrated, movement of circulating solutes into adjacent neural tissue nevertheless remains size selective and highly restricted. Larger macromolecules are retained within perivascular compartments and are rapidly internalized by CD163- and CD169-expressing macrophages, positioning BAMs as active scavengers within a multilayered molecular filtration system at CNS interfaces (Willis, Garwood & Ray, 2007). PVMs are increasingly viewed as regulators of vascular tone and hemodynamics, not just permeability or scavenging. IL-34-dependent PVMs influence vascular-cell transcriptional states and modulate cerebral blood flow and vasomotion, indicating that BAMs actively shape cerebrovascular function under physiological conditions (Van Hove et al., 2025).

3.2.2 Waste clearance and glymphatic support

PVMs also participate in CNS waste-clearance pathways. Tracer studies showed that solutes introduced into the brain parenchyma initially disperse through the interstitial space before entering vascular basement membrane pathways, where they co-localize with laminin in capillary and arterial basement membranes within minutes of injection. At later time points, tracer signal was detected within PVMs associated with both parenchymal and leptomeningeal arteries, placing these cells at the terminus of a perivascular drainage route (Carare et al., 2008). More broadly, this drainage route connects to larger CNS clearance systems, including peri-arterial and perivenous fluid exchange described in the glymphatic model and downstream meningeal lymphatic outflow (Iliff et al., 2012; Louveau et al., 2015). Recent work showed that LYVE1-positive parenchymal BAMs actively regulate CSF flow dynamics by controlling extracellular matrix composition at arterial entry points (Drieu et al., 2022). Depletion of these cells leads to extracellular matrix accumulation, impaired arterial compliance, and reduced CSF influx and efflux (Drieu et al., 2022), indicating that they are active regulators of clearance pathways rather than passive bystanders in the perivascular space.

3.2.3 Metabolic support through VEGF

CD206-positive PVMs also contribute to adaptive metabolic responses under dietary stress. In a high-fat diet model, endothelial GLUT1 levels fall early, leading to impaired brain glucose uptake (Jais et al., 2016). This is accompanied by rapid expansion and activation of perivascular CD206-positive macrophages, which upregulate VEGF as BBB GLUT1 expression recovers (Jais et al., 2016). When VEGF is deleted specifically in myeloid cells, recovery of endothelial GLUT1 and brain glucose uptake fails, and obese mice show impaired memory formation (Jais et al., 2016). These findings indicate that macrophage-derived VEGF is required for restoration of cerebral glucose metabolism under these conditions.

3.2.4 Meningeal BAMs as sentinels at the CNS border

Meningeal macrophages provide steady-state immune surveillance at CNS borders and transition into an active protective barrier during peripheral infectious challenge. During hematogenous LCMV infection, selective depletion of meningeal macrophages while sparing parenchymal microglia results in increased viral burden and fatal neuroinfection, demonstrating that these cells actively restrict viral spread. This protective function depends on interferon signaling, as macrophage-specific deletion of *Stat1* or *Ifnar* phenocopies the loss-of-protection phenotype (Rebejac et al., 2022). Age-dependent differences in this barrier are especially evident around the perivenous sinus region of the dura mater, where $MHCII^{hi}$ macrophages accumulate after birth and are required to prevent early viral propagation into the CNS. In neonates, the dural immune compartment is dominated by $CD206^{hi}$ macrophages, whereas the $MHCII^{hi}$ macrophages that accumulate around the dural venous sinuses after birth remain rare (Kim et al., 2023). This immature macrophage composition, rather than a major anatomical defect at the CNS border, is thought to underlie the heightened neonatal susceptibility to viral meningoencephalitis (Kim et al., 2023). Meningeal macrophages also respond to peripheral challenges such as LPS, SARS-CoV-2, and LCMV, indicating that their surveillance role extends beyond neurotropic viral infection to broader sensing of systemic inflammatory states (Rebejac et al., 2022). Their protective capacity is further shaped by infection history: following LCMV-induced meningitis, embryonically derived meningeal macrophages are lost and the niche is repopulated by blood-derived monocytes whose long-term properties differ from the original population and are less effective during subsequent immune challenges, indicating that meningeal macrophage identity is not fully restored by circulating precursors alone (Rua et al., 2019).

3.2.5 Choroid plexus BAMS as sensors of systemic inflammation

Choroid plexus macrophages occupy a distinct position at the blood–CSF interface, where they are among the first intracranial cells to detect and respond to systemic inflammatory signals. Following peripheral LPS challenge, choroid plexus macrophages are the primary early intracranial source of IL-1β at 1 and 4 h, preceding detectable parenchymal cytokine induction. Macrophage-derived IL-1β then acts on IL-1R1-expressing stromal cells, which upregulate *Ccl2*, *Cxcl1*, *Cxcl2*, and *Il6*, positioning choroid plexus macrophages as an initiating node in the brain response to systemic inflammation (Shimada & Hasegawa-Ishii, 2021). Under more severe inflammatory stress, such as intracerebroventricular LPS-induced meningitis, the choroid plexus mounts a coordinated multicellular response in which neutrophils and monocytes accumulate in the stroma and cross the epithelial barrier into the CSF (Xu et al., 2024). Macrophages are recruited bidirectionally from both the tissue and the CSF, where they contribute to neutrophil clearance and epithelial repair. In parallel, the choroid plexus epithelium transiently adopts a specialized state that supports immune-cell recruitment, survival, and differentiation during resolution of inflammation (Xu et al., 2024).

3.2.6 Shared trophic functions with microglia

In addition to their more specialized interface roles, BAMs share some trophic functions with microglia. One example is extracellular vesicle-mediated lipid signaling to the oligodendrocyte lineage. Endocannabinoids carried within microglia-derived extracellular vesicles promote OPC differentiation, and lipid cargo from macrophage-derived vesicles can similarly drive OPC maturation. However, intact vesicles from inflammatory macrophages do not promote differentiation and can instead inhibit it, indicating that the pro-differentiating effect depends on vesicle cargo rather than being a general property of macrophage-derived vesicles (Lombardi et al., 2019, 2024).

Together, the preceding sections show that microglia and BAMs form complementary macrophage networks that maintain CNS homeostasis across distinct anatomical compartments. Microglia are specialized for surveillance and tissue maintenance within the parenchyma, whereas BAMs regulate immune, vascular, and clearance functions at CNS borders. In neurodegenerative disease, however, these homeostatic roles are progressively reshaped by chronic exposure to protein aggregates, cellular stress, vascular dysfunction, and persistent inflammatory signaling. Under these conditions, both microglia and BAMs can shift from protective regulators of tissue integrity to active participants in disease progression, with their effects determined by anatomical niche, disease stage, and local microenvironment.

4. Alzheimer's disease (AD)

AD is a progressive neurodegenerative disorder characterized by three main pathologies: the extracellular buildup of amyloid beta (Aβ) plaques, the intracellular development of neurofibrillary tangles (composed of hyperphosphorylated tau protein), and ongoing neuroinflammation (Chen, Holtzman & Colonna, 2026). These pathological changes lead to significant synaptic damage, widespread neuronal death, gradual memory loss, and cognitive decline. Both tissue-resident microglia and distinct macrophage populations are crucial in driving this neuroinflammatory response, playing dynamic roles that vary depending on stage and region (Fig. 3).

4.1 Microglia in AD pathogenesis

The genetic architecture of late-onset AD strongly implicates immune and microglial pathways. APOE4 remains the most common and strongest genetic risk factor for late-onset AD, and the broader GWAS landscape has identified more than 20 susceptibility loci, a substantial fraction of which encode proteins preferentially or selectively expressed in microglia, including CD33, ABCA7, CR1, INPP5D, and MS4A6A (Hollingworth et al., 2012; Lambert et al., 2013; Bellenguez et al., 2022). Rare coding variants in

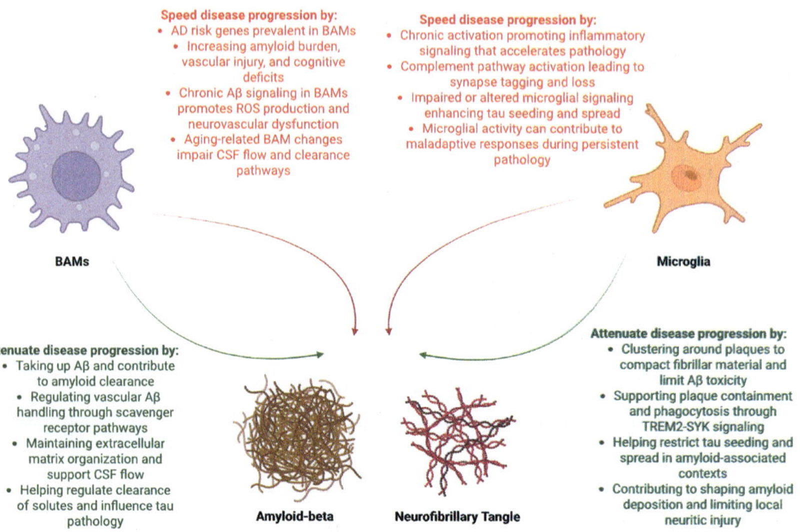

Fig. 3 Compare and contrast of microglia and BAM functions in Alzheimer's disease.

TREM2 confer risk approaching that of APOE4 and established that altered microglial state regulation is part of the core genetic architecture of the disease (Guerreiro et al., 2013; Jonsson et al., 2013). These findings shifted the field away from viewing microglial activation as a purely reactive consequence of degeneration and toward recognizing microglia as regulators of disease susceptibility and progression. Functional work has strengthened that interpretation by showing that the AD risk gene CD33 inhibits microglial uptake of Aβ, providing a direct example of how a genetic microglial pathway can impair clearance of pathogenic material (Griciuc et al., 2013).

As pathology progresses, microglia undergo major transcriptional state transitions marked by loss of homeostatic signature genes and induction of programs linked to lipid metabolism, lysosomal activity, phagocytosis, and inflammatory signaling. These states were formalized as disease-associated microglia (DAM) and the related microglial neurodegenerative phenotype (MGnD) program, with the TREM2-APOE axis emerging as a major regulator of the transition away from homeostatic identity (Keren-Shaul et al., 2017; Krasemann et al., 2017). With persistent Aβ exposure, these responses can become maladaptive. Chronic microglial activation is associated with production of inflammatory cytokines and reactive oxygen and nitrogen species. Additionally, activation of the NLRP3 inflammasome represents one defined mechanism through which microglial innate immune signaling accelerates AD pathology rather than simply reacting to it (Heneka et al., 2013). Furthermore, complement pathways that normally mediate developmental synaptic pruning become aberrantly re-engaged in AD, leading to inappropriate tagging and engulfment of synapses by microglia (Hong et al., 2016). This complement-dependent synapse loss provides a mechanistic link between amyloid-associated innate immune activation and early synaptic failure, one of the strongest correlates of cognitive decline. Human tissue studies further support this concept, showing increased ingestion of synaptic material by glia in AD brain, particularly in plaque-rich regions and in the context of APOE4 (Tzioras et al., 2023).

Microglia mount a plaque-associated response early in amyloid pathology. They cluster around the plaques and compact fibrillar material in an effort to limit exposure of adjacent neurites to plaque-associated protofibrillar Aβ42 (Condello et al., 2015). This plaque-barrier function depends in part on TREM2 as loss of TREM2 impairs microglial plaque engagement, leading to an increase in plaque-associated neuritic injury (Yuan et al., 2016). TREM2 also supports microglial metabolic fitness by sustaining mTOR-dependent anabolic programs. TREM2-deficient microglia fail to maintain energy homeostasis under the metabolic demands of chronic plaque engagement (Ulland et al., 2017). More recent mechanistic work has extended this pathway by showing that TREM2 signals through SYK to organize plaque-associated microglial responses. Microglial SYK deficiency impairs plaque encasement, reduces Aβ uptake and CD68-associated phagocytosis, resulting in worsened plaque morphology and increased dystrophic neurites (Wang et al., 2022). Importantly, the AD-risk TREM2 R47H variant fails to activate this pathway efficiently (Wang et al., 2022). In parallel, SYK has emerged as a coordinator of neuroprotective microglial responses in amyloidosis. Mice with microglia deletion of *Syk* fails to activate the DAM phenotype with an observed increased in plaque-associated pathology and behavioral deficits (Ennerfelt et al., 2022). Together, these studies place the TREM2-SYK axis at the center of plaque-associated microglial containment and state transition. However, microglial phagocytosis of plaques is also not uniformly protective, as lysosomal accumulation of APOE in microglia can bind fibrillar Aβ and promote amyloid seeding (Kaji et al., 2024). Consistent with these observations, in the case of incomplete depletion of microglia, plaques form preferentially in regions where microglia remain, indicating that surviving microglia can help seed and build parenchymal amyloid plaques (Spangenberg et al., 2019).

Microglia are also implicated in tau pathology, but their effects depend strongly on disease context. In the setting of amyloid-associated tau seeding, activated peri-plaque microglia can restrain the transition from Aβ pathology to tau pathology as both microglial depletion and TREM2 loss enhance tau seeding and spreading around plaques (Gratuze et al., 2021). Furthermore, impaired TREM2 signaling reduces microglia numbers and promotes tau seeding and propagation within plaque-associated neuronal processes, reinforcing the idea that the microglial response to amyloid is an important determinant of downstream vulnerability to tau pathology (Leyns et al., 2019). By contrast in primary tauopathy models without amyloid, microglia promote tau-mediated neurodegeneration. Early work showed that microglia depletion suppresses spread of pathogenic tau species in experimental models (Asai et al., 2015). In P301S mice expressing ApoE4, loss of TREM2 does not protect against disease. Instead, it worsens tau pathology and neurodegeneration despite reducing the usual TREM2-dependent microglial response, indicating that other microglial programs can still drive tau-mediated injury in this setting (Gratuze et al., 2023). Taken together, these findings support a stage-dependent but not purely binary model in which microglia both constrain and propagate AD pathology, with protective and pathogenic programs often operating in parallel rather than in strict sequence.

4.2 Border-associated macrophages in AD

AD-associated myeloid dysfunction extends beyond parenchymal microglia to include BAMs, particularly perivascular and leptomeningeal populations. These BAMs occupy vascular and meningeal interfaces where they regulate amyloid handling, oxidative stress, fluid dynamics, and protein clearance. Human leptomeningeal BAM subtypes express distinct AD GWAS genes that differ from microglia, with *MS4A4A*, *CD33*, *CR1*, and HLA genes enriched in various BAM subpopulations, indicating that AD genetic risk is distributed across multiple CNS macrophage compartments rather than restricted to parenchymal microglia (Adler et al., 2026). Recent work further suggests that *Maf* is an AD-linked gene required for BAM but not microglial survival. Importantly, depletion of BAMs in the 5xFAD mice increases cerebral amyloid angiopathy, total Aβ burden, and early memory deficits (Adler et al., 2026).

Perivascular macrophages (PVMs) participate in vascular Aβ control through scavenger receptor pathways including SR-BI (Thanopoulou et al., 2010). Alternatively, PVMs have also been implicated in neurovascular dysfunction during chronic amyloid exposure. Specifically, Aβ engagement of CD36–Nox2 signaling in PVMs, driving reactive oxygen production, impairing neurovascular function and worsening cerebral amyloid angiopathy (Park et al., 2017; Uekawa et al., 2023) Additionally, ApoE4 expression in BAMs is sufficient to increase susceptibility to oligemic white matter damage, identifying BAMs as active contributors to ApoE4-associated neurovascular pathology (Anfray et al., 2024).

These vascular roles intersect with another core function of arterial border compartments, the regulation of CSF flow and solute clearance. Recently, a CD163-high, LYVE1-high macrophage population that associates closely with the brain arterial tree was identified (Drieu et al., 2022). This macrophage population are essential regulators of CSF flow with depletion of these cells leading to impaired CNS perfusion and solute clearance. Importantly, single-nucleus RNA-sequencing data from patients with AD identified changes in phagocytosis, endocytosis, and interferon-γ signaling in these macrophages (Drieu et al., 2022). These are the same pathways that are altered in mouse models of AD, thus linking this macrophage population to AD-associated clearance dysfunction. Indeed, a follow-up demonstrated that depletion of this CD163-high, LYVE1-high macrophage population increased tau pathology and worsened tau-mediated neurodegeneration (Drieu et al., 2023). Taken together, these findings support a broader model in which fluid dynamics are integral to CNS homeostasis and directly relevant to neurodegeneration. Indeed, impaired meningeal lymphatic drainage worsens amyloid burden and alters neuroimmune responses in AD models. Furthermore, ablation of meningeal lymphatics in 5xFAD mice exacerbates Aβ deposition, microgliosis and behavioral impairments (Da Mesquita et al., 2018, 2021). Thus, BAMs can therefore be understood not only as local immune regulators, but also as components of a larger clearance axis linked to perivascular flow and lymphatic drainage.

BAMs also contribute directly to AD pathology through crosstalk with microglia. For instance, PVMs are the primary source of secreted SPP1/osteopontin in the hippocampal perivascular space in AD mouse models and human AD tissue (De Schepper et al., 2023) PVM-derived SPP1 results in microglia upregulation of phagocytic genes including *C1qa*, *Grn*, and *Ctsb* in the presence of amyloid-β oligomers. Importantly, *Spp1* deletion in AD mouse models dampens the SPP1-enhanced microglia phagocytosis, resulting in decreased synaptic loss (De Schepper et al., 2023). This BAM-to-microglia signaling axis represents a mechanism by which BAMs can drive parenchymal pathology. Collectively, these findings show that BAMs contribute to AD through multiple interface-specific mechanisms.

While AD remains the most prevalent neurodegenerative disorder, the second most common, Parkinson's disease (PD), shares key features of myeloid dysfunction despite distinct pathological substrates. Both diseases involve protein aggregation, chronic neuroinflammation, and impaired clearance mechanisms, yet the specific myeloid responses differ in important ways. In AD, microglia and BAMs respond primarily to Aβ and tau, whereas in PD the dominant pathological trigger is α-synuclein. The following sections examine how microglia and BAM populations contribute to PD pathogenesis.

5. Parkinson's disease

Since the 1980s, prevalence of PD has increased, with a more profound increase occurring just in the past two decades (Zhu et al., 2024). Patients with PD experience motor symptoms such as bradykinesia combined with rigidity, rest tremors, or both. Additionally, PD patients experience a combination of non-motor symptoms such as constipation, depression, cognitive decline, sleep alterations, and hyposmia (Bloem, Okun & Klein, 2021; Morris et al., 2024). The pathophysiology of PD has been hypothesized to include a combination of α -synuclein (α-syn) aggregation, mitochondrial dysfunction, lysosomal deficiencies, and synaptic transport issues, leading to neuroinflammation (Bloem, Okun & Klein, 2021; Morris et al., 2024). One hallmark of PD is the loss of dopaminergic neurons in the substantia nigra (SN) as well as the presence of Lewey bodies and other protein aggregates (Morris et al., 2024). In PD, α-syn becomes misfolded and clusters into Lewy bodies, promoting neuroinflammation that further worsens neuronal injury and advances disease progression.

5.1 Microglia in Parkinson's disease

Microglia respond to extracellular α-syn aggregates by initiating phagocytic clearance and inflammatory signaling. In both postmortem PD brains and by single-nucleus RNA-sequencing of these brains, microgliosis and reactive microglia, with a decrease in expression of homeostatic markers, have been robustly detected (McGeer et al., 1988; Smajić et al., 2022) (Fig. 4).

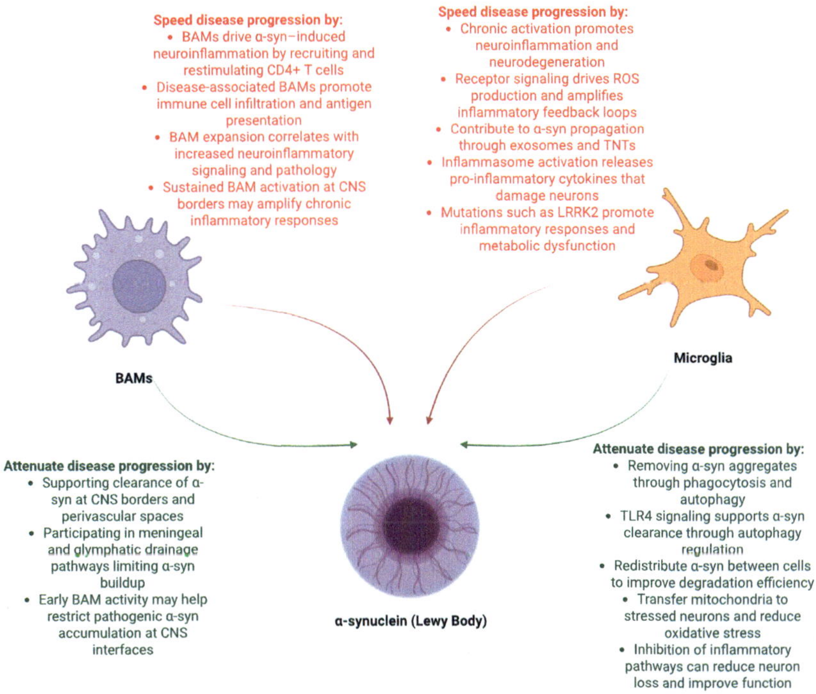

Fig. 4 Compare and contrast of microglia and BAM functions in Parkinson's disease.

Microglia detect extracellular α-syn aggregates through several innate immune receptors with the downstream response depending in part on the conformational state of the protein. Among the best characterized receptors are pattern recognition receptors (PRRs), including Toll-like receptors TLR2 and TLR4. TLR2 shows preference for oligomeric species of α-syn, while TLR4 capable of detecting multiple forms including fibrils (Kim et al., 2013). Activation of either receptor triggers the nuclear factor-κB (NF-κB) signaling pathway and pro-inflammatory cytokine production (Kim et al., 2013). TLR4 also regulates autophagy, supporting clearance of α-syn aggregates and emphasizing its dual function in PD pathology (Stefanova et al., 2011). Receptors for advanced glycation end products (RAGE) preferentially interact with fibrillar α-syn (Long et al., 2022), activating NF-κB and promoting release of pro-inflammatory cytokines and chemokines that recruit additional immune cells to sites of α-syn accumulation (Wang et al., 2020; Gasparotto et al., 2024). Cluster of differentiation 36 (CD36), a class B scavenger receptor, has also been shown to bind α-syn aggregates and activate downstream inflammatory signaling and reactive oxygen species (ROS) production (Panicker et al., 2019). Macrophage antigen complex-1 (Mac-1) similarly binds α-syn directly and stimulates NADPH oxidase activity, elevating ROS production and generating oxidative stress that damages microglia and further activates redox-sensitive pathways such as NF-κB (Zhang et al., 2007). The interaction between ROS production and NF-κB signaling forms a positive feedback cycle that intensifies neuroinflammation and increases oxidative injury to neurons.

What is less established is the role of TREM2, which have been implicated in numerous neurodegenerative conditions. Microglia have been shown to respond to α-syn aggregates through TREM2, which may regulate their activity and help limit chronic neuroinflammation (Yin et al., 2024). This response supports an adaptive state of microglial activation that promotes homeostasis and helps reduce neurotoxic effects in PD (Yin et al., 2024). However, other studies have found that a lack of TREM2 in microglia leads to increased α-syn accumulation, which heightens neuroinflammation and accelerates neurodegeneration (Guo et al., 2019; Huang et al., 2024). Additionally, an increase in NLRP3 inflammasome has been detected in microglial cells in the substantia nigra of PD patients (Gordon et al., 2018). Previous studies have reported that elevated NLRP3 inflammasome activity in microglial cells is associated with increased release of pro-inflammatory cytokines that contribute to neurodegeneration (Haque et al., 2020).

Beyond clearance, microglia actively contribute to α-syn spread through multiple mechanisms, such as through exosomes and tunneling nanotubes (TNTs). Microglia can load internalized α-syn into exosomes, which are then released into the extracellular environment and are then absorbed by nearby neurons, astrocytes, and other microglia, contributing to the spread of α-syn pathology (Guo et al., 2020). The formation of microglial TNTs can be enhanced by inflammatory stimuli, and activated microglia can transfer α-syn to nearby cells. This form of cell-to-cell communication allows the spread of α-syn aggregates, which may amplify inflammatory responses and drive the dissemination of pathology across the brain (Dieriks et al., 2017). Furthermore, the transfer of α-syn through TNTs contributes to lysosomal dysfunction and enhances microglia to microglia communication via these nanotubes (Dilsizoglu Senol et al., 2021). Conversely, microglia to microglia communication through TNTs can distribute α-syn fibrils, reducing the burden on individual cells and improving the efficiency of α-syn degradation (Scheiblich et al., 2021). Microglia exposed to α-syn fibrils establish cellular networks that transfer α-syn from overloaded cells to neighboring naive microglia, where the cargo is rapidly and effectively degraded; this distribution of burden attenuates the inflammatory profile of microglia and improves their survival (Scheiblich et al., 2021). Microglia also use TNTs to connect with α-syn-burdened or tau-burdened neurons, extracting aggregates while delivering healthy mitochondria; this reduces neuronal oxidative stress, normalizes gene expression, and rescues suppressed neuronal activity. TNT-mediated aggregate transfer and neuroprotection are impaired in microglia carrying TREM2 T66M or R47H mutations, variants that increase risk for frontotemporal dementia and Alzheimer's disease and may contribute to synucleinopathy pathogenesis (Scheiblich et al., 2021).

5.2 Border-associated macrophages in Parkinson's disease

BAMs, including perivascular and meningeal populations, are positioned at CNS interfaces where they regulate barrier-associated signaling, extracellular matrix organization, immune-cell trafficking, and clearance of material moving through perivascular and meningeal spaces. These properties place them in a strategic position to influence α-synuclein-driven neuroinflammation even though they lie outside the parenchyma itself (Faraco et al., 2016; De Vlaminck et al., 2022; Schonhoff et al., 2023) (Fig. 4). Previous studies have shown that local antigen presentation through MHCII expression is critical for the loss of dopaminergic neurons in the SN, suggesting that CNS resident macrophages may act as important antigen presenting cells that coordinate neuroinflammatory and neurodegenerative processes (Williams et al., 2018). Using an in vivo α-syn overexpression model together with single-cell profiling techniques, BAMs, rather than microglia, were shown to be responsible for recruiting and reactivating CD4+ T cell antigens required for α-syn driven neuroinflammation (Schonhoff et al., 2023). BAMs distinctly mediate the restimulation of CD4+ T cells required for α-syn driven local cytokine production and their entry into the parenchyma (Schonhoff et al., 2023). Accordingly, disease-associated BAMs were found to show high expression of genes involved in T cell recruitment (*Ccl5* and *Ccl10*), antigen processing and presentation (*H2-Aa*, *Cd74*, and *Cd274*), and extracellular matrix remodeling (*Mmp14*), indicating important roles in regulating blood brain barrier permeability, T cell restimulation, and immune cell infiltration (Schonhoff et al., 2023). Critically, depletion of BAMs reduced neuroinflammatory markers including microglial activation and peripheral immune cell infiltration, whereas conditional deletion of MHCII in microglia did not alter α-syn-induced neuroinflammation. BAMs were identified in post-mortem PD brain in close proximity to T cells, and α-syn oligomers have been detected in perivascular macrophages in human synucleinopathy brain tissue, providing pathological validation of these interactions (Schonhoff et al., 2023). Collectively, these findings position BAMs as key intermediaries between peripheral and tissue-resident immune systems and as essential contributors to neuroinflammatory processes in PD.

6. Multiple sclerosis

Multiple sclerosis (MS) is a chronic inflammatory demyelinating disease characterized by focal lesions, diffuse tissue injury, and progressive neurodegeneration within the CNS. Unlike the proteinopathies discussed above, MS is driven primarily by autoimmune mechanisms in which peripheral immune cells infiltrate the CNS and target myelin and oligodendrocytes. Within this setting, microglia occupy a central but paradoxical position: they contribute directly to lesion expansion, axonal injury, and chronic compartmentalized inflammation, yet they are also required for efficient debris clearance and remyelination. In this sense, microglia are not secondary participants in MS pathology, but major determinants of whether lesions remain destructive or transition toward repair.

6.1 Microglia in multiple sclerosis

Microglial involvement in MS is most clearly understood through lesion staging (Healy et al., 2022; Absinta, 2025). In the course of MS, there are four types of lesions, pre-active, active, chronic or smoldering, and chronic inactive. Pre-active lesions are one of the first to form in still normal-looking white matter with no overt sign of demyelination that are also characterized by clusters of HLA-DR-positive microglia (De Groot et al., 2001). Next is the active lesion stage that contain dense accumulations of activated microglia, infiltrating macrophages and lymphocytes, and high production of inflammatory cytokines throughout the lesion core (Healy et al., 2022). Chronic active or smoldering lesions, as its name indicates, are characterized by persistent inflammation. These lesions are enriched in progressive MS and are strongly associated with ongoing tissue damage, including persistent axonal injury at the lesion border (Absinta et al., 2019, 2021; Absinta, 2025). Lastly, inactive lesions are in general hypocellular but are marked by scars and gliosis.

Multiple profiling studies in rodent models and MS patients, using single-cell RNA-seq, spatial transcriptomics and imaging mass cytometry, have identify a large degree of heterogeneity in microglia profiles dependent on proximity to the lesion center or the lesion rim as well as timeline in disease progression (Ajami et al., 2018; Masuda et al., 2019; Jordão et al., 2019; Park et al., 2019; van der Poel et al., 2019). Consistent with these observations, microglia in active MS lesions downregulate homeostatic markers and acquire a pro-inflammatory phenotype characterized by increased expression of genes involved in oxidative injury and antigen presentation (Zrzavy et al., 2017). These activated microglia also amplify lesion pathology through crosstalk with astrocytes. Microglia secretion of inflammatory mediators, such as IL-1β, TNF-**α,** and C1q, transformed astrocytes into a neurotoxic phenotype (Liddelow et al., 2017; Absinta et al., 2021; Guttenplan et al., 2021). Importantly, this crosstalk is broadly extendable to other neuroinflammatory and neurodegenerative settings as well.

Despite these pathogenic roles, microglia are also indispensable for remyelination. Experimental depletion or impairment of microglia/macrophages in acute and chronic models of demyelination using cuprizone reduces debris clearance and delays remyelination, establishing phagocyte-mediated clearance as a rate-limiting step in repair (Lampron et al., 2015; Tahmasebi et al., 2019; Marzan et al., 2021). Additionally, numerous studies confirmed microglia as an essential cell type in producing signals that OPC recruitment, differentiation (Hamilton & Rome, 1994; Pang et al., 2013) and oligodendrocyte survival, including IGF-1 (Ye et al., 2002). Recent work has added an important mechanistic refinement to this reparative picture. An inducible *Clec7a*-CreERT2 system demonstrated that the disease-associated microglia (DAM) signature found in AD and other neurodegenerative diseases was also detected in demyelinating areas, induced by cuprizone administration (Barclay et al., 2024). Importantly, this DAM signature overlapped significantly with a proliferative region associated microglia state that is found during early postnatal ages in the developing white matter (Li et al., 2019). Ablation of *Clec7a*-marked DAMs significantly as these DAMs were necessary for efficient removal of myelin post-demyelination to permit remyelination to occur (Barclay et al., 2024).

An essential aspect of myelin clearance is the ability for microglia to clear and process cholesterol-rich myelin debris, and disruption of this process impairs the transition from demyelination to repair. Indeed, use of spatial transcriptomics of chronic active lesions and genetic studies discovered that inhibition of cholesterol efflux in microglia significantly increased microglial inflammatory responses. Stimulation of cholesterol efflux was able to reduce disease severity in EAE in terms of lesion number, size, and clinical score. Additionally, crosstalk between lesion remote astrocytes and microglia, through secreted matricellular protein CCN1, was essential for the lipid-storage ability of microglia and clearance of myelin debris in a spinal cord injury model (McCallum et al., 2026). Microglia expression of TREM2 is important for the accumulation of OPCs and differentiation into oligodendrocytes in the lesion (Cignarella et al., 2020).

The balance between destructive and regenerative microglial functions shifts with age. Remyelination becomes progressively less efficient in older individuals and aged mice, in part due to inefficient OPC differentiation into myelinating oligodendrocytes but also due to aged senescent microglia that are unable to clear myelin debris effectively (Ruckh et al., 2012; Rawji, Neumann & Franklin, 2023; Gross et al., 2025). The extent to which senolytic strategies can reverse this defect appears to depend on model, age, and lesion context (Gross et al., 2025). Taken together, these findings establish microglia as central arbiters of MS pathology. They contribute to lesion expansion, chronic active rim formation, axonal injury, and inflammatory amplification, but they are also indispensable for myelin debris removal, lipid handling, OPC recruitment, and remyelination. Their overall impact therefore depends on lesion stage, anatomical context, age, and the balance between inflammatory and regenerative programs active in a given lesion at a given time.

6.2 Border-associated macrophages in multiple sclerosis

Unlike neurodegenerative proteinopathies, in which BAMs encounter pathogenic proteins moving through vascular and meningeal clearance routes, MS is driven primarily by autoimmune mechanisms in which peripherally primed lymphocytes enter the CNS and require local reactivation at CNS borders before invading the parenchyma. This places BAMs, particularly perivascular and meningeal macrophages, in a position to regulate the entry, positioning, and local restimulation of autoreactive immune cells at CNS interfaces.

The canonical model of MS and EAE pathogenesis holds that myelin-reactive T cells are first primed in peripheral lymphoid organs and then migrate to CNS border compartments, where they undergo local reactivation before crossing the glia limitans into the parenchyma. Two-photon imaging directly visualized this sequence, showing that encephalitogenic CD4+ T cells arrest on leptomeningeal vessels, extravasate into perivascular spaces, and form dynamic contacts with local antigen-presenting phagocytes at the CNS surface and perivascular compartment (Bartholomäus et al., 2009; Kivisäkk et al., 2009). While a portion of meningeal macrophage express high levels of MHC-II, absence of MHC-II on meningeal macrophages and microglia did not affect T-cell mediated neurodegeneration (Wolf et al., 2018). This may be potentially due to the influx of dendritic cells, which are hugely effective at stimulating T-cells (Giles et al., 2018; Heß et al., 2020). Additional studies on perivascular macrophages and meningeal macrophages using localized depletion via chlodronate liposomes lend evidence to these macrophages providing a supporting role. Depletion of these macrophages led to a modest reduction in disease severity during the acute phase of EAE with stronger disease amelioration during the height of EAE (Polfliet et al., 2001, 2002). Taken together, the available evidence supports an important role for BAMs in shaping autoimmune inflammation at CNS borders in MS. Progress now depends on better tools tor solve these populations in space and time.

7. Other neurodegenerative conditions

Although the BAM literature is most developed in AD, PD, and MS, there is strong reason to expect that BAMs will also be relevant in other neurodegenerative diseases. This is particularly true for disorders in which disease progression involves chronic neuroinflammation, altered CNS-peripheral immune communication, or dysfunction at vascular and meningeal interfaces. At present, however, the evidence base is uneven. In diseases such as amyotrophic lateral sclerosis (ALS) and frontotemporal dementia (FTD), microglial biology has been studied in substantial depth, whereas BAM-specific contributions are only beginning to emerge.

In ALS, microglia are established contributors to disease progression, which is marked by loss of upper and lower motor neurons. In mutant SOD1 models, which mimic inherited ALS, microglia are responsible for exacerbating the later phase of disease due to their adoption of an inflammatory state coupled to increased reactive oxygen species and reduced neurotrophic support (Boillée et al., 2006). Notably, replacing mutant microglia with wild-type microglia in the SOD1 model prolongs survival

(Beers et al., 2006). As for BAMs, depletion of PVMs in SOD1^{G93A} mice preserves motor neurons and slows clinical progression due to the finding that PVMs degrade extracellular matrix, resulting in decreased integrity of the blood-spinal cord barrier (Adachi et al., 2023). These results place PVMs among the emerging non-parenchymal modifiers of ALS.

A similar argument applies to FTD. FTD is a clinically and biologically heterogeneous group of neurodegenerative disorders that most often features frontotemporal lobar degeneration. Mutations in the gene *GRN*, which encodes for progranulin, leads to low levels progranulin, a tropic factor for both microglia and neuronal health. When progranulin is lost, microglia become activated with altered lysosomal function (Lui et al., 2016; Zhang et al., 2020; Wu et al., 2021; Sung et al., 2024). In mouse models of FTD, microglia increase complement production leading to excessive pruning of inhibitory synapses resulting in neurodegeneration, behavior deficits and decreased survival (Lui et al., 2016). Additionally, loss of progranulin in microglia also promotes neuronal cytoplasmic buildup of TDP-43, an RNA processing protein that is normally sequestered in the nucleus, but in FTD, stays in the cytoplasm, forming toxic aggregates (Chang et al., 2017). Accumulation of TDP-43 is linked to broader white matter injury (Zhang et al., 2020; Wu et al., 2021). More recently, human studies showed that progranulin haploinsufficiency in microglia is itself sufficient to produce lysosomal abnormalities and promote cytoplasmic TDP-43 accumulation, strengthening the argument that myeloid dysfunction can participate directly in FTD pathogenesis (Sung et al., 2024). Taken together, these studies strongly support a role for CNS macrophage dysfunction in FTD, but almost all that evidence comes from parenchymal microglia rather than BAMs. Thus, the major gap in the field, therefore, is not whether macrophage biology matters in FTD, but what is the contribution of BAMs to disease propagation.

8. Transcriptional control of brain macrophage states in neurodegeneration

Across neurodegenerative diseases, microglia and BAMs repeatedly converge on a set of dysfunctional programs, such as inflammatory activation, altered phagocytosis, lysosomal stress, and lipid dysregulation. These shared outputs suggest that disease-associated macrophage states are coordinated by upstream gene regulatory networks in which transcription factors act on enhancers and promoters to stabilize broader cellular programs. From this perspective, identifying the transcription factors that organize these states is therefore important not only for explaining why similar macrophage programs recur across diseases, but also for revealing points of intervention that could shift maladaptive states toward more homeostatic or reparative ones. This logic is beginning to emerge most clearly in human microglial systems, where recent studies have shown that manipulation of transcription factors can indeed induce multiple gene and phenotypic programs related to those seen in neurodegeneration.

One example of this principle comes from disruption of MEF2C in human microglia. Mutations in *MEF2C* leads to MEF2C haploinsufficiency syndrome, which is neurodevelopmental disorder that is characterized by hypotonia, developmental delay, and autism spectrum disorder-like behavior features. Loss of *MEF2C* in isogenic human iPSC-derived microglia drives a broad maladaptive phenotype marked by elevated basal inflammatory cytokine secretion, impaired phagocytosis, lipid accumulation, lysosomal dysfunction, and increased reactive oxygen species, phenotypes that strongly overlaps with AD-related microglial programs (Deczkowska et al., 2017; Nguyen et al., 2025; Rahman & Bennett, 2025).

A complementary example shows that disease-relevant microglial states can also be actively induced by defined transcriptional regulators. Exposure of iPSC-derived microglia to synaptosomes, myelin debris, or synthetic amyloid-β fibrils generates states that map onto human in vivo microglial programs, including DAM-like states (Keren-Shaul et al., 2017; Dolan et al., 2023). Formation of the DAM-like state depends on TREM2 signaling, directly linking the model to AD-relevant microglial biology. Additionally, overexpression of MITF in iPSC-microglia is sufficient to drive the DAM signature (Dolan et al., 2023), providing a clear example of a transcription factor that can actively impose a neurodegeneration-relevant macrophage program rather than merely correlate with one.

Despite these advances, several fundamental questions remain unresolved. First, it is unclear what co-factors cooperate with transcription factors like MEF2C and MITF to establish or maintain these maladaptive states. Identifying these regulatory partners is essential for understanding why certain programs become stabilized during disease rather than be transiently activated. Second, the transcriptional control of disease-associated programs in BAMs remains almost entirely unexplored. BAMs occupy anatomically and functionally distinct niches from parenchymal microglia, and whether the same transcription factors drive similar neurodegenerative programs in

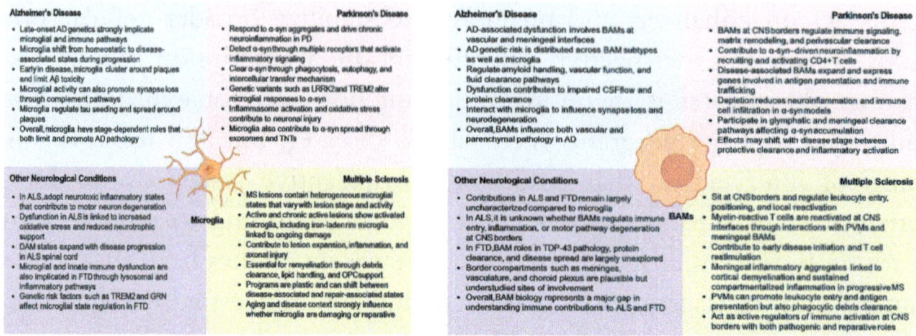

Fig. 5 Summary figure of microglia and BAM functions in neurodegeneration.

both populations, or whether BAMs rely on distinct regulatory logic, is unknown. Addressing this gap is particularly important given the growing recognition that BAMs contribute to neuroinflammation and barrier dysfunction in neurodegeneration. Defining the full regulatory architecture, such as transcription factors, co-factors, and the accessible enhancer and promoter landscape, across both microglia and BAMs will be necessary to determine which nodes are shared and therefore broadly targetable, and which are population specific.

9. Conclusions and future perspectives

Microglia and BAMs together form a distributed macrophage network that maintains CNS homeostasis across anatomically distinct compartments. Although these populations share developmental origins and core myeloid programs, they are shaped by different niche signals, exhibit distinct transcriptional identities, and make nonredundant contributions to CNS physiology and disease. A central lesson of the field is that CNS macrophages cannot be understood through a simple protective-versus-pathogenic binary. Their functions are dynamic, context-dependent, and often mixed within the same lesion or disease stage (Fig. 5).

A major obstacle to advancing our understanding of BAMs in neurodegeneration is the lack of tools that can reliably distinguish individual BAM populations from one another and from infiltrating monocyte-derived macrophages, particularly in human tissue. Perivascular macrophages, choroid plexus macrophages, and meningeal macrophages occupy distinct anatomical compartments, interface with different cellular neighborhoods, and likely perform different functions during disease, yet isolation techniques and Cre-mediated reporters are limited. Without the ability to resolve what each BAM subset is doing independently, it remains difficult to determine whether a given disease phenotype reflects the activity of one specific population or a shared response across all BAMs. Developing transgenic reporters, spatial transcriptomic strategies, and surface marker panels that can separate these populations in situ is a prerequisite for meaningful functional studies.

Equally important is the need to connect the growing catalog of disease-associated macrophage states to defined mechanistic outputs. Single-cell atlases have been valuable in identifying transcriptional programs that emerge during neurodegeneration, but in most cases the functional consequences of these states remain correlative. For example, lipid dysregulation is a recurring feature of both microglial and BAM disease states, yet it is largely unknown whether the underlying mechanisms, such as lipid uptake, storage, metabolism, and efflux, are shared between these populations or are governed by distinct molecular pathways. The same question applies to other processes implicated in disease-associated states, including phagocytic clearance, lysosomal processing, and inflammatory signaling.

A related but distinct question concerns how BAMs interact with the CNS parenchyma and whether these interactions differ fundamentally from those of microglia. Microglia are embedded within the parenchyma and maintain direct contact with neurons, synapses, and other glia. BAMs, by contrast, sit at CNS borders and are positioned to interact with the vasculature, the CSF, and peripheral immune cells. Whether BAMs influence parenchymal biology primarily through secreted signals, through regulation of barrier permeability, or through direct cellular interactions with microglia themselves is poorly understood. Clarifying these communication pathways is important because it determines whether BAMs act as independent effectors during disease or whether their impact on neurodegeneration is mediated indirectly through modulation of microglial activity or vascular function.

An additional dimension that this review has not addressed but that warrants consideration is the role of natural aging itself. Neurodegeneration overwhelmingly occurs in the context of an aging brain, and the macrophage states described throughout this review emerge against a background of age-related changes in both microglia and BAMs that are only beginning to be characterized. Aging alone alters microglial transcriptional identity, phagocytic capacity, lipid metabolism, and inflammatory tone, even in the absence of overt disease. Whether similar age-related shifts occur in BAM populations, and whether these changes predispose BAMs to adopt maladaptive states upon encountering disease-associated stimuli, is largely unknown. Equally important is the question of why some individuals age without significant neurodegeneration while others do not. Studies of cognitively resilient centenarians and superagers suggest that protective trajectories exist, but whether these trajectories involve distinct macrophage states, preserved homeostatic programs, or differences in how microglia and BAMs respond to accumulated damage has not been systematically explored. Integrating aging as a biological variable into studies of CNS macrophage will be essential for understanding the full spectrum of macrophage behavior in the human brain and for identifying what distinguishes a brain that ages with resilience from one that progresses toward neurodegeneration.

Finally, future therapeutic strategies will need to account for the spatial and temporal complexity of CNS macrophage biology. Broad immunosuppression or indiscriminate macrophage depletion risks eliminating protective functions alongside harmful ones. The challenge will be to develop approaches that can modulate specific macrophage populations or states with precision.

Acknowledgements

C.Z.H. is supported by NIH R00MHI129983 and the Brain & Behavior Research Foundation Young Investigator Grant. We also thank Washington University in St. Louis McDonnell Center for Cellular and Molecular Neurobiology and the NeuroGenomics and Informatics Center for their support. Figures made by Biorender.com.

Conflict of interest statement

We declare no conflicts of interest.

References

Absinta, M. (2025). Multiple sclerosis: A smoldering disease. *Trends in Molecular Medicine, 31*(1), 94–95. https://doi.org/10.1016/j.molmed.2024.11.005.

Absinta, M., et al. (2019). Association of chronic active multiple sclerosis lesions with disability in vivo. *JAMA Neurology, 76*(12), 1474–1483. https://doi.org/10.1001/jamaneurol.2019.2399.

Absinta, M., et al. (2021). A lymphocyte-microglia-astrocyte axis in chronic active multiple sclerosis. *Nature, 597*(7878), 709–714. https://doi.org/10.1038/s41586-021-03892-7.

Adachi, K., et al. (2023). Depletion of perivascular macrophages delays ALS disease progression by ameliorating blood-spinal cord barrier impairment in SOD1G93A mice. *Frontiers in Cellular Neuroscience, 17*, 1291673. https://doi.org/10.3389/fncel.2023.1291673.

Adler, D., et al. (2026). Functional border-associated macrophages limit Alzheimer's disease progression. *bioRxiv: The Preprint Server for Biology [Preprint]*. https://doi.org/10.64898/2026.01.31.703045.

Ajami, B., et al. (2018). Single-cell mass cytometry reveals distinct populations of brain myeloid cells in mouse neuroinflammation and neurodegeneration models. *Nature Neuroscience, 21*(4), 541–551. https://doi.org/10.1038/s41593-018-0100-x.

Amann, L., et al. (2024). Extrasinusoidal macrophages are a distinct subset of immunologically active dural macrophages. *Science Immunology, 9*(102), https://doi.org/10.1126/sciimmunol.adh1129.

Anfray, A., et al. (2024). A cell-autonomous role for border-associated macrophages in ApoE4 neurovascular dysfunction and susceptibility to white matter injury. *Nature Neuroscience, 27*(11), 2138–2151. https://doi.org/10.1038/s41593-024-01757-6.

Antony, J. M., et al. (2011). Endogenous microglia regulate development of embryonic cortical precursor cells. *Journal of Neuroscience Research, 89*(3), 286–298. https://doi.org/10.1002/jnr.22533.

Asai, H., et al. (2015). Depletion of microglia and inhibition of exosome synthesis halt tau propagation. *Nature Neuroscience, 18*(11), 1584–1593. https://doi.org/10.1038/nn.4132.

Barclay, K. M., et al. (2024). An inducible genetic tool to track and manipulate specific microglial states reveals their plasticity and roles in remyelination. *Immunity, 57*(6), 1394–1412.e8. https://doi.org/10.1016/j.immuni.2024.05.005.

Bartholomäus, I., et al. (2009). Effector T cell interactions with meningeal vascular structures in nascent autoimmune CNS lesions. *Nature, 462*(7269), 94–98. https://doi.org/10.1038/nature08478.

Bastos, J., et al. (2025). Monocytes can efficiently replace all brain macrophages and fetal liver monocytes can generate bona fide SALL1+ microglia. *Immunity, 58*(5), 1269–1288.e12. https://doi.org/10.1016/j.immuni.2025.04.006.

Beers, D. R., et al. (2006). Wild-type microglia extend survival in PU.1 knockout mice with familial amyotrophic lateral sclerosis. *Proceedings of the National Academy of Sciences of the United States of America, 103*(43), 16021–16026. https://doi.org/10.1073/pnas.0607423103.

Bellenguez, C., et al. (2022). New insights into the genetic etiology of Alzheimer's disease and related dementias. *Nature Genetics, 54*(4), 412–436. https://doi.org/10.1038/s41588-022-01024-z.

Bian, Z., et al. (2020). Deciphering human macrophage development at single-cell resolution. *Nature 2020, 582*(7813), 571–576. https://doi.org/10.1038/s41586-020-2316-7.

Bloem, B. R., Okun, M. S., & Klein, C. (2021). Parkinson's disease. *The Lancet, 397*(10291), 2284–2303. https://doi.org/10.1016/S0140-6736(21)00218-X.

Boillée, S., et al. (2006). Onset and progression in inherited ALS determined by motor neurons and microglia. *Science (New York, N. Y.), 312*(5778), 1389–1392. https://doi.org/10.1126/science.1123511.

Brioschi, S., et al. (2023). A Cre-deleter specific for embryo-derived brain macrophages reveals distinct features of microglia and border macrophages. *Immunity, 56*(5), 1027–1045.e8. https://doi.org/10.1016/j.immuni.2023.01.028.

Brioschi, S., Han, C. Z., & Colonna, M. (2025). Drivers and shapers of macrophages specification in the developing brain. *Current Opinion in Immunology, 94*, 102558. https://doi.org/10.1016/j.coi.2025.102558.

Butovsky, O., et al. (2014). Identification of a unique TGF-β–dependent molecular and functional signature in microglia. *Nature Neuroscience, 17*(1), 131–143. https://doi.org/10.1038/nn.3599.

Buttgereit, A., et al. (2016). Sall1 is a transcriptional regulator defining microglia identity and function. *Nature Immunology, 17*(12), 1397–1406. https://doi.org/10.1038/ni.3585.

Carare, R. O., et al. (2008). Solutes, but not cells, drain from the brain parenchyma along basement membranes of capillaries and arteries: Significance for cerebral amyloid angiopathy and neuroimmunology. *Neuropathology and Applied Neurobiology, 34*(2), 131–144. https://doi.org/10.1111/j.1365-2990.2007.00926.x.

Chang, M. C., et al. (2017). Progranulin deficiency causes impairment of autophagy and TDP-43 accumulation. *The Journal of Experimental Medicine, 214*(9), 2611–2628. https://doi.org/10.1084/jem.20160999.

Chen, X., Holtzman, D. M., & Colonna, M. (2026). Immunity in Alzheimer's disease: From mechanisms to therapies. *Immunity, 59*(3), 524–541. https://doi.org/10.1016/j.immuni.2026.02.004.

Cignarella, F., et al. (2020). TREM2 activation on microglia promotes myelin debris clearance and remyelination in a model of multiple sclerosis. *Acta Neuropathologica, 140*(4), 513–534. https://doi.org/10.1007/s00401-020-02193-z.

Condello, C., et al. (2015). Microglia constitute a barrier that prevents neurotoxic protofibrillar Aβ42 hotspots around plaques. *Nature Communications, 6*(1), 6176. https://doi.org/10.1038/ncomms7176.

Cugurra, A., et al. (2021). Skull and vertebral bone marrow are myeloid cell reservoirs for the meninges and CNS parenchyma. *Science (New York, N. Y.), 373*(6553), https://doi.org/10.1126/science.abf7844.

Da Mesquita, S., et al. (2018). Functional aspects of meningeal lymphatics in ageing and Alzheimer's disease. *Nature, 560*(7717), 185–191. https://doi.org/10.1038/s41586-018-0368-8.

Da Mesquita, S., et al. (2021). Meningeal lymphatics affect microglia responses and anti-Aβ immunotherapy. *Nature, 593*(7858), 255–260. https://doi.org/10.1038/s41586-021-03489-0.

Dalmau Gasull, A., et al. (2024). The niche matters: Origin, function and fate of CNS-associated macrophages during health and disease. *Acta Neuropathologica, 147*(1), 37. https://doi.org/10.1007/s00401-023-02676-9.

Dani, N., et al. (2021). A cellular and spatial map of the choroid plexus across brain ventricles and ages. *Cell, 184*(11), 3056–3074. https://doi.org/10.1016/j.cell.2021.04.003.

De Groot, C. J., et al. (2001). Post-mortem MRI-guided sampling of multiple sclerosis brain lesions: Increased yield of active demyelinating and (p)reactive lesions. *Brain: A Journal of Neurology, 124*(Pt 8), 1635–1645. https://doi.org/10.1093/brain/124.8.1635.

De Schepper, S., et al. (2023). Perivascular cells induce microglial phagocytic states and synaptic engulfment via SPP1 in mouse models of Alzheimer's disease. *Nature Neuroscience, 26*(3), 406–415. https://doi.org/10.1038/s41593-023-01257-z.

De Vlaminck, K., et al. (2022). Differential plasticity and fate of brain-resident and recruited macrophages during the onset and resolution of neuroinflammation. *Immunity, 55*(11), 2085–2102. https://doi.org/10.1016/j.immuni.2022.09.005.

Deczkowska, A., et al. (2017). Mef2C restrains microglial inflammatory response and is lost in brain ageing in an IFN-I-dependent manner. *Nature Communications, 8*(1), 717. https://doi.org/10.1038/s41467-017-00769-0.

Dick, S. A., et al. (2022). Three tissue resident macrophage subsets coexist across organs with conserved origins and life cycles. *Science Immunology,* 7(67), https://doi.org/10.1126/sciimmunol.abf7777.

Dieriks, B. V., et al. (2017). α-synuclein transfer through tunneling nanotubes occurs in SH-SY5Y cells and primary brain pericytes from Parkinson's disease patients. *Scientific Reports,* 7(1), 42984. https://doi.org/10.1038/srep42984.

Dilsizoglu Senol, A., et al. (2021). α-Synuclein fibrils subvert lysosome structure and function for the propagation of protein misfolding between cells through tunneling nanotubes. *PLoS Biology, 19*(7), e3001287. https://doi.org/10.1371/journal.pbio.3001287.

Dolan, M.-J., et al. (2023). Exposure of iPSC-derived human microglia to brain substrates enables the generation and manipulation of diverse transcriptional states in vitro. *Nature Immunology, 24*(8), 1382–1390. https://doi.org/10.1038/s41590-023-01558-2.

Drieu, A., et al. (2022). Parenchymal border macrophages regulate the flow dynamics of the cerebrospinal fluid. *Nature, 611*(7936), 585–593. https://doi.org/10.1038/s41586-022-05397-3.

Drieu, A., et al. (2023). Parenchymal border macrophages regulate tau pathology and tau-mediated neurodegeneration. *Life Science Alliance, 6*(11), https://doi.org/10.26508/lsa.202302087.

Du, S., et al. (2026). Diversity and immune dynamics of choroid plexus macrophages are shaped by distinct developmental origins. *Nature Neuroscience, 29*(3), 717–731. https://doi.org/10.1038/s41593-025-02158-z.

Ennerfelt, H., et al. (2022). SYK coordinates neuroprotective microglial responses in neurodegenerative disease. *Cell, 185*(22), 4135–4152. https://doi.org/10.1016/j.cell.2022.09.030.

Escoubas, C. C., et al. (2024). Type-I-interferon-responsive microglia shape cortical development and behavior. *Cell, 187*(8), 1936–1954. https://doi.org/10.1016/j.cell.2024.02.020.

Faraco, G., et al. (2016). Perivascular macrophages mediate the neurovascular and cognitive dysfunction associated with hypertension. *Journal of Clinical Investigation, 126*(12), 4674–4689. https://doi.org/10.1172/JCI86950.

Fixsen, B. R., et al. (2023). SALL1 enforces microglia-specific DNA binding and function of SMADs to establish microglia identity. *Nature Immunology, 24*(7), 1188–1199. https://doi.org/10.1038/s41590-023-01528-8.

Galea, I., et al. (2005). Mannose receptor expression specifically reveals perivascular macrophages in normal, injured, and diseased mouse brain. *Glia, 49*(3), 375–384. https://doi.org/10.1002/glia.20124.

Gasparotto, J., et al. (2024). Is it all the RAGE? Defining the role of the receptor for advanced glycation end products in Parkinson's disease. *Journal of Neurochemistry, 168*(8), 1608–1624. https://doi.org/10.1111/jnc.15890.

Giles, D. A., et al. (2018). CNS-resident classical DCs play a critical role in CNS autoimmune disease. *Journal of Clinical Investigation, 128*(12), 5322–5334. https://doi.org/10.1172/JCI123708.

Ginhoux, F., et al. (2010). Fate mapping analysis reveals that adult microglia derive from primitive macrophages. *Science (New York, N. Y.), 330*(6005), 841–845. https://doi.org/10.1126/science.1194637.

Ginhoux, F., & Guilliams, M. (2016). Tissue-resident macrophage ontogeny and homeostasis. *Immunity, 44*(3), 439–449. https://doi.org/10.1016/j.immuni.2016.02.024.

Ginhoux, F., et al. (2013). Origin and differentiation of microglia. *Frontiers in Cellular Neuroscience,* 7, 45. https://doi.org/10.3389/fncel.2013.00045.

Goldmann, T., et al. (2016). Origin, fate and dynamics of macrophages at central nervous system interfaces. *Nature Immunology, 17*(7), 797–805. https://doi.org/10.1038/ni.3423.

Gordon, R., Albornoz, E. A., Christie, D. C., Langley, M. R., Kumar, V., Mantovani, S., ... Woodruff, T. M. (2018). Inflammasome inhibition prevents α-synuclein pathology and dopaminergic neurodegeneration in mice. *Science Translational Medicine, 10*(465), https://doi.org/10.1126/scitranslmed.aah4066.

Gratuze, M., et al. (2021). Activated microglia mitigate Aβ-associated tau seeding and spreading. *The Journal of Experimental Medicine, 218*(8), https://doi.org/10.1084/jem.20210542.

Gratuze, M., et al. (2023). TREM2-independent microgliosis promotes tau-mediated neurodegeneration in the presence of ApoE4. *Neuron, 111*(2), 202–219.e7. https://doi.org/10.1016/j.neuron.2022.10.022.

Griciuc, A., et al. (2013). Alzheimer's disease risk gene CD33 inhibits microglial uptake of amyloid beta. *Neuron, 78*(4), 631–643. https://doi.org/10.1016/j.neuron.2013.04.014.

Gross, P. S., et al. (2025). Senescent-like microglia limit remyelination through the senescence associated secretory phenotype. *Nature Communications, 16*(1), 2283. https://doi.org/10.1038/s41467-025-57632-w.

Guerreiro, R., et al. (2013). TREM2 variants in Alzheimer's disease. *The New England Journal of Medicine, 368*(2), 117–127. https://doi.org/10.1056/NEJMoa1211851.

Guo, M., et al. (2020). Microglial exosomes facilitate α-synuclein transmission in Parkinson's disease. *Brain: A Journal of Neurology, 143*(5), 1476–1497. https://doi.org/10.1093/brain/awaa090.

Guo, Y., Wei, X., Yan, H., Qin, Y., Yan, S., Liu, J., Zhao, Y., Jiang, F., & Lou, H. (2019). TREM2 deficiency aggravates α-synuclein–induced neurodegeneration and neuroinflammation in Parkinson's disease models. *The FASEB Journal, 33*(11), 12164–12174. https://doi.org/10.1096/fj.201900992r.

Guttenplan, K. A., et al. (2021). Neurotoxic reactive astrocytes induce cell death via saturated lipids. *Nature, 599*(7883), 102–107. https://doi.org/10.1038/s41586-021-03960-y.

Hagemeyer, N., et al. (2017). Microglia contribute to normal myelinogenesis and to oligodendrocyte progenitor maintenance during adulthood. *Acta Neuropathologica, 134*(3), 441–458. https://doi.org/10.1007/s00401-017-1747-1.

Hamilton, S. P., & Rome, L. H. (1994). Stimulation of in vitro myelin synthesis by microglia. *Glia, 11*(4), 326–335. https://doi.org/10.1002/glia.440110405.

Han, C. Z., et al. (2023). Human microglia maturation is underpinned by specific gene regulatory networks. *Immunity, 56*(9), 2152–2171.e13. https://doi.org/10.1016/j.immuni.2023.07.016.

Haque, Md. E., Akther, M., Jakaria, Md, Kim, I.-S., Azam, S., & Choi, D. K. (2019). Targeting the Microglial NLRP3 Inflammasome and Its Role in Parkinson's Disease. *Movement Disorders, 35*(1), 20–33. https://doi.org/10.1002/mds.27874.

Hashimoto, D., et al. (2013). Tissue-resident macrophages self-maintain locally throughout adult life with minimal contribution from circulating monocytes. *Immunity, 38*(4), 792–804. https://doi.org/10.1016/j.immuni.2013.04.004.

Healy, L. M., et al. (2022). The role of glial cells in multiple sclerosis disease progression. *Nature Reviews. Neurology, 18*(4), 237–248. https://doi.org/10.1038/s41582-022-00624-x.

Heneka, M. T., et al. (2013). NLRP3 is activated in Alzheimer's disease and contributes to pathology in APP/PS1 mice. *Nature, 493*(7434), 674–678. https://doi.org/10.1038/nature11729.

Herisson, F., et al. (2018). Direct vascular channels connect skull bone marrow and the brain surface enabling myeloid cell migration. *Nature Neuroscience, 21*(9), 1209–1217. https://doi.org/10.1038/s41593-018-0213-2.

Heß, K., et al. (2020). Lesion stage-dependent causes for impaired remyelination in MS. *Acta Neuropathologica, 140*(3), 359–375. https://doi.org/10.1007/s00401-020-02189-9.

Hickey, W. F., & Kimura, H. (1988). Perivascular microglial cells of the CNS are bone marrow-derived and present antigen in vivo. *Science (New York, N. Y.), 239*(4837), 290–292. https://doi.org/10.1126/science.3276004.

Hickey, W. F., Vass, K., & Lassmann, H. (1992). Bone marrow-derived elements in the central nervous system: An immunohistochemical and ultrastructural survey of rat chimeras. *Journal of Neuropathology & Experimental Neurology, 51*(3), 246–256. https://doi.org/10.1097/00005072-199205000-00002.

Hoeffel, G., et al. (2015). C-Myb+ erythro-myeloid progenitor-derived fetal monocytes give rise to adult tissue-resident macrophages. *Immunity, 42*(4), 665–678. https://doi.org/10.1016/j.immuni.2015.03.011.

Hollingworth, P., et al. (2012). Genome-wide association study of Alzheimer's disease with psychotic symptoms. *Molecular Psychiatry, 17*(12), 1316–1327. https://doi.org/10.1038/mp.2011.125.

Hong, S., et al. (2016). Complement and microglia mediate early synapse loss in Alzheimer mouse models. *Science (New York, N. Y.), 352*(6286), 712–716. https://doi.org/10.1126/science.aad8373.

Huang, P., Zhang, Z., Zhang, P., Feng, J., Xie, J., Zheng, Y., ... Zhang, Y. (2024). TREM2 deficiency aggravates NLRP3 inflammasome activation and pyroptosis in MPTP-induced parkinson's disease mice and LPS-induced BV2 cells. *Molecular Neurobiology, 61*(5), 2590–2605. https://doi.org/10.1007/s12035-023-03713-0.

Hutchins, K. D., et al. (1990). Localization of morphologically distinct microglial populations in the developing human fetal brain: Implications for ontogeny. *Developmental Brain Research, 55*(1), 95–102. https://doi.org/10.1016/0165-3806(90)90109-C.

Iliff, J. J., et al. (2012). A paravascular pathway facilitates CSF flow through the brain parenchyma and the clearance of interstitial solutes, including amyloid β. *Science Translational Medicine, 4*(147), https://doi.org/10.1126/scitranslmed.3003748.

Jais, A., et al. (2016). Myeloid-cell-derived VEGF maintains brain glucose uptake and limits cognitive impairment in obesity. *Cell, 165*(4), 882–895. https://doi.org/10.1016/j.cell.2016.03.033.

Jonsson, T., et al. (2013). Variant of *TREM2* associated with the risk of Alzheimer's disease. *New England Journal of Medicine, 368*(2), 107–116. https://doi.org/10.1056/NEJMoa1211103.

Jordão, M. J. C., et al. (2019). Single-cell profiling identifies myeloid cell subsets with distinct fates during neuroinflammation. *Science (New York, N. Y.), 363*(6425), https://doi.org/10.1126/science.aat7554.

Kaji, S., et al. (2024). Apolipoprotein E aggregation in microglia initiates Alzheimer's disease pathology by seeding β-amyloidosis. *Immunity, 57*(11), 2651–2668. https://doi.org/10.1016/j.immuni.2024.09.014.

Keren-Shaul, H., et al. (2017). A unique microglia type associated with restricting development of Alzheimer's disease. *Cell, 169*(7), 1276–1290. https://doi.org/10.1016/J.CELL.2017.05.018.

Kierdorf, K., et al. (2019). Macrophages at CNS interfaces: Ontogeny and function in health and disease. *Nature Reviews. Neuroscience, 20*(9), 547–562. https://doi.org/10.1038/s41583-019-0201-x.

Kierdorf, K., Erny, D., et al. (2013). Microglia emerge from erythromyeloid precursors via Pu.1- and Irf8-dependent pathways. *Nature Neuroscience 2013, 16*(3), 273–280. https://doi.org/10.1038/nn.3318.

Kierdorf, K., Katzmarski, N., et al. (2013). Bone marrow cell recruitment to the brain in the absence of irradiation or parabiosis bias. *PLoS One, 8*(3), e58544. https://doi.org/10.1371/journal.pone.0058544.

Kim, C., et al. (2013). Neuron-released oligomeric α-synuclein is an endogenous agonist of TLR2 for paracrine activation of microglia. *Nature Communications, 4*(1), 1562. https://doi.org/10.1038/ncomms2534.

Kim, Y.-C., et al. (2023). Immaturity of immune cells around the dural venous sinuses contributes to viral meningoencephalitis in neonates. *Science Immunology, 8*(88), https://doi.org/10.1126/sciimmunol.adg6155.

Kivisäkk, P., et al. (2009). Localizing central nervous system immune surveillance: Meningeal antigen-presenting cells activate T cells during experimental autoimmune encephalomyelitis. *Annals of Neurology, 65*(4), 457–469. https://doi.org/10.1002/ana.21379.

Komori, T., et al. (2024). Brain-derived neurotrophic factor from microglia regulates neuronal development in the medial prefrontal cortex and its associated social behavior. *Molecular Psychiatry, 29*(5), 1338–1349. https://doi.org/10.1038/s41380-024-02413-y.

Kracht, L., et al. (2020). Human fetal microglia acquire homeostatic immune-sensing properties early in development. *Science (New York, N. Y.), 369*(6503), 530–537. https://doi.org/10.1126/science.aba5906.

Krasemann, S., et al. (2017). The TREM2-APOE pathway drives the transcriptional phenotype of dysfunctional microglia in neurodegenerative diseases. *Immunity, 47*(3), 566–581.e9. https://doi.org/10.1016/j.immuni.2017.08.008.

Kumaravelu, P., et al. (2002). Quantitative developmental anatomy of definitive haematopoietic stem cells/long-term repopulating units (HSC/RUs): Role of the aorta-gonad-mesonephros (AGM) region and the yolk sac in colonisation of the mouse embryonic liver. *Development (Cambridge, England), 129*(21), 4891–4899. https://doi.org/10.1242/dev.129.21.4891.

Lambert, J. C., et al. (2013). Meta-analysis of 74,046 individuals identifies 11 new susceptibility loci for Alzheimer's disease. *Nature Genetics, 45*(12), 1452–1458. https://doi.org/10.1038/ng.2802.

Lampron, A., et al. (2015). Inefficient clearance of myelin debris by microglia impairs remyelinating processes. *The Journal of Experimental Medicine, 212*(4), 481–495. https://doi.org/10.1084/jem.20141656.

Leyns, C. E. G., et al. (2019). TREM2 function impedes tau seeding in neuritic plaques. *Nature Neuroscience, 22*(8), 1217–1222. https://doi.org/10.1038/s41593-019-0433-0.

Li, Q., & Barres, B. A. (2018). Microglia and macrophages in brain homeostasis and disease. *Nature Reviews. Immunology, 18*(4), 225–242. https://doi.org/10.1038/nri.2017.125.

Li, Q., et al. (2019). Developmental heterogeneity of microglia and brain myeloid cells revealed by deep single-cell RNA sequencing. *Neuron, 101*(2), 207–223. https://doi.org/10.1016/j.neuron.2018.12.006.

Liddelow, S. A., et al. (2017). Neurotoxic reactive astrocytes are induced by activated microglia. *Nature, 541*(7638), 481–487. https://doi.org/10.1038/nature21029.

Ling, E. A., Kaur, C., & Lu, J. (1998). Origin, nature, and some functional considerations of intraventricular macrophages, with special reference to the epiplexus cells. *Microscopy Research and Technique, 41*(1), 43–56. https://doi.org/10.1002/(SICI)1097-0029(19980401)41:1<43::AID-JEMT5>3.0.CO;2-V.

Lombardi, M., et al. (2019). Detrimental and protective action of microglial extracellular vesicles on myelin lesions: Astrocyte involvement in remyelination failure. *Acta Neuropathologica, 138*(6), 987–1012. https://doi.org/10.1007/s00401-019-02049-1.

Lombardi, M., et al. (2024). Extracellular vesicles released by microglia and macrophages carry endocannabinoids which foster oligodendrocyte differentiation. *Frontiers in Immunology, 15*. https://doi.org/10.3389/fimmu.2024.1331210.

Long, H., et al. (2022). Interaction of RAGE with α-synuclein fibrils mediates inflammatory response of microglia. *Cell Reports, 40*(12), 111401. https://doi.org/10.1016/j.celrep.2022.111401.

Louveau, A., et al. (2015). Structural and functional features of central nervous system lymphatic vessels. *Nature, 523*(7560), 337–341. https://doi.org/10.1038/nature14432.

Lui, H., et al. (2016). Progranulin deficiency promotes circuit-specific synaptic pruning by microglia via complement activation. *Cell, 165*(4), 921–935. https://doi.org/10.1016/j.cell.2016.04.001.

Marsters, C. M., et al. (2020). Embryonic microglia influence developing hypothalamic glial populations. *Journal of Neuroinflammation, 17*(1), 146. https://doi.org/10.1186/s12974-020-01811-7.

Marzan, D. E., et al. (2021). Activated microglia drive demyelination via CSF1R signaling. *Glia, 69*(6), 1583–1604. https://doi.org/10.1002/glia.23980.

Mass, E., et al. (2016). Specification of tissue-resident macrophages during organogenesis. *Science (New York, N. Y.), 353*(6304), aaf4238. https://doi.org/10.1126/science.aaf4238.

Mass, E., et al. (2023). Tissue-specific macrophages: How they develop and choreograph tissue biology. *Nature Reviews. Immunology, 23*(9), 563–579. https://doi.org/10.1038/s41577-023-00848-y.

Masuda, T., et al. (2019). Spatial and temporal heterogeneity of mouse and human microglia at single-cell resolution. *Nature, 566*(7744), 388–392. https://doi.org/10.1038/s41586-019-0924-x.
Masuda, T., et al. (2022). Specification of CNS macrophage subsets occurs postnatally in defined niches. *Nature, 604*(7907), 740–748. https://doi.org/10.1038/s41586-022-04596-2.
Matcovitch-Natan, O., et al. (2016). Microglia development follows a stepwise program to regulate brain homeostasis. *Science (New York, N. Y.), 353*(6301), aad8670. https://doi.org/10.1126/science.aad8670.
Matejuk, A., & Ransohoff, R. M. (2020). Crosstalk between astrocytes and microglia: An overview. *Frontiers in Immunology, 11*. https://doi.org/10.3389/fimmu.2020.01416.
McCallum, S., et al. (2026). Lesion-remote astrocytes govern microglia-mediated white matter repair. *Nature, 649*(8098), 959–970. https://doi.org/10.1038/s41586-025-09887-y.
McGeer, P. L., et al. (1988). Reactive microglia are positive for HLA-DR in the substantia nigra of Parkinson's and Alzheimer's disease brains. *Neurology, 38*(8), https://doi.org/10.1212/WNL.38.8.1285.
McGrath, K. E., et al. (2003). Circulation is established in a stepwise pattern in the mammalian embryo. *Blood, 101*(5), 1669–1676. https://doi.org/10.1182/blood-2002-08-2531.
McKercher, S. R., et al. (1996). Targeted disruption of the PU.1 gene results in multiple hematopoietic abnormalities. *The EMBO Journal, 15*(20), 5647–5658. https://doi.org/10.1002/j.1460-2075.1996.tb00949.x.
McKinsey, G. L., et al. (2020). A new genetic strategy for targeting microglia in development and disease. *eLife, 9*. https://doi.org/10.7554/eLife.54590.
McNamara, N. B., et al. (2023). Microglia regulate central nervous system myelin growth and integrity. *Nature, 613*(7942), 120–129. https://doi.org/10.1038/s41586-022-05534-y.
Medvinsky, A. L., et al. (1993). An early pre-liver intraembryonic source of CFU-S in the developing mouse. *Nature, 364*(6432), 64–67. https://doi.org/10.1038/364064a0.
Menassa, D. A., & Gomez-Nicola, D. (2018). Microglial dynamics during human brain development. *Frontiers in Immunology, 9*, 1014. https://doi.org/10.3389/fimmu.2018.01014.
Mildenberger, W., Stifter, S. A., & Greter, M. (2022). Diversity and function of brain-associated macrophages. *Current Opinion in Immunology, 76*, 102181. https://doi.org/10.1016/j.coi.2022.102181.
Moore, M. A., & Metcalf, D. (1970). Ontogeny of the haemopoietic system: Yolk sac origin of in vivo and in vitro colony forming cells in the developing mouse embryo. *British Journal of Haematology, 18*(3), 279–296. https://doi.org/10.1111/j.1365-2141.1970.tb01443.x.
Morris, H. R., et al. (2024). The pathogenesis of Parkinson's disease. *The Lancet, 403*(10423), 293–304. https://doi.org/10.1016/S0140-6736(23)01478-2.
Moura Silva, H., et al. (2021). c-MAF–dependent perivascular macrophages regulate diet-induced metabolic syndrome. *Science Immunology, 6*(64), eabg7506. https://doi.org/10.1126/sciimmunol.abg7506.
Mrdjen, D., et al. (2018). High-dimensional single-cell mapping of central nervous system immune cells reveals distinct myeloid subsets in health, aging, and disease. *Immunity, 48*(2), 380–395.e6. https://doi.org/10.1016/j.immuni.2018.01.011.
Mundt, S., Greter, M., & Becher, B. (2022). The CNS mononuclear phagocyte system in health and disease. *Neuron, 110*(21), 3497–3512. https://doi.org/10.1016/j.neuron.2022.10.005.
Murabe, Y., & Sano, Y. (1982). Morphological studies on neuroglia. *Cell and Tissue Research, 225*(3), https://doi.org/10.1007/BF00214798.
Naito, M., Takahashi, K., & Nishikawa, S. (1990). Development, differentiation, and maturation of macrophages in the fetal mouse liver. *Journal of Leukocyte Biology, 48*(1), 27–37. https://doi.org/10.1002/jlb.48.1.27.

Nguyen, C., et al. (2025). Transcriptional and epigenetic targets of MEF2C in human microglia contribute to cellular functions related to autism risk and age-related disease. *Nature Immunology, 26*(11), 1989–2003. https://doi.org/10.1038/s41590-025-02299-0.

Nguyen, P. T., et al. (2020). Microglial remodeling of the extracellular matrix promotes synapse plasticity. *Cell, 182*(2), 388–403.e15. https://doi.org/10.1016/j.cell.2020.05.050.

Otero, A. M., & Antonson, A. M. (2025). Ontogeny and colonization of embryonic border-associated macrophages and their role in neurodevelopment. *Frontiers in cellular neuroscience, 19*, 1677414. https://doi.org/10.3389/fncel.2025.1677414.

Pang, Y., Fan, L., et al. (2013). Differential roles of astrocyte and microglia in supporting oligodendrocyte development and myelination in vitro. *Brain and Behavior, 3*(5), 503–514. https://doi.org/10.1002/brb3.152.

Panicker, N., et al. (2019). Fyn kinase regulates misfolded α-synuclein uptake and NLRP3 inflammasome activation in microglia. *Journal of Experimental Medicine, 216*(6), 1411–1430. https://doi.org/10.1084/jem.20182191.

Park, C., et al. (2019). The landscape of myeloid and astrocyte phenotypes in acute multiple sclerosis lesions. *Acta Neuropathologica Communications,* 7(1), 130. https://doi.org/10.1186/s40478-019-0779-2.

Park, L., et al. (2017). Brain perivascular macrophages initiate the neurovascular dysfunction of Alzheimer Aβ peptides. *Circulation Research, 121*(3), 258–269. https://doi.org/10.1161/CIRCRESAHA.117.311054.

Parkhurst, C. N., et al. (2013). Microglia promote learning-dependent synapse formation through brain-derived neurotrophic factor. *Cell, 155*(7), 1596–1609. https://doi.org/10.1016/j.cell.2013.11.030.

Penati, S., et al. (2025). Mechanisms and environmental factors shaping the ecosystem of brain macrophages. *Frontiers in Immunology, 16*. https://doi.org/10.3389/fimmu.2025.1539988.

Penfield, W. (1932). *Cytology & cellular pathology of the nervous system*. P.B. Hoeber Incorporated.

Perry, V. H., Hume, D. A., & Gordon, S. (1985). Immunohistochemical localization of macrophages and microglia in the adult and developing mouse brain. *Neuroscience, 15*(2), 313–326. https://doi.org/10.1016/0306-4522(85)90215-5.

Polfliet, M. M., et al. (2001). A method for the selective depletion of perivascular and meningeal macrophages in the central nervous system. *Journal of Neuroimmunology, 116*(2), 188–195. https://doi.org/10.1016/s0165-5728(01)00282-x.

Polfliet, M. M. J., et al. (2002). The role of perivascular and meningeal macrophages in experimental allergic encephalomyelitis. *Journal of Neuroimmunology, 122*(1–2), 1–8. https://doi.org/10.1016/S0165-5728(01)00445-3.

Profaci, C. P., et al. (2020). The blood–brain barrier in health and disease: Important unanswered questions. *Journal of Experimental Medicine, 217*(4), e20190062. https://doi.org/10.1084/jem.20190062.

Rahman, R. J., & Bennett, M. L. (2025). Microglial MEF2C is a uniquely human bridge between neurodevelopment and neurodegeneration. *Nature Immunology, 26*(11), 1847–1848. https://doi.org/10.1038/s41590-025-02313-5.

Rawji, K. S., Neumann, B., & Franklin, R. J. M. (2023). Glial aging and its impact on central nervous system myelin regeneration. *Annals of the New York Academy of Sciences, 1519*(1), 34–45. https://doi.org/10.1111/nyas.14933.

Rebejac, J., et al. (2022). Meningeal macrophages protect against viral neuroinfection. *Immunity, 55*(11), 2103–2117.e10. https://doi.org/10.1016/j.immuni.2022.10.005.

Rezaie, P., & Male, D. (1999). Colonisation of the developing human brain and spinal cord by microglia: A review. *Microscopy Research and Technique, 45*(6), 359–382. https://doi.org/10.1002/(SICI)1097-0029(19990615)45:6<359::AID-JEMT4>3.0.CO;2-D.

Rua, R., et al. (2019). Infection drives meningeal engraftment by inflammatory monocytes that impairs CNS immunity. *Nature Immunology, 20*(4), 407–419. https://doi.org/10.1038/s41590-019-0344-y.
Ruckh, J. M., et al. (2012). Rejuvenation of regeneration in the aging central nervous system. *Cell Stem Cell, 10*(1), 96–103. https://doi.org/10.1016/j.stem.2011.11.019.
Rustenhoven, J., & Kipnis, J. (2022). Brain borders at the central stage of neuroimmunology. *Nature, 612*(7940), 417–429. https://doi.org/10.1038/s41586-022-05474-7.
Schafer, D. P., et al. (2012). Microglia sculpt postnatal neural circuits in an activity and complement-dependent manner. *Neuron, 74*(4), 691–705. https://doi.org/10.1016/j.neuron.2012.03.026.
Scheiblich, H., et al. (2021). Microglia jointly degrade fibrillar alpha-synuclein cargo by distribution through tunneling nanotubes. *Cell, 184*(20), 5089–5106.e21. https://doi.org/10.1016/j.cell.2021.09.007.
Schonhoff, A. M., et al. (2023). Border-associated macrophages mediate the neuroinflammatory response in an alpha-synuclein model of Parkinson disease. *Nature Communications, 14*(1), 3754. https://doi.org/10.1038/s41467-023-39060-w.
Sherafat, A., et al. (2021). Microglial neuropilin-1 promotes oligodendrocyte expansion during development and remyelination by trans-activating platelet-derived growth factor receptor. *Nature Communications, 12*(1), 2265. https://doi.org/10.1038/s41467-021-22532-2.
Shimada, A., & Hasegawa-Ishii, S. (2021). Increased cytokine expression in the choroid plexus stroma and epithelium in response to endotoxin-induced systemic inflammation in mice. *Toxicology reports, 8*, 520–528. https://doi.org/10.1016/j.toxrep.2021.03.002.
Silvin, A., Qian, J., & Ginhoux, F. (2023). Brain macrophage development, diversity and dysregulation in health and disease. *Cellular & Molecular Immunology, 20*(11), 1277–1289. https://doi.org/10.1038/s41423-023-01053-6.
Smajić, S., et al. (2022). Single-cell sequencing of human midbrain reveals glial activation and a Parkinson-specific neuronal state. *Brain: a journal of neurology, 145*(3), 964–978. https://doi.org/10.1093/brain/awab446.
Spangenberg, E., et al. (2019). Sustained microglial depletion with CSF1R inhibitor impairs parenchymal plaque development in an Alzheimer's disease model. *Nature communications, 10*(1), 3758. https://doi.org/10.1038/s41467-019-11674-z.
Stefanova, N., et al. (2011). Toll-like receptor 4 promotes α-synuclein clearance and survival of nigral dopaminergic neurons. *The American Journal of Pathology, 179*(2), 954–963. https://doi.org/10.1016/j.ajpath.2011.04.013.
Stevens, B., et al. (2007). The classical complement cascade mediates CNS synapse elimination. *Cell, 131*(6), 1164–1178. https://doi.org/10.1016/j.cell.2007.10.036.
Sung, W., et al. (2024). Progranulin haploinsufficiency mediates cytoplasmic TDP-43 aggregation with lysosomal abnormalities in human microglia. *Journal of Neuroinflammation, 21*(1), 47. https://doi.org/10.1186/s12974-024-03039-1.
Tahmasebi, F., et al. (2019). Effect of the CSF1R inhibitor PLX3397 on remyelination of corpus callosum in a cuprizone-induced demyelination mouse model. *Journal of Cellular Biochemistry, 120*(6), 10576–10586. https://doi.org/10.1002/jcb.28344.
Tavian, M., & Peault, B. (2005). Embryonic development of the human hematopoietic system. *The International Journal of Developmental Biology, 49*(2–3), 243–250. https://doi.org/10.1387/ijdb.041957mt.
Tay, T. L., et al. (2017). A new fate mapping system reveals context-dependent random or clonal expansion of microglia. *Nature Neuroscience, 20*(6), 793–803. https://doi.org/10.1038/nn.4547.
Thanopoulou, K., et al. (2010). Scavenger receptor class B type I (SR-BI) regulates perivascular macrophages and modifies amyloid pathology in an Alzheimer mouse model. *Proceedings of the National Academy of Sciences of the United States of America, 107*(48), 20816–20821. https://doi.org/10.1073/pnas.1005888107.

Thion, M. S., Ginhoux, F., & Garel, S. (2018). Microglia and early brain development: An intimate journey. *Science (New York, N. Y.), 362*(6411), 185–189. https://doi.org/10.1126/science.aat0474.

Tremblay, M., Lowery, R. L., & Majewska, A. K. (2010). Microglial interactions with synapses are modulated by visual experience. *PLoS Biology, 8*(11), https://doi.org/10.1371/journal.pbio.1000527.

Tzioras, M., et al. (2023). Human astrocytes and microglia show augmented ingestion of synapses in Alzheimer's disease via MFG-E8. *Cell Reports. Medicine, 4*(9), 101175. https://doi.org/10.1016/j.xcrm.2023.101175.

Uekawa, K., et al. (2023). Border-associated macrophages promote cerebral amyloid angiopathy and cognitive impairment through vascular oxidative stress. *Molecular Neurodegeneration, 18*(1), 73. https://doi.org/10.1186/s13024-023-00660-1.

Ueno, M., et al. (2013). Layer V cortical neurons require microglial support for survival during postnatal development. *Nature Neuroscience, 16*(5), 543–551. https://doi.org/10.1038/nn.3358.

Ulland, T. K., et al. (2017). TREM2 maintains microglial metabolic fitness in Alzheimer's disease. *Cell, 170*(4), 649–663.e13. https://doi.org/10.1016/j.cell.2017.07.023.

Utz, S. G., et al. (2020). Early fate defines microglia and non-parenchymal brain macrophage development. *Cell, 181*(3), 557–573.e18. https://doi.org/10.1016/j.cell.2020.03.021.

Vainchtein, I. D., et al. (2018). Astrocyte-derived interleukin-33 promotes microglial synapse engulfment and neural circuit development. *Science (New York, N. Y.), 359*(6381), 1269–1273. https://doi.org/10.1126/science.aal3589.

van der Poel, M., et al. (2019). Transcriptional profiling of human microglia reveals grey-white matter heterogeneity and multiple sclerosis-associated changes. *Nature communications, 10*(1), 1139. https://doi.org/10.1038/s41467-019-08976-7.

Van Hove, H., et al. (2019). A single-cell atlas of mouse brain macrophages reveals unique transcriptional identities shaped by ontogeny and tissue environment. *Nature Neuroscience, 22*(6), 1021–1035. https://doi.org/10.1038/s41593-019-0393-4.

Van Hove, H., et al. (2025). Interleukin-34-dependent perivascular macrophages promote vascular function in the brain. *Immunity, 58*(5), 1289–1305.e8. https://doi.org/10.1016/j.immuni.2025.04.003.

Wake, H., et al. (2009). Resting microglia directly monitor the functional state of synapses in vivo and determine the fate of ischemic terminals. *The Journal of Neuroscience, 29*(13), 3974–3980. https://doi.org/10.1523/JNEUROSCI.4363-08.2009.

Wang, C. C., et al. (1996). Immunohistochemical study of amoeboid microglial cells in fetal rat brain. *Journal of Anatomy, 189*(Pt 3), 567–574. https://pmc.ncbi.nlm.nih.gov/articles/PMC1167699/.

Wang, S., et al. (2022). TREM2 drives microglia response to amyloid-β via SYK-dependent and -independent pathways. *Cell, 185*(22), 4153–4169. https://doi.org/10.1016/j.cell.2022.09.033.

Wang, X., et al. (2020). RAGE silencing ameliorates neuroinflammation by inhibition of p38-NF-κB signaling pathway in mouse model of Parkinson's disease. *Frontiers in Neuroscience, 14*. https://doi.org/10.3389/fnins.2020.00353.

Williams, G. P., et al. (2018). Targeting of the class II transactivator attenuates inflammation and neurodegeneration in an alpha-synuclein model of Parkinson's disease. *Journal of Neuroinflammation, 15*(1), 244. https://doi.org/10.1186/s12974-018-1286-2.

Willis, C. L., Garwood, C. J., & Ray, D. E. (2007). A size selective vascular barrier in the rat area postrema formed by perivascular macrophages and the extracellular matrix. *Neuroscience, 150*(2), 498–509. https://doi.org/10.1016/j.neuroscience.2007.09.023.

Wolf, Y., et al. (2018). Microglial MHC class II is dispensable for experimental autoimmune encephalomyelitis and cuprizone-induced demyelination. *European Journal of Immunology, 48*(8), 1308–1318. https://doi.org/10.1002/eji.201847540.

Wu, Y., et al. (2021). Microglial lysosome dysfunction contributes to white matter pathology and TDP-43 proteinopathy in GRN-associated FTD. *Cell Reports, 36*(8), 109581. https://doi.org/10.1016/j.celrep.2021.109581.

Xu, H., et al. (2024). The choroid plexus synergizes with immune cells during neuroinflammation. *Cell, 187*(18), 4946–4963. https://doi.org/10.1016/j.cell.2024.07.002.

Ye, P., et al. (2002). Myelination is altered in insulin-like growth factor-I null mutant mice. *The Journal of Neuroscience: The Official Journal of the Society for Neuroscience, 22*(14), 6041–6051. https://doi.org/10.1523/JNEUROSCI.22-14-06041.2002.

Yin, S., et al. (2024). TREM2 signaling in Parkinson's disease: Regulation of microglial function and α-synuclein pathology. *International Immunopharmacology, 143*, 113446. https://doi.org/10.1016/j.intimp.2024.113446.

Yona, S., et al. (2013). Fate mapping reveals origins and dynamics of monocytes and tissue macrophages under homeostasis. *Immunity, 38*(1), 79–91. https://doi.org/10.1016/j.immuni.2012.12.001.

Yuan, P., et al. (2016). TREM2 haplodeficiency in mice and humans impairs the microglia barrier function leading to decreased amyloid compaction and severe axonal dystrophy. *Neuron, 90*(4), 724–739. https://doi.org/10.1016/j.neuron.2016.05.003.

Zenker, D., et al. (2003). Human blood-derived macrophages enhance barrier function of cultured primary bovine and human brain capillary endothelial cells. *The Journal of Physiology, 551*(3), 1023–1032. https://doi.org/10.1113/jphysiol.2003.045880.

Zhang, J., et al. (2020). Neurotoxic microglia promote TDP-43 proteinopathy in progranulin deficiency. *Nature, 588*(7838), 459–465. https://doi.org/10.1038/s41586-020-2709-7.

Zhang, W., et al. (2007). Microglial PHOX and Mac-1 are essential to the enhanced dopaminergic neurodegeneration elicited by A30P and A53T mutant alpha-synuclein. *Glia, 55*(11), 1178–1188. https://doi.org/10.1002/glia.20532.

Zhu, J., et al. (2024). Temporal trends in the prevalence of Parkinson's disease from 1980 to 2023: A systematic review and meta-analysis. *The Lancet Healthy Longevity, 5*(7), e464–e479. https://doi.org/10.1016/S2666-7568(24)00094-1.

Zrzavy, T., et al. (2017). Loss of "homeostatic" microglia and patterns of their activation in active multiple sclerosis. *Brain: A Journal of Neurology, 140*(7), 1900–1913. https://doi.org/10.1093/brain/awx113.

CHAPTER THREE

Chemokine receptor CX3CR1 modulates microglial activity through Tau and amyloid-β interactions in Alzheimer's disease

Vaishnavi Ananathanarayana[a,1], Riddhi Upadhyay[b,1], Gouri H. Illanad[c,1], Deena Krishnan[d,1], Neha P. Bochageri[e,1], Murugan Sevanan[b], Zabin Bagewadi[c], R. Sivasamy[d], and Subashchandrabose Chinnathambi[a,*]

[a]Department of Neurochemistry, National Institute of Mental Health and Neuro Sciences Hospital (NIMHANS), Institute of National Importance, Bangalore, Karnataka, India
[b]Division of Biotechnology, Karunya Institute of Technology and Sciences (Deemed to be University), Coimbatore, Tamil Nadu, India
[c]Department of Biotechnology, KLE Technological University, Vidyanagar, Hubballi, Karnataka, India
[d]Department of Human Genetics and Molecular Biology, Bharathiar University, Coimbatore, Tamil Nadu, India
[e]School of Chemical Engineering, The University of Adelaide, Adelaide, South Australia, Australia
*Corresponding author: e-mail address: subashneuro@nimhans.ac.in

Contents

[1] These authors are equally contributed.

Advances in Immunology, Volume 171
ISSN 0065-2776, https://doi.org/10.1016/bs.ai.2025.11.002

Abstract

Alzheimer's disease is one of the most prevalent forms of dementia characterized by neurocognitive decline. Key proteins involved in the progression of disease is amyloid-β and Tau. Abnormal accumulation of amyloid-β senile plaques and Tau neurofibrillary tangles are characteristic features of AD which drives synaptic dysfunction and leads to cognitive decline. Recent studies emphasizes the importance of G-protein coupled receptors in regulating microglial cells and has diverse functions in modulating AD, particularly in the clearance of these pathological proteins. Among these GPCRs, the chemokine receptor CX3CR1 has a critical role at the intersection of pathological proteins and microglial signalling. CX3CR1 receptor mediated signalling influences interaction between microglia and neuron mediating microglial uptake and processing of Aβ and Tau. Aging is also one of the risk factors of AD which alters CX3CR1 signalling, thereby exacerbating disease progression. This review highlights the multifaceted role of CX3CR1 in Tau and Aβ pathology and outlines its signalling mechanisms. Importantly, this review emphasizes the therapeutic potential of targeting the CX3CL1-CX3CR1 axis and involved in protein clearance and reduces neuroinflammation preserving synaptic function, offering a promising way to prevent AD.

Abbreviations

AD	Alzheimer's Disease.
PD	Parkinson's Disease.
HD	Huntington's Disease.
ALS	Amyotrophic Lateral Sclerosis.
sALS	Sporadic Amyotrophic Lateral Sclerosis.
CX3CL1	Chemokine (C-X3-C motif) ligand 1/Fractalkine.
CX3CR1	Chemokine (C-X3-C motif) receptor 1.
MAPT	Microtubule-Associated Protein Tau.
α-Syn	Alpha-Synuclein.
mHTT	Mutant Huntingtin.
APP	Amyloid Precursor Protein.
Aβ	Amyloid-beta.
oAβ	Oligomeric Amyloid-beta.
NFTs	Neurofibrillary Tangles.
pTau	Phosphorylated Tau.
IL-1	Interleukin 1.
IL-1R1	Interleukin 1 Receptor Type 1.
IL-6	Interleukin 6.
IL-1β	Interleukin-1 beta.
IL-1α	Interleukin-1 alpha.
TNF	Tumor Necrosis Factor.
TGF-β	Transforming Growth Factor-beta.
DAM	Disease-Associated Microglia.
MHC	Major Histocompatibility Complex.
LPS	Lipopolysaccharide.
MPTP	1-Methyl-4-phenyl-1,2,3,6-tetrahydropyridine.
RA.40	R1.40 Alzheimer's Mouse Model.

PS19	P301S Tauopathy Mouse Model.
SVZ	Subventricular Zone.
HH	High-Altitude Hypoxia.
MAPK	Mitogen-Activated Protein Kinase.
MIP-1α	Macrophage Inflammatory Protein 1 alpha.
MSR1	Macrophage Scavenger Receptor 1.
NF-κB	Nuclear Factor kappa-light-chain-enhancer of activated B cells.
TLR4	Toll-Like Receptor 4.
TNF-α	Tumor Necrosis Factor alpha.
GSK-3β	Glycogen Synthase Kinase-3 beta.
CDK5	Cyclin-Dependent Kinase 5.

1. Introduction

Dementia is one major clinical condition characterized by persistent neurocognitive impairments, affecting around 50 million people worldwide (Livingston et al., 2020). But this estimation is projected to increase to 150 million by 2050, according to the dementia prevention, intervention, and care: 2020 report of the Lancet Commission (Livingston et al., 2020). Mainly due to the risk of global growing population and disease progression. Major dementia syndromes include Alzheimer's disease (AD), Lewy body dementia, Frontotemporal lobar degeneration and Vascular dementia these are primarily categorized as neurodegenerative dementias (Karantzoulis & Galvin, 2011). In younger adult's, Traumatic brain injury and brain tumours can also lead to dementia (Gale et al., 2018). AD is most widespread form of dementia, mainly governed by two key proteins amyloid beta which aggregates to form senile plaques, and Tau, which undergoes hyperphosphorylation and forms paired helical filaments PHFs and neurofibrillary tangles NFTs (Chinnathambi, Velmurugan, & Chandrashekar, 2024c; Creekmore et al., 2024; Dugger & Dickson, 2017; Sonawane & Chinnathambi, 2018). Over several years, thorough research has led to development of methods for early diagnosis using serum, cerebrospinal fluid and developing biomarkers for neuroimaging and clinical analysis. However, further advancements in accurate and timely diagnosis are essential (Pressman, 2025). Similarly, it's essential to develop biological therapeutic interventions required to treat and prevent the disease. Current treatments largely focus on management of symptoms, but the pressing need is to combine therapeutic strategies and exploration of novel cellular mechanisms, and to target the removal of amyloid plaques and the clearance of pathogenic extracellularly accumulated Tau (Pressman, 2025; Chinnathambi et al., 2024c; Musi et al., 2018). This marks the emergence of a new frontier for research – G-protein coupled receptors (GPCRs), are important class of cell surface receptors and are easy targets for the available drugs (Ananthanarayana et al., 2025; Chinnathambi, Velmurugan, Ananthanaraya, et al., 2025). They are mainly present on many different brain cell types such as neurons, astrocytes and microglia. In brain they regulate multiple functions such as neurotransmission, neuromodulation, neuroinflammation and maintain cellular homeostasis (Desale et al., 2021; Jong et al., 2018; Myeku et al., 2020; Sando & Südhof, 2021; Sushma & Mondal, 2019; Thathiah & De Strooper, 2011). Understanding their role in neurodegeneration and involvement in AD would open up new avenues for therapeutic developments.

1.1 GPCRs in AD

GPCRs play a vital role in regulating different cellular pathways, which mainly governs neuronal communication, synaptic plasticity, inflammation and cell survival (Huang et al., 2017; Ma et al., 2024; Thathiah & De Strooper, 2011). GPCRs interacts with multiple ligands and activates downstream signalling cascades, which in turn orchestrates intracellular signalling in AD. Prostaglandin E receptor 2 subtype EP2 (PTGER2) and orphan GPCR-GPR3 both influence γ-secretase activity, which activates the production of Aβ. These receptors bind to APP and internalize through βarr2, which promotes the production of Aβ by APP cleavage (Nelson & Sheng, 2013) as shown in Fig. 1. As a molecular pattern or damage sensor, GPR17 plays a role in both neurotoxicity and neuroinflammation. Cognitive abnormalities caused by Aβ1–42 were reversed and β-secretase 1 (BACE1) activity was decreased when cangrelor bound to GPR17. By lowering oxidative stress, neuroinflammation, and synaptic dysfunction, these effects are mediated through the Nrf2/HO-1 and NF-κB signaling pathways (Jin et al., 2021). In the presence of Aβ42, the melatonin receptor triggers the ERK pathway. Aβ40 causes an increase in the expression of serotonin receptors. In the presence of Aβ, metabolotropic glutamate receptor expression rises and inhibits the muscarinic receptor. Through the GABA receptor, Tau and Aβ modify synaptic inhibition and potentiation. Tau is internalized and interacts with the chemokine CX3CR1 receptor (Chidambaram & Chinnathambi, 2020; Chidambaram et al., 2020, 2022; Chinnathambi & Chidambaram, 2024). The purinergic P2Y12 receptor gets activated by Tau monomers, oligomers, and aggregates, which results

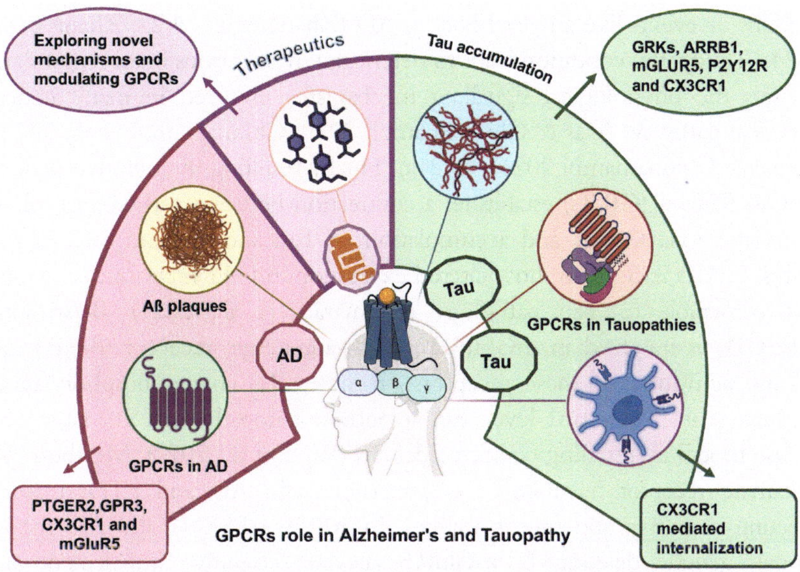

Fig. 1 GPCRs role in Alzheimer's disease and Tauopathy. This figure illustrates the role of GPCRs in Alzheimer's disease and Tauopathy. Key proteins involved in AD are Aβ and Tau proteins, the progression of disease is characterized by accumulation of these key proteins. Several GPCRs, such as PTGER2, GPR3, CX3CR1 and mGLUR5 contribute to these processes and they have diverse role in Aβ pathology. GPCRs like GRKs, ARRB1, mGLUR5, P2Y12R and CX3CR1 are involved in phosphorylation process and they are also involved in Tau internalization process particularly mediated by CX3CR1. Exploring novel GPCR pathways by targeting these receptors may offer therapeutic opportunities to reduce accumulation of pathological Tau.

in Tau internalization through the development of migratory structures (Chidambaram & Chinnathambi, 2020; Chidambaram et al., 2020, 2022; Chidambaram, Desale, Qureshi, et al., 2024a; Chidambaram, Desale, Suri, et al., 2024b; Chinnathambi & Chidambaram, 2024).

1.2 GPCRs in Tauopathy

Tauopathies cover a range of Tau associated pathological conditions, mainly due to the abnormal accumulation of Tau protein in the brain, particularly in neuron and extracellular space (Gorantla et al., 2020; Desale & Chinnathambi, 2021c; Chinnathambi et al., 2024b; Chinnathambi et al., 2025). There are more than 26 different types of Tauopathies, classified as primary and secondary tauopathies. In primary Tauopathies Tau is the central player while, in secondary Tauopathies pathology of Tau is in response to other secondary proteins or events like amyloid beta in AD (Zhang et al., 2022; Zhang et al., 2024). Tauopathy condition leads to deterioration of various brain regions and disrupts the physiological signalling mechanisms involved in many neurochemical pathways (Das & Chinnathambi, 2019; Chinnathambi et al., 2024a; Desale & Chinnathambi 2021b, 2021a). Finally resulting in cognitive deficits. GPCR Kinases (GRKs) establishes a connection between pathological phosphorylation via kinases and accumulation of Tau and amyloid beta in AD brains. GRKs 2, 5 and 6 show altered expression in CA1 hippocampal region and vulnerable to Tau pathology (Guimarães et al., 2021). β-Arrestin1 (ARRB1) is involved in mGLuR2 and β_2-adrenergic receptor (β_2AR) signalling, activation of these receptors promotes Tau hyperphosphorylation. Reduction in β-Arrestin1 levels can ameliorate tauopathy in PS19 tauopathy mouse model by rescuing cognitive deficits (Woo et al., 2022). Metabotropic glutamate receptor 5 mGluR5 is associated with AD and FTD, majorly affecting cognitive and motor abilities. In APPswe/PSEN1DE9 AD mouse model, genetic deletion of mGluR5 alleviate cognitive impairment and amyloid beta production. Antagonist 3-[(2-methyl-1,3-thiazol-4-yl)ethynyl]-pyridine (MTEP) and allosteric modulator 2 chloro-4-((2,5-dimethyl-1-(4-(trifluoromethoxy)phenyl) 1H-imidazol-4-yl)ethynyl) pyridine (CTEP) improve cognition in AD (Huang et al., 2017). In postsynaptic Tau pathology mGluR5 are associated, hippocampal mGluR5 availability is reduced in early stages of AD, thereby negatively correlating with Tau deposition (Wang et al., 2025). GPCRs also a play a dual role in disease progression, their central to Tau phosphorylation via GSK-3ß, CDK-5 and ERK signalling as well as GPCRs like CX3CR1 and P2Y12R are involved in Tau internalization process in microglial cells (Ananthanarayana et al., 2025; Chidambaram & Chinnathambi, 2024; Chidambaram et al., 2020; Chidambaram et al., 2024a, 2024b). CaS – calcium sensing receptors in astrocytes influence Tau propagation via exosomes (Chidambaram & Chinnathambi, 2020; Chidambaram et al., 2020, 2022; Chidambaram, Desale, Qureshi, et al., 2024a; Chidambaram, Desale, Suri, et al., 2024b; Chinnathambi & Chidambaram, 2024). As previously discussed, there are numerous GPCRs, glimpse of their role in Tauopathy and AD has been briefed. Among them, Class A Gi-coupled GPCR chemokine receptor stands out, particularly, during neuroinflammation or neurodegeneration, chemokines which are a subset of cytokines are produced and binds to receptor CX3CR1, potentially mediates Tau clearance. The role of CX3CR1 receptor in the area of neurodegeneration and AD is still not clear, remains to be understood. In this review, we aim to comprehensively explore the role of CX3CR1 in the context of aging and its interaction with amyloid beta and Tau. We will discuss the role of CX3CR1 and microglial activation and their interactions. Which also includes evaluating current evidences linking this receptor to Tau species clearance. Finally, we would highlight the therapeutic potential of targeting CX3CR1 in AD, with a focus on its capacity to modulate neuroinflammation and promote neuroprotection via microglial CX3CR1 mediated Tau clearance.

2. Chemokine CX3CR1 receptor and aging

The irretrievable biological process with progressive deterioration of functional capabilities in living organisms is aging, including genomic instability (DNA damage), telomere shortening, epigenetic alterations, and loss of proteostasis (Hou et al., 2019). This leads to cellular dysfunction and increased inflammation, contributing to age-related and neurodegenerative disease (ND) (Zhao et al., 2024). NDs like Alzheimer's (AD), Huntington's (HD), and Parkinson's (PD) are embodied by gradual neuronal degeneration and their functions in the central nervous system (CNS) as depicted in Fig. 2 (Muddapu et al., 2020). Central regulators of this pathology, often exacerbating neuronal damage, are the brain's resident immune cell, microglia. They maintain homeostasis through neuronal-microglial cross-talk, but their dysregulation usually drives neuroinflammation (Gao et al., 2023; Das & Chinnathambi, 2019). A crucial modulator of neuronal microglial communication is the Fractalkine (FKN, CX3CL1)/CX3C chemokine receptor 1 (CX3CR1) signaling axis, under both physiological and pathological condition (Chidambaram et al., 2020). In PD, the gradual deterioration of dopaminergic neurons and accumulation of α -Synuclein (α-Syn) protein aggregate, the CX3CR1 role demonstrate context-dependent effects. For instance, in toxin-induced (MPTP), α-Syn Over-expression, LPS–induced, or age-related models. CX3CR1 deficiency in MPTP model exacerbates the neuroinflammation (Cardona et al., 2006), and administration of CX3CL1 acts as neuroprotective by controlling macrophage polarization (Morganti et al., 2012). In contrast, CX3CR1 deficiency reduces microglial phagocytic activity and inflammatory markers but does not exacerbate α-syn–induced dopaminergic neuron loss (Thome et al., 2015). However, CX3CR1 deficiency worsens α-syn A53T-induced neurodegeneration by promoting a pro-inflammatory microglial phenotype suggesting the conflicting results (Castro-Sánchez et al., 2018). A study using Huntington mouse models demonstrated that mHTT impairs actin

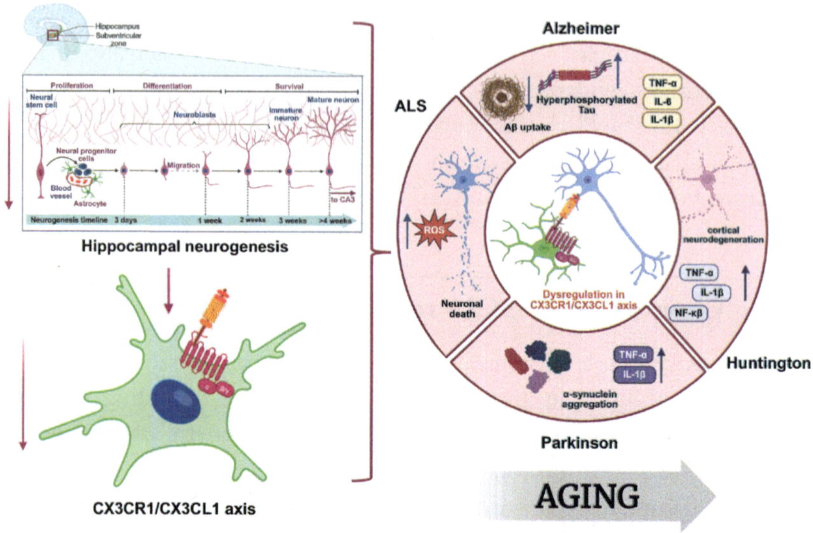

Fig. 2 Chemokine receptor CX3CR1 and aging in neurodegenerative disorders. During normal aging, reduced hippocampus neurogenesis diminishes activation of the CX3CR1/CX3CL1 axis, impairing the microglial activation and pro-inflammatory cytokines secretion, thus contributing to neurodegenerative diseases. In Alzheimer's disease, the chemokine, having a dual role, exacerbates pathology through hyperphosphorylation of the Tau protein while also offering a protective role by reducing the Aβ uptake. Huntington's and ALS progression involve chemokine-derived cortical and neuronal death, respectively. In Parkinson's, the α-synuclein aggregation exacerbates the disease, concurrently upregulating the secretion of pro-inflammatory cytokines.

remodeling, which precedes neuroinflammation and possibly drives chronic inflammation (Kwan et al., 2012). In ALS, particularly in sporadic form, genetic variations like the V249I polymorphism in CX3CR1 impair receptor function and weaken CX3CL1 binding, intensifying microglial-mediated inflammation. Unlike familial ALS, which is driven by inherited mutations, these results underscore CX3CR1's substantial influence on sALS progression and its broader implications for neurodegeneration (Lopez-Lopez et al., 2014). Aging's impact on microglial function further highlights the CX3CL1/CX3CR1 axis's significance. During normal aging, CX3CR1/FKN signaling declines, which is essential for maintaining adult hippocampal neurogenesis, resulting in increased microglial activation, elevated IL-1β, and reduced neurogenesis (Ananthanarayana et al., 2025). Age-related disruption of the signaling contributes to both normal cognitive aging and NDs (Bachstetter et al., 2011). Recent study in middle-aged mice CX3CR1 expression is upregulated, acting as a compensatory mechanism to reduce pro-inflammatory cytokines like IL-1α and IL-1β. Contrastingly, with advanced age, microglial exhibit CX3CR1 downregulation leading to sustained inflammatory response (Liu et al., 2025). Aging primarily impacts the microglial phenotype and homeostasis by downregulating immune-related genes (MHC Class II genes) and, interestingly, upregulating Adora1 and TNF, implying a premature aging transcriptome signature. Adding further complexity, environmental factors such as high-altitude hypoxia (HH) can exacerbate microglial aging-like changes. A study by Wang et al., demonstrated that HH induces M1-type microglial activation, synaptic loss, and memory impairment through CX3CL1/CX3CR1 signaling. These effects are closely related to aging, as both HH and aging share features such as microglial activation, elevated IL-1β, synaptic loss, and impaired neurogenesis (Wang et al., 2023). A recent study by Gyoneva and researchers, examined the effects of CX3CR1 deletion in mice on microglial gene expression, which accelerated the molecular aging in mice to mimic an aged phenotype. The mice exhibited reduced ramification and haploinsufficiency was evident, highlighting the CX3CR1's importance in maintain youthful microglial homeostasis (Gyoneva et al., 2019).

One of the well-known NDs is Alzheimer's disease (AD), which is marked by the build-up of amyloid-beta peptides (Aβ), and neurofibrillary tangles (NFTs) (Zhang et al., 2021). CX3CR1 acts as both a detrimental and a protective factor, depending on the disease stage, and the balance between Tau protein and amyloid-β. A striking feature of CX3CR1's role in AD is its differential impact on the two main pathological hallmarks: amyloid-β and Tau neurofibrillary tangles. CX3CR1 deficiency in APPPS1 and RA.40 Alzheimer's mouse models result in gene dose-dependent decrease in brain amyloid-β detection. This effect is attributed to enhanced microglial phagocytosis targeting amyloid-β, consequently reducing overall amyloid burden which underscores CX3CR1 modulatory influence on amyloid-β pathology (Lee et al., 2010). Although CX3CR1 deficiency clears amyloid-β, paradoxically, it worsens tau pathology. In APP/PS-1 mouse models, CX3CR1 gene ablation is associated with elevated cytokine levels and a substantial increase in tau pathology, culminating in compromised behavioral performance (Hickman et al., 2019). A recent study in 5xFAD Alzheimer's disease mice, CX3CR1 deficiency results in impaired microglial phagocytosis, escalating levels of pTau and oAβ. This induces inflammatory 'degenerative' microglia, intensifying neurodegeneration, synaptic loss, and cognitive impairments. Such effects underscore the indispensable, intricate, and stage-dependent role of CX3CR1 in modulating region-specific microglial responses and proteinopathy within Alzheimer's pathology (Puntambekar et al., 2022).

Further adding nuance, region-specific and age-related differences in microglial phenotypes also affect CX3CR1 function. One of the unique types of microglial exists in subventricular zone (SVZ) acquire a neuroprotective, DAM-like phenotype, characterized by CX3CR1 downregulation. Intriguingly, CX3CR1 haploinsufficiency specifically enhances neurogenesis in the aged SVZ, not in young mice, revealing region- and age-dependent effects. This suggests DAM-like SVZ microglia aid neurogenesis by clearing aggregates (Fritze et al., 2024). Exploring beyond CX3CR1 ablation, Overexpression of CX3CL1 in the PS19 tauopathy mouse model decreased neuronal loss and improved cognitive function by enhancing neurogenesis through the TGF-β2–3/Smad2 pathway without altering tau pathology (Fan et al., 2020).

3. Chemokine CX3CR1 receptor and amyloid beta interaction

3.1 Chemokine receptor CX3CR1 in Amyloid beta structure, function and signaling pathways

Amyloid Beta has been identified as one of the major contributors to the progression of various neurodegenerative disorders. Alzheimer's disease is one among them (Gupta et al., 2016). In AD patients, brain exhibits extensive extracellular buildup of Amyloid beta peptides, these misfold to form complex structures such as fibrils, oligomers and aggregates resulting in neurotoxicity, impairment of brain function and memory loss (Stefani, 2012) (Desale et al., 2021; Gorantla et al., 2021). Aβ plaques are identified to exert neurotoxic effect in the Alzheimer' brain with its oligomeric forms recognized to have more synaptotoxicity (Walsh et al., 2002). Amyloid fibrils stimulate increased expression of CX3CR1 in microglia (Wu et al., 2013). The CX3CR1-CX3CL1 axis acts as checkpoints and inhibits hyperneuroinflamatory actions of microglial cells in healthy brain to prevent the release of toxic chemicals as shown in Fig. 3 (Zhang et al., 2018). Different mice models used to study the role of CX3CR1 G protein receptor in Aβ clearance have produced varied results showing both positives and negatives. In normal physiological conditions amyloid precursor protein is been cleaved by α- and γ-secretases to form

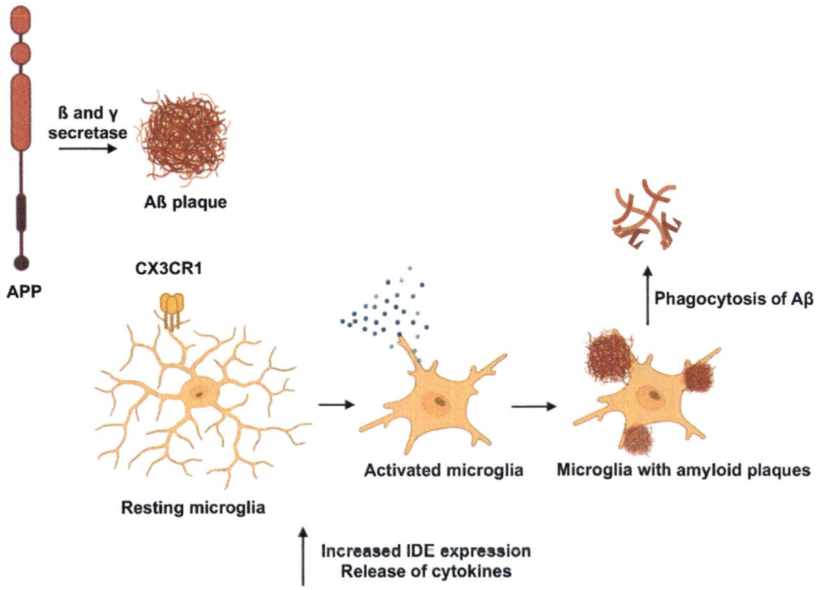

Fig. 3 Chemokine CX3CR1 receptor and Amyloid beta interaction. This scheme illustrates the process of amyloid precursor protein (APP) cleavage and Aβ plaque interaction with chemokine receptor. APP undergoes cleavage by two enzymes β and γ secretase respectively to form Aβ peptides that aggregate into plaques. following this interaction of CX3CR1 and Aβ plaques leads to increased CX3CR1 expression and subsequent microglial activation in response to Aβ. Activated microglia has a potential to increase insulin degrading enzyme (IDE) expression and releases cyto kines and chemokines, which promote the phagocytosis and directly involved in clearance of Aβ plaques. This process is critical in modulating amyloid plaque accumulation and neuroinflammation in the brain.

soluble APP. However, in AD, reduced α-secretase activity shifts processing to β- and γ-secretases activity forming insoluble Aβ (Thathiah & De Strooper, 2011). Microglial production of proteins interacting with the Aβ fibrils reduce with age leading to reduced phagocytosis. Partial deficiency of CX3CR1 in PS1-APP-CX3CR1+/- mice models have been proved to boost the expression of Aβ degrading enzyme such as IDE-Insulysin (Hickman et al., 2019). In APPPS1 mice lacking membrane-bound CX3CL1 signaling, researchers observed significantly increased activation of the p38 MAPK signaling pathway compared to APPPS1 control mice (Lee et al., 2014). This heightened activation was mainly found within microglial cells. The p38 MAPK pathway is associated with cellular stress responses, inflammation, and cytokine production (Qi et al., 2024). Its increased activity suggests that the absence of CX3CL1 signaling leads to elevated microglial reactivity and inflammatory responses. This may exacerbate neuroinflammatory processes in Alzheimer's disease, highlighting the role of CX3CL1-CX3CR1 interactions in regulating microglial behavior and maintaining neuroimmune balance (Lee et al., 2014). However, one study claims that the absence of CX3CR1 causes microglia to lose their ability to breakdown fibrillary Aβ due to interrupted cross talk signaling with receptors such as TREM2, toll like receptors and RAGE (Salminen et al., 2009).

3.2 Chemokine receptor CX3CR1 in Amyloid beta disease and clinical perspective

Eliminating CX3CR1 has been shown to impair microglial capacity to breakdown Aβ plaques, resulting in the accumulation of harmful Aβ species. It also contributes to abnormal inflammatory responses, oxidative stress and reduced TGFβ signaling causing a neurotoxic effect resulting in disease progression (Puntambekar et al., 2022). However, another study suggests CX3CR1 deficiency to have neither harmful nor protective effects on synaptic function or neuronal health in CRND8/CX3CR1-/- mice model (Liu et al., 2010). Release of various cytokines by microglial cells is observed in response to the IFNγ, IL1-β and LPS stimulation, which play a major in cell signaling, and immune response. This is predominantly influenced by CX3CR1 (Abud et al., 2017). CX3CR1 plays a crucial role in Aβ pathology in Alzheimers. Few studies reveal that the partial or complete knockout of CX3CR1 in diseased mouse model elevated the phagocytic activity of microglial cells around the Aβ plaques and Aβ fibrillary and oligomeric forms. (Dworzak et al., 2015; Hickman et al., 2019). Alternatively, studies on complete deletion of CX3CR1 have suggested to impede the microglial capacity to engulf and degrade the Aβ plaques (Puntambekar et al., 2022). In contrast, a study on 5xTg mouse model proved CX3CR1 deficiency to have no significant effect on the phagocytic function of microglia (Fuhrmann et al., 2010). CX3CR1 thus exhibits dual effects, making it a potential target for AD.

4. Chemokine CX3CR1 receptor and Tau protein interaction

Tau is an axonal microtubule-associated protein, which stabilizes microtubules and its integrity essential for axonal support (Barbier et al., 2019).

Tau enables dynamic interaction with microtubules under physiological conditions as they exist in unstructured state. Abnormal post-translational modification such as hyperphosphorylation, acetylation, ubiquitination and other PTMs leads to misfolding of Tau, finally forming NFTs in Tauopathies (Di Lorenzo, 2024). The chemokine receptor CX3CR1, a G protein-coupled receptor, with its ligand CX3CL1 in the CNS is a critical mediator influencing synaptic plasticity, activation states, and neuronal survival (Camacho-Hernández & Peña-Ortega, 2023). Recent findings reveals that external Tau, released from stressed or dying neurons, directly binds to CX3CR1 displacing CX3CL1, promoting its internalization, activation of p38 MAPK pathway which results in increased IL-6, IL-1β, TNF-α, and MIP-1α, microglial migration and proliferation in AD (Chidambaram et al., 2020). This interaction further

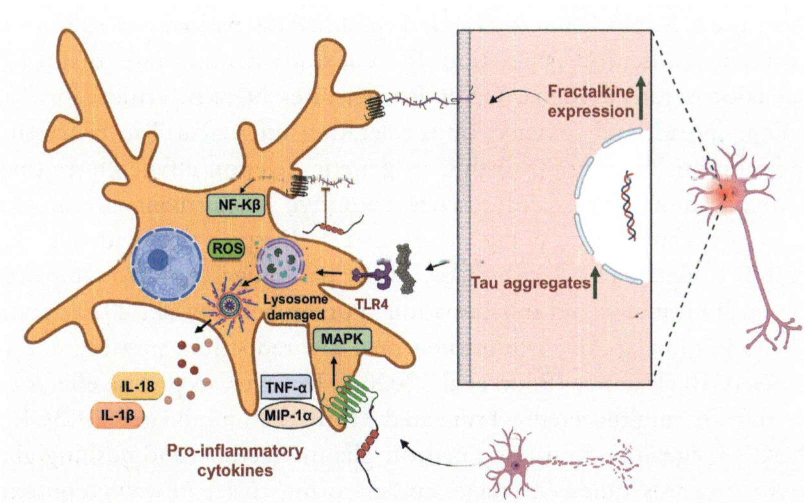

Fig. 4 Chemokine receptor CX3CR1 and Tau interaction. Tau becomes phosphorylated and forms aggregates due to aging, and oxidative stress. These toxic aggregates are internalised by microglia via TLR4, triggering NF-κB. This primes the NLRP3 inflammasome by upregulating NLRP3, pro-IL-1β, and pro-IL-18. Subsequent lysosomal rupture and ROS act as activation signals, leading to caspase-1 activation, cytokine release, and sustained neuroinflammation. When released from stressed or dying neurons, external Tau directly engages microglial CX3CR1, displacing CX3CL1 and inducing receptor internalization. This interaction instigates the activation of the p38 MAPK signaling pathway, culminating in augmented secretion of IL-6, IL-1β, TNF-α, and MIP-1α, alongside increased microglial migration and proliferation in Alzheimer's disease.

necessitates study of its downstream pathways activated by Tau-receptor engagement as shown in Fig. 4. A recent study indicates that membrane-anchored CX3CL1 loss augments microglial p38 MAPK signaling, promoting Aβ phagocytosis via MSR1, while concurrently augmenting neuronal MAPT phosphorylation, which is mediated by IL-1 and IL-6 (Lee et al., 2014). According to study by (Bhaskar et al., 2010), CX3CR1 deficiency enhances microglia-derived IL-1 signaling, activating neuronal p38 MAPK, which drives Tau (MAPT) hyperphosphorylation and aggregation. The inhibition of this effect by blocking IL-1R1 or TLR4 establishes key microglia–neuron inflammatory cascade as a central pathway in Tau-mediated neurodegeneration. A similar study by (Maphis et al., 2015) demonstrates that CX3CR1 deficiency in microglia unleashes Tau pathology, elevating IL-1 and p38 MAPK activation, and promoting Tau hyperphosphorylation and propagation. Kineret's resumption of IL-1R1 signaling reduces Tau phosphorylation, establishing the CX3CR1–microglia–IL-1–p38 MAPK pathway as a driver of Tau-mediated neurodegeneration. Recent study demonstrates that Tau's interaction with microglial CX3CR1 activates NF-κB, critical for Tau seeding, spread, and toxicity, by accelerating microglial Tau processing and secretion. In addition to this, its genetic deletion efficiently restores microglial homeostasis and rescues cognitive impairments in murine models of Tauopathy (Wang et al., 2022). Despite the evidence that CX3CR1 deficiency exacerbates Tau pathology due to impaired microglial clearance and inflammation (Puntambekar et al., 2022), some AD models (3xTg-AD) exhibit neuronal loss reduction, possibly due to increased Aβ clearance (Poon et al., 2020). However, its precise effects on tau remain multifaceted. Truncated Tau can modulate CX3CL1-CX3CR1 signaling, impacting neuron-glia interactions and pushing glial activity towards quiescent stage, underscoring this pathway's context-dependent and dynamic influence on neurodegeneration (Petra, 2024). CX3CR1 presents a promising, but complex, clinical target for tauopathies. Although there are no direct clinical interventions targeting the CX3CR1–Tau axis to date, its critical function in modulating microglial activation and neuroinflammation establishes its potential as both a diagnostic biomarker and a pharmacological target. Modulation of this pathway holds the potential to mitigate tau-induced neurotoxicity and decelerate disease progression. However, its dual protective/pathological roles demand careful timing and strategy in future research.

5. Chemokine receptor CX3CR1 activates Tau in microglia

Chemokine receptor CX3CR1 is a microglia-specific receptor in the brain and is a key regulator of neuron-microglia interactions. Fractalkine or CX3CL1 is mostly produced by neurons and is membrane-bound and soluble (Pawelec et al., 2020). Microglial homeostasis is supported by the CX3CL1-CX3CR1 signalling axis under normal physiological conditions, and the axis induces an anti-inflammatory phenotype (Szukiewicz, 2024). The interaction guarantees that microglia effectively carry out their surveillance, debris clearance, and neuroprotective functions without causing the detrimental inflammatory reactions (Gao et al., 2023). In neurodegenerative diseases like AD, the impairment of such a signalling by deletion or dysfunction of CX3CR1 changes microglial behaviour towards a reactive and pro-inflammatory state. Such a phenotype change has great implications for Tau pathology in AD (Miao et al., 2023). Microglia are important in internalizing extracellular Tau that is released by damaged neurons. Although this clearance process is neuroprotective in the early stages, its prolonged stimulation because of the loss of CX3CR1 results in a loss of microglial functionality, which causes ineffective phagocytosis and improper Tau degradation (Miao et al., 2023; Perea et al., 2020). As a result, Tau accumulates in the extracellular space, which can be taken up by adjacent neurons and so facilitate its spread across brain areas (Sonawane & Chinnathambi, 2018). CX3CR1-deficient microglia could also release internalized Tau as vesicular proteins, including exosomes, to transmit it in a prion-like manner to the adjacent cells, enhancing the frequency of Tau aggregate propagation (Chen & Yu, 2023; Perea et al., 2020).

The disappearance of CX3CR1 also causes the development of a pro-inflammatory microenvironment by increasing the expression of cytokines like IL-1β, TNF-α, and IL-6. These cytokines have been reported to stimulate various kinases that phosphorylate Tau, which include glycogen synthase kinase-3β, cyclin-dependent kinase-5, and p38 mitogen-activated protein kinase. All these kinases cause hyperphosphorylation of Tau, which leads to the development of neurofibrillary tangles, which is one of the pathological characteristics of AD (Chidambaram et al., 2020; Rawat et al., 2022; Desale & Chinnathambi, 2021). This cascade has experimental evidence, and Bhaskar et al. (2010) found that Tau transgenic mice deficient in CX3CR1 had more Tau phosphorylation, raised IL-1β 182 levels, and severe neuronal loss. On the same note, demonstrated that the lack of

CX3CR1 in microglia in Tauopathy models led to increased neurotoxicity and cognitive deficits to support the neuroprotective nature of the CX3CL1-CX3CR1 axis Castro-Sánchez et al. (2019). The same findings have been confirmed in vitro, whereby exposure of neurons to IL-1β increased Tau phosphorylation, further highlighting the direct connection between cytokines released by microglia and Tau pathology (Gao et al., 2023). Therefore, these indicate that the CX3CR1 malfunctioning participates in neuroinflammation, Tau hyperphosphorylation, inefficient clearance, and prion-like spreading of Tau aggregates (Laurent et al., 2018). CX3CL1-CX3CR1 axis is therefore a key regulatory switch point to the

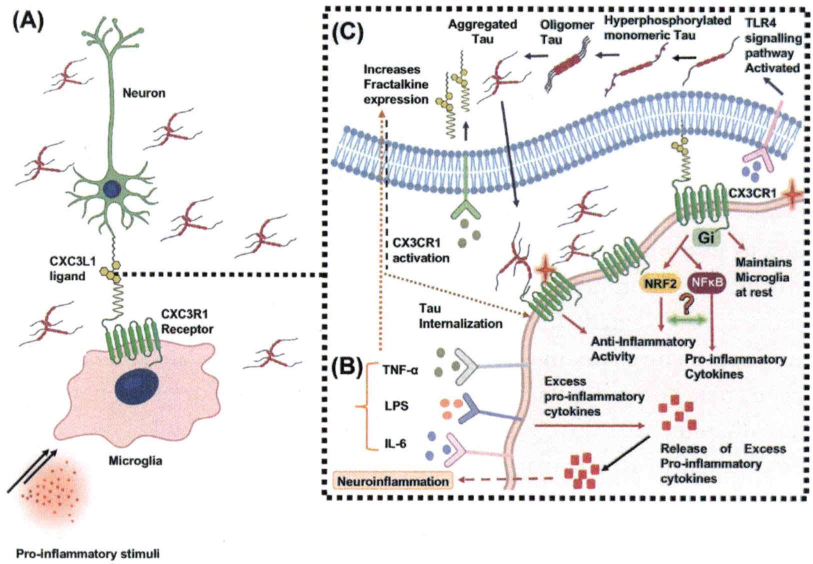

Fig. 5 Chemokine receptor CX3CR1-Tau interaction and its regulatory role in microglial activity in Alzheimer's disease. (A) Under physiological conditions, neuronal CX3CL1 (Fractalkine) interacts with microglial CX3CR1 receptors, maintaining microglia in a resting, anti-inflammatory state. This homeostatic signaling axis suppresses microglial activation in the absence of pro-inflammatory cytokines. (B) In response to pathological stimuli (e.g., LPS, TNF-α, IL-6), there is increased expression of fractalkine and activation of CX3CR1 on microglia. (C) These stimuli promote the internalization of Tau aggregates, including hyperphosphorylated and oligomeric forms, via receptor-mediated processes. This leads to microglial activation. Activated CX3CR1 signaling influences downstream pathways, including NFκB and NRF2, modulating the balance between anti-inflammatory and pro-inflammatory cytokine release. Excessive stimulation promotes Tau internalization and subsequent microglial release of pro-inflammatory cytokines, amplifying neuroinflammation in Alzheimer's disease pathology.

microglial response to neurodegenerative cascades. The reconstitution or regulation of this signaling pathway may be a promising therapeutic approach to help curb Tau-related neurotoxicity in AD as depicted in Fig. 5 (Pawelec et al., 2020).

6. Therapeutic aspects of the chemokine CX3CR1 receptor in Alzheimer's disease

Alzheimer's disease is primarily characterized by amyloid-β (Aβ) plaques, Tau tangles and microglia-induced neuroinflammation. The neuron-microglia CX3CL1(fractalkine)-CX3CR1 axis regulates microglial activation and neuroprotective homeostasis making the chemokine CX3CR1 receptor as a promising therapeutic target. This study describes how CX3CR1 regulates both Tau pathology and Aβ clearance as well as the therapeutic implications of targeting the CX3CL1/CX3CR1 axis, shown in Fig. 6. Alzheimer's disease pathogenesis includes chronic inflammation, malfunctioning microglia and protein aggregation. Microglia express the GPCR CX3CR1 which interacts with neuronal fractalkine (CX3CL1) to regulate immunological responses. CX3CR1 is a viable target since its disrupting this axis worsens neuroinflammation and causes neuronal damage. Studies in transgenic mouse models (*APP/PS1, CRND8*) show that CX3CR1 deletion enhances Aβ clearance by increasing microglial phagocytosis (Lee et al., 2010; Lee et al., 2010). However, excessive microglial activation in complete CX3CR1 knockouts may worsen inflammation. Partial inhibition (heterozygous deletion) appears more beneficial, reducing amyloid burden while preserving immune homeostasis (Hickman et al., 2013). In CX3CR1-deficient animals, Tau pathology intended due to higher IL-1β and TNF-α levels which leads to hyperphosphorylation and neuronal death (Bhaskar et al., 2010; Maphis et al., 2015). The overexpression of soluble fractalkine mitigates Tau-induced neurotoxicity and enhances synaptic function (Nash et al., 2013).

6.1 CX3CR1 in neuroinflammation & synaptic dysfunction

Microglial quiescence is maintained by CX3CL1/CX3CR1. Cognitive impairments, synaptic pruning and increased pro-inflammatory cytokines are the results of disruption (Paolicelli et al., 2014). Through epigenetic modifications Aβ upregulates CX3CR1 and due to that it reinforces the microglial activation and also CX3CR1-silencing undoes these effects (Chen et al., 2016).

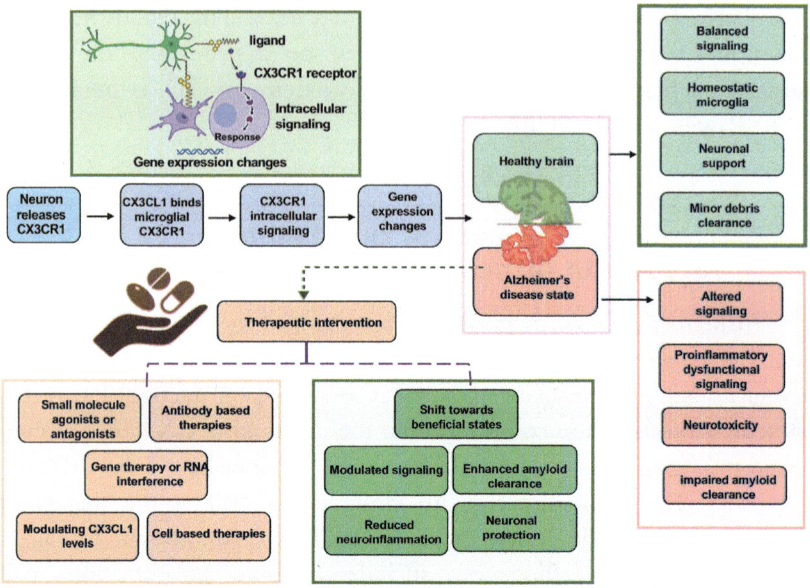

Fig. 6 Therapeutic aspects of the chemokine CX3CR1 receptor in Alzheimer's disease. This scheme outlines the interaction between receptor CX3CR1 in microglial signalling and its therapeutic potential in AD. CX3CL1, ligand is released by neurons which binds to microglial receptor CX3CR1, leading to initiation of intracellular signalling and resulting in gene expression changes. CX3CL1-CX3CR1 signalling maintains balanced microglial activity, neuronal support and enhanced clearance of minor debris. But in AD, altered signalling leads to proinflammatory signals, neurotoxicity and impaired amyloid clearance. Therapeutic interventions include small molecule agonists/antagonists, antibody-based therapies, gene therapy, RNA interference, cell-based therapies and modulating CX3CL1-CX3CR1 signalling axis. These strategies are beneficial to reduce neuroinflammation, improving amyloid and Tau clearance, neuronal protection and overall shift towards homeostatic microglial function.

6.2 Therapeutic strategies

- CX3CR1 Modulation: Partial inhibition improves Aβ clearance without exacerbating tau pathology (Fonseca et al., 2017)
- CX3CL1-Based Therapies: In tauopathy models, neuronal survival is restored by viral vector-mediated CX3CL1 expression (Rogers et al., 2011)
- CX3CR1 Antagonists: Small molecules like AZD8797 exhibit anti-inflammatory effects and warrant exploration in AD (Ridderstad et al., 2022)
- Epigenetic modulators: CX3CR1 expression is influenced by histone acetylation; addressing epigenetic enzymes may help to reestablish equilibrium (Zhou et al., 2018).

- Cell-Based Therapies: CX3CR1-transduced Tregs reduce neuroinflammation in AD models (Zhao et al., 2023).

V249I and T280M polymorphisms in CX3CR1 affects receptor function and AD susceptibility (Faure et al., 2000). Because the advantages of CX3CR1 modulation it may vary depending on the stage of the disease because of that stage-specific therapies are essential. Particularly, CX3CL1-CX3CR1 axis serves as the key regulator for microglial activation in AD. Precise tuning is necessary for therapeutic modulation to strike a balance between Aβ clearance and Tau-related neuroinflammation reduction. Its therapeutic potential could be unlocked by tailored strategies depending on the disease specificity and genetic background.

7. Conclusion

GPCRs are highly relevant class of regulators in AD, but their role in regulating and modulating disease progression are still underexplored. Among them, chemokine CX3CR1 receptor emerges as a unique receptor that bridges communication between microglia and neuron which influences Aβ, Tau protein interaction and regulates signalling pathways. Evidences suggest that CX3CR1 receptor is involved in uptake and degradation of Tau leading to attenuation of neuroinflammation. Despite this normal physiological function, due to associated risk factors like age, leads to dysfunction of CX3CR1 biology in AD. Considering the degradative capacity via CX3CR1 targeting this receptor would offer a novel therapeutic way to enhance microglia mediated Tau clearance and reduces neuroinflammation providing synaptic integrity. However, a precise mechanistic signalling mechanism and age associated roles remain essential to translate these findings into effective clinical interventions.

8. Future directions

- The precise signalling pathways downstream of CX3CR1 activation requires deeper investigation particularly, those involving PI3K/AKT, NF-kβ, mTOR and AMPK
- Impact of ageing and genetic variability of CX3CR1 on its functional outcomes in microglial cells needs to be investigated

- To develop CX3CR1 as a bridge between mechanistic and therapeutic intervention, advanced invitro models, such as iPSc-derived microglia from AD and non-AD controls would be necessary to provide valuable insights
- Future research should explore and provide the basis of combinational therapy for CX3CR1 modulation and this would give comprehensive insights to tackle AD pathology

References

Abud, E. M., Ramirez, R. N., Martinez, E. S., Healy, L. M., Nguyen, C. H. H., Newman, S. A., Yeromin, A. V., Scarfone, V. M., Marsh, S. E., Fimbres, C., Caraway, C. A., Fote, G. M., Madany, A. M., Agrawal, A.., Kayed, R., Gylys, K. H., Cahalan, M. D., Cummings, B. J., Antel, J. P., Mortazavi, A., Carson, M. J., Poon, W. W., & Blurton-Jones, M. (2017). iPSC-Derived Human Microglia-like Cells to Study Neurological Diseases. *Neuron, 94*(2), 278–293.e9. https://doi.org/10.1016/j.neuron.2017.03.042.

Ananthanarayana, V., Chidamabram, H., Periyasamy, G., Kalyan, V., & Chinnathambi, S. (2025). Mechanisms and routes of G-protein coupled receptor-mediated Tau degradation in Alzheimer's disease. *Cytokine & Growth Factor Reviews*. https://doi.org/10.1016/j.cytogfr.2025.07.003.

Bachstetter, A. D., Morganti, J. M., Jernberg, J., Schlunk, A., Mitchell, S. H., Brewster, K. W., ... Gemma, C. (2011). Fractalkine and CX3CR1 regulate hippocampal neurogenesis in adult and aged rats. *Neurobiology of Aging, 32*(11), 2030–2044. https://doi.org/10.1016/j.neurobiolaging.2009.11.022.

Barbier, P., Zejneli, O., Martinho, M., Lasorsa, A., Belle, V., Smet-Nocca, C., ... Landrieu, I. (2019). Role of Tau as a microtubule-associated protein: Structural and functional aspects. *Frontiers in Aging Neuroscience, 11*. https://doi.org/10.3389/fnagi.2019.00204.

Bhaskar, K., et al. (2010). Microglial responses to tau pathology are regulated by fractalkine signaling. *Journal of Neuroscience, 30*(50), 17015–17025. https://doi.org/10.1523/JNEUROSCI.3930-10.2010.

Bhaskar, K., Konerth, M., Kokiko-Cochran, O. N., Cardona, A., Ransohoff, R. M., & Lamb, B. T. (2010). Regulation of Tau pathology by the microglial fractalkine receptor. *Neuron, 68*(1), 19–31. https://doi.org/10.1016/j.neuron.2010.08.023.

Bhaskar, K., Konerth, M., Kokiko-Cochran, O. N., Cardona, A., Ransohoff, R. M., & Lamb, B. T. (2010). Regulation of Tau pathology by the microglial fractalkine receptor. *Neuron, 68*(1), 19–31. https://doi.org/10.1016/j.neuron.2010.08.023.

Camacho-Hernández, N. P., & Peña-Ortega, F. (2023). Fractalkine/CX3CR1-dependent modulation of synaptic and network plasticity in health and disease. *Neural Plasticity, 2023*, 1–17. https://doi.org/10.1155/2023/4637073.

Cardona, A. E., Pioro, E. P., Sasse, M. E., Kostenko, V., Cardona, S. M., Dijkstra, I. M., ... Ransohoff, R. M. (2006). Control of microglial neurotoxicity by the fractalkine receptor. *Nature Neuroscience, 9*(7), 917–924. https://doi.org/10.1038/nn1715.

Castro-Sánchez, S., García-Yagüe, Á. J., Kügler, S., & Lastres-Becker, I. (2019). CX3CR1-deficient microglia shows impaired signalling of the transcription factor NRF2: Implications in tauopathies. *Redox Biology, 22*, 101118. https://doi.org/10.1016/j.redox.2019.101118.

Castro-Sánchez, S., García-Yagüe, Á. J., López-Royo, T., Casarejos, M., Lanciego, J. L., & Lastres-Becker, I. (2018). Cx3cr1-deficiency exacerbates alpha-synuclein-A53T induced neuroinflammation and neurodegeneration in a mouse model of Parkinson's disease. *Glia, 66*(8), 1752–1762. https://doi.org/10.1002/glia.23338.

Chen, Y., & Yu, Y. (2023). Tau and neuroinflammation in Alzheimer's disease: Interplay mechanisms and clinical translation. *Journal of Neuroinflammation, 20*(1), 165.

Chen, P., Zhao, W., Gu, H., Li, J., Feng, Y., Li, H., et al. (2016). Silencing of CX3CR1 ameliorates synaptic deficits and improves cognitive function in Alzheimer's disease. *Scientific Reports, 6*, 33125. https://doi.org/10.1038/srep33125.

Chidambaram, H., & Chinnathambi, S. (2020). G-Protein coupled receptors and Tau-different roles in Alzheimer's disease. *Neuroscience, 438, 198–214*. https://doi.org/10.1016/j.neuroscience.2020.04.019.

Chidambaram, H., & Chinnathambi, S. (2024). LC3-associated endocytosis facilitates extracellular Tau aggregate internalization and degradation in microglia. *bioRxiv, 2024*. https://doi.org/10.1101/2024.12.06.627303.

Chidambaram, H., Das, R., & Chinnathambi, S. (2020). Interaction of Tau with the chemokine receptor, CX3CR1 and its effect on microglial activation, migration and proliferation. *Cell BioSciences, 10, 109*. https://doi.org/10.1186/s13578-020-00474-4.

Chidambaram, H., Das, R., & Chinnathambi, S. (2022). G-protein coupled purinergic P2Y12 receptor interacts and internalizes Tau(RD)-mediated by membrane-associated actin cytoskeleton remodeling in microglia. *European Journal of Cell Biology, 101*(2), 151201. https://doi.org/10.1016/j.ejcb.2022.151201.

Chidambaram, H., Desale, S. E., Qureshi, T., & Chinnathambi, S. (2024). Microglial uptake of extracellular tau by actin-mediated phagocytosis. In S. K. Ray (Ed.). *Neuroprotection: Method and protocols* (pp. 231–243) Springer US. https://doi.org/10.1007/978-1-0716-3662-6_16.

Chidambaram, H., Desale, S. E., Suri, K., Murugan N, A., & Chinnathambi, S. (2024). Microglia undergoes chemokine receptor, CX3CR1-mediated internalization of extracellular Tau. *bioRxiv*. https://doi.org/10.1101/2024.12.03.626734.

Chinnathambi, S., Adithyan, A., & Chandrashekar, M. (2024a). Lipid role in synapse and nuclear envelope-associated endocytic pathways in Tauopathy. *Advances in Protein Chemistry and Structural Biology*. https://doi.org/10.1016/bs.apcsb.2024.08.002.

Chinnathambi, S., & Chidambaram, H. (2024). G-protein coupled receptors regulates Tauopathy in neurodegeneration. *Advances in Protein Chemistry and Structural Biology, 141*, 467–493. https://doi.org/10.1016/bs.apcsb.2024.04.001.

Chinnathambi, S., Malik, S., Kumarappan, M., & Chandrashekar, M. (2024b). Modifiable chemical risk factors for amyloid-β and Tau protein in Alzheimer's disease. *Advances in Protein Chemistry and Structural Biology*. https://doi.org/10.1016/bs.apcsb.2024.10.005.

Chinnathambi, S., Velmurugan, G., Ananthanaraya, V., Chandrashekar, M., & Rangappa, N. (2025). G-protein coupled receptors (GPCRs) interacts with Tau protein in Alzheimer's disease. *Adv Protein Chem Struct Biol, 147*, 259–273.

Chinnathambi, S., Velmurugan, G., & Chandrashekar, M. (2024c). Tau protein structure and dynamics. https://doi.org/10.1016/bs.apcsb.2024.09.002.

Creekmore, B. C., Watanabe, R., & Lee, E. B. (2024). Neurodegenerative disease Tauopathies. *Annual Review of Pathology, 19*, 345–370. https://doi.org/10.1146/annurev-pathmechdis-051222-120750.

Das, R., & Chinnathambi, S. (2019). Microglial priming of antigen presentation and adaptive stimulation in Alzheimer's disease. *Cellular and Molecular Life Sciences: CMLS, 76*(19), 3681–3694. https://doi.org/10.1007/s00018-019-03132-2.

Desale, S. E., Chidambaram, H., & Chinnathambi, S. (2021). G-protein coupled receptor, PI3K and Rho signaling pathways regulate the cascades of Tau and amyloid-beta in Alzheimer's disease. *Molecular Biomedicine, 2*(1), *17*. https://doi.org/10.1186/s43556-021-00036-1.

Desale, S. E., & Chinnathambi, S. (2021). Phosphoinositides signaling modulates microglial actin remodeling and phagocytosis in Alzheimer's disease. *Cell Communication and Signaling: CCS, 19*(1), 28. https://doi.org/10.1186/s12964-021-00715-0.

Desale, S. E., & Chinnathambi, S. (2021a). Alpha- Linolenic acid modulates phagocytosis and endosomal pathways of extracellular Tau in microglia. *Cell Adhesion & Migration, 15*(1), 84–100. https://doi.org/10.1080/19336918.2021.1898727.

Desale, S. E., & Chinnathambi, S. (2021b). Alpha-linolenic acid induces clearance of Tau seeds via Actin-remodeling in microglia. *Molecular Medicine, 2*(1), 4. https://doi.org/10.1186/s43556-021-00028-1.

Desale, S. E., & Chinnathambi, S. (2021c). Phosphoinositides signaling modulates microglial actin remodeling and phagocytosis in Alzheimer's disease. *Cell Communication and Signaling: CCS, 19*(1), 28. https://doi.org/10.1186/s12964-021-00715-0.

Di Lorenzo, D. (2024). TAU protein and Tauopathies: Exploring Tau protein–protein and microtubule interactions, cross-interactions and therapeutic strategies. *ChemMedChem, 19*(21), https://doi.org/10.1002/cmdc.202400180.

Dugger, B. N., & Dickson, D. W. (2017). Pathology of neurodegenerative diseases. *Cold Spring Harbor Perspectives in Biology, 9*(7), https://doi.org/10.1101/cshperspect.a028035.

Dworzak, J., Renvoisé, B., Habchi, J., Yates, E. V., Combadière, C., Knowles, T. P., Dobson, C. M., Blackstone, C., Paulsen, O., & Murphy, P. M. (2015). Neuronal Cx3cr1 Deficiency Protects against Amyloid β-Induced Neurotoxicity. *PLOS ONE, 10*(6), e0127730. https://doi.org/10.1371/journal.pone.0127730.

Fan, Q., He, W., Gayen, M., Benoit, M. R., Luo, X., Hu, X., & Yan, R. (2020). Activated CX3CL1/Smad2 signals prevent neuronal loss and Alzheimer's Tau pathology-mediated cognitive dysfunction. *The Journal of Neuroscience, 40*(5), 1133–1144. https://doi.org/10.1523/JNEUROSCI.1333-19.2019.

Faure, S., Meyer, L., Costagliola, D., Vaneensberghe, C., Genin, E., Autran, B., et al. (2000). Rapid progression to AIDS in HIV+ individuals with a structural variant of the chemokine receptor CX3CR1. *Science (New York, N. Y.), 287*(5461), 2274–2277. https://doi.org/10.1126/science.287.5461.2274.

Fonseca, M. I., Ager, R. R., Chu, S. H., Yazan, O., Sanderson, S. D., Laferla, F. M., & Tenner, A. J. (2017). Treatment with a C5aR antagonist decreases pathology and enhances behavioral performance in murine models of Alzheimer's disease. *Journal of Neuroinflammation, 14*(1), 53. https://doi.org/10.1186/s12974-017-0815-2.

Fritze, J., Muralidharan, C., Stamp, E., & Ahlenius, H. (2024). Microglia undergo disease-associated transcriptional activation and CX3C motif chemokine receptor 1 expression regulates neurogenesis in the aged brain. *Developmental Neurobiology, 84*(3), 128–141. https://doi.org/10.1002/dneu.22939.

Fuhrmann, M., et al. (2010). Microglial Cx3cr1 knockout prevents neuron loss in a mouse model of Alzheimer's disease. *Nature Neuroscience, 13*(4), 411–413. https://doi.org/10.1038/nn.2511.

Gale, S. A., Acar, D., & Daffner, K. R. (2018). Dementia. *The American Journal of Medicine, 131*(10), 1161–1169. https://doi.org/10.1016/j.amjmed.2018.01.022.

Gao, C., Jiang, J., Tan, Y., & Chen, S. (2023). Microglia in neurodegenerative diseases: Mechanism and potential therapeutic targets. *Signal Transduction And Targeted Therapy, 8*(1), 359. https://doi.org/10.1038/s41392-023-01588-0.

Gao, C., Jiang, J., Tan, Y., & Chen, S. (2023). Microglia in neurodegenerative diseases: Mechanism and potential therapeutic targets. *Signal Transduction and Targeted Therapy, 8*(1), 359. https://doi.org/10.1038/s41392-023-01588-0.

Gorantla, N. V., Das, R., Balaraman, E., & Chinnathambi, S. (2020). Transition metal nickel prevents Tau aggregation in Alzheimer's disease. *International Journal of Biological Macromolecules, 156*, 1359–1365. https://doi.org/10.1016/j.ijbiomac.2019.11.176.

Gorantla, N. V., Sunny, L. P., Rajasekhar, K., Nagaraju, P. G., Cg, P. P., Govindaraju, T., & Chinnathambi, S. (2021). Amyloid-beta-derived peptidomimetics inhibits Tau aggregation. *ACS Omega, 6*(17), 11131–11138. https://doi.org/10.1021/acsomega.9b03497.

Guimarães, T. R., Swanson, E., Kofler, J., & Thathiah, A. (2021). G protein-coupled receptor kinases are associated with Alzheimer's disease pathology. *Neuropathology and Applied Neurobiology, 47*(7), *942–957*. https://doi.org/10.1111/nan.12742.

Gupta, V., Gupta, V. B., Chitranshi, N., Gangoda, S., Vander Wall, R., Abbasi, M., Golzan, M., Dheer, Y., Shah, T., Avolio, A., Chung, R., Martins, R., & Graham, S. (2016). One protein, multiple pathologies: multifaceted involvement of amyloid β in neurodegenerative disorders of the brain and retina. *Cellular and Molecular Life Sciences, 73*(22), 4279–4297. https://doi.org/10.1007/s00018-016-2295-x.

Gyoneva, S., Hosur, R., Gosselin, D., Zhang, B., Ouyang, Z., Cotleur, A. C., ... Ransohoff, R. M. (2019). Cx3cr1-deficient microglia exhibit a premature aging transcriptome. *Life Science Alliance, 2*(6), e201900453. https://doi.org/10.26508/lsa.201900453.

Hickman, S. E., Allison, E. K., Coleman, U., Kingery-Gallagher, N. D., & El Khoury, J. (2019). Heterozygous CX3CR1 deficiency in microglia restores neuronal β-Amyloid clearance pathways and slows progression of Alzheimer's like-disease in PS1-APP mice. *Frontiers in Immunology, 10*. https://doi.org/10.3389/fimmu.2019.02780.

Hickman, S. E., Kingery, N. D., Ohsumi, T. K., Borowsky, M. L., Wang, L. C., Means, T. K., & El Khoury, J. (2013). The microglial sensome revealed by direct RNA sequencing. *Neuron,* 77(5), 1023–1037. https://doi.org/10.1016/j.neuron.2013.01.006.

Hou, Y., Dan, X., Babbar, M., Wei, Y., Hasselbalch, S. G., Croteau, D. L., & Bohr, V. A. (2019). Ageing as a risk factor for neurodegenerative disease. *Nature Reviews Neurology, 15*(10), 565–581. https://doi.org/10.1038/s41582-019-0244-7.

Huang, Y., Todd, N., & Thathiah, A. (2017). The role of GPCRs in neurodegenerative diseases: Avenues for therapeutic intervention. *Current Opinion in Pharmacology, 32*, 96–110. https://doi.org/10.1016/j.coph.2017.02.001.

Jin, S., Wang, X., Xiang, X. T., Wu, Y. M., Hu, J., Li, Y. Y., Lin Dong, Y., Tan, Y. Q., & Wu, X. (2021). Inhibition of GPR17 with cangrelor improves cognitive impairment and synaptic deficits induced by Aβ1–42 through Nrf2/HO-1 and NF-κB signaling pathway in mice. *International Immunopharmacology, 101*, 108335. https://doi.org/10.1016/j.intimp.2021.108335.

Jong, Y. I., Harmon, S. K., & O'malley, K. L. (2018). Intracellular GPCRs play key roles in synaptic plasticity. *ACS Chemical Neuroscience, 9*(9), 2162–2172. https://doi.org/10.1021/acschemneuro.7b00516.

Karantzoulis, S., & Galvin, J. E. (2011). Distinguishing Alzheimer's disease from other major forms of dementia. *Expert Review of Neurotherapeutics, 11*(11), 1579–1591. https://doi.org/10.1586/ern.11.155.

Kwan, W., Träger, U., Davalos, D., Chou, A., Bouchard, J., Andre, R., ... Muchowski, P. J. (2012). Mutant huntingtin impairs immune cell migration in Huntington disease. *Journal of Clinical Investigation, 122*(12), 4737–4747. https://doi.org/10.1172/JCI64484.

Laurent, C., Buee, L., & Blum, D. (2018). Tau and neuroinflammation: What impact for Alzheimer's Disease and Tauopathies? *Biomedical Journal, 41*(1), 21–33. https://doi.org/10.1016/j.bj.2018.01.003.

Lee, S., et al. (2010). CX3CR1 deficiency alters microglial activation and reduces beta-amyloid deposition in two Alzheimer's disease mouse models. *Journal of Neuroscience, 30*(14), 5059–5066. https://doi.org/10.1523/JNEUROSCI.6069-09.2010.

Lee, S., Varvel, N. H., Konerth, M. E., Xu, G., Cardona, A. E., Ransohoff, R. M., & Lamb, B. T. (2010). CX3CR1 deficiency alters microglial activation and reduces beta-amyloid deposition in two Alzheimer's disease mouse models. *American Journal of Pathology, 177*(5), 2549–2562. https://doi.org/10.2353/ajpath.2010.100265.

Lee, S., Varvel, N. H., Konerth, M. E., Xu, G., Cardona, A. E., Ransohoff, R. M., & Lamb, B. T. (2010). CX3CR1 deficiency alters microglial activation and reduces beta-amyloid deposition in two Alzheimer's disease mouse models. *The American Journal of Pathology, 177*(5), 2549–2562. https://doi.org/10.2353/ajpath.2010.100265.

Lee, S., Xu, G., Jay, T. R., Bhatta, S., Kim, K.-W., Jung, S., ... Lamb, B. T. (2014). Opposing effects of membrane-anchored CX3CL1 on amyloid and Tau pathologies via the p38 MAPK pathway. *The Journal of Neuroscience, 34*(37), 12538–12546. https://doi.org/10.1523/JNEUROSCI.0853-14.2014.

Liu, Z., Condello, C., Schain, A., Harb, R., Deane, R., & Friedman, B. (2010). CX3CR1 knockout exacerbates the microglial activation and neurodegeneration in a tauopathy mouse model. *Neurobiology of Aging, 31*(12), 2103–2114. https://doi.org/10.1016/j.neurobiolaging.2008.11.005.

Liu, J., Sun, Z., Liu, X., Chiu, K., Ma, L., & Wanj, J. (2025). CX3CR1 upregulation modulates microglial activation and preserves synapse in the hippocampus and frontal cortex of middle-aged mice. *Frontiers in Aging, 6*, https://www.frontiersin.org/journals/aging/articles/10.3389/fragi.2025.1549848/abstract.

Livingston, G., Huntley, J., Sommerlad, A., Ames, D., Ballard, C., Banerjee, S., ... Mukadam, N. (2020). Dementia prevention, intervention, and care: 2020 report of the lancet commission. *Lancet, 396*(10248), *413–446.* https://doi.org/10.1016/s0140-6736(20)30367-6.

Lopez-Lopez, A., Gamez, J., Syriani, E., Morales, M., Salvado, M., Rodríguez, M. J., ... Vidal-Taboada, J. M. (2014). CX3CR1 Is a modifying gene of survival and progression in amyotrophic lateral sclerosis. *PLoS One, 9*(5), e96528. https://doi.org/10.1371/journal.pone.0096528.

Ma, C., Campbell, K., Kovalenko, A., Sandusky-Beltran, L. A., Liang, H., Hunt, J. B., ... Lee, D. C. (2024). Nutrient sensing receptor GPRC6A regulates mTORC1 signaling and Tau biology. *bioRxiv*. https://doi.org/10.1101/2024.03.24.586459.

Maphis, N., Xu, G., Kokiko-Cochran, O. N., Jiang, S., Cardona, A., Ransohoff, R. M., ... Bhaskar, K. (2015). Reactive microglia drive tau pathology and contribute to the spreading of pathological tau in the brain. *Brain, 138*(6), 1738–1755. https://doi.org/10.1093/brain/awv081.

Maphis, N., Xu, G., Kokiko-Cochran, O. N., Jiang, S., Cardona, A., Ransohoff, R. M., & Lamb, B. T. (2015). Reactive microglia drive tau pathology and contribute to the spreading of pathological tau in the brain. *Journal of Neuroscience, 35*(12), 5294–5305. https://doi.org/10.1523/JNEUROSCI.4067-14.2015.

Miao, J., Ma, H., Yang, Y., Liao, Y., Lin, C., Zheng, J., ... Lan, J. (2023). Microglia in Alzheimer's disease: Pathogenesis, mechanisms, and therapeutic potentials. *Frontiers in Aging Neuroscience, 15*, 1201982. https://doi.org/10.3389/fnagi.2023.1201982.

Morganti, J. M., Nash, K. R., Grimmig, B. A., Ranjit, S., Small, B., Bickford, P. C., & Gemma, C. (2012). The soluble isoform of CX3CL1 is necessary for neuroprotection in a mouse model of Parkinson's disease. *The Journal of Neuroscience, 32*(42), 14592–14601. https://doi.org/10.1523/JNEUROSCI.0539-12.2012.

Muddapu, V. R., Dharshini, S. A. P., Chakravarthy, V. S., & Gromiha, M. M. (2020). Neurodegenerative diseases – Is metabolic deficiency the root cause? *Frontiers in Neuroscience, 14*. https://doi.org/10.3389/fnins.2020.00213.

Musi, N., Valentine, J. M., Sickora, K. R., Baeuerle, E., Thompson, C. S., Shen, Q., & Orr, M. E. (2018). Tau protein aggregation is associated with cellular senescence in the brain. *Aging Cell, 17*(6), e12840. https://doi.org/10.1111/acel.12840.

Myeku, N., Schaler, A. W., Runyan, A. M., Fowler, S. L., Figueroa, H. Y., Shioda, S., ... Duff, K. E. (2020). GPCR-mediated clearance of tau in post-synaptic compartments attenuates tau pathology in vivo. *Cold Spring Harbor.*

Nash, K. R., Moran, P., Finneran, D. J., Hudson, C., Robinson, J., Morgan, D., & Gordon, M. N. (2013). Fractalkine overexpression suppresses tau pathology in a mouse model of tauopathy. *Neurobiology of Aging, 34*(6), 1540–1548. https://doi.org/10.1016/j.neurobiolaging.2012.11.025.

Nelson, C. D., & Sheng, M. (2013). Gpr3 stimulates Aβ production via interactions with APP and β-arrestin2. *PLoS One, 8*, e74680.

Paolicelli, R. C., Bolasco, G., Pagani, F., Maggi, L., Scianni, M., Panzanelli, P., et al. (2014). Synaptic pruning by microglia is necessary for normal brain development. *Journal of Neuroscience, 34*(6), 2114–2123. https://doi.org/10.1523/JNEUROSCI.2314-13.2014.

Pawelec, P., Ziemka-Nalecz, M., Sypecka, J., & Zalewska, T. (2020). The impact of the CX3CL1/CX3CR1 axis in neurological disorders. *Cells, 9*(10), 2277. https://doi.org/10.3390/cells9102277.

Perea, J. R., Bolós, M., & Avila, J. (2020). Microglia in Alzheimer's disease in the context of Tau pathology. *Biomolecules, 10*(10), 1439. https://doi.org/10.3390/biom10101439.

Petra, M. (2024). Truncated tau modulates neuron-glia signaling through CX3CL1-CX3CR1 and CD47-SIRP-α pathways. https://www.researchsquare.com/article/rs-4868529/v1.

Poon, C. H., Wang, Y., Fung, M.-L., Zhang, C., & Lim, L. W. (2020). Rodent models of amyloid-beta feature of Alzheimer's disease: Development and potential treatment implications. *Aging and Disease, 11*(5), 1235. https://doi.org/10.14336/AD.2019.1026.

Pressman, P. S. (2025). Alzheimer's disease. In J. D. England (Ed.). *Encyclopedia of the neurological sciences* (pp. 504–510)(Third ed.). Academic Press. https://doi.org/10.1016/B978-0-323-95702-1.00119-6.

Puntambekar, S. S., Moutinho, M., Lin, P. B., Jadhav, V., Tumbleson-Brink, D., Balaji, A., ... Lamb, B. T. (2022). CX3CR1 deficiency aggravates amyloid driven neuronal pathology and cognitive decline in Alzheimer's disease. *Molecular Neurodegeneration, 17*, 47. https://doi.org/10.1186/s13024-022-00545-9.

Puntambekar, S. S., Moutinho, M., Lin, P. B.-C., Jadhav, V., Tumbleson-Brink, D., Balaji, A., ... Lamb, B. T. (2022). CX3CR1 deficiency aggravates amyloid driven neuronal pathology and cognitive decline in Alzheimer's disease. *Molecular Neurodegeneration, 17*(1), 47. https://doi.org/10.1186/s13024-022-00545-9.

Qi, Z., Peng, J., Wang, H., Wang, L., Su, Y., Ding, L., ... Yang, J. J. (2024). Modulating neuroinflammation and cognitive function in postoperative cognitive dysfunction via CCR5-GPCRs-Ras-MAPK pathway targeting with microglial EVs. *CNS Neuroscience & Therapeutics, 30*(8), e14924. https://doi.org/10.1111/cns.14924.

Rawat, P., Sehar, U., Bisht, J., Selman, A., Culberson, J., & Reddy, P. H. (2022). Phosphorylated Tau in Alzheimer's disease and other Tauopathies. *International Journal of Molecular Sciences, 23*(21), 12841. https://doi.org/10.3390/ijms232112841.

Ridderstad Wollberg, A., Ericsson-Dahlstrand, A., Jureus, A., Ekerot, P., Simon, S., Nilsson, M., et al. (2022). Pharmacological inhibition of the chemokine receptor CX3CR1 attenuates neuroinflammation and improves outcomes in CNS disease models. *Frontiers in Pharmacology, 13*, 899654. https://doi.org/10.3389/fphar.2022.899654.

Rogers, J. T., Morganti, J. M., Bachstetter, A. D., Hudson, C. E., Peters, M. M., Grimmig, B. A., et al. (2011). CX3CR1 deficiency leads to reduced tau phosphorylation and loss of synaptic proteins in a tauopathy model. *Molecular Therapy, 19*(9), 1640–1649. https://doi.org/10.1038/mt.2011.128.

Salminen, A., Ojala, J., Kauppinen, A., Kaarniranta, K., & Suuronen, T. (2009). Inflammation in Alzheimer's disease: Amyloid-β oligomers trigger innate immunity defence via pattern recognition receptors. *Progress in Neurobiology, 87*(3), 181–194.

Sando, R., & Südhof, T. C. (2021). Latrophilin GPCR signaling mediates synapse formation. *Elife, 10*. https://doi.org/10.7554/eLife.65717.

Sonawane, S. K., & Chinnathambi, S. (2018). Prion-like propagation of post-translationally modified Tau in Alzheimer's disease: A hypothesis. *Journal of Molecular Neuroscience: MN, 65*(4), 480–490. https://doi.org/10.1007/s12031-018-1111-5.

Sushma, & Mondal, A. C. (2019). Role of GPCR signaling and calcium dysregulation in Alzheimer's disease. *Molecular and Cellular Neurosciences, 101*, 103414. https://doi.org/10.1016/j.mcn.2019.103414.

Szukiewicz, D. (2024). CX3CL1 (Fractalkine)-CX3CR1 axis in inflammation-induced angiogenesis and tumorigenesis. *International Journal of Molecular Sciences, 25*(9), 4679. https://doi.org/10.3390/ijms25094679.

Thathiah, A., & De Strooper, B. (2011). The role of G protein-coupled receptors in the pathology of Alzheimer's disease. *Nature Reviews. Neuroscience, 12*(2), 73–87. https://doi.org/10.1038/nrn2977.

Thome, A. D., Standaert, D. G., & Harms, A. S. (2015). Fractalkine signaling regulates the inflammatory response in an α-synuclein model of Parkinson disease. *PLoS One, 10*(10), e0140566. https://doi.org/10.1371/journal.pone.0140566.

Walsh, D. M., Klyubin, I., Fadeeva, J. V., Cullen, W. K., Anwyl, R., Wolfe, M. S., Rowan, M. J., & Selkoe, D. J. (2002). Naturally secreted oligomers of amyloid β protein potently inhibit hippocampal long-term potentiation in vivo. *Nature, 416*(6880), 535–539. https://doi.org/10.1038/416535a.

Wang, C., Fan, L., Khawaja, R. R., Liu, B., Zhan, L., Kodama, L., ... Gan, L. (2022). Microglial NF-κB drives tau spreading and toxicity in a mouse model of tauopathy. *Nature Communications, 13*(1), 1969. https://doi.org/10.1038/s41467-022-29552-6.

Wang, Y., Wang, J., Chen, X., Lin, Z., You, Z., He, K., ... Xie, F. (2025). Tau pathology is associated with postsynaptic metabotropic glutamate receptor 5 (mGluR5) in early Alzheimer's disease in a sex-specific manner. *Alzheimer's & Dementia: the Journal of the Alzheimer's Association, 21*(2), e70004. https://doi.org/10.1002/alz.70004.

Wang, X., Xie, Y., Niu, Y., Wan, B., Lu, Y., Luo, Q., & Zhu, L. (2023). CX3CL1/CX3CR1 signal mediates M1-type microglia and accelerates high-altitude-induced forgetting. *Frontiers in Cellular Neuroscience, 17*. https://doi.org/10.3389/fncel.2023.1189348.

Woo, J.-A., Yan, Y., Kee, T. R., Cazzaro, S., Mcgill Percy, K. C., Wang, X., ... Kang, D. E. (2022). β-Arrestin1 promotes tauopathy by transducing GPCR signaling, disrupting microtubules and autophagy. *Life Science Alliance, 5*(3), e202101183. https://doi.org/10.26508/lsa.202101183.

Wu, J., Bie, B., Yang, H., Xu, J. J., Brown, D. L., & Naguib, M. (2013). Suppression of central chemokine fractalkine receptor signaling alleviates amyloid-induced memory deficiency. *Neurobiology of Aging, 34*(12), 2843–2852. https://doi.org/10.1016/j.neurobiolaging.2013.06.003.

Zhang, X., Wang, J., Zhang, Z., & Ye, K. (2024). Tau in neurodegenerative diseases: Molecular mechanisms, biomarkers, and therapeutic strategies. *Transl Neurodegener, 13*(1), 40. https://doi.org/10.1186/s40035-024-00429-6.

Zhang, H., Wei, W., Zhao, M., Ma, L., Jiang, X., Pei, H., ... Li, H. (2021). Interaction between Aβ and Tau in the pathogenesis of Alzheimer's Disease. *International Journal of Biological Sciences, 17*(9), 2181–2192. https://doi.org/10.7150/ijbs.57078.

Zhang, Y., Wu, K. M., Yang, L., Dong, Q., & Yu, J. T. (2022). Tauopathies: New perspectives and challenges. *Molecular Neurodegeneration, 17*(1), 28. https://doi.org/10.1186/s13024-022-00533-z.

Zhang, L., Xu, J., Gao, J., Wu, Y., Yin, M., & Zhao, W. (2018). CD200-, CX3CL1-, and TREM2-mediated neuron-microglia interactions and their involvements in Alzheimer's disease. *Reviews in the Neurosciences, 29*(8), 837–848.

Zhao, J., Han, Z., Ding, L., Wang, P., He, X., & Lin, L. (2024). The molecular mechanism of aging and the role in neurodegenerative diseases. *Heliyon, 10*(2), e24751. https://doi.org/10.1016/j.heliyon.2024.e24751.

Zhao, Y., Xin, Y., He, Z., Hu, Z., Lin, C., Chen, L., et al. (2023). Adoptive transfer of CX3CR1-transduced regulatory T cells improves neuroinflammation and cognition in an Alzheimer's disease mouse model. *Brain, Behavior, and Immunity, 105*, 1–11. https://doi.org/10.1016/j.bbi.2023.02.004.

Zhou, T., Zheng, Y., Sun, L., Badea, A., Jin, Y., Liu, Y., et al. (2018). Histone deacetylase inhibitors suppress CX3CR1 expression and prevent hippocampal synaptic dysfunction in Alzheimer's disease. *Epigenetics: Official Journal of the DNA Methylation Society, 13*(10-11), 1078–1089. https://doi.org/10.1080/15592294.2018.1532304.

CHAPTER FOUR

Human-induced pluripotent stem cells in psychiatric disorders: An inflammatory perspective

Varsha Vishnu, Ashitha Siddappa Niranjana Murthy, and Biju Viswanath*
Department of Psychiatry, National Institute of Mental Health, and Neuroscience (NIMHANS), Centre for Brain and Mind, Bengaluru, India
*Corresponding author. e-mail address: bijuv1@gmail.com

Contents

Abstract

Psychiatric disorders have long been associated with inflammation- either as prolonged mental illnesses leading to immune dysregulations or as psychiatric conditions arising from systemic inflammation. Physiologically, inflammation is one of the responses to bodily stress, however, the degree of inflammation depends on the type and duration of the stressor. Here, we focus on understanding both- inflammation-induced brain cellular response alterations and neuroinflammation caused by an underlying psychiatric condition. Apart from post-mortem brains, the closest approach by which one can recreate

Advances in Immunology, Volume 171
ISSN 0065-2776, https://doi.org/10.1016/bs.ai.2026.04.004

both these phenomena are by using patient-derived induced pluripotent stem cells (IPSCs), as the brain tissue is inaccessible. Therefore, we focus on studies using IPSC-derived brain cells from patients to model inflammation across psychiatric conditions. Unlike any other available model system, IPSCs hold a major advantage of carrying patients' genetic background that is crucial to understand disorders as complex and enigmatic as psychiatric disorders. When knowledge on patients' genetic risks and environmental exposures are integrated into patient iPSC-derived brain cellular models, it holds enormous potential to delineate psychiatry related pathophysiology from other comorbidities. Therefore, understanding the cellular responses to inflammation and treatment helps us refine the existing therapeutic strategies and initiate early interventions to better manage psychiatric disorders.

1. Introduction

Psychiatric disorders are clinically characterized through significant disturbances in cognition, mood, behaviour, emotion, and perception (Trivedi, Goel & Resident, 2006). These disorders are diagnosed in accordance with psychiatric manuals such as the International Classification of Diseases (ICD) by the World Health Organization (WHO) and the Diagnostic and Statistical Manual of Mental Disorders (DSM) by the American Psychiatric Association (APA) (Aboraya et al., 2006). Some of the most commonly occurring psychiatric disorders include Schizophrenia (SCZ), bipolar disorder (BD)(Roser, Ritchie & Spooner, 2021), Autism (ASD), Major Depressive Disorder (MDD), Attention-deficit/Hyperactivity disorder (ADHD), and obsessive-compulsive disorder (OCD). They remain one of the major burdens of non-communicable diseases worldwide, following cardiovascular disorders, respiratory disorders, and cancer. The Lancet's 2025 publication presents the latest findings from the Global Burden of Disease Study (GBD), incorporating data up to 2023. They report that psychiatric disorders accounted for 5.4 % of the total global disease burden in 2021, with over 155 million Disability Adjusted Life Years (DALYs) (Schumacher et al., 2024).

Research in psychiatric disorders has led to significant advances in diagnosis and treatment through the development of targeted interventions and has contributed to reducing the stigma associated with mental illnesse (Tanaka & Vécsei, 2024). Despite these advances, the pathophysiology of most psychiatric disorders remains poorly understood. Among the numerous studies conducted, there has been consistent evidence on the involvement of neuroinflammation across mental illness since the 1970s, with the first study showing that depressive patients also had chronic Hepatitis C infection (Renault et al., 1987). Since then, research has further described the roles of peripheral immune systems in psychiatric illness, demonstrating bidirectional communication between the cells of the central nervous system (CNS), and mental stress induced systemic immune response mechanisms (Limanaqi et al., 2019).

As the central hub for consciousness and involuntary control, any minor change in the homeostasis of the CNS can be manifested as a systemic condition in no time. Chronic stress is sensed by the Hypothalamic-pituitary-adrenal (HPA) axis in the brain (Chen et al., 2017). It responds by increasing the cortisol levels, thereby shifting the body to fight or flight mode. An immediate measure for such a response can be detected by blood-based biomarkers for inflammation, such as cytokines or acute-phase proteins that are elevated during inflammation (Belvederi Murri et al., 2016). A more direct measure of CNS inflammation can be detected by using neuroimaging (Albrecht et al., 2016), Cerebrospinal fluid (CSF) (Gracias et al., 2022), and cervical lymph nodes (Giff et al., 2026).

Additionally, post-mortem brain studies also provided initial proof of inflammatory manifestations of psychiatric disorders (Liu et al., 2022). These studies showed a variety of brain pathologies, such as differences in glial cell numbers, white and grey matter abnormalities, and brain size and structure. Therefore, there is piling evidence suggesting inflammation as a key mechanism of pathogenesis in many psychiatric disorders.

Importantly, patients with high cytokine levels are not likely to respond to medications (Haroon et al., 2018). Therefore, there is an urgent need for research to delineate the specific roles of neuroinflammation in psychiatric manifestations and find alternative therapeutic strategies targeting inflammatory mechanisms. This chapter focuses on understanding neuroinflammatory studies using IPSC-derived model systems for psychiatric conditions.

2. Modelling neuroinflammation in psychiatric disorders using IPSC

Neuroinflammation is a condition in which the cells of the brain respond to stress by initiating neuroprotective mechanisms (Shabab et al., 2017). For example, neurons respond by secreting neurotrophic factors, clear cellular debris, and secrete cytokines and chemokines. While glial cells respond by getting activated and multiplying to perform immunological functions like phagocytosis, cytokine secretion, activation of secondary messengers, oxidative stress response, and maintaining homeostasis (Yang & Zhou, 2019). These cells do not respond independently; instead, they respond by communicating with the other cell types in the brain- like Microglia and Astrocytes- primary immune cells that respond to an external stimuli (Yang & Zhou, 2019). Hence, neuroinflammation is not a condition involving a single cell type, as modelled by most studies. Instead, it is a complex reaction involving numerous cell types, and hence it is ideal to model it by increasing the culture complexity (Yang & Zhou, 2019).

Owing to the lack of availability of brain tissue, human IPSCs provide the best opportunity to model neuroinflammation in vitro (Hong et al., 2023). IPSCs are cells that have the ability to regenerate and can be differentiated into any desired cell type. It is an invaluable tool to understand cellular response in a more personalized manner, as the individual's genetic makeup is preserved. IPSC-derived cells can be used to understand their direct response to stressors, effects of treatment, immunomodulatory functions of various molecules and model genetic alterations. Despite the limitation that IPSC-derived models represent a foetal or developmental aspect and not a model to represent the adult brain (Upthegrove et al., 2025), it is important to understand how each cell type responds to inflammation in an accurate manner to dissect its interactions with other cell types.

Studies thus far have utilised one of the following three approaches to model neuroinflammation using iPSCs. Firstly, majority of these studies have focused on understanding brain cellular response by treating them individually with stressors to replicate the in vivo inflammation in psychiatric conditions (Upthegrove et al., 2025). Some commonly used stressors include Lipopolysaccharide (LPS), polyinosine- polycytidylic and pro-inflammatory cytokines such as IL-1β, IL-6, IL-8, Tumour Necrosis Factor-alpha (TNFα), and Interferon gamma (IFN-ɣ) (Stöberl et al., 2023). These inflammatory stressors further activate and translocate nuclear factor kappa-light chain enhancer of activated B-cell (NFκB) to the nucleus and elicit a pro-inflammatory response.

Secondly, since cells are in constant communication and contact with the surrounding cells during an inflammatory response, some studies either used conditioned media (CM) from one cell type to test the response of other cell types, or used a third approach- that is to co-culture cells in close physical proximity (Cardozo et al., 2025). Several studies modelled neuroinflammation by co-culturing neurons with a glial cell type -either microglia or astrocytes as they are primary responders to immune dysregulation in the brain and also produce pro-inflammatory response on detecting damage/pathogen associated molecular patterns (DAMS/PAMS) (Stöberl et al., 2023) (Fig. 1). We observed that there are limited number of

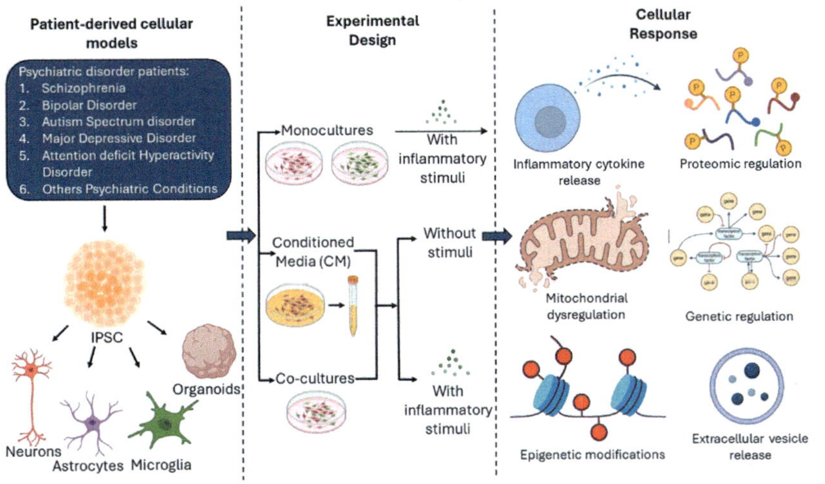

Fig. 1 A sequential illustration of modelling neuroinflammation in psychiatry using IPSC patient-derived brain cells and their responses with and without stimuli.

iPSC-based studies that focused on understanding epigenetic modulations like differential methylation patterns, miRNA, and others, that occur as a consequence of neuroinflammation in psychiatric disorders (Mostafavi Abdolmaleky et al., 2024).

Overall, this chapter gives a brief overview on recent research trends and knowledge gained from these studies that modelled neuroinflammation in psychiatric patient derived IPSC brain cells (Fig. 1). We have excluded studies that modelled cytokine response in control IPSC-astrocytes and microglia as they lacked a disease context.

3. Schizophrenia

Schizophrenia (SCZ) is a serious mental health condition characterized primarily by psychosis and functional decline (Luvsannyam et al., 2022). It is a condition in which contact with external reality is lost, and the patient is unable to distinguish between reality and illusion (Rantala et al., 2022). It presents as a combination of positive symptoms (hallucinations, delusions, disorganized speech and thought), and negative symptoms (anhedonia, alogia, avolition, social withdrawal), as well as cognitive impairment (Luvsannyam et al., 2022). As rendered by DSM, SCZ is diagnosed by the occurrence of at least two of the above-mentioned symptoms with occupational and socio-functional dysregulation (Luvsannyam et al., 2022). According to the Lancet GBD 2017 study on mental disorders across Indian states, SCZ had a prevalence of 0.3 % and contributed 9.8 % to the total DALYs due to mental disorders (Sagar et al., 2020). A person with SCZ has about 5–10 % chance of mortality by suicide (Hjorthøj et al., 2017). Antipsychotics, being the first line of SCZ treatment, fail to treat negative symptoms. These drugs have a 30 % chance of side effects. Therefore, therapeutic approaches typically include antipsychotics in combination with psychotherapy and rehabilitation (Patel et al., 2014).

Although SCZ is genetically highly heritable, it does not follow a mendelian pattern of inheritance and has a highly complex genetic architecture (Salleh, 2004). Besides, multiple post-mortem studies point towards an elevated inflammatory profile. According to the neurodevelopmental hypothesis of SCZ, immune dysregulation during early neurodevelopment could lead to hyper synaptic pruning (Howes & Onwordi, 2023) by microglia, known to disrupt neurodevelopment. Consistent with this, there have been numerous studies exploring the inflammatory aspect of SCZ from a neurodevelopmental perspective using patient IPSC-derived model systems. This section of the chapter aims to brief on the inflammatory modulations that contribute to schizophrenia aetiology.

3.1 Cellular response to cytokine treatment in SCZ

A simple model to study neuroinflammation using IPSC is by 2-Dimension (2D) monocultures. Monocultures are a single population of cells differentiated from IPSCs (Summers et al., 2024). The most frequently used strategy to understand neuroinflammation in monocultures is to treat them with a stimulant and check for cellular responses (Table 1). For example, upon TNF-α stimulation, SCZ IPSC-derived Astrocytes (IPSC-Astrocytes) responded differently when compared to healthy controls. They showed a higher pro-inflammatory response with notable high expression of IL-6 and IL-8, and a decrease in the P65 subunit of NF-κB (Trindade, Nascimento, Bárbara S Casas, et al., 2023). This decrease in NF-κB subunit was confirmed in SCZ postmortem prefrontal cortex samples. NF-κB acts by translocating inside the nucleus and induces the transcription of the NOD-, LRR- and pyrin domain-containing protein 3 (NLRP3) complex and induces 1L1b secretion.

In line with the previous findings, a study by Szabo et al. (2025) found that SCZ astrocytes express lower levels of NLRP3 complex (Szabo et al., 2025). When SCZ IPSC-Astrocytes were treated with Lysophophatidylcholine (LPC), they exhibited high caspase activity, but lower NLRP3

Table 1 Varying concentrations of stimulants used to study neuroinflammation in IPSC-derived cellular models in psychiatry.

S no	Disorder	Stimulant used	Concentration	Duration	IPSC- patient-derived cell type	Method of cytokine detection	Measure of inflammation	Summary	References
1	SCZ	TNFa	10ng/ml	24 h	Astrocyte	Bead-based multiplex immunoassays	Increase in IL-1β, IL-2, IL-4, IL-6, IL-8, TNF-α, IL-10, IL-13, BDNF interferon (IFN)-γ	Astrocytes from SCZ patients exhibit a pro-inflammatory profile with increased IL8 and impaired NFkb signalling that affects vascularization	Trindade et al. (2023)
2	SCZ	TNFa	10ng/ml	24 h	Astrocyte	RT-qPCR	Increase in CCL5, TNF-α, IL-1α, IL-1β, IL-6, and IL-8, CX3CL8	SCZ astrocytes expressed high levels of CX3CL1, which caused a premature aging phenotype in microglia characterized by reduced migration and impaired phagocytosis	Cardozo et al. (2025)
						ELISA	Increase in CX3CL1, IL6, IL8		

(continued)

Table 1 Varying concentrations of stimulants used to study neuroinflammation in IPSC-derived cellular models in psychiatry. (*cont'd*)

S no	Disorder	Stimulant used	Concentration	Duration	IPSC- patient-derived cell type	Method of cytokine detection	Measure of inflammation	Summary	References
3	SCZ	IFNg	25 ng/ml	24 h	Neurons	RT-qPCR	Increase in C4A, HLA-B, STAT1	SCZ neurons, upon stimulation, showed an increase in expression of MHC-I genes and a decrease in synaptic marker expression, implying a compromised synaptic integrity	Pavlinek et al. (2022)
4	SCZ	Lysophos-phatidyl-choline	25–100 μm	6 h	Astrocyte	ELISA	Increase in IL-1β, IL-18, Decrease in IL-6, IL-8/CXCL8	SCZ astrocytes exhibit a hyper-inflammatory profile that, when triggered, releases high levels of IL1b, which impairs microglial phagocytosis and T-cell recruitment	Szabo et al. (2025)

5	SCZ	IL1b	0.1–10 ng/ml	4 h	Astrocyte	RT-qPCR	Decrease in CCL20, HILPDA1, HILPDA2	Dysregulation in the CCL20 response upon stimulation in SCZ astrocytes that leads to impaired recruitment of anti-inflammatory T-cells	Akkouh et al. (2020)
						ELISA	Decrease in CCL20		
6	SCZ	IL1b	1 ng/ml	24 h	Neurons	RT-qPCR	Increase in C4A, No increase in C4B	The CSF levels of C4A in FEP SCZ patients were high; a similar trend was observed in patient-derived neurons, linking the genetic risk of the C4A locus to direct immune-mediated protein change in vivo	Gracias et al. (2022)
		IL6	1 ng/ml			Bead-based multiplex immunoassays	Increase in C4A, no increase in C4B in CSF		

(continued)

Table 1 Varying concentrations of stimulants used to study neuroinflammation in IPSC-derived cellular models in psychiatry. (*cont'd*)

S no	Disorder	Stimulant used	Concentration	Duration	IPSC- patient-derived cell type	Method of cytokine detection	Measure of inflammation	Summary	References
7	BD	IL1b	10 ng/ml	5 h and 24 h	Astrocytes	Dot blot	Increase in IL6, IL8, CXCL1, MIF, Serpin	BD astrocytes had an increased IL6 secretion that led to dysregulation in the neuronal activity	Vadodaria et al. (2021)
		TNFa	50 ng/ml			Flowcytometry	Increase in IL6, No difference in IL8		
8	SCZ	TNFa	10 ng/ml	24 h	Astrocyte	ELISA	Increase in IL6, TNFα, IL1β in iMG	Antipsychotics like Clozapine and Olanzapine modulate microglial phagocytosis and motility via astrocyte-derived extracellular vesicles	Yeh et al. (2026)
		IL1b	10 ng/ml						
		IFNg	10 ng/ml						

9	BD	LPS	100 ng/ml	24 h	Microglia	ELISA	No difference in IL6, TNFα, IL10, IL8, an increase in IL12P70	The kynurenine pathway is inhibited by lithium, thereby causing a decrease in IDO1 expression and tryptophan metabolism and an increase in anti-inflammatory cytokine secretion	Göttert et al. (2022)
		IFNg	20 ng/ml						

and ASC (Apoptosis-associated Speck-like protein containing a CARD)- an adaptor protein that aid in the formation of NLRP3 complex- expression and higher expression of pro-inflammatory cytokines, implying dysregulation in the inflammasome complex . A similar pattern of NLRP3 and ASC downregulation was observed in postmortem prefrontal cortex region of SCZ patients. They also observed reduced mitochondrial gly-colysis and glutamate uptake, which did not show any difference post LPC stimulation. On specific NLRP3 inflammasome activation, SCZ Astrocytes showed impaired Th1/Th17 lymphocyte activation capacity. Together, they provide evidence for NLRP3-dependent dysregulation of innate and adaptive immune mechanisms in SCZ astrocytes. To check if these NLRP3-mediated signalling affects adaptive immunity, they co-cultured control T-cells with stimulated and unstimulated IPSC-astrocytes from SCZ or healthy controls. They found that response of T-cells cultured with SCZ unstimulated astrocytes was comparable to unstimulated healthy control astrocytes, but when cultured with stimulated SCZ astrocytes, T-cells showed a heightened response, more responsive than the control stimulated astrocytes. These studies suggest that SCZ patients have a heightened inflammatory profile alongside NF-κB and inflammasome dysregulation. Such an inflammatory profile also abnormally triggers the adaptive systemic response upon stimulation.

To model cellular response and communication during inflammation, studies have used CM from one cell type cultured for a stipulated amount of time. CM or spent media contains secreted growth factors, small molecules, cytokines, and other components secreted by the cells in culture (Fadilah, Fauzi & Maarof, 2024). CM is a valuable source to study inter-cellular response under inflammatory conditions . In neuroinflammation, it is widely used to study the response of neurons or other peripheral immune cells to glial cell derived CM. To exemplify this, Cardozo et al. (2025) showed that Peripheral Blood Mononuclear Cells (PBMC)-derived microglial (piMG) cells had abnormal levels of ligand *CX3CL1* when exposed to CM of TNFα-treated SCZ IPSC-Astrocytes (Cardozo et al., 2025). Despite a significant increase in *CX3CL1* levels, which is a frac-talkine ligand that helps in microglial motility, it did not induce piMG motility. This is possibly due to the reactive astrocytes reducing the membrane-bound *CX3CR1* expression- that aids in cellular adherence to a substrate- in piMG cells exposed to CM of SCZ IPSC-Astrocytes, thereby hindering migration. Additionally, they also observed a noticeable decrease in piMG phagocytic ability.

A similar migratory impairment was seen by Akkouh et al (2020), when SCZ IPSC-Astrocytes were stimulated with IL-1β for 4 h (Akkouh et al., 2020). Transcriptionally, following IL-1β exposure, three genes appeared to be significantly downregulated in SCZ IPSC-Astrocytes, namely *HILPDA1, HILPDA2,* and *CCL20.* It is known that astrocytes can induce a migratory effect, especially on T-regulatory (T-reg) cells that express *CCR6*, a chemoattractant receptor for *CCL20.* Hence, when a transwell migration assay was performed to validate this, stimulated SCZ IPSC-Astrocytes CM showed a weaker chemotactic effect on T-reg cells than controls. Further to corroborate their findings, SCZ patients' blood was used to check *FOXP3*, a T-reg cell marker. Its expression in patient blood had plummeted, implying an impaired T-cell regulation and chemotaxis in SCZ, which affects the peripheral immune cell recruitment. Like in the previous study there might have been altered *CX3CL* levels that also could have contributed to the reduced chemotactic behaviour. However, the CX3CL level were not measure in the present study. Overall, these studies suggest that astrocytic interactions play a crucial role in disease pathophysiology of SCZ.

To closely study the established astrocytic intercellular interactions that might be responsible for the SCZ predisposition, a study by Yeh et al. (2026) focused on astrocytic Extracellular Vesicles (EVs). EVs are membrane-bound vesicles that carry lipids, proteins, and amino acids to aid cellular communications (Yeh et al., 2026). To mimic the inflammatory phenotype, SCZ IPSC-Astrocytes were treated with IL-1β and Adenosine triphosphate (ATP) separately. When Yeh et al. (2025) exposed piMG to these astrocytic EVs they had an anti-inflammatory response, whereas SCZ IPSC-Astrocytic EVs without any treatment gave a pro-inflammatory cytokine response. Remarkably, ATP stimulated SCZ IPSC-Astrocytes EVs were bigger in size compared to untreated SCZ IPSC-Astrocytes. This proves that the differential effects observed in microglia are influenced by the distinct stimulators of astrocytes. Further, to understand how antipsychotic medications modulate these cellular interactions, EVs from primary astrocytes exposed to Clozapine (CLOZ), Norclozapine (NR), or Olanzapine (OLAN) were given to piMG. It was observed that EVs from OLAN and NR-exposed astrocytes alone increased the phagocytosis of microglia. An increase in the migratory ability was also observed only in piMG treated with CLOZ. These results suggest that the contents of the EVs are highly dependent on the antipsychotic exposure given to astrocytes.

Astrocytes are located mainly at the blood-brain barrier (BBB) to ensure integrity and facilitate communication between neurons and blood vessels

(Cabezas et al., 2014). Hence, they influence the vascular architecture of the BBB with their response during neuroinflammation. Upon proteomic analysis of those SCZ IPSC-Astrocytes, they revealed dysregulations in the angiogenic proteins and related pathways (Trindade, Nascimento, Bárbara S. Casas, et al., 2023). To validate the proteomic data, a chick Chorioallantoic membrane (CAM) assay, was performed to check the vascularization capacity of SCZ IPSC-Astrocytes CM. It induces the formation of more blood vessels than control astrocyte CM. However, the control astrocytic CM was also able to induce more vessel formation upon IL-8 treatment, suggesting that this ability to induce vessel formation is via IL-8 signalling.

Astrocytes not only play a vital role in immune regulation, but they also help in maintaining homeostasis in neurons by maintaining the glutamate levels (Beekhuis-Hoekstra et al., 2022). When SCZ IPSC-Astrocytes with high Polygenic Risk Score (PRS) were co-cultured with SCZ IPSC-Neurons, there was a decrease in the Vesicular glutamate transporter/vesicular GABA transporter (VGLUT/VGAT) ratio. VGLUT and VGAT are transporter proteins that load neurotransmitters into synaptic vesicles before their release. This reduction in the glutamate transporters points towards an excitatory inhibitory imbalance mediated by astrocytes that might contribute to one of the SCZ pathophysiologies. Additionally, another study by Gracias et al. (2022) immune challenged IPSC-derived neurons from First Episode Psychosis (FEP) SCZ patients with IL-1β and IL-6. They observed elevated levels of C4A mRNA (Gracias et al., 2022). C4A is a complement protein that is involved in the tagging of underused synapses, thereby marking them for microglial synaptic pruning (Yilmaz et al., 2021). This process traditionally should occur during brain development. However, over-tagging of these synapses leads to synaptic over-pruning, thereby leading to SCZ. Correspondingly, the CSF of the same FEP SCZ patients also had higher levels of C4A (Gracias et al., 2022). To substantiate the above study further, another study by (Pavlinek et al., 2022) showed that even in the control of IPSC-derived Neural Stem cells (NSCs), IFN-γ exposure elevated the expression of *C4A* . It should be noted that in both studies, irrespective of cytokine used, it led to an increase in C4A levels. This could be because, SCZ's strongest common genetic association involves variation in the major histocompatibility complex (MHC) locus containing many structurally diverse alleles of the C4 genes that affects expression of *C4A* in the brain (Sekar et al., 2016). These findings suggest that inflammation along with neurodevelopmental abnormalities associated with SCZ risk factors contribute to the SCZ predisposition.

3.2 Mitochondrial dysregulation in SCZ

Mitochondrial dysregulation is one of the hallmarks of inflammation, as inflammatory stimulants damage mitochondria, triggering a release of DAMPs in the form of mitochondrial DNA (mtDNA), cardiolipin, ATP, and Reactive oxygen Species (ROS) (Nesci, Spagnoletta & Oppedisano, 2023). These signals can activate the NLRP3 inflammasome, leading to cellular death. Numerous studies show an inherent mitochondrial dysregulation in SCZ IPSC-derived models. One such study by Ni et al. (2020) showed that mitochondrial Oxidative phosphorylation (OXPHOS) is among the most affected pathways in the transcriptome analysis of IPSC-derived Cortical Inter neurons (cIN) from SCZ patients (Ni et al., 2020). There was a significant downregulation of a gene encoding mitochondrial complex I, suggesting dysregulation of fundamental processes such as the Electron Transport chain (ETC). It was interesting to note that such mitochondrial pathway dysregulation was not observed in IPSC-derived Glutamatergic neurons from the same patients, implying a cell-type-specific dysregulation. To validate this, a bioenergetics assay was performed. A decrease in mitochondrial respiration and maximum reserve capacity was observed in patient-derived cIN. Additionally, mitochondrial enzyme, Nicotinamide adenine dinucleotide (NAD), was also found to be significantly reduced, and the overall mitochondria were oxidatively stressed. To mitigate this, they found that when these cells were exposed to Alpha Lipoic Acid/Acetyl-L-Carnitine (ALA/ALC), these dysregulated mitochondrial phenotypes were rescued.

In line with the previous study, proteomic analysis of SCZ patient derived NSCs and neurons revealed that OXPHOS pathway proteins were differentially expressed (Zuccoli et al., 2023). In particular, proteins involved in ATP synthase activity and the pyruvate dehydrogenase complex were altered in patient-derived cells. In addition, proteins related to DNA damage, mRNA translation, cell cycle, and RNA stability were also differentially expressed in nuclear proteome analysis. These were validated by performing a mitochondrial bioenergetic assay on patient derived NSCs that showed altered mitochondrial function with increased ROS. Conclusively, these studies suggest that SCZ patient-derived cells exhibit inflammatory abnormalities in the form of mitochondrial dysregulations, however these are dependent on a specific cell type and might not be present in other cell type of a patient brain.

3.3 Epigenetic modifications in SCZ

Epigenetic modification is the influence of environmental factors on DNA modulators like the histone proteins and Cytosine phosphate Guanine (CpG) islands. They also include microRNA (miRNAs) that are involved in the regulation of gene expression by tagging to the non-coding end of mRNA (Yang et al., 2025). There are ample studies suggesting abnormal histone modification in SCZ samples. However, recent IPSC-derived studies explore the influence of miRNA on SCZ. In a study by Akkouh et al. (2020), when SCZ IPSC-derived astrocytes were tested for a panel of global miRNA, there was a baseline decrease in four miRNAs (Akkouh et al., 2021). When the expression for the target genes of these four miRNAs were checked in the blood of SCZ and control patients, three genes, *LAMTOR4, IL23R*, and *ERBB3*, were minimally expressed. These genes are involved in the neuro-immune response, suggesting an immune dysregulation in SCZ. Upon IL-1β stimulation, there was a significant difference in the expression of miR-146a-3p, miR-146a- 5p, and miR-4485–3p in control IPSC-Astrocytes, while no such difference was observed in these miRNAs in SCZ IPSC-Astrocytes, implying an inability to respond to immune activators during stress.

Likewise, the previously discussed study by Yen et al. (2025) showed that when the antipsychotic exposed EVs were characterized for the common miRNA panel, miRNA23a was differentially expressed across different antipsychotics. miRNA23a is a known target of the inflammasome axis and microglial motility by binding to CXCR4 (Yeh et al., 2026).

Collectively, these studies suggest that inflammation contributes to the SCZ pathology by the systemic increase of pro-inflammatory cytokines, mitochondrial dysregulation, and epigenetic modifications. However, there are no studies with IPSC-derived oligodendrocytes that explore these cells under inflammatory conditions. Given the complexity of the neuroinflammatory process, these limitations need to be addressed to fully recapitulate the in vivo interactions in a psychiatric conditions under an inflammatory influence.

4. Bipolar disorder

Bipolar Disorder (BD) is a mood disorder characterised by episodes of mania and depression in affected individuals (Singh et al., 2025). BD often co-exists with other psychiatric illnesses and comorbidities, with frequent suicides leading to an increase in mortality rate among BD patients, causing a substantial economic burden (Biazus et al., 2023). In the United States (US) alone, BD was estimated to have an economic burden of more than $195 billion annually (McGrath et al., 2023). With a prevalence of 0.6 % among other psychiatric disorders in India, about 44.9 million Indians were estimated to be diagnosed with BD in 2017 (Sagar et al., 2020).

There are two types of BD: BD-I manifests with alternating episodes of mania and depression, and BD-II with episodes of depression and hypomanic state (Goes, 2023). Commonly prescribed medications are mood stabilizers like Lithium (Li), divalproate, and carbamazepine. However, above 40 % of BD patients do not respond to Li, referred to as Li non-responders (LNRs), and are hence prescribed other mood stabilizers (Papiol, Schulze & Heilbronner, 2022). Often, clinicians combine anti-psychotics and psychosocial interventions with a mood stabilizer to effectively manage the disorder (Ljubic et al., 2021). Unlike SCZ, BD has no direct genetic implications; instead, it is highly polygenic, with overlapping genetic variations with other psychiatric and neurodevelopmental disorders (O'Connell & Coombes, 2021). However, due to the lack of a definitive brain pathology, it is challenging to model BD in a dish.

IPSC models are often used in mood disorders, mostly to test drug responsiveness, but there is accumulating evidence from recent studies showing neurodevelopmental abnormalities in BD patient-derived brain organoids (Phalnikar et al., 2024). Also, repeated fluctuations between states of mania and depression can activate the HPA axis, leading to irregular cortisol levels (Belvederi Murri et al., 2016). Chronic exposure to fluctuating levels of cortisol might trigger systemic inflammation (Chen et al., 2017). While systemic pro-inflammatory phenotypes are frequently reported across the literature, they are contradicted by an equal number of studies showing minimal inflammation in BD patients (Vega-núñez et al., 2022). This inconsistency might be due to the lack of patient stratification and difference in the time of blood draw, as previous studies have reported an increased inflammation during mania and depressive phases and reduced inflammation in the euthymic phase (Özdin & Usta, 2021). Also, differences in the genetic makeup, early exposure to drugs, infections, environmental changes, and other factors might influence immune profiles (Robinson & Bergen, 2021). Therefore, it is essential to understand patient-specific responses in mood disorders and address the differential responses observed across patients. Here, we discuss studies that used IPSC-derived models to understand the effect of neuroinflammation on BD.

4.1 Cellular response to cytokine exposure in BD

Several studies in BD report elevated pro-inflammatory cytokines and chemokines in blood and CSF, thereby implicating both the central and peripheral immune systems (Sayana et al., 2017). These cytokines levels, especially in CSF might be a response to BD induced CNS neuroinflammation that dissipate to the peripheral system too. These are mostly secreted by microglia and astrocytes that interact with neurons in response to inflammation. BD patient IPSCs-derived neurons and astrocytes have been mostly studied to determine the effects of cytokines on these cells.

When BD IPSC-Astrocytes were stimulated with IL-1β and co-cultured with control IPSC-derived neurons, a reduction in the neuronal mean firing rate and spike numbers was observed when compared with stimulated control astrocytes (Vadodaria et al., 2021). This implies that inflamed BD IPSC-Astrocytes affect the neuronal excitability. These stimulated BD IPSC-Astrocytes also showed an increased IL-6 and IL-8 secretion in their CM. To delineate which among these cytokines were responsible for such impaired response, they blocked the cytokine transport from the Endoplasmic Reticulum to ensure it accumulate inside the cells. They found that IL-1β treated cells had a higher percentage of IL-6-positive cells, while IL-8-positive cells were not different from control. To validate that the impaired neuronal activity was due to an increase in IL-6, they treated stimulated BD IPSC-Astrocytes CM with control IPSC-derived glutamatergic neurons and saw a similar ablation in their firing. They additionally pre-treated IPSC-atrocytes with Li, then exposed them to IL-1β, but no significant results were found. This study suggests that the inflammatory profile of BD patient astrocytes affects their mood via IL-6 mediated neuronal hyperexcitability.

In contrast to the previous finding where Li was unable to rescue the inflammatory phenotype observed in neurons, a study by Gottert et al. (2022) showed that, upon LPS and IFN-ɣ stimulation, control IPSC-derived microglial cells had increased *IDO1* mRNA expression (Göttert et al., 2022). *IDO1* gene is responsible for the synthesis of Indoleamine 2,3 dioxygenase 1 (IDO1). It is an enzyme involved in the kynurenine pathway to metabolize tryptophan. Usually, in homeostatic microglia, IDO1 takes tryptophan away from serotonin biosynthesis to produce kynurenine. By inhibiting IDO1, Li maintains the serotonin levels, contributing to mood stability. Li does this by increasing inhibitory phosphorylation of GSK-3β. This leads to a reduction in the phosphorylation of the transcriptional regulators STAT1 and STAT3, thereby blocking their translocation into the nucleus, and inhibiting inflammation-induced gene transcription. This suggests an anti-inflammatory mechanism of lithium via reducing the activity of the IDO1 enzyme.

Altogether, these studies suggest that cellular responses during inflammation play a critical role in the symptom manifestation of BD, especially glial cell responses. These cells communicate within the brain via secreting paracrine signals that, upon inflammation, might be pro-inflammatory. It is also evident from the above studies that Li can reverse some of these negative effects and exerts an anti-inflammatory phenotype.

4.2 Altered Lithium responsiveness in BD

Lithium is the mainstay drug of choice for BD; however, not every patient will respond to lithium administration. About 40 %–50 % of patients with BD require alternatives to Li due to partial response or no response (Lin et al., 2021). To understand the cellular mechanism underlying these responses during inflammation, studies have derived astrocytes and neurons from both Li Responder (LR) and LNR. One such study by Osete et al. (2021) derived IPSC-derived NSC from three LR and three LNR (Osete et al., 2021). Transcriptomic analysis revealed differentially expressed genes (DEGs) that were mostly involved in mitochondrial genes and spliceosome-associated genes. They also found mitochondrial abnormalities that were rescued by Li only in LR lines but not in LNR.

Likewise, a similar finding by Baek et al. (2025) was made. They derived IPSC-Astrocytes from LR and LNR, both groups showed an increased dependence on glycolytic proton efflux rate than OXPHOS, and an increase in cellular glutamate uptake in astrocytes (Baek et al., 2025). Traditionally, mitochondria generate energy through the OXPHOS pathway, only during stress or when there is a high energy demand, mitochondria switches to glycolysis. Here, dependence on glycolytic pathways implies an inherent inflammation or stress in BD cells. But, in contrast with the previous study, here Li did not rescue these bioenergetic variations. However, when lipid droplet accumulation was checked, as they serve as a reservoir to supply fatty acids to fuel OXPHOS in mitochondria, they observed an increase in lipid droplets in both the LR and LNR groups. This lipid droplet accumulation was reduced by Li treatment only in the LR group, suggesting a selective restoration of the phenotype. To validate this, a lipid uptake assay was done by co-culturing IPSC-Astrocytes with neurons, as astrocytes are known to take up lipids from neurons. It was observed that LNR astrocytes take up

Table 2 Mitochondrial dysregulation phenotypes observed across IPSC-derived models in psychiatry.

S no	Disorder	Sample numbers/ patient information	IPSC- patient-derived cell type	Mitochondrial readout	Findings	References
1	SCZ	N = 18 (9 Healthy controls, 9 SCZ patients)	Cortical interneurons	Sea Horse	SCZ interneurons had hyperfunctioning of mitochondria, with reduced ATP production and basal respiration	Ni et al. (2020)
				DCFDA	Higher ROS in SCZ interneurons	
				NAD Assay	Reduced total NAD content in SCZ interneurons	
				RT-PCR	Decreases in the expression of NADH Dehydrogenase complex (ND) in SCZ interneurons	
2	SCZ	N = 5 (3 healthy controls, 2 SCZ patients)	NSC and neurons	LC/MS	Dysregulation in proteins involved in the Krebs cycle and the electron transport chain in SCZ NSCs	Zuccoli et al. (2023)
				Sea Horse	SCZ NSCs had reduced maximal respiration and spare respiratory capacity, and the cells were unable to meet the increased energy demand by reduced basal respiration and ATP-linked respiration	
				DCFDA	Increased ROS levels in SCZ NSCs	
3	BD	N = 9 (3 Healthy controls, 6 patients)	NPCs	Mitophagy assay	Lithium NR had increased mitophagy, and lithium did not rescue it	Osete et al. (2021)
				Sea Horse	Lithium increased the mitochondrial respiration in LR but not in NR	

4	BD	N = 9 (3 healthy control, 3 LR, 3 LNR)	Astrocytes	Sea Horse	Decrease in the ATP production, mitochondria proton efflux rate (PER), and basal respiration in BD Astrocytes	Baek et al. (2025)
				JC1	No significant difference in the mitochondrial membrane potential between BD astrocytes and healthy controls	
				DCFDA	Decrease in the intracellular ROS of BD astrocytes	
5	BD	N = 10 (5 healthy controls, 5 BD patients)	Cerebral organoids	Mito tracker green	No significant difference in the mitochondrial mass between the case and the control	El Soufi El Sabbagh et al. (2025)
				Mito Tracker Red	Mitochondria in the control organoids were more hyperpolarized and healthier compared to BD organoids	
				JC1	Decreased MMP in BD organoids when compared to controls	
				TEM	BD organoids had more round mitochondria than the elongated ones when compared to the control	
				DCFDA	Increase in the extracellular ROS in BD organoids when compared to the control	
				RT-qPCR	BD organoids had a higher amount of cell-free mitochondrial DNA than control organoids	

more lipid droplets than LR astrocytes. To also understand the effect of astrocytic interaction with neurons, a multielectrode array (MEA) was performed. There were a greater number of spikes in neurons cultured with LNR IPSC-Astrocytes than in the Control or LR groups. This study suggests an altered cellular metabolic dysregulation and varied endophenotypes in the developing astrocytes that are manifested as altered Li responses over time, contribute to the pathophysiology of BD.

4.3 Mitochondria-linked neuroinflammation in BD

Mitochondrial dysregulation has been the most consistently observed pathology in BD patients' derived brain cells (Osete et al., 2021), (Baek et al., 2025). It was also observed in cerebral organoid models by Soufi El Sabbagh D E et al (2025) (El Soufi El Sabbagh et al., 2025). This study showed that cerebral organoids derived from BD patients showed elevated mitochondrial membrane potential, ROS, and higher levels of cell-free mtDNA, implying an inflamed state compared to control organoids. Additionally, BD organoids have higher ASC specks in them compared to controls. ASC is one among the components of the inflammasome; upon activation, it assembles with other components to form the NLRP3 complex. They also showed reduced ATP levels in BD organoids. These results suggest a mitochondrial and metabolic dysregulation in BD during the developmental phase. To date, this is the only study that has shown mitochondrial abnormalities in BD organoid models. Despite BD being manifested in adulthood, it is essential to acknowledge these intrinsic dysregulations to design therapeutic approaches to prevent or delay the symptom onset. Table 2 gives a more detailed experimental findings of mitochondrial dysregulation in IPSC-derived cells from psychiatric patients.

5. Autism spectrum disorder

Autism Spectrum disorder (ASD) is a neurodevelopmental disorder characterized by difficulties in social communication and restrictive, repetitive behaviours and interests, with a plausible genetic aetiology (Joon, Kumar & Parle, 2021). ASD individuals exhibit a spectrum of highly heterogeneous symptoms and genetic causes. ASD is often misdiagnosed as Attention Deficit/Hyperactivity Disorder (ADHD) due to similar clinical presentations, leading to a lot of misrepresentation in their epidemiology (Sagar et al., 2020). Remarkably, ASD is about 4 times more prevalent among males.

The cost of treating ASD in the USA and UK is estimated to be around \$2.4 million and \$2.2 million, respectively, for a child (Buescher et al., 2014). The financial burden is deeply concerning, underscoring the necessity for research to aid in and improve diagnosis. Commonly used medications to treat ASD comorbities include selective serotonin reuptake inhibitors (SSRIs), mood stabilizers, anti-psychotics, along with social skill training, and applied behaviour analysis (Aishworiya et al., 2022).

ASD can be influenced mainly by (i) genetic risk factors like heritability, or presence of a novel, de novo genetic variation in an ASD child that is absent in the parents. Genes such as *SHANK3, CHD8, SCN2A*, or large structural Copy Number Variations (CNVs) like deletions or insertions in chromosomal positions 16p11.2, 22q11.2, 15q11-q13 are strongly implicated in ASD (Rylaarsdam & Guemez-Gamboa, 2019), (ii) prenatal factors like maternal infections, stress, pre-gestational metabolic disorders and extreme preterm birth and birth weight, (Wang et al., 2017) and (iii) environmental factors, such as early-life stress, toxins, heavy metals, and pollution (Carter & Blizard, 2016). Postmortem brain tissue expression studies have consistently shown that high-risk ASD genes are expressed predominantly in the neocortex during prenatal stages.

Inflammation has been implicated in ASD in the following conditions-material immune activation, genetic factors, environmental factors like heavy metal exposure and maternal predispositions, such as gestational diabetes and other metabolic abnormalities (Freitas et al., 2018). All these causes convergently lead to a common characteristic of difference in the number of synapses during foetal development that, in turn, is manifested as ASD during the developmental years of a child. For these reasons, IPSC systems are best suited to recapitulate these early neurodevelopmental perturbations in patient-derived brain cells. Here, we discuss the IPSC based studies that have used ASD patient-derived cells to elucidate the inflammatory mechanisms in ASD.

5.1 Glia neuron crosstalk in ASD

In the developing human brain, the neurons and glial cells should work in synchrony to ensure the proper sequential occurrence of developmental events (Jäntti et al., 2026). Loss of a programmed interplay between these cells can lead to neurodevelopmental abnormalities implicated in ASD. IPSC-derived models are critical to understand such interactions, especially in the case of non-syndromic ASD. This interplay is well studied by Russo F B et al (2018), where IPSC-derived NSCs from three non-syndromic

ASD patients were studied (Russo et al., 2018). They found that ASD NSC had a decrease in the expression of synaptogenic markers, dysregulated neural activity, and decreased glutamate production. When astrocytes were derived from these patients, they showed an increase in the ROS levels, glutamate secretion, and increased IL-6 secretion. When ASD astrocytes were co-cultured with control neurons, the neurons showed a decrease in the synaptic puncta, implying a decreased synaptogenesis. They also confirmed that this decrease in synaptogenesis is due to ASD astrocytes via IL-6, by blocking IL-6 in neurons for two weeks, which rescued this effect by showing an increase in the synaptic puncta. This study underscored the importance of neuron glia interaction that contributes to the excess synaptogenesis happening in the developing brain. They also prove that IL-6 plays a major role in accelerating the ASD pathogenesis.

These collective interactions across cells were also observed in organoid models by Ilieva M et al (2022). In this study, four idiopathic ASD patient-derived cerebral organoids were assessed for proliferation, metabolism, and proteome (Ilieva et al., 2022). They found that ASD organoids had higher cell proliferation, mitochondrial respiration, and differential expression of proteins associated with cell cycle and cell adhesion. Unlike the previous study, here they do not pinpoint a specific cause of these dysregulations in the ASD organoid. However, they prove that these dysregulations are consistently observed in a dish model, despite them being asymptomatic in certain cases.

5.2 Genetic risks of neuroinflammation in ASD

Genetic and environmental determinants being a leading cause of ASD, modelling it through IPSC helps understand ASD's molecular pathology, and having IPSC lines from patients with a specific endophenotype like macrocephaly can be informative (Qin et al., 2024). For example, when the disease phenotype of patients with ASD carrying bi-allelic *NRXN1a* deletion was modelled using IPSC, they showed neural circuit dysregulations (Bose et al., 2025). *NRXN1a* is a presynaptic cell adhesion protein crucial for synaptic organization. When microglia were derived from patients carrying these mutations, they had morphological abnormalities with increased activated cells, and secreted more IL-6. IPSC-derived Neuroepithelial-like cells (NES) from these patients also showed variation in their differentiation capacities. When these control IPSC-derived NES that were induced for spontaneous differentiation to neurons were co-cultured with ASD microglia, they showed reduced firing activity. Additionally, by experimenting with the addition of IL-6 in the co-cultures, they were able to show a direct link between IL-6 and abnormal neuronal activity. This study affirms the involvement of IL-6 in ASD and emphasizes modelling patient-specific mutations.

Mansur et al (2021) found that IPSC-derived astrocytes from non-symptomatic ASD patients had a decrease in the expression and protein concentration of Complement protein C4 (Mansur et al., 2021). As C4 proteins are involved in synaptic pruning, a decrease in C4 is correlated with defective synaptic pruning, thereby supporting enhanced brain connectivity observed in ASD patient brains. An opposing effect of an increase in complement-mediated synaptic pruning has been observed in SCZ (Yilmaz et al., 2021). Hence, it makes sense that these disorders have overlapping genetic risk factors.

5.3 Epigenetic regulations in ASD

There is substantial evidence to support that epigenetic alterations contribute to ASD predisposition. Few studies in ASD patient-derived cells have examined the implications of differentially methylated regions (DMRs) for disease physiology (Khogeer, Abomansour & Mohammed, 2022). The changes in the DMR contribute to the disorder by affecting the promoter CpG regions, thereby controlling the respective gene expression. Using IPSC-derived NSCs, neurons, and astrocytes from idiopathic ASD patients Abdolmaleky H M et al (2024) found DMRs in ASD inflammatory risk genes (Mostafavi Abdolmaleky et al., 2024). They found increased expression of the *IL-6, TGFβ1, TGFβ2,* and *IFI16* genes in IPSC-Astrocytes from these patients. Correspondingly, the *TGFβ1* promoter was almost completely unmethylated in ASD IPSC-Astrocytes. In neurons, *IL-6* and *HAP1* were hyper expressed. Epigenetically, in these neurons, they observed a hypomethylated pattern in the *HAP1* genes, while other genes like *IFI16* and *SCL1A3* were hypermethylated. The risk genes of ASD that are hypomethylated were highly expressed which contribute to ASD pathophysiology. They also observed an abnormal morphology of IPSC astrocytes derived from ASD patients. This epigenetic pattern was also observed in post-mortem brains of ASD patients. Thereby, the study reiterates the association of IL-6 in ASD and supports that IPSC models mimic the in vivo epigenetic regulations observed in patient blood and post-mortem studies.

6. Additional psychiatric disorders

Apart from the above-mentioned psychiatric disorders, there are many other psychiatric disorders that remain relatively underexplored, particularly in the context of IPSC-based models. Disorders such as obsessive-compulsive disorders (OCD), Anxiety and panic disorders, etc., are yet to be modelled in a petri dish. This section highlights some emerging studies in other psychiatric conditions, including Major Depressive Disorder (MDD) and ADHD. Additionally, Table 3 summarizes existing IPSC-derived models for psychiatric disorders that have received comparatively limited research attention.

6.1 IPSC research in major depressive disorder

Major Depressive Disorder (MDD) is a mood disorder in which a common emotion, depression, is felt for a chronic duration despite the absence of any external stimuli (Otte et al., 2016). It is characterized by a persistent feeling of sadness, loss of interest, and low self-esteem affecting cognition, neurovegetative functions, and psychomotor activities (Fava & Kendler, 2000). Treatment for MDD includes Tricyclic antidepressants, SSRIs, serotonin-norepinephrine reuptake inhibitors (SNRIs) in combination with dietary adjustments, exercise, sleep improvement, and social interventions (Cui et al., 2024). Most studies in MDD have been done in animal models, in which the behavioural phenotypes have been replicated. However, animal brains do not have the structural complexity observed in human brains, and we cannot model the genetic make-up of an MDD patient in animal systems. This necessitates the need to use, human IPSC-based models to elucidate the cellular and molecular phenotype of MDD patients.

A study by Cardon et al. (2025) showed that IPSC-derived NSCs from MDD patients showed reduced mitochondrial respiration rates and differences in basal calcium levels (Cardon et al., 2024). Neurons derived from these patients showed reduced standard membrane potential and elevated neuronal firing. The higher neural activity might be due to a compensatory mechanism that the cells acquire during the process of differentiation. Although, this study does not report mitochondrial activity in neurons, it showed that cellular functions are altered in MDD IPSC-derived cells, which may be rooted to a genetic cause.

In mood disorders, there is always a subset of patients who do not respond to mood stabilizers due to abrupt discontinuation of the medications or genetic liabilities (Papiol, Schulze & Heilbronner, 2022). (Triebelhorn, 2024) showed

Table 3 IPSC-derived models in other psychiatric disorders.

S no	Disorder	Model system	Source IPSC	Summary	References
1.	Anorexia Nervosa (AN)	IPSC-derived neurons	4 adolescent females with AN and 4 healthy female controls	The study identifies a novel transcriptional disruption of the tachykinin system, specifically the upregulation of the *TACR1* gene, as a potential driver of the disorder's molecular pathophysiology	Negraes et al. (2017)
2	Anorexia Nervosa (AN)	IPSC-derived neurons	4 adolescent females with AN and 4 healthy female controls	Transcriptomic analysis of neurons derived from anorexia nervosa patients reveals a signature of differentially expressed genes, such as *TACR1* and *CALCB*, that are uniquely enriched in microglia and subcortical appetitive circuits like the lateral parabrachial nucleus	Howard et al. (2020)
3	PTSD	IPSC-derived glutamatergic neurons	19 donors with a PTSD diagnosis and 20 combat-exposed controls without PTSD	PTSD-derived neurons exhibit a unique glucocorticoid hypersensitivity, characterized by diagnosis-specific transcriptomic signatures that significantly overlap with patterns found in postmortem PTSD brain tissue	Seah et al. (2022)

(continued)

Table 3 IPSC-derived models in other psychiatric disorders. (*cont'd*)

S no	Disorder	Model system	Source IPSC	Summary	References
4	PTSD/MDD	IPSC-derived cortical neurons	11 PTSD, 10 MDD, and 11 neurotypical controls	By exposing hiPSC-derived neurons to glucocorticoids, this study demonstrates that the resulting transcriptomic changes positively correlate with the gene expression signatures found in PTSD patients but show an opposite direction of regulation compared to MDD, particularly within excitatory neurons	Chatzinakos et al. (2023)
5	Tourette's syndrome(TS)	IPSC-derived neurons	2 TS affected, 1 unaffected family member, 1 unrelated unaffected subject	A rare nonsense mutation in TS-patient-derived neurons causes nonsense-mediated decay of the brain-enriched *PNKD* long isoform, leading to a significant reduction of both PNKD (L) and its synaptic partner RIMS1	Sun et al. (2018)
6	Tourette's syndrome	IPSC-derived basal ganglia organoids	5 TS affected, 11 healthy unaffected subjects	TS-derived basal ganglia organoids exhibit early developmental mispatterning and a deficit in GABAergic and cholinergic interneurons driven by cilia dysfunction and the over-activation of GLI repressor proteins within the Sonic Hedgehog signaling pathway	Brady et al. (2022)

that such patients respond to neurotransmitters like serotonin by altering gene expression in MDD patient-derived neurons and astrocytes- especially genes related to mitochondrial respiration. This underpins the findings of previous study on mitochondrial dysregulation (Triebelhorn et al., 2024). Direct serotonin treatment of astrocytes was able to mildly influence the ATP and mitochondrial respiration; however, it was not significant. More importantly, they showed that neurons from non-responder patients had an increase in the excitatory transmission when they were exposed to serotonin. This implies that even though the non-responder does not respond to medication, they can respond to neurotransmitters like serotonin, thus addressing the "serotonin hypothesis" which states that deficiency or decrease in serotonin activity in the brain causes depression (Bremshey et al., 2024).

6.2 IPSC research in attention-deficit/ hyperactivity disorder

Attention-deficit/Hyperactivity disorder (ADHD) is a behavioural disorder often observed in children that might also persist into adulthood (Núñez-Jaramillo, Herrera-Solís & Herrera-Morales, 2021). It is presented by hyperactivity, impulsiveness, and inattention. As reported by the WHO, adult ADHD affects 2.8 % of the global population, with a greater prevalence in high-income countries and a notable correlation with lower educational attainment (Fayyad et al., 2017). Causes of ADHD include brain anatomical changes, heavy metal exposure, premature delivery, substance use during pregnancy, and genetics (Sapkale & Sawal, 2023). Treatment for ADHD includes psychostimulants like Methylphenidate and Amphetamine derivatives, and antidepressants, among others. At times, behavioural therapies with or without stimulants and cognitive training are also recommended (Caye et al., 2019). Maternal immune activation, allergic reactions, and autoimmune activations have been associated with the inflammatory pathophysiology of ADHD.

Additionally, decreases in essential fatty acids have also been a risk factor for ADHD, where ADHD symptoms were negatively correlated with Docosahexaenoic Acid (DHA) levels in the blood of ADHD children (Pei-Chen Chang, 2021). To check if the supplementation of essential fatty acids can rescue ADHD phenotype in cellular models, a study by Walter NM et al (2025) used IPSC-derived NSCs from ADHD patients. Firstly, to check if an inflammatory phenotype is manifested, they checked for mtDNA in patient-derived cortical neurons and their saliva, and they found increased mtDNA concentration in patient-derived cortical neurons (Walter et al., 2025). As they also showed an increase in superoxide, the patient-derived cells were treated with omega-3 fatty acids – DHA, and Eicosapentaenoic Acid (EPA), and Omega-6 fatty acid – Archidonic Acid (AA). They found that EPA had a positive influence on superoxide levels but without a statistically significant change. Further, they reported that when ADHD neurons were cultured with their respective astrocytes, IL-6 secretion increased compared to cultures containing only neurons. They found a negative correlation with IL-6 secretion and NSC proliferation. However, omega-3 fatty acids were unable to rescue these effects. This study proves that manifestation of ADHD involves a neuron-glia crosstalk and that omega-3 fatty acids were not enough to rescue these effects.

These challenges the findings of a double-blinded study where 103 ADHD children were given omega-3 supplements that reduced inflammation in the peripheral blood of children with ADHD (Hariri et al., 2012). This also implies that there is a distinct difference in the observations made in the peripheral and the CNS in ADHD, that there is a need for further research.

7. Conclusion

This chapter underscores the importance of using patient derived IPSC brain cells to model neuroinflammation in psychiatric disorders. Several studies have used different cytokines to mimic inflammatory environment or used neuron-glial co-culture system to produce neuro-immune interaction mimicking their cellular environment and responses in the brain. These patient derived cells exhibit an inflammatory phenotype primarily in the form of cytokine and chemokine release, mitochondrial dysregulations, altered neuronal activity and epigenetic modifications. The above-mentioned phenotypes have been studied mostly in IPSC-derived neurons, astrocytes, and microglia, with oligodendrocytes and other cell types of the brain still under-represented. Besides, there are certain limitations in using IPSC models as they do not accurately model adult brain (Hong et al., 2023). There is also heterogeneity that stems from the use of different differentiation protocol that might alter cellular response and influence epigenetic makeup of the cell. Despite these, IPSC remains an extremely valuable resource as it counteracts the problem of brain tissue inaccessibility.

There are also certain experimental caveats that needs to be addressed in future studies to substantiate the findings. Firstly, in most psychiatric disorders, peripheral inflammatory markers have been studied extensively compared to CSF markers (Carvalho et al., 2020). This is understandable as obtaining CSF is an invasive technique. However, studying the important CNS markers from CSF would provide a better understanding of brain's microenvironment that is the closest representation of the diseased brain. Moreover, analysis of peripheral systemic markers has several drawbacks- they are variable and hence may not be a direct representation of the disorder of interest.

Secondly, with regards to the cellular experimental models of neuroinflammation, there are inconsistencies in the type, concentration of the stimulant and the duration of exposure (Table 1). There are ample evidence showing the differential responses of cells with respect to the duration of cytokine stimulation. For example, in this study, Vadodaria et al. (2021) showed higher concentration of IL-8 in the initial 5 h of IL-1β treatment using dot blots, while it reduced after 24h (Vadodaria et al., 2021). In some cases, where the concentration of a cytokine was considered cytotoxic, the similar concentration in another study showed a minimal response. Hence, to mitigate this disparity, researchers should try to set a range that should be considered standard for each cell type or use a commercial stimulant like the cell stimulation cocktails to ensure fewer experimental variants.

Thirdly, IPSCs cannot model the behavioural dynamics of psychiatric disorders. For instance, in mood disorders like BD it is important to acknowledge that the level of peripheral cytokines might be influenced by the specific symptom presented by the patient (e.g.: mania, depression or euthymia). Most studies do not account for these differences in their study design leading to counterintuitive findings. Also, these phases of BD presentation cannot be accurately models in IPSC systems.

Finally, there were additional studies that used healthy IPSC brain cells to model neuroinflammation as a proof of concept. However, it is essential to study them in the background of patients' genetic make-up. Additionally, mutation studies must show phenotype reversal on gene correction that is essential for disease-specific risk gene assessment.

Overall, this chapter underpins the importance of modelling neuroinflammation using IPSC-derived cellular models, highlights the molecular and cellular convergence across psychiatric disorders, and brain cell-type-specific differential inflammatory responses. Considering the complexity of these disorders and the brain structure and function, further refinement, and advancement in all aspects of this technology is essential- including modelling other brain cell types and regions using 3D organoid systems- to accurately recapitulate psychiatric disease phenotypes in a dish.

References

Aboraya, A., Rankin, E., France, C., El-Missiry, A., & John, C. (2006). The Reliability of Psychiatric Diagnosis Revisited: The Clinician's Guide to Improve the Reliability of Psychiatric Diagnosis. *Psychiatry (Edgmont), 3*(1), 41–50. PMID: 21103149; PMCID: PMC2990547.

Aishworiya, R., et al. (2022). An update on psychopharmacological treatment of autism spectrum disorder. *Neurotherapeutics: the Journal of the American Society for Experimental NeuroTherapeutics, 19*(1), 248–262. https://doi.org/10.1007/s13311-022-01183-1.

Akkouh, I. A., Ueland, T., Hansson, L., Inderhaug, E., Hughes, T., Steen, N. E., ... Djurovic, S. (2020). Decreased IL-1β-induced CCL20 response in human iPSC-astrocytes in schizophrenia: Potential attenuating effects on recruitment of regulatory T cells. *Brain, Behavior, and Immunity, 87*, 634–644. https://doi.org/10.1016/j.bbi.2020.02.008.

Akkouh, I. A., et al. (2020). Decreased IL-1β-induced CCL20 response in human iPSC-astrocytes in schizophrenia: Potential attenuating effects on recruitment of regulatory T cells. *Brain, Behavior, and Immunity, 87*, 634–644. https://doi.org/10.1016/j.bbi.2020.02.008.

Akkouh, I. A., et al. (2021). Transcriptome analysis reveals disparate expression of inflammation-related miRNAs and their gene targets in iPSC-astrocytes from people with schizophrenia. *Brain, Behavior, and Immunity, 94*, 235–244. https://doi.org/10.1016/j.bbi.2021.01.037.

Albrecht, D. S., et al. (2016). Vivo imaging of human neuroinflammation. *ACS Chemical Neuroscience,* 7(4), 470–483. https://doi.org/10.1021/acschemneuro.6b00056.

Baek, G. H., Kim, D., Son, G., Do, H., Yeon, G. B., Lee, M. J., ... Han, J. (2025). Differential effects of lithium on metabolic dysfunctions in astrocytes derived from bipolar disorder patients. *Molecular Psychiatry, 30*(12), 5833–5848. https://doi.org/10.1038/s41380-025-03176-w.

Baek, G. H., et al. (2025). Differential effects of lithium on metabolic dysfunctions in astrocytes derived from bipolar disorder patients. *Molecular Psychiatry, 30*(12), 5833–5848. https://doi.org/10.1038/s41380-025-03176-w.

Beekhuis-Hoekstra, S., et al. Patient iPSC-derived astrocytes with high polygenic risk for schizophrenia reveals a role for mitochondrial glutamate carrier SLC25A18 2022. https://doi.org/10.21203/rs.3.rs-1811182/v1.

Belvederi Murri, M., et al. (2016). The HPA axis in bipolar disorder: Systematic review and meta-analysis. *Psychoneuroendocrinology,* 327–342. https://doi.org/10.1016/j.psyneuen.2015.10.014.

Biazus, T. B., et al. (2023). All-cause and cause-specific mortality among people with bipolar disorder: A large-scale systematic review and meta-analysis. *Molecular Psychiatry,* 2508–2524. https://doi.org/10.1038/s41380-023-02109-9.

Bose, R., et al. (2025). Bi-allelic NRXN1α deletion in microglia derived from iPSC of an autistic patient increases interleukin-6 production and impairs supporting function on neuronal networking. *Brain, Behavior, and Immunity, 123*, 28–42. https://doi.org/10.1016/j.bbi.2024.09.001.

Brady, M. V., Mariani, J., Koca, Y., Szekely, A., King, R. A., Bloch, M. H., ... Vaccarino, F. M. (2022). Mispatterning and interneuron deficit in tourette syndrome basal ganglia organoids. *Molecular Psychiatry, 27*(12), 5007–5019. https://doi.org/10.1038/s41380-022-01880-5.

Bremshey, S., et al. (2024). The role of serotonin in depression—A historical roundup and future directions. *Journal of Neurochemistry,* 1751–1779. https://doi.org/10.1111/jnc.16097.

Buescher, A. V. S., et al. (2014). Costs of autism spectrum disorders in the United Kingdom and the United States. *JAMA Pediatrics, 168*(8), 721–728. https://doi.org/10.1001/jamapediatrics.2014.210.

Cabezas, R., et al. (2014). Astrocytic modulation of blood brain barrier: Perspectives on Parkinson's disease. *Frontiers in Cellular Neuroscience.* https://doi.org/10.3389/fncel.2014.00211 Frontiers Research Foundation.

Cardon, I., et al. (2024). Serotonin effects on human iPSC-derived neural cell functions: From mitochondria to depression. *Molecular Psychiatry, 29*(9), 2689–2700. https://doi.org/10.1038/s41380-024-02538-0.

Cardozo, P. L., Lee, C. Y., Lacerda, J. P. S., Fahel, J. S., Trindade, P., Vitória, G., ... Ribeiro, F. M. (2025). hiPSC-derived astrocytes from individuals with schizophrenia induce a dystrophic phenotype in microglial-like cells. *Glia*. https://doi.org/10.1002/glia.70085.

Cardozo, P. L., et al. (2025). hiPSC-derived astrocytes from individuals with schizophrenia induce a dystrophic phenotype in microglial-like cells. *GLIA [Preprint]*. https://doi.org/10.1002/glia.70085.

Carter, C. J., & Blizard, R. A. (2016). Autism genes are selectively targeted by environmental pollutants including pesticides, heavy metals, bisphenol A, phthalates and many others in food, cosmetics or household products. *Neurochemistry International*, 83–109. https://doi.org/10.1016/j.neuint.2016.10.011.

Carvalho, A. F., et al. (2020). Evidence-based umbrella review of 162 peripheral biomarkers for major mental disorders. *Translational Psychiatry, 10*(1), 152. https://doi.org/10.1038/s41398-020-0835-5.

Caye, A., et al. (2019). Treatment strategies for ADHD: An evidence-based guide to select optimal treatment. *Molecular Psychiatry*, 390–408. https://doi.org/10.1038/s41380-018-0116-3.

Chatzinakos, C., Pernia, C. D., Morrison, F. G., Iatrou, A., McCullough, K. M., Schuler, H., ... Daskalakis, N. P. (2023). Single-nucleus transcriptome profiling of dorsolateral prefrontal cortex: Mechanistic roles for neuronal gene expression, including the 17q21.31 locus, in PTSD stress response. *The American Journal of Psychiatry, 180*(10), 739–754. https://doi.org/10.1176/appi.ajp.20220478.

Chen, X., et al. (2017). HPA-axis and inflammatory reactivity to acute stress is related with basal HPA-axis activity. *Psychoneuroendocrinology, 78*, 168–176. https://doi.org/10.1016/j.psyneuen.2017.01.035.

Cui, L., et al. (2024). Major depressive disorder: Hypothesis, mechanism, prevention and treatment. *Signal Transduction and Targeted Therapy*. https://doi.org/10.1038/s41392-024-01738-y Springer Nature.

El Soufi El Sabbagh, D., et al. (2025). iPSC-derived cerebral organoids reveal mitochondrial, inflammatory and neuronal vulnerabilities in bipolar disorder. *Translational Psychiatry, 15*(1), https://doi.org/10.1038/s41398-025-03529-7.

Fadilah, N. I. M., Fauzi, M. B., & Maarof, M. (2024). Effect of multiple-cycle collections of conditioned media from different cell sources towards fibroblasts in in vitro wound healing model. *Pharmaceutics, 16*(6), https://doi.org/10.3390/pharmaceutics16060767.

Fava, M., & Kendler, K. S. (2000). Review major depressive disordertions in "first-world" countries such as the United States. *Neuron*.

Fayyad, J., et al. (2017). The descriptive epidemiology of DSM-IV Adult ADHD in the World Health Organization World Mental Health Surveys. *ADHD Attention Deficit and Hyperactivity Disorders, 9*(1), 47–65. https://doi.org/10.1007/s12402-016-0208-3.

Freitas, B. C., et al. (2018). Modeling inflammation in autism spectrum disorders using stem cells. *Frontiers in Pediatrics*. https://doi.org/10.3389/fped.2018.00394 Frontiers Media S.A.

Giff, A. E., et al. (2026). Deep cervical lymph node analysis in central nervous system inflammatory disease. *Frontiers in Immunology*. https://doi.org/10.3389/fimmu.2026.1747114 Frontiers Media SA.

Goes, F. S. (2023). Diagnosis and management of bipolar disorders. *British Medical Journal*. https://doi.org/10.1136/bmj-2022-073591.

Göttert, R., et al. (2022). Lithium inhibits tryptophan catabolism via the inflammation-induced kynurenine pathway in human microglia. *Glia, 70*(3), 558–571. https://doi.org/10.1002/glia.24123.

Gracias, J., et al. (2022). Cerebrospinal fluid concentration of complement component 4A is increased in first episode schizophrenia. *Nature Communications, 13*(1), https://doi.org/10.1038/s41467-022-33797-6.

Hariri, M., et al. (2012). Effect of n-3 supplementation on hyperactivity, oxidative stress and inflammatory mediators in children with attention-deficit-hyperactivity disorder. *Malaysian Journal of Nutrition, 18*, 329–335.

Haroon, E., et al. (2018). Antidepressant treatment resistance is associated with increased inflammatory markers in patients with major depressive disorder. *Psychoneuroendocrinology, 95*, 43–49. https://doi.org/10.1016/j.psyneuen.2018.05.026.

Hjorthøj, C., et al. (2017). Years of potential life lost and life expectancy in schizophrenia: A systematic review and meta-analysis. *The Lancet Psychiatry, 4*(4), 295–301. https://doi.org/10.1016/S2215-0366(17)30078-0.

Hong, Y., et al. (2023). Opportunities and limitations for studying neuropsychiatric disorders using patient-derived induced pluripotent stem cells. *Molecular Psychiatry*, 1430–1439. https://doi.org/10.1038/s41380-023-01990-8.

Howard, D., Negraes, P., Voineskos, A. N., Kaplan, A. S., Muotri, A. R., Duvvuri, V., & French, L. (2020). Molecular neuroanatomy of anorexia nervosa. *Scientific Reports, 10*(1), https://doi.org/10.1038/s41598-020-67692-1.

Howes, O. D., & Onwordi, E. C. (2023). The synaptic hypothesis of schizophrenia version III: A master mechanism. *Molecular Psychiatry, 28*(5), 1843–1856. https://doi.org/10.1038/s41380-023-02043-w.

Ilieva, M., et al. (2022). Proteomic phenotype of cerebral organoids derived from autism spectrum disorder patients reveal disrupted energy metabolism, cellular components, and biological processes. *Molecular Psychiatry, 27*(9), 3749–3759. https://doi.org/10.1038/s41380-022-01627-2.

Jäntti, H., et al. (2026). Non-neuronal mechanisms in autism spectrum disorder (ASD): Microglia and astrocytes at the crossroads with neurons. *Brain, Behavior, and Immunity, 133*, 106275. https://doi.org/10.1016/j.bbi.2026.106275.

Joon, P., Kumar, A., & Parle, M. (2021). What is autism? *Pharmacological Reports*, 1255–1264. https://doi.org/10.1007/s43440-021-00244-0.

Khogeer, A. A., Abomansour, I. S., & Mohammed, D. A. (2022). The role of genetics, epigenetics, and the environment in ASD: A mini review. *Epigenomes*. https://doi.org/10.3390/epigenomes6020015 MDPI.

Limanaqi, F., et al. (2019). A sentinel in the crosstalk between the nervous and immune system: The (immuno)-proteasome. *Frontiers in Immunology*. https://doi.org/10.3389/fimmu.2019.00628 Frontiers Media S.A.

Lin, Y., et al. (2021). Clinical predictors of non-response to lithium treatment in the pharmacogenomics of bipolar disorder (PGBD) study. *Bipolar Disorders, 23*(8), 821–831. https://doi.org/10.1111/bdi.13078.

Liu, S. H., et al. (2022). Glial cell abnormalities in major psychiatric diseases: A systematic review of postmortem brain studies. *Molecular Neurobiology*, 1665–1692. https://doi.org/10.1007/s12035-021-02672-8.

Ljubic, N., et al. (2021). Treatment of bipolar disorders in older adults: a review. *Annals of General Psychiatry*. https://doi.org/10.1186/s12991-021-00367-x BioMed Central Ltd.

Luvsannyam, E., et al. (2022). Neurobiology of schizophrenia: A comprehensive review. *Cureus [Preprint]*. https://doi.org/10.7759/cureus.23959.

Luvsannyam, E., Jain, M. S., Pormento, M. K. L., Siddiqui, H., Balagtas, A. R. A., Emuze, B. O., & Poprawski, T. (2022). Neurobiology of Schizophrenia: A Comprehensive Review. *Cureus, 14*(4), e23959. https://doi.org/10.7759/cureus.23959 PMID: 35541299; PMCID: PMC9080788.

Mansur, F., et al. (2021). Complement c4 is reduced in ipsc-derived astrocytes of autism spectrum disorder subjects. *International Journal of Molecular Sciences, 22*(14), https://doi.org/10.3390/ijms22147579.

McGrath, J. J., et al. (2023). Age of onset and cumulative risk of mental disorders: A cross-national analysis of population surveys from 29 countries. *The Lancet Psychiatry, 10*(9), 668–681. https://doi.org/10.1016/S2215-0366(23)00193-1.

Mostafavi Abdolmaleky, H., et al. (2024). iPSC-derived astrocytes and neurons replicate brain gene expression, epigenetic, cell morphology and connectivity alterations found in autism. *Cells, 13*(13), https://doi.org/10.3390/cells13131095.

Negraes, P. D., Cugola, F. R., Herai, R. H., Trujillo, C. A., Cristino, A. S., Chailangkarn, T., ... Duvvuri, V. (2017). Modeling anorexia nervosa: Transcriptional insights from human iPSC-derived neurons. *Translational Psychiatry,* 7(3), https://doi.org/10.1038/tp.2017.37.

Nesci, S., Spagnoletta, A., & Oppedisano, F. (2023). Inflammation, mitochondria and natural compounds together in the circle of trust. *International Journal of Molecular Sciences*. https://doi.org/10.3390/ijms24076106.

Ni, P., et al. (2020). iPSC-derived homogeneous populations of developing schizophrenia cortical interneurons have compromised mitochondrial function. *Molecular Psychiatry, 25*(11), 2873–2888. https://doi.org/10.1038/s41380-019-0423-3.

Ni, P., Noh, H., Park, G. H., Shao, Z., Guan, Y., Park, J. M., ... Chung, S. (2020). iPSC-derived homogeneous populations of developing schizophrenia cortical interneurons have compromised mitochondrial function. *Molecular Psychiatry, 25*(11), 2873–2888. https://doi.org/10.1038/s41380-019-0423-3.

Núñez-Jaramillo, L., Herrera-Solís, A., & Herrera-Morales, W. V. (2021). Adhd: Reviewing the causes and evaluating solutions. *Journal of Personalized Medicine,* 1–25. https://doi.org/10.3390/jpm11030166.

O'Connell, K. S., & Coombes, B. J. (2021). Genetic contributions to bipolar disorder: Current status and future directions. *Psychological medicine*. Cambridge University Press, 2156–2167. https://doi.org/10.1017/S0033291721001252.

Osete, J. R., Akkouh, I. A., de Assis, D. R., Szabo, A., Frei, E., Hughes, T., ... Djurovic, S. (2021). Lithium increases mitochondrial respiration in iPSC-derived neural precursor cells from lithium responders. *Molecular Psychiatry, 26*(11), 6789–6805. https://doi.org/10.1038/s41380-021-01164-4.

Osete, J. R., et al. (2021). Lithium increases mitochondrial respiration in iPSC-derived neural precursor cells from lithium responders. *Molecular Psychiatry, 26*(11), 6789–6805. https://doi.org/10.1038/s41380-021-01164-4.

Otte, C., et al. (2016). Major depressive disorder. *Nature Reviews Disease Primers*. https://doi.org/10.1038/nrdp.2016.65 Nature Publishing Group.

Özdin, S., & Usta, M. B. (2021). A comparison of inflammatory markers in manic and euthymic states of bipolar disorder. *Nordic Journal of Psychiatry, 75*(2), 124–129. https://doi.org/10.1080/08039488.2020.1807048.

Papiol, S., Schulze, T. G., & Heilbronner, U. (2022). Lithium response in bipolar disorder: Genetics, genomics, and beyond. *Neuroscience Letters, 785*, 136786. https://doi.org/10.1016/j.neulet.2022.136786.

Patel, K. R., Cherian, J., Gohil, K., & Atkinson, D. (2014). Schizophrenia: overview and treatment options. *P T, 39*(9), 638–645. PMID: 25210417; PMCID: PMC4159061.

Pavlinek, A., Matuleviciute, R., Sichlinger, L., Dutan Polit, L., Armeniakos, N., Vernon, A. C., & Srivastava, D. P. (2022). Interferon-γ exposure of human iPSC-derived neurons alters major histocompatibility complex I and synapsin protein expression. *Front Psychiatry, 13*, 836217. https://doi.org/10.3389/fpsyt.2022.836217 PMID: 36186864; PMCID: PMC9515429.

Pei-Chen Chang, J. (2021). Personalised medicine in child and adolescent psychiatry: Focus on omega-3 polyunsaturated fatty acids and ADHD. *Brain, Behavior, and Immunity - Health, 16*. https://doi.org/10.1016/j.bbih.2021.100310.

Phalnikar, K., et al. (2024). Altered neuroepithelial morphogenesis and migration defects in iPSC-derived cerebral organoids and 2D neural stem cells in familial bipolar disorder. *Oxford Open Neuroscience, 3*. https://doi.org/10.1093/oons/kvae007.

Qin, L., et al. (2024). New advances in the diagnosis and treatment of autism spectrum disorders. *European Journal of Medical Research,* 322. https://doi.org/10.1186/s40001-024-01916-2.

Rantala, M. J., et al. (2022). Schizophrenia: The new etiological synthesis. *Neuroscience & Biobehavioral Reviews, 142*, 104894. https://doi.org/10.1016/j.neubiorev.2022.104894.

Renault, P. F., et al. (1987). Psychiatric complications of long-term interferon alfa therapy. *Archives of Internal Medicine, 147*(9), 1577–1580. https://doi.org/10.1001/archinte.1987.00370090055011.

Robinson, N., & Bergen, S. E. (2021). Environmental risk factors for schizophrenia and bipolar disorder and their relationship to genetic risk: Current knowledge and future directions. *Frontiers in Genetics*. https://doi.org/10.3389/fgene.2021.686666 Frontiers Media S.A.

Roser, M., Ritchie, H., & Spooner, F. (2021). Burden of disease. *Our World in Data* ([Preprint]).

Russo, F. B., et al. (2018). Modeling the interplay between neurons and astrocytes in autism using human induced pluripotent stem cells. *Biological Psychiatry, 83*(7), 569–578. https://doi.org/10.1016/j.biopsych.2017.09.021.

Rylaarsdam, L., & Guemez-Gamboa, A. (2019). Genetic causes and modifiers of autism spectrum disorder. *Frontiers in Cellular Neuroscience*. https://doi.org/10.3389/fncel.2019.00385 Frontiers Media S.A.

Sagar, R., et al. (2020). The burden of mental disorders across the states of India: The Global Burden of disease study 1990–2017. *The Lancet Psychiatry,* 7(2), 148–161. https://doi.org/10.1016/S2215-0366(19)30475-4.

Salleh, M. R. (2004). The genetics of schizophrenia. *Malays J Med Sci, 11*(2), 3–11. PMID: 22973121; PMCID: PMC3433970.

Sapkale, B., & Sawal, A. (2023). Attention deficit hyperactivity disorder (ADHD) causes and diagnosis in adults: A review. *Cureus [Preprint]*. https://doi.org/10.7759/cureus.49144.

Sayana, P., et al. (2017). A systematic review of evidence for the role of inflammatory biomarkers in bipolar patients. *Journal of Psychiatric Research, 92*, 160–182. https://doi.org/10.1016/j.jpsychires.2017.03.018.

Schumacher, A. E., et al. (2024). Global age-sex-specific mortality, life expectancy, and population estimates in 204 countries and territories and 811 subnational locations, 1950–2021, and the impact of the COVID-19 pandemic: A comprehensive demographic analysis for the Global Burden of Disease Study 2021. *The Lancet, 403*(10440), 1989–2056. https://doi.org/10.1016/S0140-6736(24)00476-8.

Seah, C., Breen, M. S., Rusielewicz, T., Bader, H. N., Xu, C., Hunter, C. J., ... Yehuda, R. (2022). Modeling gene × environment interactions in PTSD using human neurons reveals diagnosis-specific glucocorticoid-induced gene expression. *Nature Neuroscience, 25*(11), 1434–1445. https://doi.org/10.1038/s41593-022-01161-y.

Sekar, A., et al. (2016). Schizophrenia risk from complex variation of complement component 4. *Nature, 530*(7589), 177–183. https://doi.org/10.1038/nature16549.

Shabab, T., et al. (2017). Neuroinflammation pathways: A general review. *International Journal of Neuroscience, 127*(7), 624–633. https://doi.org/10.1080/00207454.2016.1212854.

Singh, B., et al. (2025). Bipolar disorder. *The Lancet,* 963–978. https://doi.org/10.1016/S0140-6736(25)01140-7.

Stöberl, N., et al. (2023). Human iPSC-derived glia models for the study of neuroinflammation. *Journal of Neuroinflammation*. https://doi.org/10.1186/s12974-023-02919-2 BioMed Central Ltd.

Summers, R. A., et al. (2024). Novel human iPSC models of neuroinflammation in neurodegenerative disease and regenerative medicine. *Trends in Immunology, 45*(10), 799–813. https://doi.org/10.1016/j.it.2024.08.004.

Sun, N., Nasello, C., Deng, L., Wang, N., Zhang, Y., Xu, Z., ... Tischfield, J. A. (2018). The PNKD gene is associated with tourette disorder or Tic disorder in a multiplex family. *Molecular Psychiatry, 23*(6), 1487–1495. https://doi.org/10.1038/mp.2017.179.

Szabo, A., et al. (2025). NLRP3 inflammasome mediates astroglial dysregulation of innate and adaptive immune responses in schizophrenia. *Brain, Behavior, and Immunity, 124*, 144–156. https://doi.org/10.1016/j.bbi.2024.11.030.

Szabo, A., Akkouh, I., Osete, J. R., de Assis, D. R., Kondratskaya, E., Hughes, T., ... Djurovic, S. (2025). NLRP3 inflammasome mediates astroglial dysregulation of innate and adaptive immune responses in schizophrenia. *Brain, Behavior, and Immunity, 124*, 144–156. https://doi.org/10.1016/j.bbi.2024.11.030.

Tanaka, M., & Vécsei, L. (2024). From lab to life: Exploring cutting-edge models for neurological and psychiatric disorders. *Biomedicines*. https://doi.org/10.3390/biomedicines12030613.

Triebelhorn, J., et al. (2024). Induced neural progenitor cells and iPS-neurons from major depressive disorder patients show altered bioenergetics and electrophysiological properties. *Molecular Psychiatry, 29*(5), 1217–1227. https://doi.org/10.1038/s41380-022-01660-1.

Trindade, P., Nascimento, J. M., Casas, B. S., Monteverde, T., Gasparotto, J., Ribeiro, C. T., ... Rehen, S. K. (2023). Induced pluripotent stem cell-derived astrocytes from patients with schizophrenia exhibit an inflammatory phenotype that affects vascularization. *Molecular Psychiatry, 28*(2), 871–882. https://doi.org/10.1038/s41380-022-01830-1.

Trindade, P., Nascimento, J. M., Casas, B. S., et al. (2023). Induced pluripotent stem cell-derived astrocytes from patients with schizophrenia exhibit an inflammatory phenotype that affects vascularization. *Molecular Psychiatry, 28*(2), 871–882. https://doi.org/10.1038/s41380-022-01830-1.

Trivedi, J. K., Goel, D., & Resident, J. (2006). What psychiatry means to us. *Mens Sana Monographs*.

Upthegrove, R., et al. (2025). Current position and future direction of inflammation in neuropsychiatric disorders: A review. *JAMA Psychiatry, 82*(10), 1030–1046. https://doi.org/10.1001/jamapsychiatry.2025.1369.

Upthegrove, R, Corsi-Zuelli, F, Couch, ACM, Barnes, NM, & Vernon, AC (2025). Current Position and Future Direction of Inflammation in Neuropsychiatric Disorders: A Review. *JAMA Psychiatry, 82*(10), 1030–1046. https://doi.org/10.1001/jamapsychiatry.2025.1369.

Vadodaria, K. C., Mendes, A. P. D., Mei, A., Racha, V., Erikson, G., Shokhirev, M. N., ... Gage, F. H. (2021). Altered neuronal support and inflammatory response in bipolar disorder patient-derived astrocytes. *Stem Cell Reports, 16*(4), 825–835. https://doi.org/10.1016/j.stemcr.2021.02.004.

Vega-núñez, A., et al. (2022). Clinical value of inflammatory and neurotrophic biomarkers in bipolar disorder: A systematic review and meta-analysis. *Biomedicines*. https://doi.org/10.3390/biomedicines10061368 MDPI.

Walter, N. M., et al. (2025). Investigating the impact of omega-3 fatty acids on oxidative stress and pro-inflammatory cytokine release in iPSC-derived forebrain cortical neurons from ADHD patients. *Journal of Psychiatric Research, 182*, 257–269. https://doi.org/10.1016/j.jpsychires.2025.01.020.

Wang, C., et al. (2017). Prenatal, perinatal, and postnatal factors associated with autism: A meta-analysis. *Medicine (United States)*. https://doi.org/10.1097/MD.0000000000006696 Lippincott Williams and Wilkins.

Yang, H., et al. (2025). Epigenetics factors in schizophrenia: Future directions for etiologic and therapeutic study approaches. *Annals of General Psychiatry*. https://doi.org/10.1186/s12991-025-00557-x BioMed Central Ltd.

Yang, Q., & Zhou, J. (2019). Neuroinflammation in the central nervous system: Symphony of glial cells. *Glia, 67*(6), 1017–1035. https://doi.org/10.1002/glia.23571.

Yeh, H., et al. (2026). Atypical antipsychotics alter microglial functions via astrocyte-derived extracellular vesicles. *Brain, Behavior, and Immunity, 131*. https://doi.org/10.1016/j.bbi.2025.106132.

Yilmaz, M., et al. (2021). Overexpression of schizophrenia susceptibility factor human complement C4A promotes excessive synaptic loss and behavioral changes in mice. *Nature Neuroscience, 24*(2), 214–224. https://doi.org/10.1038/s41593-020-00763-8.

Zuccoli, G. S., Nascimento, J. M., Moraes-Vieira, P. M., Rehen, S. K., & Martins-de-Souza, D. (2023). Mitochondrial, cell cycle control and neuritogenesis alterations in an iPSC-based neurodevelopmental model for schizophrenia. *European Archives of Psychiatry and Clinical Neuroscience, 273*(8), 1649–1664. https://doi.org/10.1007/s00406-023-01605-x.

Zuccoli, G. S., et al. (2023). Mitochondrial, cell cycle control and neuritogenesis alterations in an iPSC-based neurodevelopmental model for schizophrenia. *European Archives of Psychiatry and Clinical Neuroscience, 273*(8), 1649–1664. https://doi.org/10.1007/s00406-023-01605-x.

CHAPTER FIVE

G-Protein coupled receptor-mediated internalization and endosomal sorting of Tau-GPCR complex in microglia

Hariharakrishnan Chidamabram, Vaishnavi Ananathanarayana, and Subashchandrabose Chinnathambi*

Department of Neurochemistry, National Institute of Mental Health and Neuro Sciences Hospital (NIMHANS), Institute of National Importance, Bangalore, Karnataka, India

*Corresponding author: e-mail address: subashneuro@nimhans.ac.in

Contents

Abstract

Microglia are the resident immune cells of the central nervous system (CNS), which are in constant surveillance of the brain microenvironment to maintain tissue homeostasis. Microglia play significant role both in the physiological and pathological conditions of the brain. Alzheimer's Disease (AD) is a neurodegenerative disease that

Advances in Immunology, Volume 171
ISSN 0065-2776, https://doi.org/10.1016/bs.ai.2025.11.003

includes progressive dementia and cognitive deficits. The two main culprits of AD are extracellular amyloid-β plaques and neurofibrillary tangles formed by Tau protein. In AD brain, intrinsically disordered Tau undergoes rapid oligomerization and self-aggregates to form filamentous species. Clearance of these toxic species is mainly performed by microglia, which can sense through various receptors such as Toll-like receptors (TLRs), G-Protein coupled receptor (GPCRs), purinergic receptors, *etc.* One such receptor is P2Y12R, a purinergic receptor whose expression is restricted to microglia in CNS. In this review, we envisioned providing an insight into the involvement of P2Y12R, a purinergic cell surface receptor that facilitates the internalization of Tau along with the other mechanisms of Tau clearance in microglia. Exploring these receptors and elucidating the mechanisms underlying Tau 'transmission could pave the way for the development of innovative therapeutic approaches aimed at impeding the spread of Tau pathology in neurodegenerative diseases.

Abbreviations

SCARA-1	Scavenger receptor class A member 1.
MACRO	macrophage receptor with collagenous structure.
SCARB-1	Scavenger Receptor Class B, Member 1.
TREM-2	Triggering receptor expressed on myeloid cells 2.
FRP-2	N-formyl peptide receptor 2.
CMKLR1	Chemokine like receptor 1.
TLR	Toll-like receptor.
KO	Knock-out.
LAMP2A	Lysosome-associated membrane protein-2A.
GRKs	G protein-coupled receptor kinases.
ADP	Adenosine diphosphate.
ALA	α-linolenic acid.

1. Background

In neurodegenerative diseases, the brain microglia plays a multifaceted role in both minimizing and progressing the disease conditions (Chinnathambi, 2024c; Chidambaram et al., 2024c). Alzheimer's disease, the most common type of dementia that leads to neuronal damage, and cognitive decline mostly in people at an age of 65 years and above (Qureshi & Chinnathambi, 2022; Chidambaram et al., 2020; Gorantla et al., 2020; Chinnathambi et al., 2023; Sonawane et al., 2021). The two major pathological hallmarks of Alzheimer's disease, Tau filaments and Amyloid-β plaques are actively phagocytosed and cleared by microglia at early stages of AD pathology. Upon disease progression, impaired phagocytic capability, endosomal dysfunction and enhanced pro-inflammatory activation of microglia leads to synaptic engulfment, neuronal dysfunction and neurodegeneration (Desale & Chinnathambi, 2021b; Das et al., 2020c; Gorantla et al., 2021; Dubey & Chinnathambi, 2019; Chinnathambi & Dubey, 2024; Dubey et al., 2023b; Das et al., 2020a; Chinnathambi, 2024b). The Microtubule-Associated Protein Tau (MAPT or Tau) is an intrinsically disordered protein that, under pathological conditions, undergoes aggregation and forms filamentous inclusions referred to as neurofibrillary tangles (NFTs) (Desale et al., 2021b) shown in Fig. 1. Despite having a well-characterized composition and structure, the in vivo process of Tau aggregation still needs to be better understood. The presence of NFTs is a defining feature of several human diseases collectively known as Tauopathies (Chinnathambi & Chidambaram, 2024; Chinnathambi, 2024a). The propagation of protein aggregates is a prominent feature in several neurodegenerative disorders, including Parkinson's disease, Huntington's disease, and amyotrophic lateral sclerosis (Balmik & Chinnathambi, 2021). The successive spread and deposition of protein aggregates in a predictable manner that corresponds with clinical severity characterize the progression of these disorders. The transmission of Tau to naïve cells, where it simulates misfolding and aggregation, has revealed that Tau can propagate in a prion-like fashion (Rauch et al., 2018).

In Tauopathies, such as Alzheimer's disease (AD), the progression of NFT pathology follows a predictable pattern throughout the brain, explicitly affecting regions associated with learning and memory. This sequential advancement of NFT pathology is closely associated with cognitive decline in patients and enables the neuropathological classification of individuals at different stages of AD (Dubey et al., 2023a; Dubey et al., 2019; Dubey et al., 2020). While the precise mechanisms underlying the intercellular spread of aggregates, specifically Tau protein in Alzheimer's disease, remain incompletely understood, emerging evidence suggests that pathogenic or misfolded Tau aggregates are released, taken up, and transported between synaptically connected neurons (Chinnathambi et al., 2024a). These misfolded Tau species act as seeds that recruit soluble Tau, leading to the formation of aggregates (Chidambaram & Chinnathambi, 2020; Kapoor & Chinnathambi, 2023; Sonawane et al., 2019; Chidambaram et al., 2022a; Das et al., 2020b; Balmik et al., 2021). However, studies have presented conflicting findings regarding the specific forms of Tau that can be internalized, with some indicating monomeric or oligomeric Tau, while others suggesting only oligomeric or fibrillar Tau. Further investigations are required to reconcile these discrepancies and gain a deeper understanding of the cellular processes involved in the transmission of Tau aggregates (Chidambaram et al., 2024b;

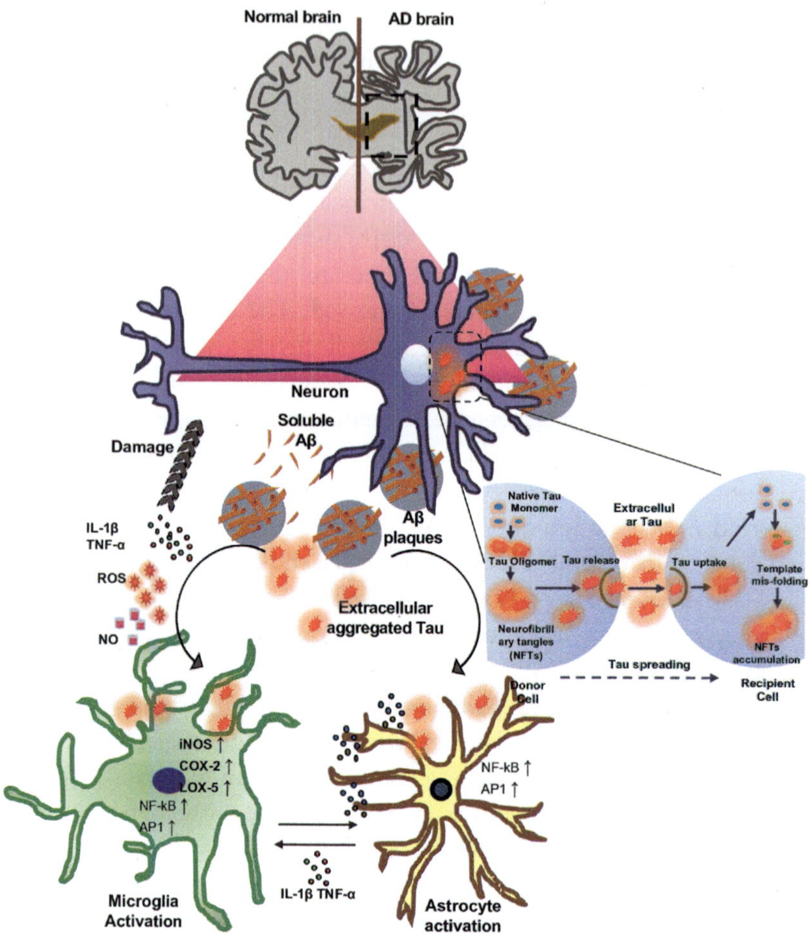

Fig. 1 Overview of Tauopathy in Alzheimer's disease. Alzheimer's disease is a neurodegenerative disease with progressive loss of memory, ultimately leading to brain atrophy and dementia. At cellular level, neurons undergo severe neurodegeneration leading to impaired neuronal signalling. Microtubule associated protein Tau and Amyloid-β fragments forms intracellular and extracellular aggregates respectively. Tau aggregates are released from damaged neurons to extracellular space as neurofibrillary tangles which propagates Tau aggregation in healthy neurons. Microglia undergoes over activation, migration, astrocyte activation and phagocytosis of neuronal cells in addition to extracellular deposits that further worsens the disease condition.

Chinnathambi, 2024c; Desale et al., 2024b; Chinnathambi & Desale, 2024; Chidambaram & Chinnathambi, 2020; Desale et al., 2024a; Chidambaram et al., 2022a).

Main.

2. Microglia modulates key proteins in Alzheimer's disease

Microglia are the brain resident immune cells of hematopoietic origin which are in constant surveillance of the brain microenvironment and constitute ~10–15 % of the brain cell population. Besides their well-documented role in the immune system and tissue homeostasis, they possess ramified processes that enable them to perform endocytic clearance of apoptotic vesicular material (Napoli & Neumann, 2009; Nanjundaiah et al., 2021; Chinnathambi & Das, 2023; Desale & Chinnathambi, 2021c; Desale & Chinnathambi, 2020; Desale & Chinnathambi, 2021a; Desale et al., 2021a; Das & Chinnathambi, 2021; Ramakrishnan et al., 2024; Chidambaram et al., 2024a). Under physiological conditions, microglia are present in resting

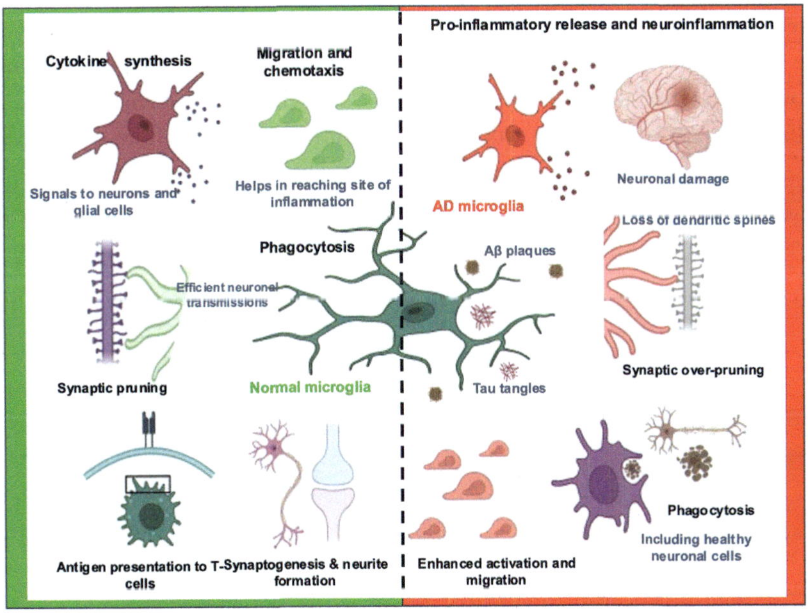

Fig. 2 Physiological and pathological role of microglia in Alzheimer's disease. In the brain, microglial cells play several vital roles that include scavenging brain microenvironment for dead cells, debris, misfolded proteins, microbes, etc. by activation and chemotactic migration. Microglia is also involved in cytokine synthesis, antigen presentation to T-cells, neuronal synaptic pruning, synaptogenesis and neurite formation. In AD conditions, microglia is over activated to phagocytose Amyloid-β plaques and Tau filaments. Enhanced activation and migration lead to synaptic over-pruning, loss of dendritic spines, and even phagocytosis of healthy neurons ultimately leading to neuroinflammation and brain atrophy.

phenotype with small cell body and highly ramified branching processes shown in Fig. 2. At the pathogen invasion or injury site, microglia transformed into an active state with retracted processes and "amoeboid" morphology (Koizumi et al., 2013). Microglia senses amyloid-β plaques through a wide variety of surface receptors that include surface receptors such as SCARA-1, MACRO, SCARB-1, TREM-2, G-protein coupled receptors such as FRP-2 and CMKLR1, toll-like receptors such as TLR2 and TLR4 shown in Fig. 3. These receptors are majorly involved in inducing inflammatory response and phagocytosis of Aβ upon interaction. Similarly, Tau proteins are sensed by G-protein coupled receptors such as purinergic P2Y12 receptor, P2Y12R; muscarinic acetylcholine receptor, M1mAChR; and chemokine receptor, CX3CR1 shown in Fig. 4. (Bolós et al., 2017; Das & Chinnathambi, 2021; Gómez-Ramos et al., 2006; Gómez-Ramos et al., 2009; Chidambaram et al., 2022a). Bolos et al. (2017) showed enhanced Tau internalization upon microglial CX3CR1 interaction. The author proved the hypothesis by using CX3CR1 KO primary microglial cultures that showed no Tau internalization upon its extracellular exposure. The internalization was observable only after 60 min exposure which was again

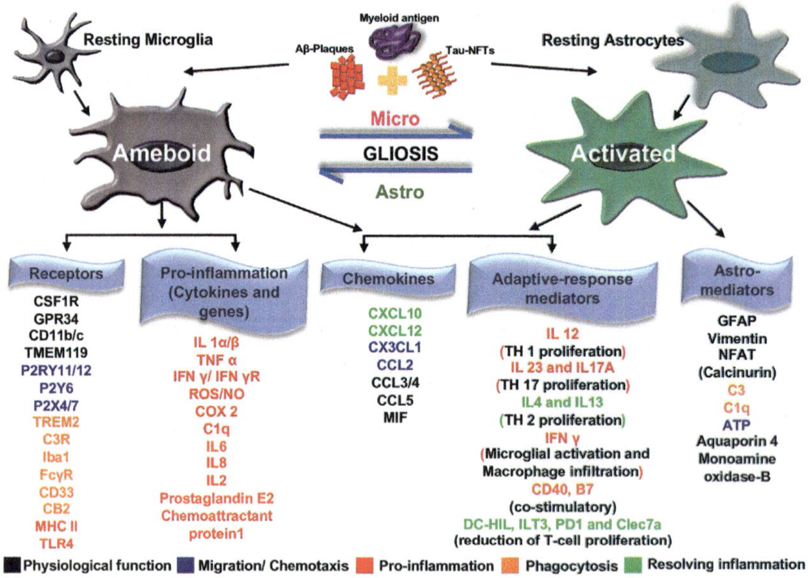

Fig. 3 Micro-astroglial receptors in Alzheimer's disease. Extracellular Tau and amyloid-β activate resting microglia and astrocytes. Activated microglia and astrocytes express several surface receptors which are involved in regulating cellular proliferation, migration/ chemotaxis, inflammation and phagocytosis.

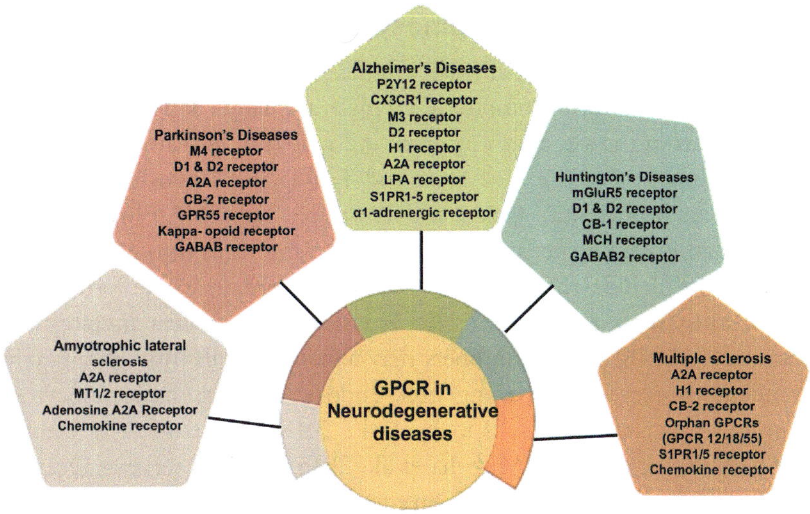

Fig. 4 G-protein coupled receptors (GPCRs) in neurodegenerative diseases. Schematic representation of various G-protein coupled receptors reported in different neurodegenerative diseases such as Alzheimer's disease, Parkinson's disease, amyotrophic lateral sclerosis, Huntington's disease, multiple sclerosis, etc.

significantly low as compared to wild-type cells. This is interesting to know that Tau is internalized upon binding to microglial CX3CR1 receptor. Further research should be carried-out at this particular mechanism, i.e. the receptor-mediated endocytosis of extracellular Tau by microglia.

3. Signalling pathways of endocytosis in Tauopathy

Endocytosis is essential for organismal homeostasis that involves the internalization of nutrients, antigen presentation, regulation of cell-surface receptor expression, cellular cholesterol homeostasis, maintenance of cell polarity, and removal of pathogens, among other functions (Mukherjee et al., 1999; Chinnathambi et al., 2024c). Any endocytic process underlays a standard mechanism that begins at coated invaginations of the plasma membrane, progresses through several endosomal compartments, and culminates in lysosomes. Several mechanisms are involved in the cellular uptake of different materials by the cells; apart from the classical clathrin-dependent pathway, other pathways include the caveolar pathway and fluid-phase endocytosis (Chinnathambi et al., 2024c).

3.1 GPCR-mediated macropinocytosis in Tauopathy

The clathrin-independent pathway engulfs extracellular fluid in a non-selective way and forms pinosome, which are large endocytic vacuolar compartments of the size that vary from 0.2 to 10 μm in diameter. Dextran, another hallmark of bulk endocytosis, and Tau aggregates co-localize, while cholera toxin B does not. This result shows that rather than breaching the cell membrane, Tau aggregates are internalized into cells through endocytic pathways that include engulfment by the cell membrane in the form of tiny invaginations (Frost et al., 2009). According to more recent investigations (Evans et al., 2018), Tau monomers may also enter cells through an actin-dependent process encompassing bulk-endocytosis and macropinocytosis. According to many studies (Rauch et al., 2018; Christianson & Belting, 2014; Holmes et al., 2013; Mirbaha et al., 2015), HSPGs serve as receptors for Tau endocytosis in neurons during macropinocytosis.

3.2 GPCR-mediated phagocytosis in Tauopathy

Phagocytosis usually refers to engulfing large particles of size > 0.5 μ in diameter. Macrophages and neutrophils exhibit this first line of defense internalization property as a part of an innate immune response. The majority of the brain's macrophages are microglia. In the internalization of oligomeric Tau, peripheral macrophages and microglia display phagocytic activity (Bolós et al., 2016; Majerova et al., 2014). In microglia, upon Tau phagocytosis, the extracellular Tau is taken through the endosomal compartments for its degradation by lysosomal fusion. Desale et al. (2021) clearly elucidated the endosomal trafficking of internalized Tau protein in N9 microglial cells and the role of ALA in promoting its internalization and degradation shown in Fig. 5. The immunofluorescence microscope analysis shows colocalization of internalized Tau species with early and late endosomal markers, Rab5 and Rab7 respectively. Following this, internalized Tau species also colocalized with lysosomal marker, LAMP2A demonstrating the lysosomal degradation of Tau species by microglia (Desale & Chinnathambi, 2021d).

A number of mechanisms mediate the microglial phagocytosis of Tau. The CX3CL1/CX3CR1 axis is one of them, and it is crucial for the interaction between microglia and neurons. Microglia express the CX3CR1 receptor, which binds to CX3CL1 shown in Fig. 6. Bolos et al. (2017) state that CX3CR1 may secure monomeric Tau and facilitate their internalization. The phosphorylation of Tau has an impact on phagocytosis as well because phosphorylated Tau has a lesser affinity for CX3CR1 than non-phosphorylated Tau shown in Fig. 7.

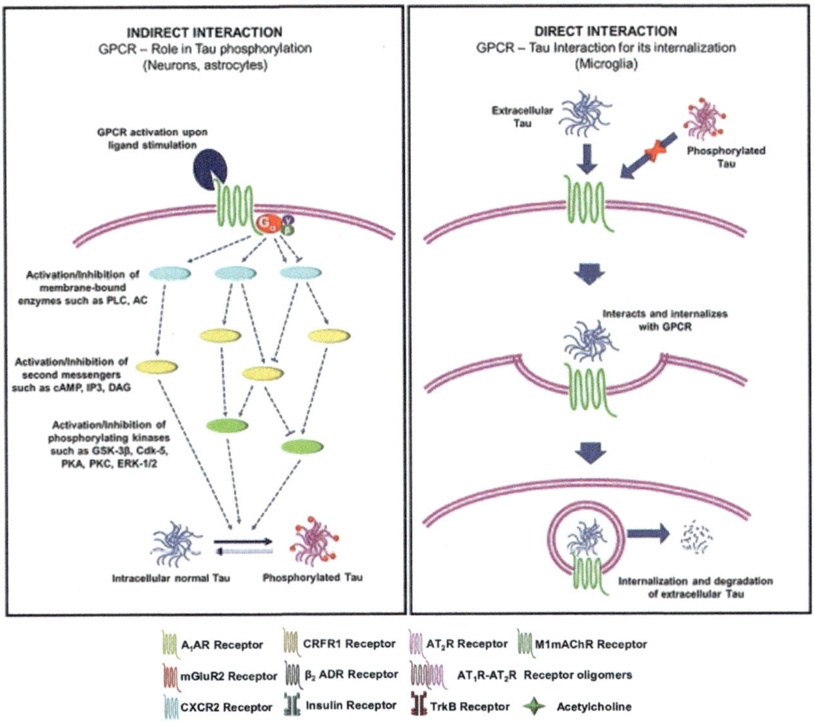

Fig. 5 GPCRs in Alzheimer's disease. This figure illustrates the principal pathological proteins of Alzheimer's disease, which interact with and modify cellular signaling through G-protein coupled receptors (GPCRs). Amyloid beta protein, particularly its Aβ40, Aβ42, and Aβ oligomers, and Tau protein, including its monomer, oligomer, aggregates, and pseudophosphorylated form, are observed to interact with various GPCRs and contribute to disease progression. Full-length Tau protein and pseudophosphorylated Tau protein interact with muscarinic receptors, reducing neurite outgrowth by increasing cytoplasmic calcium levels. Aβ and its oligomers phosphorylate Tau protein via GSK3β and JNK by interacting with adrenergic β2 receptors. The melatonin receptor activates the ERK pathway in the presence of Aβ42. Serotonin receptor expression increases in the presence of Aβ40. Metabotropic glutamate receptor expression increases and inhibits the muscarinic receptor in the presence of Aβ. Tau and Aβ alter synaptic potentiation and inhibition through the GABA receptor. Tau interacts with the chemokine CX3CR1 receptor and undergoes internalization. Tau monomers, oligomers, and aggregates interact with the purinergic P2Y12 receptor, leading to Tau internalization and the formation of migratory structures.

Researchers have also suggested lipid raft-dependent endocytosis as an additional endocytic pathway for Tau internalization. Clathrin independence, dynamin independence, and sensitivity to cholesterol depletion are the characteristics that distinguish lipid raft-dependent endocytosis. Tunnelling

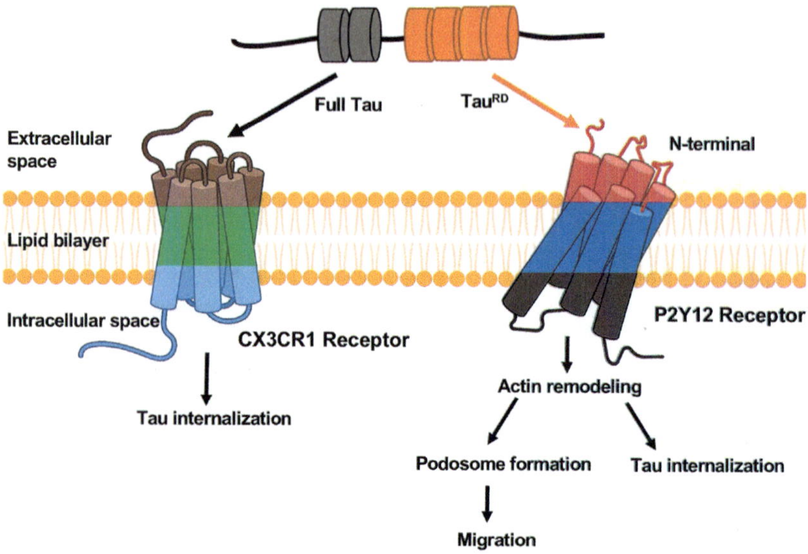

Fig. 6 Tau interacts with purinergic and chemokine receptors. This figure delineates the interaction between the Tau protein and microglial purinergic and chemokine receptors. The purinergic receptor P2Y12 and the chemokine receptor CX3CR1 are GPCRs, classified under ligand-gated receptors. These receptors feature seven transmembrane domains that form a binding pocket for ligand interactions. The full-length Tau protein, comprising 441 amino acids, interacts with the CX3CR1 receptor and undergoes internalization within the cell. The repeat domain of Tau engages with the N-terminal region of the P2Y12 receptor, initiating downstream signaling that culminates in actin remodeling. Actin remodeling via the P2Y12R-Tau interaction facilitates podosome formation, thereby promoting cell migration and contributing to Tau internalization.

nanotubes (TNTs) are a kind of cell-cell communication that acts as a route for the transportation of materials between cells. TNTs transport parts of the plasma membrane across distant cells in both directions, including actin. Actin abundance, tubulin negativity, and myosin 10 protein content are all shared characteristics of TNTs. TNTs can internalize prions and prion-like proteins, such as Tau. A 2.6-fold increase in the proportion of cells establishing TNTs has been observed, instead of the number of TNTs per cell, when exposed to Tau fibrils.

3.3 GPCR-derived clathrin-mediated endocytosis

Receptor-mediated endocytosis is one of the most important processes with which viruses and bioparticles can enter or leave an animal cell. The first mammalian Rab proteins localized to the endocytic pathway were

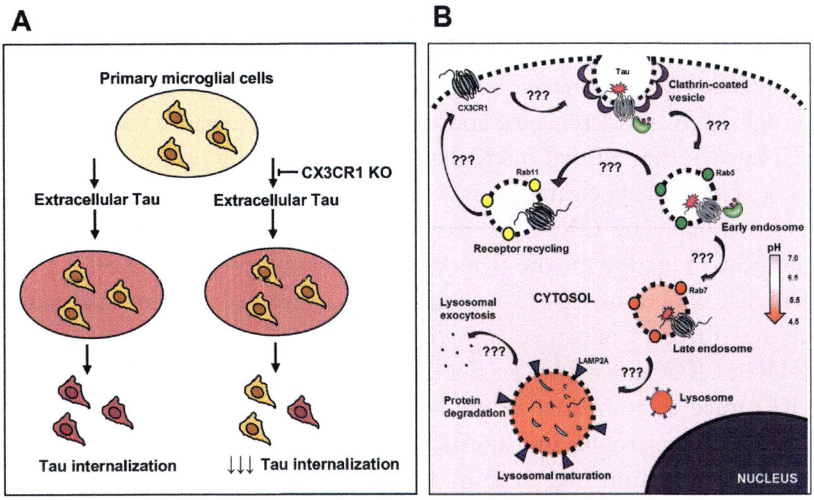

Fig. 7 CX3CR1-mediated Tau endocytosis and degradation in microglia. (A) Primary microglial cells uptake extracellular Tau in the presence of the chemokine receptor, CX3CR1. (B) Tau pathospecies such as oligomers and aggregates undergo endosomal sorting upon microglial phagocytosis that ultimately fuses with lysosomes for its degradation. Would Tau undergoes receptor-mediated endocytosis by microglia? Would Tau species act as ligand to CX3CR1 and Tau-bound CX3CR1 undergo clathrin-mediated endocytosis followed by endosomal sorting?.

Rab5, which sequentially regulate the cargo uptake into early endosomes (Vitelli et al., 1997). Rab7 acts downstream from Rab5 to regulate transport from early to late endosomes and lysosomes (Vitelli et al., 1997; Gutierrez et al., 2004). Rab4 and Rab11 regulates the recycling of receptors and other transport machinery. Genome-wide association studies (GWAS) have identified BIN1, which is likewise implicated in Tau endocytosis and is considered to be an additional AD risk factor besides PICALM. According to Franzmeier et al. (2019), BIN1 deficiency contributes to the pathophysiology of Tau (Franzmeier et al., 2019). Neuronal-specific BIN1 has a lower protein level in the brains of late-onset AD patients. The endosomal small guanosine triphosphatase (GTPase) Rab5 is induced by a reduction in BIN1, which increases the flow to the endosome (Calafate et al., 2016). In individuals with late-onset AD, the expression level of BIN1 is downregulated, which upregulates the CME (Calafate et al., 2016). As a result, in late-onset AD, this endocytic pathway of extracellular Tau may be increased and serve to seed the aggregation of soluble Tau.

4. Chemokine-receptor mediated internalization of Tau

In 2017, Bolos *et al.* stated for the first time that Tau binds to microglial CX3CR1 receptor and competes with its ligand, fractalkine. As it is a known the fact that microglia internalize Tau by several mechanisms and degrades for its clearance in AD environment, they have determined the Tau uptake by CX3CR1 KO microglia as compared to control. A significant reduction in the Tau uptake was observed in CX3CR1 KO microglia, which showed its importance in microglial Tau internalization. This was further confirmed in-vivo by stereotaxically injecting Tau into the DG of KO and wild-type mice. Tau intensity was significantly higher in KO mice as compared to wild-type proving the impaired Tau internalization by microglia and in-efficient clearance from the brain. Further, microglial activation measured by CD68 expression was impaired in KO microglia as compared to wild-type group. CD68 expression increased with Tau treatment in wild-type groups, whereas the expression remained the same in CX3CR1 KO microglia (Bolós et al., 2017). This study signifies the importance of CX3CR1 receptor in microglial activation, Tau internalization and degradation shown in Fig. 7B.

Following this, the author showed that Tau can interact with CX3CR1 receptor by in vitro binding assay. In the affinity chromatography, total Tau bound to CX3CR1 receptor coupled to CN-sepharose. Chemokine domain of fractalkine was considered as positive control that also bound to CX3CR1, whereas the negatively charged C-terminal of Tau protein did not bind to the receptor acted as a negative control. In Alzheimer's disease, Tau protein undergoes hyperphosphorylation that misfolds and forms filamentous structures. Bolos *et al.* also tested the binding of phosphorylated Tau to this receptor by GSK-3β Tau phosphorylation. Tau protein bound to the column containing CX3CR1 irrespective of its phosphorylation state but with a weaker binding affinity for phosphorylated Tau as compared to total Tau. In immunofluorescence assay, impaired phagocytosis was observed with microglia treated with phosphorylated Tau as compared to total Tau. As the level of phosphorylated Tau increases with Braak-Tau stages, this could be a possible reason for the down regulated microglial internalization and clearance of extracellular pathological Tau in AD. Upon addition of fractalkine, Tau competes to bind CX3CR1 and shows reduced internalization which is proved by affinity chromatography and immunofluorescence assay respectively (Bolós et al., 2017). This again indicates the possible mechanism for reduced Tau interaction and internalization at later stages of disease progression as the levels of fractalkine also increases with Braak-Tau stage shown in Fig. 7A. As stated by Bolos et al. 2017, the CX3CR1-Tau interaction mediated internalization could be further studied for Tau-CX3CR1 distribution in endosomal compartments of microglial cells. In this context of receptor-mediated endocytosis of extracellular Tau by microglial GPCRs such as P2Y12R and CX3CR1, further research should be carried out to study the GPCR activation, desensitization followed by endosomal sorting to either receptor recycling or degradation. This could possibly unravel the mechanisms of receptor-mediated endocytosis of extracellular Tau and its spreading in AD microglia.

As we know, post-transnationally modified Tau self-aggregates to form filaments and neurofibrillary tangles which are predominant in the later stages of AD. According to recent studies, Tau undergoes a complex oligomeric conformation which promotes self-assembly of Tau monomers to form filamentous structures. These oligomeric species are toxic and are capable of causing neurodegeneration in the brain. Hence, these pathospecies of Tau protein are considered as key players in neuroinflammation and neuronal damage (Das & Chinnathambi, 2021). Though there are several surface receptors identified for Tau monomers that could interact and signal-through or internalize via receptor-mediated endocytosis and transmit to neighbouring healthy cells (Bolós et al., 2017; Das & Chinnathambi, 2021). It would be interesting to find receptors for Tau oligomers and aggregates that could aid/aggravate in neurodegenerative conditions. The alternative GPCR downstream signalling upon Tau species interaction could be studied to interpret the impaired GPCR signalling mechanisms in disease pathology. Further research has to be performed and interpreted whether these receptors are capable of interacting with Tau pathospecies, oligomers and aggregates which would shed some light in understanding the molecular mechanisms involved in Tau spreading in AD shown in Fig. 7B.

5. Signaling pathways of microglial purinergic receptors in Tauopathy

The advent of high-throughput technologies such as single-cell RNA analysis of CNS cells in Alzheimer's disease and diverse other neurodegenerative conditions revealed the transcriptome signature of microglia and the transition from homeostatic microglia to disease-associated microglia, governed by changes in gene expression levels. Microglia express a wide array of receptors suited to the detection of a range of stimuli. Microglia show chemotaxis properties as they can re-orient their actin-associated cytoskeletal network towards the area of damage (Das & Chinnathambi, 2019). There are various powerful chemoattractant designated as 'find-me' signals released by apoptotic cells that help initiate phagocytosis. The well-documented find me signals are ATP, ADP, and adenosine. Microglia expresses a wide array of receptors suited to the detection of a range of find me signals that include purinergic receptors P2×4 and P2×7 or P2Y6 and P2Y12 and various adenosine receptors A1R, A3R, and A2AR which are expressed by microglia shown in Fig. 8 (Das & Chinnathambi, 2020). Overexpression of P2Y12R has been reported upon cargo interaction (Haynes et al., 2006; Koizumi et al., 2013;

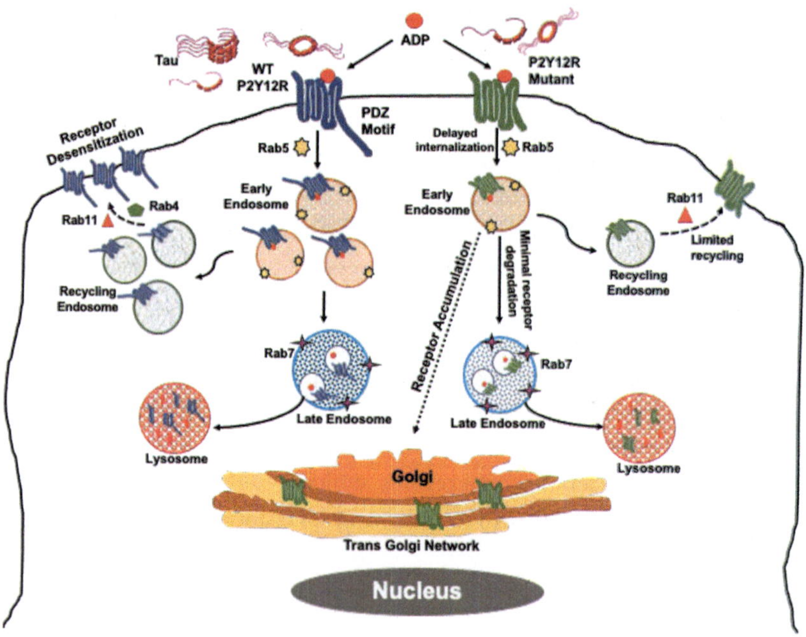

Fig. 8 P2Y12 receptor in endocytosis. Upon extracellular Tau interaction with P2Y12 receptor, the ligand-bound complex is driven by endocytosis and vesicular trafficking through early (Rab5+), late (Rab7+) and recycling endosomes (Rab4+ and Rab11+). The internalized Tau undergoes lysosomal degradation (LAMP+). P2Y12 receptor mutation at ligand binding site delays receptor internalization, limits receptor recycling and degradation, and ultimately promotes receptor accumulation at the endosomes.

Ohsawa et al., 2007). The role of P2Y12R in the periphery has been known for decades. Still, its expression and importance in the central nervous system (CNS), where it is expressed exclusively on microglia – the first responders to brain insults and neurodegeneration, was least explored.

In comparison with the classical identifiers of microglia such as Iba1, CD68, or MHCII, investigation on the expression of P2Y12 in human brain tissue showed P2Y12-positive parenchymal microglia and the absence of P2Y12 expression from perivascular or meningeal macrophages shown in Fig. 8. In physiological conditions, P2Y12 expression is stable throughout human brain development, including fetal phases (Mildner et al., 2017). The P2 receptors, classified into two families—the ionotropic P2X receptors with seven members and the metabotropic P2Y receptors with eight members identified—are sensitive to the nucleosides triphosphate and diphosphate. Among them, the receptors P2×4, P2×7, P2Y1, P2Y2, P2Y4, P2Y6, P2Y12, and P2Y13 are expressed by microglial cells shown in Fig. 9 (Puerto et al., 2013).

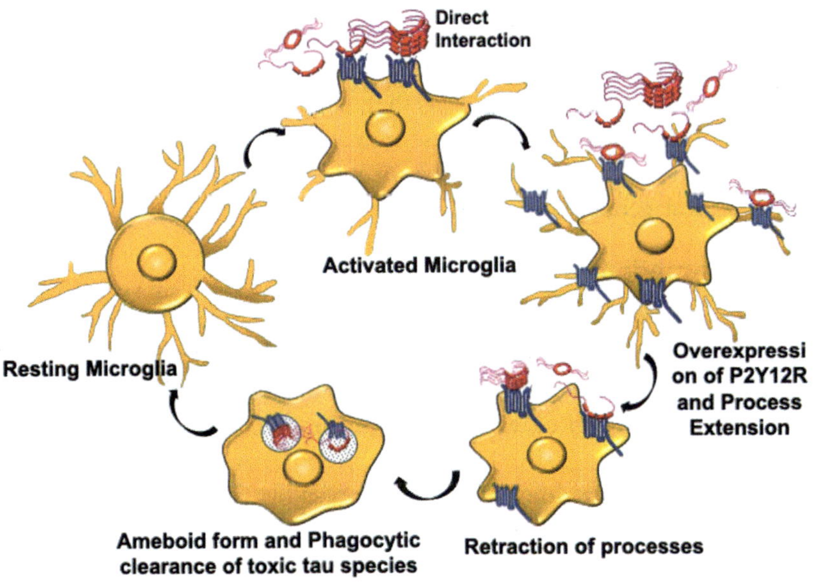

Fig. 9 Microglial activation and phagocytic clearance of toxic Tau species. Under physiological conditions, microglial cells are maintained at rest (ramified). Extracellular Tau activates microglia (amoeboid), and promotes Tau clearance by active phagocytosis. Tau oligomers and aggregates promotes P2Y12 receptor overexpression, retraction of actin-extensions that further leads to microglial activation and phagocytic clearance of toxic Tau species.

The Tg2576, a transgenic AD mouse model expressing human APP and studies conducted with human AD brains, showed the upregulation of P2×7 in close proximity to Aβ plaques in correlation with the Aβ load (Mclarnon et al., 2006; Parvathenani et al., 2003). Various studies have explored the behaviour of several metabotropic receptors in AD by using mouse models. For example, In APPPS1 mice, Reichenbach et al. (2018) reported the association of P2Y1 expression with astrocyte hyperactivity and spatial learning and memory (Reichenbach et al., 2018). In the TgCRND8 mouse brain that expresses Swedish and Indiana mutations in APP, observed that P2Y2R is critical for the recruitment and activation of microglial cells. They also showed that loss of the P2Y2R can hasten the establishment of an AD-like phenotype in the TgCRND8 mice. These findings suggest that the P2Y2R may regulate neuroprotective processes through microglia-mediated clearance of Aβ (Ajit et al., 2014).

Alzheimer's disease and non-Alzheimer's disease Tauopathy patient's brains and mice model displayed the down-regulation of microglial P2Y12 receptor levels in areas intimately abundant in Tau inclusions, with an increase in the total microglial population, rather than amyloid-β neuritic plaques, which account as a sensitive index for neuroinflammatory responses (Maeda et al., 2021). Together, these studies signify that P2Y12 can act as a useful marker in the discrimination of activated microglia and infiltrating myeloid cells from quiescent microglia in Alzheimer's disease-related neurodegenerative processes.

5.1 GPCR-mediated Tau internalization in AD

The internalization of Tau is a complex but critical step in Tau propagation (Zhao et al., 2021). Recent shreds of evidence suggest that microglia participate in the internalization and degradation of pathological Tau (insoluble) in vitro and ex vivo, although the precise mechanisms remain unclear (Funk et al., 2015; Luo et al., 2015). For example, one study showed the internalization of human extracellular Tau in three models, namely primary microglia culture exposed to Tau as the in vitro model, C57Bl/6 mice stereotaxically injected with Tau, and human tissues from AD patients and control subjects for the in vivo studies. Later, Das et al. (2021) and Chidambaram et al. showed P2Y12R-mediated Tau internalization and degradation upon extracellular repeat-Tau exposure. Chidambaram et al. showed a time-dependent internalization of repeat-domain of Tau by N9 microglial cells upto 6 h. Tau internalization reduced significantly upon P2Y12 receptor inhibition with clopidogrel. Moreover, the authors found that all Tau species including monomer, oligomer and aggregate species to be interacting with P2Y12 receptor by co-immunoprecipitation Fig. 9 (Das & Chinnathambi, 2021). In specific, the interaction of repeat-domain of Tau with extracellular P2Y12 receptor was supported by molecular modelling, docking and MD-simulation analysis by building POPC membrane around the Tau-P2Y12R complex. The charged amino acid residues of repeat-Tau including D252, E269, K331, K343, and H330 majorly contributed to the extracellular P2Y12 receptor interaction. The valine and proline residues of Tau has contributed to the hydrophobic interaction. Further the surface electrostatic potential analysis proved that repeat-Tau majorly binds to the negatively charged region of extracellular P2Y12 receptor.

They observed membrane-associated actin remodelling and filopodia formation, which indicates microglial migration and phagocytosis of extracellular Tau (Qureshi et al., 2024). Next, the most interesting part of the study is the lysosomal degradation of internalized repeat-Tau which is mediated by P2Y12 receptor. P2Y12R-mediated lysosomal degradation is studied by immunofluorescence assay of N9 microglial cells extracellularly exposed to Tau in the presence and absence of P2Y12R inhibitor, clopidogrel. In clopidogrel exposed group, the associated of Tau with the lysosomal marker, LAMP2A was found to be reduced compared to Tau-treated groups which is quantified by Pearson's colocalization co-efficient (Chinnathambi, 2022; Das & Chinnathambi, 2021). Hereby, this experiment again provides the possible mechanism of receptor-mediated endocytosis of P2Y12 and extracellular Tau.

5.2 Endosomal sorting of P2Y12 receptor upon ligand binding

Upon ligand binding, any GPCR undergoes activation and binds to G_α-proteins for further downstream signalling. The ligand itself determines the ability of any given GPCR to differentially regulate activation and desensitization. Following ligand binding and activation, most of the GPCRs undergo the process of desensitization. The active GPCR is phosphorylated by GRKs that leads to β-arrestin recruitment. β-arrestin binding prevents further binding of G-proteins and activation of downstream signalling pathways, eventually follows receptor internalization. Upon clathrin-mediated endocytosis of β-arrestin bound GPCRs, the fate of GPCR to sort to lysosomes or recycled back to membrane by resensitization is regulated by several factors such as binding affinity of β-arrestin, class of GPCRS, nature of ligand binding (reversible/irreversible), *etc* (L Mohan et al., 2012) (Fig. 10). In 2013, Cunningham et al., demonstrated the endosomal sorting of a purinergic GPCR, P2Y12R upon its ligand binding (ADP). ADP activates P2Y12 receptor and undergoes clathrin- and dynamin-dependent internalization for the endosomal trafficking. First, author showed the Rab5-dependent internalization by live cell confocal microscopy and colocalization studies by coexpressing HA-WT P2Y12 and GFP-Rab5. Colocalization between P2Y12R and Rab5 was observed within 5 min time interval after ADP exposure. Next, the author identified the P2Y12 resensitization and the recycling endosomal compartments. P2Y12 receptor undergoes endosomal sorting and recycling via Rab4 and Rab11 endosomal compartments. This has been proved using cell surface ELISA that detects the expression of P2Y12 expressed on cell surface. ADP treatment to microglial cells for

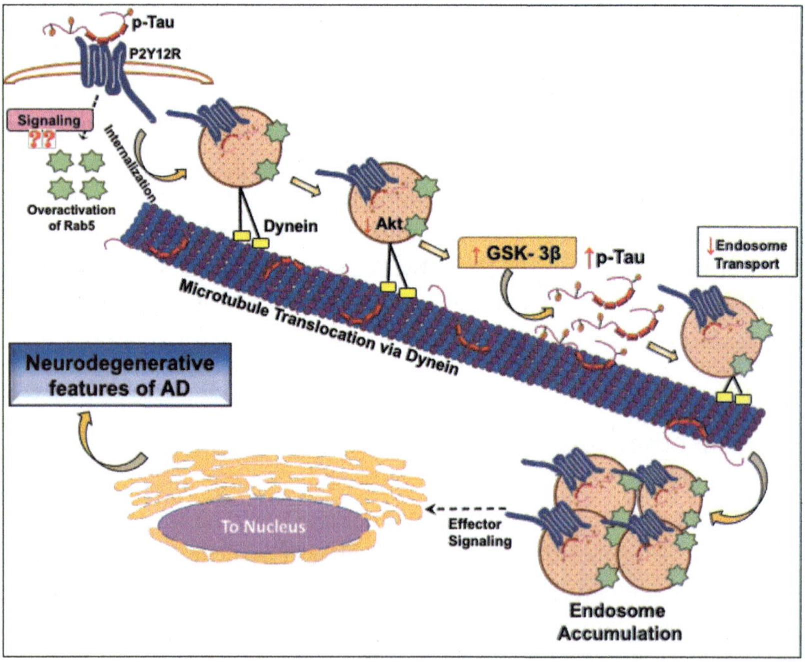

Fig. 10 P2Y12R-mediated purinergic signalling partakes in endosomal dysfunction. In Alzheimer's Disease, endosomal dysfunction and impaired vesicular transport is observed that promotes Tau accumulation in cells. Rab5 is overexpressed and activated on endosomes of AD brain. P2Y12 receptor signalling upon Tau binding could promote Rab5 overactivation in disease conditions. Abnormal AKT signalling and overactivation of GSK-3b is also observed that ultimately promotes Tau hyperphophorylation and microtubule destabilization in AD.

30 min promoted endocytosis which is followed by apyrase addition that removes excess residual ADP and leads to receptor recycling. Inability of P2Y12 receptor to recycle back to the membrane was observed in cells with Rab4 and Rab11 siRNAs individually. Hence, Cunningham et al. 2013 proved the endosomal trafficking of P2Y12 receptor through Rab5 early endosomal compartments and its recycling back to membrane via Rab4 and Rab11 endosomes (Cunningham et al., 2013). It is interesting to study and explore the endosomal sorting machineries of individual G-protein coupled receptors upon ligand binding and factors that regulate endosomal sorting in cells (Desale & Chinnathambi, 2021b).

5.3 GPCR-mediated endosomal dysfunction in Alzheimer's disease

In light of the endosome's role as an integrator of inter-cellular communication, signalling, and metabolism inside the cell, it is readily envisaged how even minuscule form of endocytic malfunction might negatively impair brain function and induce neurodegeneration. In Alzheimer's disease (AD), endosome abnormalities are among the first neuropathologic traits to emerge and have recently been strongly related to genetic risk factors for AD, including APP triplication in Trisomy 21 (Down syndrome, DS) and ApoE4 genotype in sporadic AD. Moreover, evidence is accumulating indicating vesicular transport is disrupted in neurons in AD and in AD animal models (Terwel et al., 2002; Nixon, 2005; Chinnathambi et al., 2024b). In sporadic AD, endosome dysfunction signals the early aberrant elevations in AB levels (Cataldo et al., 2000). The hallmark growth of rab5 endosomes that has been identified in AD is not a feature of normal brain aging or other major neurodegenerative disorders as far examined and is different from changes in late endosome size that are created experimentally to imitate other diseases shown in Fig. 10 (Cataldo et al., 2000). Rab5 is aberrantly overactivated on endosomes in AD and DS (Kim et al., 2016; Xu et al., 2016). Pensalfini, A., et al. studied the direct Rab5 overexpression, separately from APP-βCTF in the PA-Rab5 mouse model. They found out that Rab5 overactivation alone recapitulates numerous prodromal and degenerative aspects of AD. PA-Rab5 mice exhibit abnormal AKT Signalling and Tau hyperphosphorylation via overactivated Glycogen Synthase Kinase-3b (GSK-3b) (Pensalfini et al., 2020). Expected repercussions of rab5 overactivation are found in DS fibroblasts, including substantially faster endocytosis rates, enhanced fusion and swelling of early endosomes and abnormal endosomal signalling shown in Fig. 10. Moreover, transgenic mice that overexpress rab5 in neurons demonstrate abnormalities in synaptic plasticity and memory as expected given the known synaptic activities of rab5. Pathologic Rab5 activation that promotes endocytic dysfunction in AD severely influences LTP and long-term depression (LTD), 2 elements of synaptic plasticity that are intimately connected with learning and memory (Kessels & Malinow, 2009). Endosomal disruption in microglia has been postulated as a possible contribution to Alzheimer's disease, however the specific pathways and causal variables are currently under research.

5.4 P2Y12R-mediated purinergic signalling partakes in endosomal dysfunction

There are evidence suggesting a relationship between purinergic signalling and endosomal dysfunction in various cellular processes. Purinergic signalling involves releasing and recognizing extracellular nucleotides, such as ATP and adenosine, which act as signalling molecules by binding to specific purinergic receptors on the cell surface. Research has shown that purinergic signalling pathways play a role in regulating endosomal trafficking and function. ATP, as a key component of purinergic signalling, has been implicated in the modulation of endosomal acidification, fusion, and recycling processes. It can affect the activity of ATPase proton pumps in endosomal acidification, influencing the pH environment necessary for proper endosomal function. Furthermore, studies have demonstrated that aberrant purinergic signalling can disrupt endosomal trafficking and contribute to pathological conditions. Dysregulation of purinergic receptors or impaired ATP release can lead to altered endosomal function, affecting the sorting and clearance of cellular components shown in Fig. 11. This disruption in endosomal processes may have implications for various diseases, including neurodegenerative disorders. In the context of neurodegenerative diseases, emerging evidence suggests that purinergic signalling dysfunction and endosomal abnormalities are interconnected. For example, in Alzheimer's disease, altered purinergic signalling has been linked to impaired endosomal function and amyloid-beta accumulation. Dysfunctional purinergic receptors may influence endosomal processes involved in the clearance of amyloid-beta, leading to its accumulation and subsequent neurodegenerative processes.

As P2Y12R is also a mediator of purinergic signalling inside the cell, we hypothesize the linkage between P2Y12R and Tau interaction could lead

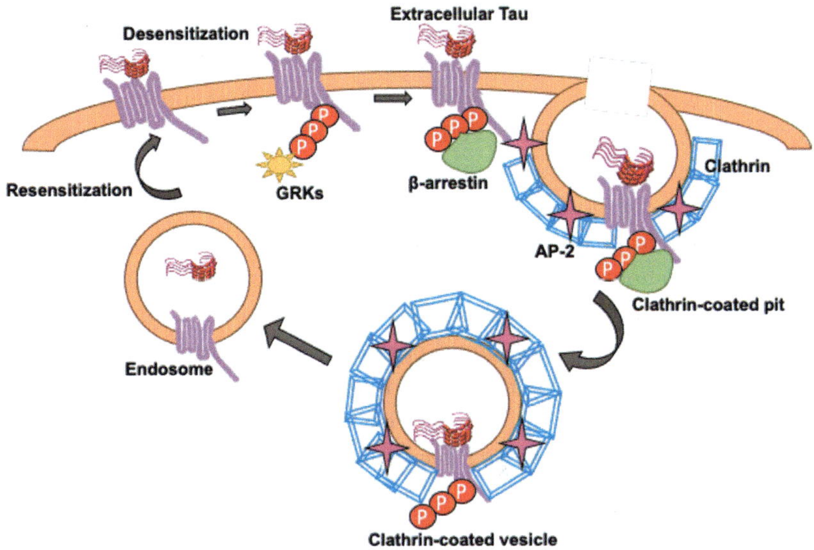

Fig. 11 GPCR-mediated endosomal dysfunction in Alzheimer's disease. Diagrammatic representation of Tau species binding to G-Protein coupled receptor, receptor activation, GPCR receptor kinases (GRKs) recruitment, receptor phosphorylation, β-arrestin recruitment, and Clathrin-mediated endocytosis that leads to vesicular trafficking of GPCRs to either recycling or degradation.

to aberrant increase in Rab5 expression followed by endosomal dysfunction in the context of neurodegenerative diseases, particularly Alzheimer's disease. Further research is needed to elucidate the specific molecular mechanisms underlying this relationship and explore the potential of targeting the P2Y12 receptor as a therapeutic approach for endosomal dysfunction-related disorders (Das & Chinnathambi, 2021; Chinnathambi & Chidambaram, 2024; Chidambaram et al., 2024a; Desale & Chinnathambi, 2021b; Chinnathambi & Das, 2023; Chidambaram et al., 2022a; Chidambaram et al., 2024b).

6. Conclusion

In this review, we have emphasized the significance of microglial P2Y12R/CX3CR1 and Tau interaction that leads to the clearance of Tau. P2Y12R can be a useful marker in discriminating activated microglia and infiltrating myeloid cells from quiescent microglia. P2Y12R can be seen as a potential therapeutic approach to halt the prion-like propagation of Tau from cell to cell. Advent in high throughput technologies gave us an insight into targeting endosomal dysfunction for early detection of various neurodegenerative illnesses with a particular focus on Alzheimer's disease. As per emerging evidence, we have delineated the interconnection between purinergic signalling dysfunction and endosomal abnormalities. Thus, this review suggests the possible engulfment ability of microglial P2Y12R and their downstream purinergic signalling can be modulated in various therapeutic approaches for the clearance of Tau. We are further interested in delineating various degradation mechanisms after Tau internalization escorted by P2Y12R, which could provide a better understanding of Tau propagation in AD. Further research is needed to elucidate the specific molecular mechanisms underlying this relationship and explore the potential of targeting the P2Y12 receptor as a therapeutic approach.

Acknowledgements

We are grateful to Chinnathambi's lab members for their scientific discussions, helpful suggestions and critical reading of the manuscript. We also greatly acknowledge internal support from the Department of Neurochemistry, National Institute of Mental Health and Neuro Sciences (NIMHANS), Institute of National Importance, Bangalore.

Funding

This project is supported in part by grant from India ENIGMA Initiative for Global Aging & Mental Health grant R01AG060610 and under National Institute of Aging/National Institute of Health (NIA/NIH), USA.

Ethics declarations

Ethics approval and consent to participate.
Not applicable.

CRediT authorship contribution statement

Subashchandrabose Chinnathambi: Literature collection, Writing -review & editing, Supervision.

Hariharakrishnan Chidambaram: Editing. Vaishnavi Ananathanarayana and Madhura Chandrashekar: Literature collection.

Consent for publication

Not applicable.

Competing interest

The authors declare that they have no competing interests.

References

Ajit, D., Woods, L. T., Camden, J. M., Thebeau, C. N., El-Sayed, F. G., Greeson, G. W., ... Sun, G. Y. (2014). Loss of P2Y 2 nucleotide receptors enhances early pathology in the TgCRND8 mouse model of Alzheimer's disease. *Molecular Neurobiology, 49*, 1031–1042.

Balmik, A. A., & Chinnathambi, S. (2021). Methylation as a key regulator of Tau aggregation and neuronal health in Alzheimer's disease. *Cell Communication and Signaling: CCS, 19*, 51.

Balmik, A. A., Sonawane, S. K., & Chinnathambi, S. (2021). The extracellular HDAC6 ZnF UBP domain modulates the actin network and post-translational modifications of Tau. *Cell Communication and Signaling: CCS, 19*, 49.

Bolós, M., Llorens-Martín, M., Jurado-Arjona, J., Hernández, F., Rábano, A., & Avila, J. (2016). Direct evidence of internalization of tau by microglia in vitro and in vivo. *Journal of Alzheimer's Disease, 50*, 77–87.

Bolós, M., Llorens-Martín, M., Perea, J. R., Jurado-Arjona, J., Rábano, A., Hernández, F., & Avila, J. (2017). Absence of CX3CR1 impairs the internalization of Tau by microglia. *Molecular Neurodegeneration, 12*, 59.

Calafate, S., Flavin, W., Verstreken, P., & Moechars, D. (2016). Loss of Bin1 promotes the propagation of tau pathology. *Cell Reports, 17*, 931–940.

Cataldo, A. M., Peterhoff, C. M., Troncoso, J. C., Gomez-Isla, T., Hyman, B. T., & Nixon, R. A. (2000). Endocytic pathway abnormalities precede amyloid β deposition in sporadic Alzheimer's disease and down syndrome: Differential effects of APOE genotype and presenilin mutations. *The American Journal of Pathology, 157*, 277–286.

Chidambaram, H., & Chinnathambi, S. (2020). G-Protein coupled receptors and Tau-different Roles in Alzheimer's disease. *Neuroscience, 438*, 198–214.

Chidambaram, H., Das, R., & Chinnathambi, S. (2020). Interaction of Tau with the chemokine receptor, CX3CR1 and its effect on microglial activation, migration and proliferation. *Cell BioSciences, 10*, 109.

Chidambaram, H., Das, R., & Chinnathambi, S. (2022a). G-protein coupled purinergic P2Y12 receptor interacts and internalizes Tau(RD)-mediated by membrane-associated actin cytoskeleton remodeling in microglia. *European Journal of Cell Biology, 101*, 151201.

Chidambaram, H., Desale, S. E., & Chinnathambi, S. (2024a). Interaction of Tau with G-Protein-coupled purinergic P2Y12 receptor by molecular docking and molecular dynamic simulation. *Methods in Molecular Biology, 2754*, 33–54.

Chidambaram, H., Desale, S. E., & Chinnathambi, S. (2024b). Purinergic receptor P2Y12-mediated Tau internalization in microglia. *Methods in Molecular Biology, 2754*, 457–470.

Chidambaram, H., Desale, S. E., Qureshi, T., & Chinnathambi, S. (2024c). Microglial uptake of extracellular Tau by actin-mediated phagocytosis. *Methods in Molecular Biology, 2761*, 231–243.

Chinnathambi, S. (2022). Role of cysteines in accelerating Tau filament formation. *Journal of Biomolecular Structure and Dynamics, 40*(10), 4366–4375. https://doi.org/10.1080/07391102.2020.1856720.

Chinnathambi, S. (2024a). Heat shock proteins regulates Tau protein aggregation in Alzheimer's disease. *Advances in Protein Chemistry and Structural Biology, 146*, 161–178. https://doi.org/10.1016/bs.apcsb.2024.08.003 2025.

Chinnathambi, S. (2024b). Histone deacetylase's regulates Tau function in Alzheimer's disease. *Advances in Protein Chemistry and Structural Biology, 143*, 339–361. https://doi.org/10.1016/bs.apcsb.2024.09.008 2025.

Chinnathambi, S. (2024c). α-Linolenic acid vesicles-mediated Tau internalization in microglia. *Methods in Molecular Biology, 2816*, 117–128. https://doi.org/10.1007/978-1-0716-3902-3_11.

Chinnathambi, S., Adithyan, A., & Chandrashekar, M. (2024). Lipid role in synapse and nuclear envelope-associated endocytic pathways in Tauopathy. *Advances in Protein Chemistry and Structural Biology, 143*, 387–409. https://doi.org/10.1016/bs.apcsb.2024.08.002.

Chinnathambi, S., & Chidambaram, H. (2024). G-protein coupled receptors regulates Tauopathy in neurodegeneration. *Advances in Protein Chemistry and Structural Biology, 141*, 467–493. https://doi.org/10.1016/bs.apcsb.2024.04.001.

Chinnathambi, S., & Das, R. (2023). Microglia degrade Tau oligomers deposit via purinergic P2Y12-associated podosome and filopodia formation and induce chemotaxis. *Cell BioSciences, 13*, 95.

Chinnathambi, S., Das, R., & Desale, S. E. (2023). Tau aggregates improve the purinergic receptor P2Y12-associated podosome rearrangements in microglial cells. *Biochimica et Biophysica Acta (BBA) - Molecular Cell Research, 1870*, 119477.

Chinnathambi, S., & Desale, S. E. (2024). The crosstalk between extracellular matrix proteins and Tau. *Advances in Protein Chemistry and Structural Biology, 141*, 447–466.

Chinnathambi, S., & Dubey, T. (2024). Photo-excited dyes: Emerging technique against Tau protein aggregation. *Methods in Molecular Biology, 2754*, 105–116.

Chinnathambi, S., Kumarappan, M., & Chandrashekar, M. (2024b). The cross-talk between ApoE and Tau protein in Alzheimer's disease.

Chinnathambi, S., Selvakumar, S., & Chandrashekar, M. (2024c). Lipids modulates Tau and amyloid-β proteins in Alzheimer's disease.

Christianson, H. C., & Belting, M. (2014). Heparan sulfate proteoglycan as a cell-surface endocytosis receptor. *Matrix Biology, 35*, 51–55.

Cunningham, M. R., Nisar, S. P., Cooke, A. E., Emery, E. D., & Mundell, S. J. (2013). Differential endosomal sorting of a novel P2Y12 purinoreceptor mutant. *Traffic (Copenhagen, Denmark), 14*, 585–598.

Das, R., Balmik, A. A., & Chinnathambi, S. (2020a). Effect of melatonin on Tau aggregation and Tau-mediated cell surface morphology. *International Journal of Biological Macromolecules, 152*, 30–39.

Das, R., Balmik, A. A., & Chinnathambi, S. (2020b). Melatonin reduces GSK3β-mediated Tau phosphorylation, enhances Nrf2 nuclear translocation and anti-inflammation. *ASN Neuro, 12*, 1759091420981204.

Das, R., Balmik, A. A., & Chinnathambi, S. (2020c). Phagocytosis of full-length Tau oligomers by actin-remodeling of activated microglia. *Journal of Neuroinflammation, 17*, 10.

Das, R., & Chinnathambi, S. (2019). Microglial priming of antigen presentation and adaptive stimulation in Alzheimer's disease. *Cellular and Molecular Life Sciences*, 1–14.

Das, R., & Chinnathambi, S. (2020). Actin-mediated microglial chemotaxis via G-protein coupled purinergic receptor in Alzheimer's disease. *Neuroscience, 448*, 325–336.

Das, R., & Chinnathambi, S. (2021). Microglial remodeling of actin network by Tau oligomers, via G protein-coupled purinergic receptor, P2Y12R-driven chemotaxis. *Traffic (Copenhagen, Denmark), 22*, 153–170.

Desale, S. E., Chidambaram, H., & Chinnathambi, S. (2021a). G-protein coupled receptor, PI3K and Rho signaling pathways regulate the cascades of Tau and amyloid-β in Alzheimer's disease. *Molecular Biomedicine, 2*, 17.

Desale, S. E., Chidambaram, H., & Chinnathambi, S. (2024a). α-Linolenic acid induces microglial activation and extracellular Tau internalization. *Methods in Molecular Biology, 2754*, 471–481.

Desale, S. E., Chidambaram, H., Qureshi, T., & Chinnathambi, S. (2024b). Internalization and endosomal trafficking of extracellular Tau in microglia improved by α-linolenic acid. *Methods in Molecular Biology, 2761*, 245–255.

Desale, S. E., & Chinnathambi, S. (2020). Role of dietary fatty acids in microglial polarization in Alzheimer's disease. *Journal of Neuroinflammation, 17*, 93.

Desale, S. E., & Chinnathambi, S. (2021a). Phosphoinositides signaling modulates microglial actin remodeling and phagocytosis in Alzheimer's disease. *Cell Communication and Signaling: CCS, 19*, 28.

Desale, S. E., & Chinnathambi, S. (2021b). α- Linolenic acid modulates phagocytosis and endosomal pathways of extracellular Tau in microglia. *Cell Adhesion & Migration, 15*, 84–100.

Desale, S. E., & Chinnathambi, S. (2021c). α-Linolenic acid induces clearance of Tau seeds via actin-remodeling in microglia. *Molecular Biomedicine, 2*, 4.

Desale, S. E., & Chinnathambi, S. (2021d). α–Linolenic acid modulates phagocytosis and endosomal pathways of extracellular Tau in microglia. *Cell Adhesion & Migration, 15*, 84–100.

Desale, S. E., Dubey, T., & Chinnathambi, S. (2021b). α-Linolenic acid inhibits Tau aggregation and modulates Tau conformation. *International Journal of Biological Macromolecules, 166*, 687–693.

Dubey, T., & Chinnathambi, S. (2019). Brahmi (Bacopa monnieri): An ayurvedic herb against the Alzheimer's disease. *Archives of Biochemistry and Biophysics, 676*, 108153.

Dubey, T., Gorantla, N. V., Chandrashekara, K. T., & Chinnathambi, S. (2019). Photoexcited toluidine blue inhibits Tau Aggregation in Alzheimer's disease. *ACS Omega, 4*, 18793–18802.

Dubey, T., Gorantla, N. V., Chandrashekara, K. T., & Chinnathambi, S. (2020). Photodynamic exposure of Rose-Bengal inhibits Tau aggregation and modulates cytoskeletal network in neuronal cells. *Scientific Reports, 10*, 12380.

Dubey, T., Kushwaha, P., Thulasiram, H. V., Chandrashekar, M., & Chinnathambi, S. (2023a). Bacopa monnieri reduces Tau aggregation and Tau-mediated toxicity in cells. *International Journal of Biological Macromolecules, 234*, 123171.

Dubey, T., Sonawane, S. K., Mannava, M. C., Nangia, A. K., Chandrashekar, M., & Chinnathambi, S. (2023b). The inhibitory effect of curcumin-artemisinin co-amorphous on Tau aggregation and Tau phosphorylation. *Colloids and Surfaces. B, Biointerfaces, 221*, 112970.

Evans, L. D., Wassmer, T., Fraser, G., Smith, J., Perkinton, M., Billinton, A., & Livesey, F. J. (2018). Extracellular monomeric and aggregated tau efficiently enter human neurons through overlapping but distinct pathways. *Cell Reports, 22*, 3612–3624.

Franzmeier, N., Rubinski, A., Neitzel, J., Kim, Y., Damm, A., Na, D. L., ... Finsterwalder, S. (2019). Functional connectivity associated with tau levels in ageing, Alzheimer's, and small vessel disease. *Brain, 142*, 1093–1107.

Frost, B., Jacks, R. L., & Diamond, M. I. (2009). Propagation of tau misfolding from the outside to the inside of a cell. *Journal of Biological Chemistry, 284*, 12845–12852.

Funk, K. E., Mirbaha, H., Jiang, H., Holtzman, D. M., & Diamond, M. I. (2015). Distinct therapeutic mechanisms of tau antibodies: Promoting microglial clearance versus blocking neuronal uptake. *Journal of Biological Chemistry, 290*, 21652–21662.

Gómez-Ramos, A., Díaz-Hernández, M., Cuadros, R., Hernández, F., & Avila, J. (2006). Extracellular tau is toxic to neuronal cells. *FEBS Letters, 580*, 4842–4850.

Gómez-Ramos, A., Díaz-Hernández, M., Rubio, A., Díaz-Hernández, J. I., Miras-Portugal, M. T., & Avila, J. (2009). Characteristics and consequences of muscarinic receptor activation by tau protein. *European Neuropsychopharmacology, 19*, 708–717.

Gorantla, N. V., Das, R., Balaraman, E., & Chinnathambi, S. (2020). Transition metal nickel prevents Tau aggregation in Alzheimer's disease. *International Journal of Biological Macromolecules, 156*, 1359–1365.

Gorantla, N. V., Sunny, L. P., Rajasekhar, K., Nagaraju, P. G., Cg, P. P., Govindaraju, T., & Chinnathambi, S. (2021). Amyloid-β-derived peptidomimetics inhibits Tau aggregation. *ACS Omega, 6*, 11131–11138.

Gutierrez, M. G., Munafó, D. B., Berón, W., & Colombo, M. I. (2004). Rab7 is required for the normal progression of the autophagic pathway in mammalian cells. *Journal of Cell Science, 117*, 2687–2697.

Haynes, S. E., Hollopeter, G., Yang, G., Kurpius, D., Dailey, M. E., Gan, W.-B., & Julius, D. (2006). The P2Y12 receptor regulates microglial activation by extracellular nucleotides. *Nature Neuroscience, 9*, 1512–1519.

Holmes, B. B., Devos, S. L., Kfoury, N., Li, M., Jacks, R., Yanamandra, K., ... Bagchi, D. P. (2013). Heparan sulfate proteoglycans mediate internalization and propagation of specific proteopathic seeds. *Proceedings of the National Academy of Sciences, 110*, E3138–E3147.

Kapoor, M., & Chinnathambi, S. (2023). TGF-β1 signalling in Alzheimer's pathology and cytoskeletal reorganization: A specialized Tau perspective. *Journal of Neuroinflammation, 20*, 72.

Kessels, H. W., & Malinow, R. (2009). Synaptic AMPA receptor plasticity and behavior. *Neuron, 61*, 340–350.

Kim, S., Sato, Y., Mohan, P. S., Peterhoff, C., Pensalfini, A., Rigoglioso, A., ... Nixon, R. A. (2016). Evidence that the rab5 effector APPL1 mediates APP-βCTF-induced dysfunction of endosomes in down syndrome and Alzheimer's disease. *Molecular Psychiatry, 21*, 707–716.

Koizumi, S., Ohsawa, K., Inoue, K., & Kohsaka, S. (2013). Purinergic receptors in microglia: Functional modal shifts of microglia mediated by P2 and P1 receptors. *Glia, 61*, 47–54.

Mohan, M. L., Vasudevan, N. T., Gupta, M. K., Martelli, E. E., & Naga Prasad, S. V. (2012). G-protein coupled receptor resensitization-appreciating the balancing act of receptor function. *Current Molecular Pharmacology, 5*, 350–361.

Luo, W., Liu, W., Hu, X., Hanna, M., Caravaca, A., & Paul, S. M. (2015). Microglial internalization and degradation of pathological tau is enhanced by an anti-tau monoclonal antibody. *Scientific Reports, 5*, 11161.

Maeda, J., Minamihisamatsu, T., Shimojo, M., Zhou, X., Ono, M., Matsuba, Y., ... Akatsu, H. (2021). Distinct microglial response against Alzheimer's amyloid and tau pathologies characterized by P2Y12 receptor. *Brain Communications, 3*, fcab011.

Majerova, P., Zilkova, M., Kazmerova, Z., Kovac, A., Paholikova, K., Kovacech, B., ... Novak, M. (2014). Microglia display modest phagocytic capacity for extracellular tau oligomers. *Journal of Neuroinflammation, 11*, 1–12.

Mclarnon, J. G., Ryu, J. K., Walker, D. G., & Choi, H. B. (2006). Upregulated expression of purinergic P2×7 receptor in Alzheimer disease and amyloid-β peptide-treated microglia and in peptide-injected rat hippocampus. *Journal of Neuropathology & Experimental Neurology, 65*, 1090–1097.

Mildner, A., Huang, H., Radke, J., Stenzel, W., & Priller, J. (2017). P2Y12 receptor is expressed on human microglia under physiological conditions throughout development and is sensitive to neuroinflammatory diseases. *Glia, 65*, 375–387.

Mirbaha, H., Holmes, B. B., Sanders, D. W., Bieschke, J., & Diamond, M. I. (2015). Tau trimers are the minimal propagation unit spontaneously internalized to seed intracellular aggregation. *Journal of Biological Chemistry, 290*, 14893–14903.

Mukherjee, S., Soe, T. T., & Maxfield, F. R. (1999). Endocytic sorting of lipid analogues differing solely in the chemistry of their hydrophobic tails. *The Journal of Cell Biology, 144*, 1271–1284.

Nanjundaiah, S., Chidambaram, H., Chandrashekar, M., & Chinnathambi, S. (2021). Role of microglia in regulating cholesterol and Tau pathology in Alzheimer's disease. *Cellular and Molecular Neurobiology, 41*, 651–668.

Napoli, I., & Neumann, H. (2009). Microglial clearance function in health and disease. *Neuroscience, 158*, 1030–1038.

Nixon, R. A. (2005). Endosome function and dysfunction in Alzheimer's disease and other neurodegenerative diseases. *Neurobiology of Aging, 26*, 373–382.

Ohsawa, K., Irino, Y., Nakamura, Y., Akazawa, C., Inoue, K., & Kohsaka, S. (2007). Involvement of P2×4 and P2Y12 receptors in ATP-induced microglial chemotaxis. *Glia, 55*, 604–616.

Parvathenani, L. K., Tertyshnikova, S., Greco, C. R., Roberts, S. B., Robertson, B., & Posmantur, R. (2003). P2×7 mediates superoxide production in primary microglia and is up-regulated in a transgenic mouse model of Alzheimer's disease. *Journal of Biological Chemistry, 278*, 13309–13317.

Pensalfini, A., Kim, S., Subbanna, S., Bleiwas, C., Goulbourne, C. N., Stavrides, P. H., ... Pawlik, M. (2020). Endosomal dysfunction induced by directly overactivating Rab5 recapitulates prodromal and neurodegenerative features of Alzheimer's disease. *Cell Reports, 33*.

Puerto, A. D., Wandosell, F., & Garrido, J. J. (2013). Neuronal and glial purinergic receptors functions in neuron development and brain disease. *Frontiers in Cellular Neuroscience, 7*, 197.

Qureshi, T., Chandrashekar, M., Ananthanarayana, V., Kumarappan, M., Rangappa, N., Velmurugan, G., & Chinnathambi, S. (2024). Nuclear podosomes regulates cellular migration in Tau and Alzheimer's disease.

Qureshi, T., & Chinnathambi, S. (2022). Histone deacetylase-6 modulates Tau function in Alzheimer's disease. *Biochimica et Biophysica Acta (BBA) - Molecular Cell Research, 1869*, 119275.

Ramakrishnan, S., Arshad, F., Bs, K., Pon, A. G., Bosco, S., Kumar, S., ... Alladi, S. (2024). Primary microgliopathy presenting as degenerative dementias: A case series of novel gene mutations from India. *Dementia and Geriatric Cognitive Disorders Extra, 14*, 14–28.

Rauch, J. N., Chen, J. J., Sorum, A. W., Miller, G. M., Sharf, T., See, S. K., ... Kosik, K. S. (2018). Tau internalization is regulated by 6-O sulfation on heparan sulfate proteoglycans (HSPGs). *Scientific Reports, 8*, 6382.

Reichenbach, N., Delekate, A., Breithausen, B., Keppler, K., Poll, S., Schulte, T., ... Blank, N. (2018). P2Y1 receptor blockade normalizes network dysfunction and cognition in an Alzheimer's disease model. *Journal of Experimental Medicine, 215*, 1649–1663.

Sonawane, S. K., Balmik, A. A., Boral, D., Ramasamy, S., & Chinnathambi, S. (2019). Baicalein suppresses repeat Tau fibrillization by sequestering oligomers. *Archives of Biochemistry and Biophysics, 675*, 108119.

Sonawane, S. K., Uversky, V. N., & Chinnathambi, S. (2021). Baicalein inhibits heparin-induced Tau aggregation by initializing non-toxic Tau oligomer formation. *Cell Communication and Signaling: CCS, 19*, 16.

Terwel, D., Dewachter, I., & Van Leuven, F. (2002). Axonal transport, tau protein, and neurodegeneration in Alzheimer's disease. *Neuromolecular Medicine, 2*, 151–165.

Vitelli, R., Santillo, M., Lattero, D., Chiariello, M., Bifulco, M., Bruni, C. B., & Bucci, C. (1997). Role of the small GTPase Rab7 in the late endocytic pathway. *Journal of Biological Chemistry, 272*, 4391–4397.

Xu, W., Weissmiller, A. M., White, J. A., Fang, F., Wang, X., Wu, Y., ... Chen, S. (2016). Amyloid precursor protein–mediated endocytic pathway disruption induces axonal dysfunction and neurodegeneration. *The Journal of Clinical Investigation, 126*, 1815–1833.

Zhao, J., Wu, H., & Tang, X.-Q. (2021). Tau internalization: A complex step in tau propagation. *Ageing Research Reviews, 67*, 101272.

CHAPTER SIX

iPSC-derived neurospheres: A cellular platform for Tau and Alzheimer's disease immunotherapy

Subashchandrabose Chinnathambi*, Anusree Adityan, Madhura Chandrashekar, and Gowshika Velmurugan
Department of Neurochemistry, National Institute of Mental Health and Neuro Sciences Hospital (NIMHANS), Institute of National Importance, Bangalore, Karnataka, India
*Corresponding author: e-mail address: subashneuro@nimhans.ac.in

Contents

Advances in Immunology, Volume 171
ISSN 0065-2776, https://doi.org/10.1016/bs.ai.2025.11.001

Abstract

Alzheimer's disease is the most prevalent type of dementia, which is characterized by a progressive loss of memory and cognitive impairment. The internalization of extracellular Tau and Amyloid-β-induced pluripotent stem cells plays a crucial role in understanding the AD pathology. iPSC-derived neuron, microglia, and astrocyte are used as models to study the spreading of pathological proteins and their contribution in the disease progression. iPSC-derived neurons serve as an essential model for studying AD, particularly in relation to Tau aggregation, prion-like propagation, and the toxic effects of oligomeric amyloid beta. Extracellular Tau, along with oligomeric amyloid beta, enters neurons via endocytosis and macropinocytosis, leading to cellular abnormalities, oxidative stress, and dysfunction in neurons. Additionally, iPSC-derived microglia provide insights into neuroinflammatory responses and neurotoxic effects of Tau aggregation and Amyloid-β, highlighting their combined role in Alzheimer's pathology. Extracellular Tau internalization by microglia involves phagocytosis and exhibits activation response to Tau aggregates, releasing cytokines and undergoing calcium homeostasis. iPSC-derived astrocytes demonstrated a reactive state and disruption in calcium homeostasis upon the exposure of the pathological proteins, contributing to neurodegeneration. Further, the mechanisms of Tau and Amyloid-β internalization in iPSC-derived cells provide insights into disease progression and highlights potential therapeutic targets for neurodegenerative disease.

Abbreviations

AD Alzheimer's disease.
ALS Amyotrophic lateral sclerosis.
α7nAChR α subunit that contains the nicotinic acetylcholine receptor.
β-AR β-adrenergic receptor.
CK1ε Casine kinase 1.
c-Myc cytoplasmic Myc gene.
COPI coatomer complex proteins.
CNS Central nervous system.
CRMPs collapsin response mediator protein.
CX3CL1 C motif chemokine ligand1.
DPYL5 dihydropyrimidinase-related protein 5.
EphR erythropoietin-producing hepatoma cell line receptor.
ESCs Embryonic stem cells.
FUMH fumarate hydratase.
EV extracellular vesicle.
HD Huntington disease.
hnRNP heterogeneous nuclear ribonucleoprotein.
HSPG Heparan sulfate proteoglycan.
IL Interleukin.
iMGs in vitro microglia.
LRP lipoprotein receptor-related protein.

oMGs	organoid microglia.
iPSC	Induced pluripotent stem cell.
iPSC MG	iPSC derived microglia.
Klf4	Krüppel-like factor 4.
mGluR5	metabotropic glutamate receptors.
NMDAR	N-methyl-D-aspartic acid receptor.
NFTs	Neurofibrillary tangles.
NPC	Neural progenitor cell.
oAβ	Aβ oligomers.
Oct4	octamer-binding transcription factor 4.
PrPc	cellular prion protein.
PSC	Pluripotent stem cell.
P75NRT	p75 neurotrophin receptor.
SGTA	small glutamine-rich tetratricopeptide repeat-containing protein alpha.
sEPSC	spontaneous excitatory postsynaptic current.
Sox2	SRY-box containing gene 2.
TDP43	TAR DNA binding protein43.
TTBK	Tau-tubulin kinases.
TMEM119	Trans membrane protein 119.
xMGs	xenotransplanted microglia.
γH2AX	Gamma histone family member X.

1. Introduction

Alzheimer's disease (AD) is an age-related neurodegenerative illness characterized by two primary features: intracellular neurofibrillary tangles (NFTs) of aberrantly hyperphosphorylated tau and extracellular amyloid plaques composed of Amyloid-β (Aβ) (Qureshi & Chinnathambi, 2022; Gu & Liu, 2020; Gorantla et al., 2017). It progresses with duration and has been associated with cognitive decline, memory loss, and spatial disorientation (Medeiros et al., 2011; Das & Chinnathambi, 2019; Sonawane & Chinnathambi, 2018). Stem cell differentiates into various types of tissues and it shows the capacity of self-renewal. Based on their differentiation capacity these are divided into pluripotent stem cells such as iPSCs – induced pluripotent stem cells (iPSC) and embryonic stem cells (ESCs), and multipotent stem cells (adult stem cells) (Chang et al., 2019; Melton et al., 2009). Yamanaka was first one to develop the iPSCs, using mice in 2006. Following that, in 2007, human iPSCs were developed. With the expression of particular exogenous genes or proteins, iPSCs are generated from somatic cells of the adult body and have many characteristics with ESCs in terms of morphology, antigens, and phenotype. Comparing iPSCs to ESCs produced from blastocysts indicates the following similarities: (1) the cell's morphology and development speed are similar. (2) Chromatin modification patterns and gene expression are similar. The expression of transcription factors like Oct4, Klf4 and Sox2 is required for somatic cell reprogramming in iPSC cells (Ye et al., 2013). iPSCs are used in the following applications: (1) development of disease-specific autologous cell therapy, (2) disease models to evaluate underlying mechanisms, and (3) drug screening and toxicity tests. Human iPSCs-derived from the somatic tissue of living donors and human tissue harvesting require extensive ethical and legal considerations regarding the dissemination of results and potential commercial benefit to donors for clinical translation. The following uses are possible with iPSCs: (1) developing an autologous cell treatment specific to a particular disease; (2) disease models to assess underlying mechanisms; and (3) Toxicity tests and screening of drugs (Kiskinis & Eggan, 2010). Significant ethical and legal considerations concerning the disclosure of data and potential financial benefits to donors for therapeutic translation are necessary for utilizing human iPSCs produced from the somatic cells of living donors and human tissue harvesting (Okano et al., 2013). iPSC-generated neural progenitors undergo further growth to develop terminally differentiated neurons (Klincumhom et al., 2012). Utilizing induced pluripotent stem cells (iPSCs), human microglia-like cells (iMGLs) are generated to investigate this function in neurological conditions like Alzheimer's disease. The impact of brain-derived Tau oligomers and Aβ fibrils on the expression of genes linked to AD was examined using iMGLs, along with the mechanisms underlying synaptic pruning (Schwartz et al., 2015). Astrocytes, the most numerous glial cells in the brain, also play a vital role in maintaining neuronal health and have been effectively modeled using iPSCs. iPasts gene expression profile mimics that of human primary astrocytes, and their functionality has been established in multiple domains, such as glucose metabolism, neural synapse formation, glutamate absorption, and calcium dynamics (Leventoux et al., 2020). Thus, iPSC-derived neural cells, including neurons, microglia, and astrocytes, offer promising tools for understanding the mechanisms of neurodegenerative diseases and developing therapeutic strategies, providing invaluable insights into the cellular and molecular pathways involved in diseases like AD (Fig. 1).

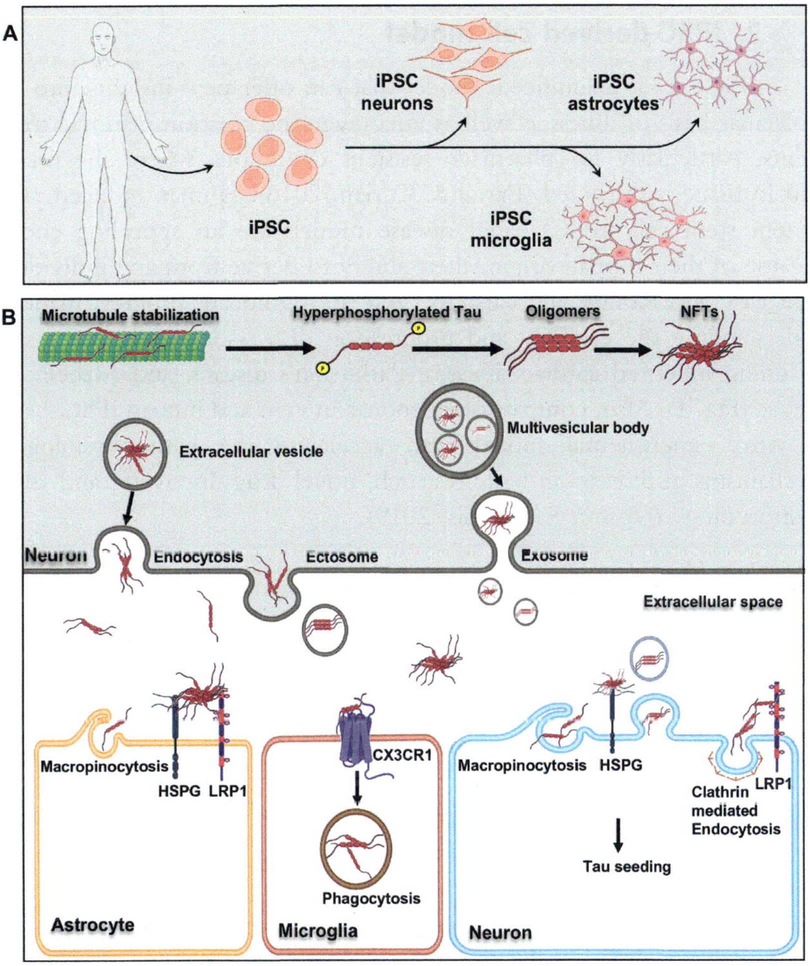

Fig. 1 iPSC and extracellular Tau internalization. (A) The derivation of induced pluripotent stem cells (iPSCs) from adult human cells. These iPSCs are then differentiated into three types of brain cells: iPSC neurons, iPSC microglia, and iPSC astrocytes showcasing the potential for studying neurodegenerative diseases and developing targeted therapies. (B) Internalization pathways of extracellular Tau proteins, focusing on the progression from neuronal release to uptake by astrocytes, microglia, and neurons. Initially Tau proteins stabilize microtubules within neurons; however, upon hyper phosphorylation, they form oligomers and eventually form neurofibrillary tangles (NFTs). Diseased neurons release these hyperphosphorylated Tau proteins into the extracellular space *via* extracellular vesicles like ectosomes and exosomes. Astrocytes internalize extracellular tau through macropinocytosis, utilizing receptors such as heparan sulfate proteoglycans (HSPG) and low-density lipoprotein receptor-related protein 1 (LRP1). Microglia, engage in phagocytosis mediated by the CX3C chemokine receptor 1 (CX3CR1) to uptake Tau. Healthy neurons internalize extracellular Tau through macropinocytosis, HSPG receptors, and clathrin-mediated endocytosis involving LRP1, leading to Tau seeding and further propagation of Tau pathology.

2. iPSC-derived cell model

iPSCs are a magnificent model that can offer new insights into the molecular basis of illness as well as encourage the creation of novel treatments, particularly for pharmaco-resistant conditions where the use of human tissue is restricted (Barral & Kurian, 2016). Human induced pluripotent stem cell (iPSC)-based disease models are an appealing choice because of their human origin, their ability to derive from any individual, their easy accessibility and capacity, and the significant progress made in understanding the etiology and progression of a wide range of diseases, including inherited cardiac diseases, Parkinson's disease, and Alzheimer's disease (Fig. 1). Also, comparison of mouse in vivo and human iPSC-based in vitro experimental models can accelerate the pathophysiological mechanisms of diseases in basic research, novel drug discovery, and safety pharmacology (Doss & Sachinidis, 2019).

2.1 iPSC-derived neuronal cell model

Pluripotent stem cells that may be produced from somatic cells are induced pluripotent stem cells, or iPSCs (Bell et al., 2019). Neural progenitors generated from iPSC were further developed into terminally differentiated neurons (Klincumhom et al., 2012). iPSC can be divided into many specific neurons such as GABAergic neuron, cortical neuron, dopaminergic neuron, dopaminergic neuron, serotonergic neuron, sensory neuron and motor neuron (Farkhondeh et al., 2019). A recent study that tested the chemical R33, which stabilizes the retromer, on neurons produced from human induced pluripotent stem cells (hiPSCs) and it also shown that retromer stabilization offers a prospective path for therapeutic development against sporadic AD (sAD) (Young et al., 2018). Peripheral sensory neurons derived from iPSCs have a wide range of applications for studying disease mechanisms and individual or group therapy development. iPSC-derived sensory neurons provide a personalized therapeutic strategy that can be useful in determining whether medications are particularly effective for a specific patient. An FDA-approved medication was found to be an efficient in vitro therapy preferred for that particular patient with the assistance of iPSC-derived sensory neurons (Lampert et al., 2020). Many of the cellular phenotypes associated with amyloid precursor protein (APP), presenilin, or SORL1 mutation that are linked to the processing of amyloid precursor proteins are also present in IPSC-derived neurons. These protein dysfunction may result in abnormalities related to γ-secretase activity, endoplasmic reticulum and oxidative stress with tau protein hyperphosphorylation, and amyloid β peptide (Aβ) accumulation. (Nicholson et al., 2022).

2.2 iPSC-derived microglial cell model

Microglia are the innate immune cells of the brain (Desale et al., 2021). They provide a various supporting functions in the maturing, adult, and aging brain, including neuroinflammation modulation, clearing out dead cells and other detritus, and pruning synapses (Penney et al., 2020). iPSC-derived microglia (iPSC-MG) and human primary microglia were shown to have significant similarities in gene expression and cytokine release analyses (Douvaras et al., 2017). Human microglia like cells (iMGLs) are derived from induced pluripotent stem cells (iPSC) to examine this role in neurological disorders such as Alzheimer's disease. iMGLs were used to investigate the effects of brain derived Tau oligomers and Aβ fibrils on the expression of genes associated with AD and also to study the mechanisms involved in synaptic pruning. Moreover, iMGLs are implanted into human brain organoids and transgenic mice which mimics microglia in vivo. To study neurotoxicity, human iPSC microglia were cocultured with neurons in three dimensions (3D) (Schwartz et al., 2015). iMGL cells are a potential model system for the development of neurodegenerative therapy because of their complex transcriptional profile and reactivity, which are similar to those of in vivo microglia (Ramaswami et al., 2023). TARDP/TDP-43 gene removal in microglia specifically highlights the importance of microglia in neurodegeneration and shows the necessity for human iPSC microglia co-cultures to investigate prevention strategies for this synapse loss (Haenseler & Rajendran, 2019). The transcription factors, protein profiles, and gene expression of microglia are shown by iPSC-derived microglia-like cells. The microglial marker TMEM119 was expressed by the majority of the microglial cells generated from iPSC and these cells showed comparable microglial gene expression patterns (Ihnatovych et al., 2020). This demonstration shows that iMGLs are used to study the function of microglia and also provides a new understanding of neurological disease in humans (Abud et al., 2017).

2.3 iPSC-derived astrocytes cell model

In the human brain, astrocytes are the most numerous and largest glial cells. Adult somatic cells are used to develop induced pluripotent stem cells (iPSCs) by specific transcription factors including Oct3/4, Sox2, Klf4, and c-Myc (Supakul et al., 2024). The iPSCs have pluripotent and proliferative characteristics with embryonic stem cells (ESCs). The differentiation of human induced pluripotent stem cells (iPSCs) into neural progenitor cells (NPCs) and subsequently into astrocytes (Gordillo-Sampedro et al., 2024). Understanding the processes of pathogenesis using iPSC-based disease modeling holds considerable promise, particularly for neurodegenerative disorders where patient-derived disease-susceptible cells are typically unavailable. iPSC-derived astrocytes (iPasts) showed glutamate absorption activity and calcium kinetics similar to human main astrocytes (Leventoux et al., 2020). The functioning of iPasts was validated in several areas' glucose metabolism, neural synapse formation, glutamate uptake, and calcium dynamics. Their gene expression profile was also shown to be consistent with human primary astrocytes. iPasts therefore include important physiological characteristics of human primary astrocytes. Given the increasing social and financial costs associated with neurodegenerative illnesses in aging populations, iPasts provide a valuable new resource for understanding the astrocyte-related processes underlying neurodegeneration. By addressing the role that astrocytes play in the emergence of neurodegenerative illnesses, iPasts will pave the way for the initial testing of potential medications in an in vitro setting before creating in vivo models (Leventoux et al., 2020).

3. Extracellular Tau internalization and its role in iPSC-derived cells

Tau aggregates can spread Tau pathology throughout many brain regions in a prion-like way by transferring from one cell to another and by causing templated misfolding and aggregation of healthy Tau molecules in prior healthy cells. After entering the extracellular space, Tau aggregates can be taken up by nearby neuronal and other glial cells through various process such as phagocytosis, micropinocytosis, and endocytosis (Fig. 1).

3.1 iPSC-derived neurons and Tau internalization mechanisms

Human-induced pluripotent stem cell (iPSC) neurons are vehicles for the aggregation and spread of Tau through human exosomes (Podvin et al., 2020). Tau aggregates can spread throughout many brain regions in a prion-like way by transferring from one cell to another and by causing templated misfolding and aggregation of Tau in previously healthy cells (Chinnathambi & Desale, 2024; Gorantla et al., 2019; Brunello et al., 2020). Endocytosis and micropinocytosis are the two ways that extracellular Tau protein enters human iPSC neurons (Fig. 2). Macropinocytosis is a brief process that requires actin and results in the internalization of fluid, membrane, and other particles into enormous vacuoles (Zeineddine & Yerbury, 2015; Chidambaram et al., 2022). Human iPSC neurons are predominantly accessed via endocytosis of Tau aggregates (Evans et al., 2018). Tau aggregate uptake is mostly dynamin dependent and unaffected

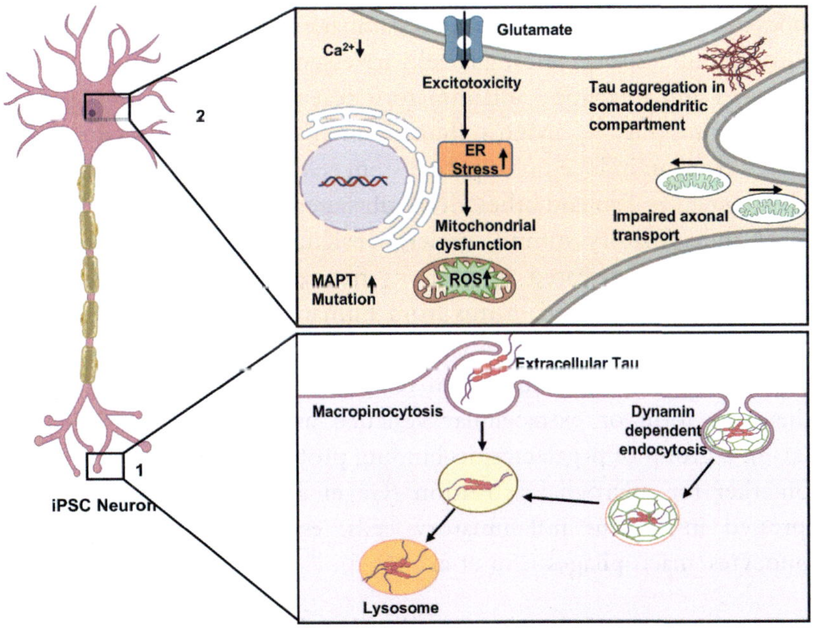

Fig. 2 Extracellular Tau internalization and role in iPSC Neuron. Extracellular Tau internalized into iPSC Neuron through Macropinocytosis and Dynamin dependent endocytosis. Elevated Tau phosphorylation leads to mislocalization of Tau and also increases insolubility of Tau, Tau in iPSC neurons increases susceptibility to oxidative stress and altered axonal transport. MAPT mutation causes the dysregulation in calcium signaling and upregulation of cell stress [including mitochondrial stress and increases markers of stress granules] and this confirms ability of Tau mutation to induce neuronal dysfunction. Tau overexpression in iPSC derived neurons results in cell death through Tau aggregation. Extracellular Tau also leads to mislocalization of Tau to the somatodendritic compartment, glutamate induced excitotoxicity and ER stress.

by actin polymerization (Sonawane & Chinnathambi, 2021; Balmik & Chinnathambi, 2021; Evans et al., 2018). Monomeric free Tau and Tau aggregates can be internalized by rapid dynamin-dependent endocytosis (Merezhko et al., 2020). In many AD iPSC models, elevated Tau phosphorylation (Balmik et al., 2022), mislocalization, and enhanced Tau insolubility have been described (Wray, 2017).

3.2 Mechanism of Tau internalization by iPSC derived microglia

Microglia are activated in Alzheimer's disease to phagocytose the extracellular Tau deposits and the damaged neurons. There are several ways for microglia to internalize Tau, including receptor-mediated endocytosis, pinocytosis, and phagocytosis (Chidambaram et al., 2024; Desale & Chinnathambi, 2021). Microglia cells are essential for both phagocytosing pathogens and mediating inflammatory reactions to stimuli (Ma et al., 2023). From (Fig. 3) iMGLs (human microglial-like cells) are differentiated from an induced pluripotent stem cells (iPSC), iMGLs phagocyte the extracellular Tau and other CNS substrates, and also secrete cytokines due to inflammatory stimuli, undergo calcium transients (Abud et al., 2017). Gal3 was released in both its free and extracellular vesicular-associated (EV-associated) forms from human induced pluripotent stem cell-derived microglia in response to phosphorylated Tau. Pathogenic Tau is abundantly accumulated in recipient cells as Gal3 is released in either free form or extracellular vesicular associated (EV). Galectin-3 (Gal-3), a group of β-galactoside-binding proteins has been an important biomarker for microglial activation (Ge et al., 2022) and it is widely expressed in various inflammatory cells, especially in microglia and monocytes/macrophages (Liu et al., 1995).

3.3 Mechanism of Tau internalization by iPSC derived astrocyte

From (Fig. 4) The neurotoxic extracellular free Tau is internalized by astrocytes using heparin sulphate proteoglycan (HSPG). Upon Tau exposure Alzheimer's disease (AD) astrocytes demonstrate specific GFAP overexpression and morphological rearrangement, which are indicative of a reactive state. Non-AD astrocytes do not exhibit this reaction. In AD astrocytes, Tau is processed and then degraded in the endo-lysosomal compartment. The unique pathophysiological function of AD astrocytes in Tau processing and clearance is highlighted by this specific

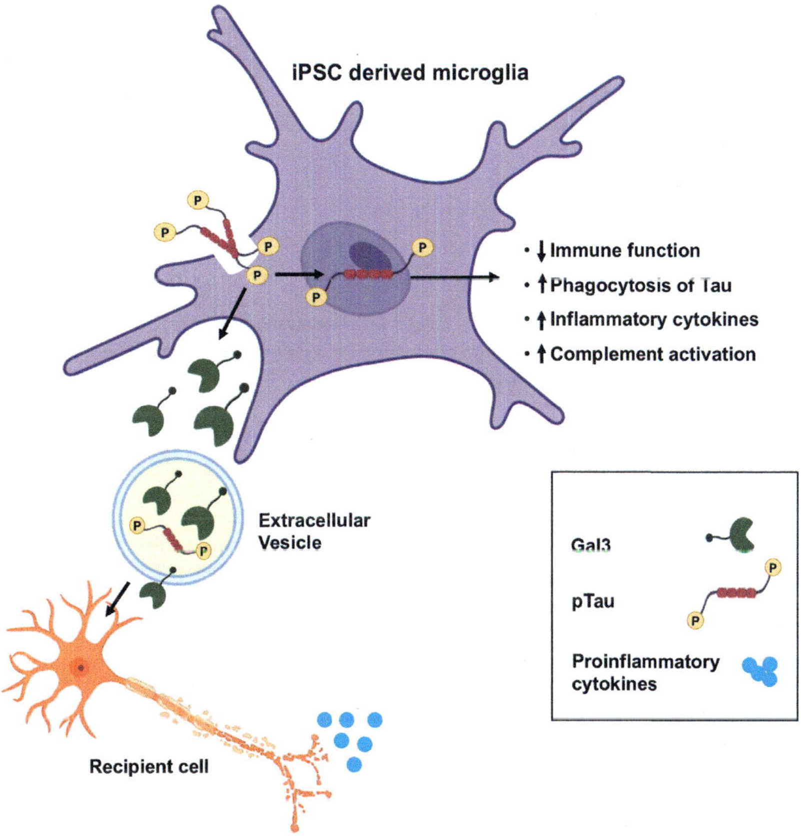

Fig. 3 Extracellular Tau internalization and its role in iPSC derived microglia. Phosphorylated Tau is internalized into iPSC derived microglia through phagocytosis, pTau triggers the release of Gal3 from iPSC microglia in both extracellular vesicles associated forms and its free form. Gal3 (Galectin-3) increases the accumulation of pathogenic Tau in recipient cells and the binding of Gal3 pTau enhances Tau fibrillation. pTau also induces production of inflammatory cytokines, increases complement activation, and decreases immune function.

response Calcium hemostasis is disrupted in astrocytes produced from iPSCs (Brezovakova et al., 2022). Long-term neurodegeneration is further facilitated by changes in astrocyte vesicle flow, which alters the signaling landscape of these cells and impairs astroglial Ca^{2+} (Sonawane et al., 2022; Vardjan et al., 2017). iPSC derived astrocytes are significantly impacted by neuronal Ca^{2+} response to glutamate activation (Brawek & Garaschuk, 2014).

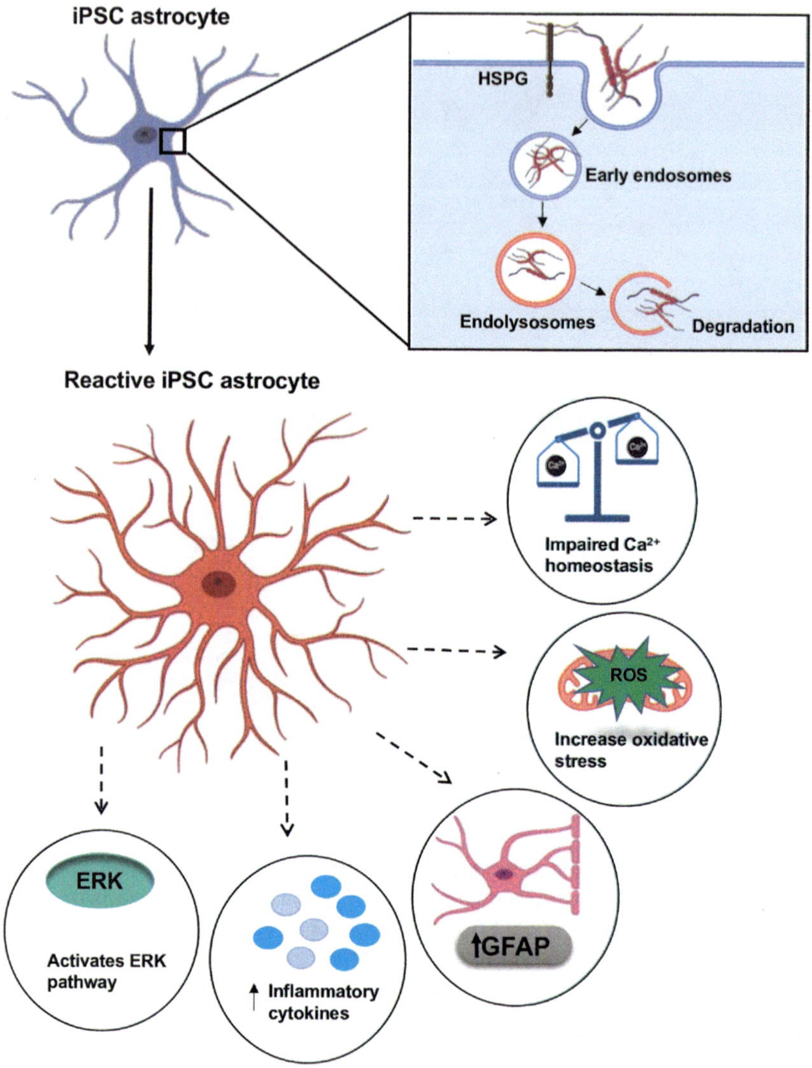

Fig. 4 Extracellular Tau internalization and its role in iPSC derived astrocyte. Extracellular Tau which is neurotoxic is taken up by astrocyte via heparin sulphate proteoglycan (HSPG) and Tau is further processed in the endo-lysosomal compartment and it gets degraded. In the presence of extracellular Tau astrocytes gets activated and upon Tau exposure astrocytes exhibit GFAP regulation, also glutamate increases and induces the calcium transient in presence of extracellular Tau. Activated astrocytes involve increase in oxidative stress, impaired calcium homeostasis and also increase inflammatory cytokines. Uptake of Tau activates the ERK pathway.

4. Effects of internalized Tau on iPSC derived neuroglial cells function

Hyperphosphorylated Tau species or mutated Tau are prone to aggregation and can cause neuronal dysfunction and cell death (Das et al., 2020) (Penney et al., 2020). Tau alterations lead to cellular abnormalities, including increased oxidative stress sensitivity (Kondo et al., 2013), aberrant endosomes, and altered axonal transport in iPSC neurons (Lacovich et al., 2017). Altered ROS concentration damages vital macromolecules including DNA, RNA, and proteins (Bartolome et al., 2022). The MAPT gene encodes with microtubule-associated protein Tau (Dubey & Chinnathambi, 2021), which plays an important role in the pathogenesis of neurodegenerative diseases (Chandrashekar & Chinnathambi, 2020; Sonawane et al., 2020; Verheyen et al., 2018). Misfolded Tau protein accumulation and aberrant Tau phosphorylation levels are linked to MAPT mutations (Chinnathambi & Chidambaram, 2024; Dubey et al., 2023). These abnormalities can spread between neurons and eventually result in cell death (Balmik et al., 2022; Cheng et al., 2021). Mutations in the Tau-encoding MAPT gene can directly result in neurodegeneration (Strang et al., 2019). A disruption in calcium homeostasis was supported by the marked reduction of calcium levels in MAPT mutant neurons (Minaya et al., 2023). Tau fibrils induce distinct Tau pathology in human iPSC-derived neurons (Mothes et al., 2023). MAPT mutation causes Tau mislocalization to the somatodendric compartment (Sonawane et al., 2022; Fong et al., 2013), glutamate-induced excitotoxicity (Kühn et al., 2021), elevated oxidative stress and ROS generation (Esteras et al., 2017), and endoplasmic reticulum stress (García-León et al., 2018). Microglia associated with Gal3 exhibit modified cellular mechanisms linked to dementia and neurodegeneration, such as enhanced immunological and inflammatory reactions (Siew et al., 2024). iPSC microglia can be activated by Tau aggregates and it undergoes morphological changes and releases a variety of chemicals, including complement proteins like C1q, once they are activated. Complement receptors CR1, CR3, C3aR, and C5aR1 are expressed by microglia (Batista et al., 2024). Inflammatory factors are continuously released when microglia are activated which also increases proinflammatory cytokines, and the activated iPSC microglia decrease the immune function. (Qu et al., 2023). The uptake of Tau activates the ERK pathway in iPSC derived astrocytes (Webster et al., 2006; Brawek & Garaschuk, 2014). The neuroinflammatory signaling pathway is activated, which induces the release of proinflammatory cytokines (Chinnathambi & Das, 2023; Kühn et al., 2021) (Fig. 5).

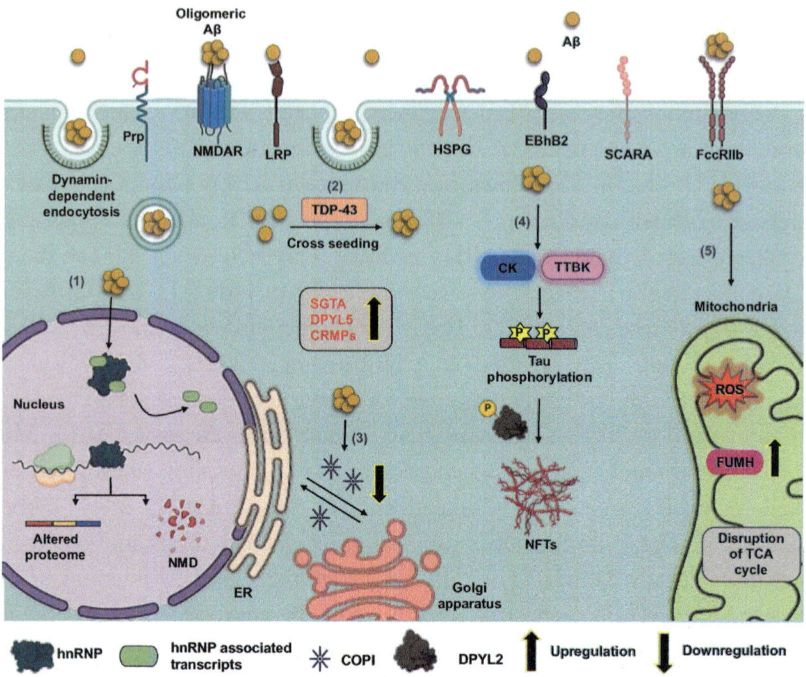

Fig. 5 Mechanism of oligomeric Amyloid beta toxicity in iPSC-derived neuron. This illustration depicts the effect of extracellular oligomeric Amyloid-β in the iPSC-derived neurons. Amyloid-β and its oligomer internalized into neuronal cell through various cellular pathway including, dynamin-dependent endocytosis and receptor-mediated endocytosis. (Bates et al., 2009) The internalization it triggers mRNA processing protein hnRNP-F and dissociates hnRNP-associated transcripts and leads mRNA to form altered proteome or it undergoes non-sense mediated decay (NMD). (Kraus et al., 2019) TAR DNA-binding protein 43 causes cross seeding between Aβ and results in oligomer formation. (Murphy & Levine, 2010) oAβ decreases the activity of COPI, which involved in trafficking mechanism between ER and Golgi apparatus (Bates et al., 2009) oAβ also tends to trigger hyperphosphorylation of Tau through casein kinase and Tau Tubulin kinase. DPYL2 phosphorylated by oAβ and implicated in the formation of NFTs. (5) In mitochondria they have an impact on the TCA cycle and upregulating FUMH (Fumarate hydratase) that increases oxidative stress. Due to the effect of oligomeric Amyloid-β several protein complexes also got upregulated including, SGTA, DPYL5 and CRMPs.

5. Mechanism of oligomeric amyloid beta toxicity in iPSC-derived neuron

Amyloid-β a histopathological hallmark in AD (Chinnathambi et al., 2023; Chinnathambi et al., 2024b; Chinnathambi et al., 2024a), accumulates extracellularly in neuronal cells. Investigations in their internalization mechanism provide a significant consideration in the study of AD pathology and its therapeutic approaches (Chidambaram & Chinnathambi, 2020). Studies indicate that low molecular weight Aβ oligomers (oAβ) and protofibrils play a role in initiating an accumulation of naïve Aβ, causing neurotoxicity, and are also associated with cognitive impairment. Currently, iPSCs can differentiate into all main brain cell types, particularly neurons, astrocytes, microglia, and oligodendrocytes, which are important for investigating Alzheimer's disease (AD). Advanced co-culture systems may now recreate AD-relevant brain environments, allowing for the study of key aspects such as amyloid-beta accumulation, Tau protein aggregation, and neuroinflammation. These models enable in-depth studies of cellular interactions in Alzheimer's disease pathogenesis and serve as an effective platform for evaluating possible treatment approaches in a human-derived system (Gallo et al., 2024). iPSC-derived neuronal cells are used to mimic many of the cellular processes disrupted in Alzheimer's disease in vitro, and co-culture platforms are starting to shed light on the intricate relationships that develop between different types of brain cells and pathogenic proteins underlying neurodegeneration (Ghatak et al., 2024). Comparatively among the Amyloid-β species, oligomeric forms result in high neurotoxicity in the brain (Johansson et al., 2024). These species efficiently internalized through various cellular mechanisms, including dynamin-dependent endocytosis and receptor-mediated endocytosis. The extracellular buildup of Amyloid-β in neuritic plaques and its binding to various receptors are the key feature of Alzheimer's disease (Sonawane et al., 2020). The binding of Amyloid-β to the various types of receptors have been claimed as the catalyst for the neuronal toxicity (Nazere et al., 2022). Soluble oligomeric Aβ exhibits toxicity, by binding to different types of receptors, such as the low-density lipoprotein receptor-related protein (LRP), cellular prion protein (PrPc), metabotropic glutamate receptors (mGluR5). It also interacts with α subunit that contains the nicotinic acetylcholine receptor (α7nAChR), N-methyl-D-aspartic acid receptor (NMDAR), the β-adrenergic receptor (β-AR), and the erythropoietin-producing hepatoma cell line receptor (EphR) p75 neurotrophin receptor (P75NRT) (Chen et al., 2017; Konings et al., 2024). It is hypothesized that the interactions between Aβ and Aβ receptors produce and transmit neurotoxic impulses into neurons, leading to cellular abnormalities such as mitochondrial malfunction and the ER stress response (Dubey & Chinnathambi, 2019). Proteome analysis revealed 42 prominently up- and down-regulated proteins in iPSC-derived neurons after the effective internalization of Amyloid-β (Sackmann & Hallbeck, 2020). OAβ impacts translation and alternative splicing by causing a reduction in the mRNA processing protein like hnRNP-DF. The affected hnRNP results in the production of an altered proteome, or the mRNA undergoes non-sense-mediated decay (Gaminde-Blasco et al., 2024). TDP-43, TAR DNA-binding protein, increases the level of oligomeric amyloid beta by cross-seeding Aβ monomers. The toxic oAβ also has a crucial effect on Tau protein and developing into neurofibrillary tangles (NFTs) (Gatch & Ding, 2024). oAβ triggers Casein kinase 1 (CK1ε) and Tau-tubulin kinases (TTBK1 and TTBK2), and this causes Tau to phosphorylate at serine 208 (Purushothaman et al., 2024). Further, it has been demonstrated that AD is associated with a substantial elevation of casein kinase 1, which in turn promotes the development of Aβ (Sackmann & Hallbeck, 2020; Ko et al., 2024). Furthermore, phosphorylation of DPLY2 (dihydropyrimidinase-related protein 5) protein has been implicated in the formation of neurofibrillary tangles (Sackmann & Hallbeck, 2020). On the other hand, oAβ disrupts trafficking between ER and Golgi bodies by downregulating coatomer complex proteins (COPI) (Arab et al., 2024; Li et al., 2024). By upregulating the FUMH (fumarate hydratase) protein and thereby raising ROS, they triggered the TCA cycle in the mitochondria (Sackmann & Hallbeck, 2020). SGTA (small glutamine-rich tetratricopeptide repeat-containing protein alpha), DPYL5 (dihydropyrimidinase-related protein 5), and CRMPs (collapsin response mediator protein) are upregulated following exposure to oligomeric Aβ (Sackmann & Hallbeck, 2020) (Fig. 6).

5.1 Neurotoxic impact of amyloid beta on iPSC-derived astrocyte

Astrocytes play a critical role in preserving synaptic function and alteration of synaptic signaling, neurotransmitter recycling, control of the blood-brain-barrier (BBB), and lymphatic clearance, and they are also closely linked to the a etiology of AD (Brandebura et al., 2023). Research findings indicates that astrocytes uptake significant quantities of accumulated Amyloid-β. However instead of degrading this toxic protein, astrocyte store it within their cells. This buildup of Amyloid-β can cause significant stress and impairment in astrocytes, potentially contributing to the progression of AD. Reactive astrocytes are mostly located around the Aβ-plaques in the AD brain and tend to generate elevated levels of Aβ, which exacerbates AD disease (Sonawane et al., 2021; Das & Chinnathambi, 2019). After the significant internalization of Amyloid-β through endocytosis, they begin to develop as an oligomeric form (Desale et al., 2021).

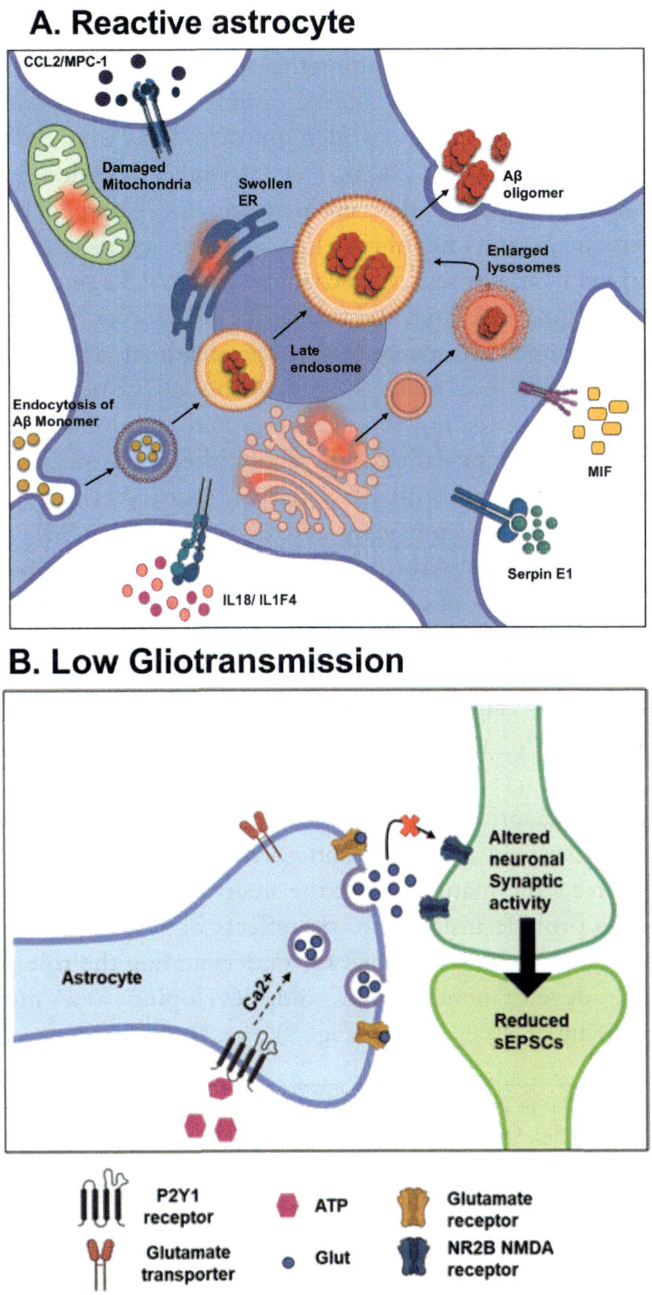

Fig. 6 Neurotoxic impact of Amyloid beta on iPSC-derived astrocyte. This illustration shows the impact of Amyloid-β over iPSC-derived astrocytes. (A) Reactive astrocytes. With the exposure of the Amyloid-β in astrocytes through endocytosis,

With increasing exposure of the Aβ, the astrocyte turns into a reactive state. This exposed Aβ starts invading the organelles and results in severe damage to the astrocyte. They altered double membranous organelles, which results in abnormally swollen mitochondria and endoplasmic reticulum (Johansson et al., 2024). Recent studies revealed that exposure of Aβ into the iPSC-derived astrocyte has enlarged lysosomes, which carry oAβ, amyloid fibrils. In particular, extracellular vesicles (EVs)- derived from astrocytes exposed to soluble Aβ aggregates caused synaptic loss, axonal swelling, and formation of vacuoles in the neuronal cells. These changes ultimately led to the death of neurons through apoptosis. (Konstantinidis et al., 2023b). Although astrocytes are highly secretory cells, investigating the cytokines and chemokines they produce might reveal important details about their inflammatory status. Interestingly, Aβ treated with iPSC-derived astrocytes secreted larger amounts of the pro-inflammatory cytokines, including MIF, CCL2/MCP-1, and Serpin E1/PAI-1 (Santos et al., 2017; Konstantinidis et al., 2023a). In cases of synaptic activity, there is a reduction in the gliotransmission in the astrocyte (Santello et al., 2012). Numerous substances, like glutamate, D-serine, ATP, and other growth factors, are known to improve synaptic transmission and can be released by astrocytes (Lei et al., 2024). Remarkably, after repeated exposure to Aβ, iPSC-derived astrocytes showed a substantial decrease in spontaneous excitatory postsynaptic current (sEPSC) frequency. sEPSC reduction leads to the decreased or less synaptic activity in neurons. This effect ultimately affects the maturation of the neuronal cells (Ju et al., 2024). These studies provide insight into the effects of long-term Aβ deposition on astrocytes, which is crucial for understanding the role glial cells play in the development of AD and developing new therapeutic approaches (Kumar et al., 2022) (Fig. 7).

---

they develop into large abnormal lysosomes. This lysosome contains the developed oligomeric Amyloid-β, which causes neurotoxicity to the astrocyte and invades internal organelles. Amyloid-β affects the double membrane organelles, including mitochondria, ER, and golgi bodies, where they are abnormally swollen and damaged. Reactive astrocytes tend to release several proinflammatory cytokines in response to amyloid beta, including MIF, CCL2/MCP-1, and Serpin E1/PAI-1. (B) Low gliotransmission. Amyloid-β, impacts synaptic transmission by causing a reduction in gliotransmission. This results in a loss of maturation and development of neurons. Low gliotransmission ultimately causes altered or reduced sEPSCs.

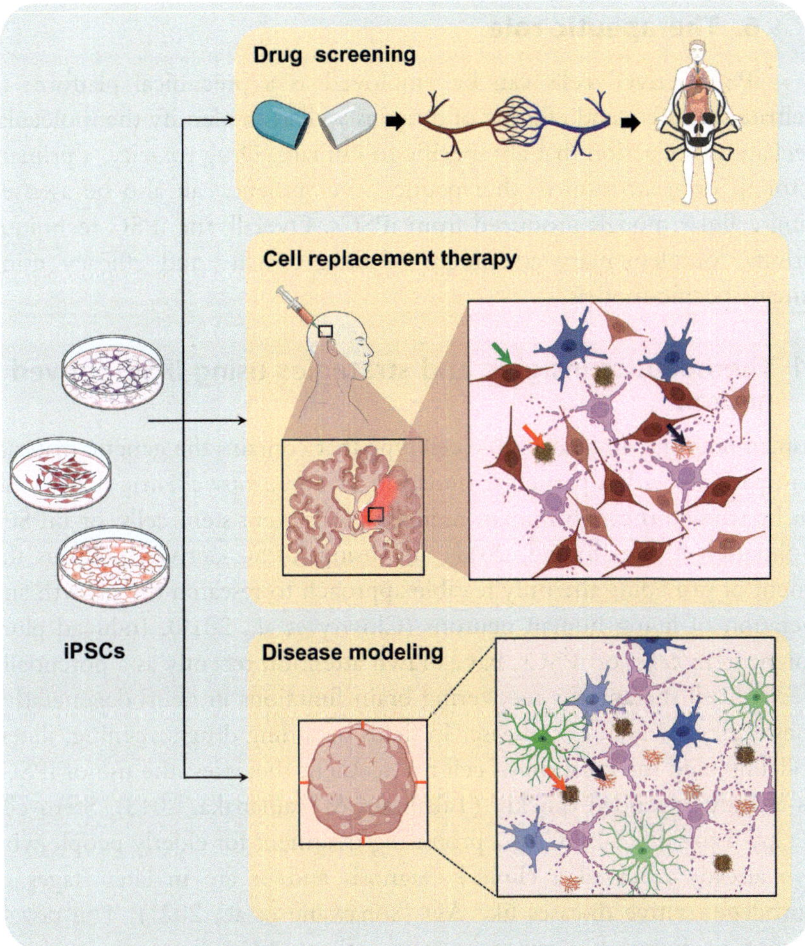

Fig. 7 iPSCs: AD therapeutic role. Induced pluripotent stem cells (iPSCs) are important in developing therapeutic interventions for Alzheimer's disease (AD). iPSCs are utilized in drug screening to study absorption, circulation, and toxicity, aiding in identifying a compound's effectiveness. iPSCs also play a crucial role in cell replacement therapy for AD patients, showing significant symptom reduction and memory improvement. Additionally, iPSCs are used to create disease models, including 2D cultures and 3D organoids, which serve as in vitro replicas of the AD patient's brain. These models provide valuable insights into the disease's pathology, and helps to explore mechanisms and test potential treatments.

6. Therapeutic role

iPSC-derived cells can be employed as a preclinical platform to evaluate the safety and efficacy of drugs as well as to identify the molecular mechanisms of action that are specific to humans. Drug toxicity, a primary factor in drug attrition in therapeutic development, can also be assessed using cellular models produced from iPSCs. Overall, the iPSC technique permits complementary assessment of drug toxicity and efficacy using human-specific models.

6.1 Therapeutics insights and strategies using iPSC-derived neuron

Human neurons, an inaccessible cell type that contains the genetic material from patients with a particular mutation or a neuropsychiatric illness, this can be studied through human induced pluripotent stem cells, or hiPSCs (Dolmetsch & Geschwind, 2011) and using hiPSC-derived neurons the benefit of providing the only feasible approach to research the growth and operation of living human neurons (Clowry et al., 2010). Induced pluripotent stem cells, or iPSCs, have drawn attention recently as a potentially effective cell therapy for recovering brain functions in neurodegenerative illnesses like Alzheimer's disease. In fields including drug screening, illness modeling, and the creation of cell replacement therapies, the use of iPSCs has already expanded quickly (Takahashi & Yamanaka, 2013). Stem cell therapy using iPSC-NPCs is a promising treatment for elderly people who have already received a clinical diagnosis and/or are in later stages of neurodegenerative diseases like AD (Sonawane et al., 2021). The development of induced pluripotent stem cells (iPSCs) from the patient's somatic cells has made patient-specific stem cells conceivable, and this has been proposed as a new, revolutionary step toward personalized medicine (Robinton & Daley, 2012). Docosahexaenoic acid therapy was found to be able to reduce the related stress responses in a study using iPSC-derived neurons from AD patients. Another study shown that using a drug screening platform, certain anti-Aβ compounds could inhibit Aβ plaque deposition in patient-derived cortical neurons (Nicholson et al., 2022).

6.2 Therapeutics insights and strategies using iPSC derived microglia

Recent developments in the production of microglia from human induced pluripotent stem cells (iPSCs) have opened up fascinating new approaches to studying and understanding the biology of microglia. Through these methods, a novel scientific understanding of the genetics and functionality of human microglia is being developed. Therefore, three distinct "flavors" of iPSC-derived microglia are accessible for researchers as a toolset: in vitro microglia (iMGs), organoid microglia (oMGs), and xeno-transplanted microglia (xMGs) (Hasselmann & Blurton-Jones, 2020). In vitro, in vivo, and toxicity studies are used to evaluate drugs designed for various targets in order to get useful preclinical data (Lee et al., 2020). Though their acceptability and safety for human use are sometimes uncertain, iPSCs derived from AD patients are certainly a strong platform for discovering novel medicines and intriguing targets. The iPSC model holds scientific value for aspects of drug discovery (Marei et al., 2023).

6.3 Therapeutics insights and strategies in iPSC astrocytes

Human astrocytes produced from patient fibroblasts mirror the characteristics of many neurodegenerative disorders including AD, ALS, HD, and fragile X syndrome, advances in iPSC technology are essential to adapting astrocyte research to translational studies. iPSC-derived astrocytes containing the p.Glu693Asp or p.Val717Leu mutations of the amyloid precursor protein were obtained from three AS patients: two with familial AD and one with sporadic AD. They discovered that astrocytes derived from AD iPSCs had an excessive build-up of Aβ oligomers. They also assessed the application of docosahexaenoic acid as a symptom-prevention medicinal agent (Kondo et al., 2013). The majority of these investigations revealed that AD patients had elevated Aβ42 secretion using iPSC-derived neuronal and glial cells (Yagi et al., 2011). According to this research, astrocytes play a major role in the pathophysiology of AD. Hence, AD patient iPSC-derived astrocytes can be utilized as a testing platform to identify the best pharmacological course of treatment. There are still few studies using iPSC-derived astrocytes from AD patients, despite the fact that they are instructive. The identification and advancement of human iPSC technologies offer a novel and accurate platform for human neurodegenerative disease modeling. iPSC-derived astrocytes with gene mutations unique to the illness might be a useful tool for in vitro comprehension of the cellular and molecular pathways underlying various diseases. These models have the potential to provide insight into the role that astrocytes play in neurological and neurodegenerative illnesses, as well as help discover novel treatments that can slow the progression of these debilitating diseases (Kumar et al., 2022).

7. Conclusion

The pathophysiology of neurodegenerative disorders such as Alzheimer's and Tauopathies is significantly influenced by the extracellular function of Tau and amyloid beta in neurons, microglia, and astrocytes. Tau interacts with neighboring cells, which causes neuroinflammation, neuronal damage, and cellular dysfunction. Extracellular Tau is internalized by neurons, which leads to intracellular aggregation and the spread of Tau disease. In response to Tau, astrocytes absorb Tau fibrils, which causes cellular malfunction and neurotoxicity. Likewise, Amyloid beta, another significant hallmark of AD, accumulates extracellularly, causing plaque formation and further exacerbating neuroinflammation. The combination of Amyloid-β and Tau pathologies accelerates neuronal death, loss of synapse and the overall progression of neurodegenerative diseases. In case of microglia, they initiate inflammatory pathways and contribute to neuroinflammation. Induced pluripotent stem cell (iPSC) derived neurons on aggregation and propagation of Tau, contribute to neurodegeneration in conditions like Alzheimer's disease. Understanding the mechanisms underlying propagation, internalization, and subsequent cellular responses of Tau and amyloid beta is crucial for developing targeted therapeutic interventions aimed at mitigating the neurotoxic effects of extracellular Tau, prevent amyloid beta accumulation, and halting the progression of Tauopathies.

Acknowledgements

We are grateful to Chinnathambi's lab members for their scientific discussions, helpful suggestions and critical reading of the manuscript. We greatly acknowledge Swathi for preparing the schemes and diagrams. We also greatly acknowledge internal support from the Department of Neurochemistry, National Institute of Mental Health and Neuro Sciences (NIMHANS), Institute of National Importance, Bangalore.

Ethical approval and consent to participate

Not applicable.

Funding

This project is supported in part by National Institute of Mental Health and Neuro Sciences (NIMHANS), Institute of National Importance, Hosur Road, Bangalore −560029, Karnataka, India.

Data availability

All the data have been included in the manuscript.

Author contributions

SBC conceived, designed, supervised, initial draft, review editing and wrote the paper.

Declarations

Competing interest

The authors declare no competing interests.

Consent for publication

Not applicable.

References

Abud, E. M., Ramirez, R. N., Martinez, E. S., Healy, L. M., Nguyen, C. H., Newman, S. A., ... Fimbres, C. (2017). iPSC-derived human microglia-like cells to study neurological diseases. *Neuron, 94*, 278–293.e9.

Arab, M., Chen, T., & Lowe, M. (2024). Mechanisms governing vesicle traffic at the Golgi apparatus. *Current Opinion in Cell Biology, 88*, 102365.

Balmik, A. A., & Chinnathambi, S. (2021). Methylation as a key regulator of Tau aggregation and neuronal health in Alzheimer's disease. *Cell Communication and Signaling: CCS, 19*, 51.

Balmik, A. A., Das, R., Sonawane, S. K., & Chinnathambi, S. (2022). Aggregation species of amyloid-β and Tau oligomers in Alzheimer's disease: Role in therapeutics and diagnostics. In T. Govindaraju (Ed.). *Alzheimer's disease: Recent findings in pathophysiology, diagnostic and therapeutic modalities*. The Royal Society of Chemistry.

Barral, S., & Kurian, M. A. (2016). Utility of induced pluripotent stem cells for the study and treatment of genetic diseases: Focus on childhood neurological disorders. *Frontiers in Molecular Neuroscience, 9*.

Bartolome, F., Carro, E., & Alquezar, C. (2022). Oxidative stress in tauopathies: From cause to therapy. *Antioxidants (Basel), 11*.

Bates, K., Verdile, G., Li, Q., Ames, D., Hudson, P., Masters, C., & Martins, R. (2009). Clearance mechanisms of Alzheimer's amyloid-β peptide: Implications for therapeutic design and diagnostic tests. *Molecular Psychiatry, 14*, 469–486.

Batista, A. F., Khan, K. A., Papavergi, M.-T., & Lemere, C. A. (2024). The importance of complement-mediated immune signaling in Alzheimer's disease pathogenesis. *International Journal of Molecular Sciences, 25*, 817.

Bell, S., Hettige, N. C., Silveira, H., Peng, H., Wu, H., Jefri, M., ... Ernst, C. (2019). Differentiation of human induced pluripotent stem cells (iPSCs) into an effective model of forebrain neural progenitor cells and mature neurons. *Bio-Protocol, 9*, e3188.

Brandebura, A. N., Paumier, A., Onur, T. S., & Allen, N. J. (2023). Astrocyte contribution to dysfunction, risk and progression in neurodegenerative disorders. *Nature Reviews. Neuroscience, 24*, 23–39.

Brawek, B., & Garaschuk, O. (2014). Network-wide dysregulation of calcium homeostasis in Alzheimer's disease. *Cell and Tissue Research, 357*, 427–438.

Brezovakova, V., Sykova, E., & Jadhav, S. (2022). Astrocytes derived from familial and sporadic Alzheimer's disease iPSCs show altered calcium signaling and respond differently to misfolded protein Tau. *Cells, 11*.

Brunello, C. A., Merezhko, M., Uronen, R. L., & Huttunen, H. J. (2020). Mechanisms of secretion and spreading of pathological tau protein. *Cellular and Molecular Life Sciences: CMLS, 77*, 1721–1744.

Chandrashekar, M., & Chinnathambi, S. (2020). Protein misfolding and aggregation of Tau protein in Alzheimer's disease. In R. Vyas (Ed.). *Advances in bioengineering. Singapore.* Singapore: Springer.

Chang, E. A., Jin, S. W., Nam, M. H., & Kim, S. D. (2019). Human induced pluripotent stem cells: Clinical significance and applications in neurologic diseases. *Journal of Korean Neurosurgical Society, 62*, 493–501.

Chen, G. F., Xu, T. H., Yan, Y., Zhou, Y. R., Jiang, Y., Melcher, K., & Xu, H. E. (2017). Amyloid beta: Structure, biology and structure-based therapeutic development. *Acta Pharmacologica Sinica, 38*, 1205–1235.

Cheng, C., Reis, S. A., Adams, E. T., Fass, D. M., Angus, S. P., Stuhlmiller, T. J., ... Haggarty, S. J. (2021). High-content image-based analysis and proteomic profiling identifies Tau phosphorylation inhibitors in a human iPSC-derived glutamatergic neuronal model of tauopathy. *Scientific Reports, 11*, 17029.

Chidambaram, H., & Chinnathambi, S. (2020). G-Protein coupled receptors and Tau-different roles in Alzheimer's disease. *Neuroscience, 438*, 198–214.

Chidambaram, H., Das, R., & Chinnathambi, S. (2022). G-protein coupled purinergic P2Y12 receptor interacts and internalizes Tau(RD)-mediated by membrane-associated actin cytoskeleton remodeling in microglia. *European Journal of Cell Biology, 101*, 151201.

Chidambaram, H., Desale, S. E., Qureshi, T., & Chinnathambi, S. (2024). Microglial uptake of extracellular tau by actin-mediated phagocytosis. In S. K. Ray (Ed.). *Neuroprotection: Method and protocols.* New York, NY: Springer US.

Chinnathambi, S., Adithyan, A., Suresh, S., Velmurugan, G., Chandrashekar, M., Sahu, S., & Mishra, M. (2024a). *Nuclear transport protein suppresses Tau neurodegeneration. Advances in protein chemistry and structural biology.* Academic Press.

Chinnathambi, S., & Chidambaram, H. (2024). G-protein coupled receptors regulates Tauopathy in neurodegeneration. *Advances in Protein Chemistry and Structural Biology, 141*, 467–493.

Chinnathambi, S., & Das, R. (2023). Microglia degrade Tau oligomers deposit via purinergic P2Y12-associated podosome and filopodia formation and induce chemotaxis. *Cell & Bioscience, 13*, 95.

Chinnathambi, S., Das, R., & Desale, S. E. (2023). Tau aggregates improve the purinergic receptor P2Y12-associated podosome rearrangements in microglial cells. *Biochimica et Biophysica Acta (BBA) - Molecular Cell Research, 1870*, 119477.

Chinnathambi, S., & Desale, S. E. (2024). The crosstalk between extracellular matrix proteins and Tau. *Advances in Protein Chemistry and Structural Biology, 141*, 447–466.

Chinnathambi, S., Velmurugan, G., Suresh, S., Adithyan, A., & Chandrashekar, M. (2024b). *Nuclear Tau accumulation in Alzheimer's disease. Advances in protein chemistry and structural biology.* Academic Press.

Clowry, G., Molnar, Z., & Rakic, P. (2010). Renewed focus on the developing human neocortex. *Journal of Anatomy, 217*, 276–288.

Das, R., Balmik, A. A., & Chinnathambi, S. (2020). Melatonin reduces GSK3β-mediated Tau phosphorylation, enhances Nrf2 nuclear translocation and anti-inflammation. *ASN Neuro, 12*, 1759091420981204.

Das, R., & Chinnathambi, S. (2019). Microglial priming of antigen presentation and adaptive stimulation in Alzheimer's disease. *Cellular and Molecular Life Sciences: CMLS, 76*, 3681–3694.

Desale, S. E., & Chinnathambi, S. (2021). Phosphoinositides signaling modulates microglial actin remodeling and phagocytosis in Alzheimer's disease. *Cell Communication and Signaling: CCS, 19*, 28.

Desale, S. E., Dubey, T., & Chinnathambi, S. (2021). α-Linolenic acid inhibits Tau aggregation and modulates Tau conformation. *International Journal of Biological Macromolecules, 166*, 687–693.

Dolmetsch, R., & Geschwind, D. H. (2011). The human brain in a dish: The promise of iPSC-derived neurons. *Cell, 145*, 831–834.

Doss, M. X., & Sachinidis, A. (2019). Current challenges of iPSC-based disease modeling and therapeutic implications. *Cells, 8*.

Douvaras, P., Sun, B., Wang, M., Kruglikov, I., Lallos, G., Zimmer, M., ... Fossati, V. (2017). Directed differentiation of human pluripotent stem cells to microglia. *Stem Cell Reports, 8*, 1516–1524.

Dubey, T., & Chinnathambi, S. (2019). Brahmi (Bacopa monnieri): An ayurvedic herb against the Alzheimer's disease. *Archives of Biochemistry and Biophysics, 676*, 108153.

Dubey, T., & Chinnathambi, S. (2021). Photodynamic sensitizers modulate cytoskeleton structural dynamics in neuronal cells. *Cytoskeleton, 78*, 232–248.

Dubey, T., Kushwaha, P., Thulasiram, H. V., Chandrashekar, M., & Chinnathambi, S. (2023). Bacopa monnieri reduces Tau aggregation and Tau-mediated toxicity in cells. *International Journal of Biological Macromolecules, 234*, 123171.

Esteras, N., Rohrer, J. D., Hardy, J., Wray, S., & Abramov, A. Y. (2017). Mitochondrial hyperpolarization in iPSC-derived neurons from patients of FTDP-17 with 10+16 MAPT mutation leads to oxidative stress and neurodegeneration. *Redox Biology, 12*, 410–422.

Evans, L. D., Wassmer, T., Fraser, G., Smith, J., Perkinton, M., Billinton, A., & Livesey, F. J. (2018). Extracellular monomeric and aggregated Tau efficiently enter human neurons through overlapping but distinct pathways. *Cell Reports, 22*, 3612–3624.

Farkhondeh, A., Li, R., Gorshkov, K., Chen, K. G., Might, M., Rodems, S., ... Zheng, W. (2019). Induced pluripotent stem cells for neural drug discovery. *Drug Discovery Today, 24*, 992–999.

Fong, H., Wang, C., Knoferle, J., Walker, D., Balestra, M. E., Tong, L. M., ... Huang, Y. (2013). Genetic correction of tauopathy phenotypes in neurons derived from human induced pluripotent stem cells. *Stem Cell Reports, 1*, 226–234.

Gallo, L. H., Akanda, N., Autar, K., Patel, A., Cox, I., Powell, H. A., ... Guo, X. (2024). A functional aged human iPSC-cortical neuron model recapitulates Alzheimer's disease, senescence, and the response to therapeutics. *Alzheimer's & Dementia.*

Gaminde-Blasco, A., Senovilla-Ganzo, R., Balantzategi, U., Garcia-Moreno, F., Matute, C., Baleriola, J., & Alberdi, E. (2024). Amyloid-beta increases MBP and MOBP translation in oligodendrocytes through dysregulation of hnRNP A2 dependent RNA dynamics. *bioRxiv* 2024.04. 19.590214.

García-León, J. A., Cabrera-Socorro, A., Eggermont, K., Swijsen, A., Terryn, J., Fazal, R., ... Verfaillie, C. M. (2018). Generation of a human induced pluripotent stem cell-based model for tauopathies combining three microtubule-associated protein TAU mutations which displays several phenotypes linked to neurodegeneration. *Alzheimer's & Dementia: the Journal of the Alzheimer's Association, 14*, 1261–1280.

Gatch, A. J., & Ding, F. (2024). TDP-43 promotes amyloid-beta toxicity by delaying fibril maturation via direct molecular interaction. *Biophysical Journal, 123*, 73a–74a.

Ge, M. M., Chen, N., Zhou, Y. Q., Yang, H., Tian, Y. K., & Ye, D. W. (2022). Galectin-3 in microglia-mediated neuroinflammation: Implications for central nervous system diseases. *Current Neuropharmacology, 20*, 2066–2080.

Ghatak, S., Diedrich, J. K., Talantova, M., Bhadra, N., Scott, H., Sharma, M., ... Lipton, S. A. (2024). Single-cell patch-clamp/proteomics of human Alzheimer's disease iPSC-derived excitatory neurons versus isogenic wild-type controls suggests novel causation and therapeutic targets. *Advanced Science,* 2400545.

Gorantla, N. V., Das, R., Mulani, F. A., Thulasiram, H. V., & Chinnathambi, S. (2019). Neem derivatives inhibits Tau aggregation. *Journal of Alzheimer's Disease & Reports, 3*, 169–178.

Gorantla, N. V., Khandelwal, P., Poddar, P., & Chinnathambi, S. (2017). Global conformation of Tau protein mapped by Raman spectroscopy. *Methods in Molecular Biology, 1523*, 21–31.

Gordillo-Sampedro, S., Antounians, L., Wei, W., Mufteev, M., Lendemeijer, B., Kushner, S. A., ... Ellis, J. (2024). iPSC-derived healthy human astrocytes selectively load miRNAs targeting neuronal genes into extracellular vesicles. *Molecular and Cellular Neuroscience, 129*, 103933.

Gu, J.-L., & Liu, F. (2020). Tau in Alzheimer's disease: Pathological alterations and an attractive therapeutic target. *Current Medical Science, 40*, 1009–1021.

Haenseler, W., & Rajendran, L. (2019). Concise review: Modeling neurodegenerative diseases with human pluripotent stem cell-derived microglia. *Stem Cells, 37*, 724–730.

Hasselmann, J., & Blurton-Jones, M. (2020). Human iPSC-derived microglia: A growing toolset to study the brain's innate immune cells. *Glia, 68*, 721–739.

Ihnatovych, I., Birkaya, B., Notari, E., & Szigeti, K. (2020). iPSC-derived microglia for modeling human-specific DAMP and PAMP responses in the context of Alzheimer's disease. *International Journal of Molecular Sciences, 21*.

Johansson, L., Sandberg, A., Nyström, S., Hammarström, P., & Hallbeck, M. (2024). Amyloid beta 1-40 and 1-42 fibril ratios and maturation level cause conformational differences with minimal impact on autophagy and cytotoxicity. *Journal of Neurochemistry*.

Ju, Y. H., Cho, J., Park, J.-Y., Kim, H., Hong, E.-B., Lee, C. J., ... Nam, M.-H. (2024). Tonic excitation by astrocytic GABA causes neuropathic pain by augmenting neuronal activity and glucose metabolism. *Experimental & Molecular Medicine*, 1–13.

Kiskinis, E., & Eggan, K. (2010). Progress toward the clinical application of patient-specific pluripotent stem cells. *The Journal of Clinical Investigation, 120*, 51–59.

Klincumhom, N., Pirity, M. K., Berzsenyi, S., Ujhelly, O., Muenthaisong, S., Rungarunlert, S., ... Dinnyes, A. (2012). Generation of neuronal progenitor cells and neurons from mouse sleeping beauty transposon-generated induced pluripotent stem cells. *Cell Reprogram, 14*, 390–397.

Ko, V. I., Ong, K., Cleveland, D. W., Yu, H., & Ravits, J. M. (2024). CK1δ/ε kinases regulate TDP-43 phosphorylation and are therapeutic targets for ALS-related TDP-43 hyperphosphorylation. *Neurobiology of Disease, 196*, 106516.

Kondo, T., Asai, M., Tsukita, K., Kutoku, Y., Ohsawa, Y., Sunada, Y., ... Inoue, H. (2013). Modeling Alzheimer's disease with iPSCs reveals stress phenotypes associated with intracellular Aβ and differential drug responsiveness. *Cell Stem Cell, 12*, 487–496.

Konings, S. C., Nyberg, E., Martinsson, I., Torres-Garcia, L., Klementieva, O., Guimas Almeida, C., & Gouras, G. K. (2024). Correction: Apolipoprotein E intersects with amyloid-beta within neurons. *Life Sci Alliance*, 7.

Konstantinidis, E., Dakhel, A., Beretta, C., & Erlandsson, A. (2023a). Long-term effects of amyloid-beta deposits in human iPSC-derived astrocytes. *Molecular and Cellular Neurosciences, 125*, 103839.

Konstantinidis, E., Portal, B., Mothes, T., Beretta, C., Lindskog, M., & Erlandsson, A. (2023b). Intracellular deposits of amyloid-beta influence the ability of human iPSC-derived astrocytes to support neuronal function. *Journal of Neuroinflammation, 20*, 3.

Kraus, A., Saijo, E., Metrick, M. A., 2nd, Newell, K., Sigurdson, C. J., ... Caughey, B. (2019). Seeding selectivity and ultrasensitive detection of tau aggregate conformers of Alzheimer disease. *Acta Neuropathologica, 137*, 585–598.

Kühn, R., Mahajan, A., Canoll, P., & Hargus, G. (2021). Human induced pluripotent stem cell models of frontotemporal dementia with Tau pathology. *Frontiers in Cell and Developmental Biology, 9*, 766773.

Kumar, M., Nguyen, N. T. P., Milanese, M., & Bonanno, G. (2022). Insights into human-induced pluripotent stem cell-derived astrocytes in neurodegenerative disorders. *Biomolecules, 12*.

Lacovich, V., Espindola, S. L., Alloatti, M., Pozo Devoto, V., Cromberg, L. E., Čarná, M. E., ... Falzone, T. L. (2017). Tau Isoforms Imbalance Impairs the axonal transport of the amyloid precursor protein in human neurons. *The Journal of Neuroscience, 37*, 58–69.

Lampert, A., Bennett, D. L., Mcdermott, L. A., Neureiter, A., Eberhardt, E., Winner, B., & Zenke, M. (2020). Human sensory neurons derived from pluripotent stem cells for disease modelling and personalized medicine. *Neurobiology of Pain, 8*, 100055.

Lee, C., Willerth, S. M., & Nygaard, H. B. (2020). The use of patient-derived induced pluripotent stem cells for Alzheimer's disease modeling. *Progress in Neurobiology, 192*, 101804.

Lei, L., Wang, Y.-F., Chen, C.-Y., Wang, Y.-T., & Zhang, Y. (2024). Novel insight into astrocyte-mediated gliotransmission modulates the synaptic plasticity in major depressive disorder. *Life Sciences*, 122988.

Leventoux, N., Morimoto, S., Imaizumi, K., Sato, Y., Takahashi, S., Mashima, K., ... Okano, H. (2020). Human astrocytes model derived from induced pluripotent stem cells. *Cells, 9*.

Li, X., Zhang, J., Xiao, Y., Song, H., Li, Y., Li, W., ... Wang, C. (2024). Chemoproteomics enables identification of coatomer subunit zeta-1 targeted by a small molecule for enterovirus A71 inhibition. *MedComm, 5*, e587.

Liu, F.-T., Hsu, D. K., Zuberi, R. I., Kuwabara, I., Chi, E. Y., & Henderson Jr, W. R. (1995). Expression and function of galectin-3, a beta-galactoside-binding lectin, in human monocytes and macrophages. *The American Journal of Pathology, 147*, 1016.

Ma, W., Zhao, L., Xu, B., Fariss, R. N., Michael Redmond, T., Zou, J., ... Li, W. (2023). Human iPSC-derived microglia cells integrated into mouse retina and recapitulated features of endogenous microglia cells. *Cold Spring Harbor Laboratory*.

Marei, H. E., Khan, M. U. A., & Hasan, A. (2023). Potential use of iPSCs for disease modeling, drug screening, and cell-based therapy for Alzheimer's disease. *Cellular & Molecular Biology Letters, 28*, 98.

Medeiros, R., Baglietto-Vargas, D., & Laferla, F. M. (2011). The role of tau in Alzheimer's disease and related disorders. *CNS Neuroscience & Therapeutics, 17*, 514–524.

Melton, D., Cowen, C., & Lanza, R. (2009). *Essentials of stem cell biology*. Oxford: Academic Press.

Merezhko, M., Uronen, R. L., & Huttunen, H. J. (2020). The cell biology of Tau secretion. *Frontiers in Molecular Neuroscience, 13*, 569818.

Minaya, M. A., Mahali, S., Iyer, A. K., Eteleeb, A. M., Martinez, R., Huang, G., ... Karch, C. M. (2023). Conserved gene signatures shared among MAPT mutations reveal defects in calcium signaling. *Frontiers in Molecular Biosciences, 10*, 1051494.

Mothes, T., Portal, B., Konstantinidis, E., Eltom, K., Libard, S., Streubel-Gallasch, L., ... Erlandsson, A. (2023). Astrocytic uptake of neuronal corpses promotes cell-to-cell spreading of tau pathology. *Acta Neuropathologica Communications, 11*, 97.

Murphy, M. P., & Levine, H., 3RD (2010). Alzheimer's disease and the amyloid-beta peptide. *Journal of Alzheimer's Disease: JAD, 19*, 311–323.

Nazere, K., Takahashi, T., Hara, N., Muguruma, K., Nakamori, M., Yamazaki, Y., ... Maruyama, H. (2022). Amyloid beta is internalized via macropinocytosis, an HSPG- and lipid raft-dependent and Rac1-mediated process. *Frontiers in Molecular Neuroscience, 15*, 804702.

Nicholson, M. W., Ting, C.-Y., Chan, D. Z. H., Cheng, Y.-C., Lee, Y.-C., Hsu, C.-C., ... Hsieh, P. C. H. (2022). Utility of iPSC-derived cells for disease modeling, drug development, and cell therapy. *Cells, 11*, 1853.

Okano, H., Nakamura, M., Yoshida, K., Okada, Y., Tsuji, O., Nori, S., ... Miura, K. (2013). Steps toward safe cell therapy using induced pluripotent stem cells. *Circulation Research, 112*, 523–533.

Penney, J., Ralvenius, W. T., & Tsai, L.-H. (2020). Modeling Alzheimer's disease with iPSC-derived brain cells. *Molecular Psychiatry, 25*, 148–167.

Podvin, S., Jones, A., Liu, Q., Aulston, B., Ransom, L., Ames, J., ... Hook, V. (2020). Dysregulation of exosome Cargo by mutant tau expressed in human-induced pluripotent stem cell (iPSC) neurons revealed by proteomics analyses. *Molecular & Cellular Proteomics: MCP, 19*, 1017–1034.

Purushothaman, K., Sivasankar, E., Krishnamoorthy, M., Karunakaran, K., & Muniyan, R. (2024). Computational identification of potential tau tubulin kinase 1 (TTBK1) inhibitors: A structural analog approach. *Silico pharmacology, 12*, 1–11.

Qu, W., Canoll, P., & Hargus, G. (2023). Molecular insights into cell type-specific roles in Alzheimer's disease: Human induced pluripotent stem cell-based disease modelling. *Neuroscience, 518*, 10–26.

Qureshi, T., & Chinnathambi, S. (2022). Histone deacetylase-6 modulates Tau function in Alzheimer's disease. *Biochimica et Biophysica Acta (BBA)-Molecular Cell Research, 1869*, 119275.

Ramaswami, G., Yuva-Aydemir, Y., Akerberg, B., Matthews, B., Williams, J., Golczer, G., ... Bumcrot, D. (2023). Transcriptional characterization of iPSC-derived microglia as a model for therapeutic development in neurodegeneration. *bioRxiv* 2023.03.09.531934.

Robinton, D. A., & Daley, G. Q. (2012). The promise of induced pluripotent stem cells in research and therapy. *Nature, 481*, 295–305.

Sackmann, C., & Hallbeck, M. (2020). Oligomeric amyloid-beta induces early and widespread changes to the proteome in human iPSC-derived neurons. *Sci Rep, 10*, 6538.

Santello, M., Cali, C., & Bezzi, P. (2012). Gliotransmission and the tripartite synapse. *Advances in Experimental Medicine and Biology, 970*, 307–331.

Santos, R., Vadodaria, K. C., Jaeger, B. N., Mei, A., Lefcochilos-Fogelquist, S., Mendes, A. P. D., ... Gage, F. H. (2017). Differentiation of inflammation-responsive astrocytes from glial progenitors generated from human induced pluripotent stem cells. *Stem Cell Reports, 8*, 1757–1769.

Schwartz, M. P., Hou, Z., Propson, N. E., Zhang, J., Engstrom, C. J., Costa, V. S., ... Thomson, J. A. (2015). Human pluripotent stem cell-derived neural constructs for predicting neural toxicity. *Proceedings of the National Academy of Sciences, 112*, 12516–12521.

Siew, J. J., Chen, H. M., Chiu, F. L., Lee, C. W., Chang, Y. M., Chen, H. L., ... Chern, Y. (2024). Galectin-3 aggravates microglial activation and tau transmission in tauopathy. *The Journal of Clinical Investigation, 134*.

Sonawane, S. K., Chidambaram, H., Boral, D., Gorantla, N. V., Balmik, A. A., Dangi, A., ... Chinnathambi, S. (2020). EGCG impedes human Tau aggregation and interacts with Tau. *Scientific Reports, 10*, 12579.

Sonawane, S. K., & Chinnathambi, S. (2018). Prion-like propagation of post-translationally modified Tau in Alzheimer's disease: A hypothesis. *Journal of Molecular Neuroscience: MN, 65*, 480–490.

Sonawane, S. K., & Chinnathambi, S. (2021). Epigallocatechin-3-gallate modulates Tau post-translational modifications and cytoskeletal network. *Oncotarget, 12*, 1083–1099.

Sonawane, S. K., Dubey, T., Balmik, A. A., Das, R., & Chinnathambi, S. (2022). Alzheimer's disease pathology: A Tau perspective. In T. Govindaraju (Ed.). *Alzheimer's disease: Recent findings in pathophysiology, diagnostic and therapeutic modalities*. The Royal Society of Chemistry.

Sonawane, S. K., Uversky, V. N., & Chinnathambi, S. (2021). Baicalein inhibits heparin-induced Tau aggregation by initializing non-toxic Tau oligomer formation. *Cell Communication and Signaling: CCS, 19*, 16.

Strang, K. H., Golde, T. E., & Giasson, B. I. (2019). MAPT mutations, tauopathy, and mechanisms of neurodegeneration. *Laboratory Investigation; a Journal of Technical Methods and Pathology, 99*, 912–928.

Supakul, S., Murakami, R., Oyama, C., Shindo, T., Hatakeyama, Y., Itsuno, M., ... Okano, H. (2024). Mutual interaction of neurons and astrocytes derived from iPSCs with APP V717L mutation developed the astrocytic phenotypes of Alzheimer's disease. *Inflammation and Regeneration, 44*, 8.
Takahashi, K., & Yamanaka, S. (2013). Induced pluripotent stem cells in medicine and biology. *Development (Cambridge, England), 140*, 2457–2461.
Vardjan, N., Verkhratsky, A., & Zorec, R. (2017). Astrocytic pathological calcium homeostasis and impaired vesicle trafficking in neurodegeneration. *International Journal of Molecular Sciences, 18*.
Verheyen, A., Diels, A., Reumers, J., Van Hoorde, K., Van Den Wyngaert, I., Van Outryve D'ydewalle, C., ... Peeters, P. J. (2018). Genetically engineered iPSC-derived FTDP-17 MAPT neurons display mutation-specific neurodegenerative and neurodevelopmental phenotypes. *Stem Cell Reports, 11*, 363–379.
Webster, B., Hansen, L., Adame, A., Crews, L., Torrance, M., Thal, L., & Masliah, E. (2006). Astroglial activation of extracellular-regulated kinase in early stages of Alzheimer disease. *Journal of Neuropathology & Experimental Neurology, 65*, 142–151.
Wray, S. (2017). Modeling tau pathology in human stem cell derived neurons. *Brain Pathology (Zurich, Switzerland), 27*, 525–529.
Yagi, T., Ito, D., Okada, Y., Akamatsu, W., Nihei, Y., Yoshizaki, T., ... Suzuki, N. (2011). Modeling familial Alzheimer's disease with induced pluripotent stem cells. *Human Molecular Genetics, 20*, 4530–4539.
Ye, L., Swingen, C., & Zhang, J. (2013). Induced pluripotent stem cells and their potential for basic and clinical sciences. *Current Cardiology Reviews, 9*, 63–72.
Young, J. E., Fong, L. K., Frankowski, H., Petsko, G. A., Small, S. A., & Goldstein, L. S. (2018). Stabilizing the retromer complex in a human stem cell model of Alzheimer's disease reduces TAU phosphorylation independently of amyloid precursor protein. *Stem Cell Reports, 10*, 1046–1058.
Zeineddine, R., & Yerbury, J. J. (2015). The role of macropinocytosis in the propagation of protein aggregation associated with neurodegenerative diseases. *Frontiers in Physiology, 6*, 277.

CHAPTER SEVEN

Harnessing neuromodulation to target microglial activity in neurodegenerative diseases

Venkata Chaitanya Chirumamilla[a] **and Muthuraman Muthuraman**[b,c,*]
[a]The Zickler Family Prenatal Pediatrics Institute, Children's National Hospital, Washington, DC, United States
[b]Department of Neurology, University Hospital Würzburg, Würzburg, Germany
[c]Institute of Computer Science, University Augsburg, Augsburg, Germany
*Corresponding author. e-mail address: muthuramanm10@gmail.com

Contents

Abstract

Neurodegenerative diseases are increasingly understood as conditions of disrupted neuroimmune homeostasis in which microglia play an important, dynamic, and state-dependent role. Beyond their immune functions, microglia continuously monitor neuronal activity, participate in synaptic remodeling, and contribute to neural circuit regulation in ways that vary across brain regions, disease types, and stages of neurodegeneration. In parallel, neuromodulation can modify neural activity patterns, thereby influencing downstream cellular responses and immune-related signaling within the central nervous system. Accumulating experimental evidence suggests that neuromodulatory interventions can influence microglial state, morphology, and function through activity-dependent neuron–microglia interactions and modulation of inflammatory signaling pathways. By synthesizing findings from both experimental animal models and translational human studies, this chapter presents a mechanistic framework for examining how neuromodulation may be leveraged to modulate microglial activity in neurodegenerative diseases. This approach integrates current understanding of microglial heterogeneity, neuromodulation mechanisms, biomarker strategies, and key translational challenges, with the goal of positioning microglia as measurable and biologically grounded therapeutic targets.

Advances in Immunology, Volume 171
ISSN 0065-2776, https://doi.org/10.1016/bs.ai.2026.06.002

1. Neuroimmune dysregulation in neurodegenerative diseases

Neurodegenerative diseases, such as Alzheimer's disease, Parkinson's disease, and amyotrophic lateral sclerosis (ALS), are characterized by progressive neuronal dysfunction and loss within specific regions of the central nervous system (CNS) (Fołta et al., 2025). Traditionally, these disorders were viewed primarily as neuron-centered pathologies driven by abnormal protein aggregation, mitochondrial dysfunction, and synaptic degeneration. However, growing evidence indicates that disturbances in the interaction between the nervous system and the immune system play a crucial role in disease onset and progression (Chen et al., 2025). As a result, neurodegenerative diseases are increasingly recognized as conditions involving disrupted neuroimmune homeostasis. It is now clear that the nervous and immune systems maintain continuous bidirectional communication that is essential for maintaining brain homeostasis. Neural activity can influence immune responses through neurotransmitters, neuropeptides, and neuroendocrine signaling pathways, while immune mediators can directly affect neuronal activity and synaptic function (Zang et al., 2022). Neurotransmitters such as norepinephrine, dopamine, and acetylcholine regulate immune cell activity by acting on receptors expressed by immune cells. These signals influence immune cell migration, proliferation, and cytokine production. However, cytokines such as tumor necrosis factor-α (TNF-α), interleukin-1β (IL-1β), and interleukin-6 (IL−6) alter neuronal excitability and synaptic transmission. Through these interactions, immune signaling participates in processes such as synaptic plasticity, neurogenesis, and adaptive responses to injury. Under physiological conditions, these neuroimmune interactions contribute to maintaining CNS homeostasis and coordinating protective responses to tissue damage or infection (Mason & McGavern, 2022).

1.1 Neuroimmune communication and microglial function

Within CNS, microglia serve as the primary innate immune cells and are central regulators of neuroimmune communication. Microglia originate from embryonic yolk-sac progenitors and populate the brain early in development, remaining within the CNS throughout life (Scheiblich et al., 2020). In the healthy brain, microglia exhibit a surveillant phenotype characterized by highly motile processes that continuously monitor the neural microenvironment for signs of injury or infection. Microglia also contribute to synaptic remodeling, regulate neuronal connectivity, and remove cellular debris and apoptotic cells (Borst et al., 2021). During development, microglia play a critical role in synaptic pruning, a process that refines neural circuits by eliminating excess synapses. Microglia also interact with neural stem cells and influence neurogenesis, highlighting their role in maintaining brain plasticity and structural integrity. In response to injury or pathological stimuli, microglia become activated and undergo morphological and transcriptional changes (Godeanu & Cătălin, 2025). Activated microglia release cytokines, chemokines, and other signaling molecules that coordinate immune responses within the CNS. Although these initial responses promote tissue repair and pathogen clearance, sustained activation can cause inflammatory signals and neuronal dysfunction (Adamu et al., 2024).

1.2 Neuroinflammation and therapeutic implications

Chronic neuroinflammation is now recognized as a common pathological feature across multiple neurodegenerative diseases. In neurodegenerative disorders, inflammatory signaling is frequently initiated by the accumulation of abnormal proteins such as amyloid-β or α-synuclein. These proteins can act as danger-associated molecular patterns that activate innate immune receptors on microglia and astrocytes. Activation of glial cells leads to the release of pro-inflammatory cytokines, chemokines, and reactive oxygen species that disrupt synaptic function and increase oxidative stress within neural tissue (Kempuraj et al., 2016). Over time, persistent inflammatory signaling creates a chronic inflammatory environment that accelerates neuronal injury and degeneration. Importantly, recent research suggests that neuroinflammation may arise early in disease progression rather than appearing solely as a secondary consequence of neuronal damage (Chen et al., 2016). Since microglia regulate inflammatory signaling, they play a critical role in shaping disease trajectories. Dysregulated microglial responses can amplify inflammation and disrupt neural circuits, yet microglia also possess protective functions such as clearing pathological protein aggregates and supporting tissue repair (De Marchi et al., 2023). This functional dichotomy suggests that modulation of microglial phenotypes, rather than non-specific immune suppression, represents a potent therapeutic paradigm for decelerating the trajectory of neurodegenerative pathologies.

2. Microglial heterogeneity across brain states, regions, and disease trajectories

Microglia are increasingly recognized as a highly heterogeneous population of immune cells whose phenotypes and functions vary across brain regions, developmental stages, and disease states. Early studies considered microglia a relatively uniform cell population. However, the advances in transcriptomic and single-cell technologies have revealed substantial diversity in their molecular signatures, morphology, and functional roles across the CNS (De Schepper et al., 2021). This heterogeneity arises from both intrinsic factors such as genetic background, developmental origin, as well as extrinsic influences including the local neuronal environment, aging, microbiota, and pathological stimuli. Regional differences in microglial abundance, cellular morphology, gene expression profiles, and functional properties have been reported across different brain areas, suggesting that microglia adapt their phenotype to the specific neural circuits in which they reside (Tan et al., 2020). In neurodegenerative diseases, microglial heterogeneity becomes even more pronounced, with multiple activation states emerging in response to pathological protein accumulation, neuronal injury, and inflammatory signaling (Wang, 2021). Single-cell transcriptomic analyses have identified numerous disease-associated microglial states, including transcriptionally distinct populations that appear at different stages of disorders such as Alzheimer's disease, reflecting dynamic changes in gene expression and regulatory networks during disease progression (Sun et al., 2023). Importantly, these microglial states can exert both protective and detrimental effects. For example, microglia may initially contribute to the clearance of pathological protein aggregates and support neuronal homeostasis. However, persistent activation can promote chronic neuroinflammation and neuronal damage (Gao et al., 2023). Underscoring this functional heterogeneity, neuroimaging observations in the prodromal phases of Alzheimer's disease reveal a striking correlation between microglial activation and the preservation of gray matter volume. Such evidence suggests a biphasic trajectory, wherein microglia initially adopt a neuroprotective posture to safeguard neural integrity before ultimately transitioning into the destructive, chronic inflammatory state that defines advanced neurodegeneration (Femminella et al., 2019). Collectively, these findings show that microglia are not a single, uniform group of cells. Instead, they exist along a spectrum of different states that change depending on their location in the brain, the stage of life, and the specific disease. Understanding this diversity is essential for developing better treatments. Rather than simply shutting down all inflammation, future therapies must be precise enough to target harmful microglial behaviors while supporting their protective roles.

3. Regulating neuron-microglia interactions using neuromodulation

Communication between neurons and microglia is essential for maintaining CNS homeostasis, regulating synaptic plasticity, and coordinating neural circuit function. Under physiological conditions, neurons regulate microglial activation through inhibitory pathways involving molecules such as fractalkine (CX3CL1), CD200, and transforming growth factor-β, which help maintain microglia in a surveillant state and prevent excessive inflammatory activation. Through these interactions, microglia contribute to synaptic remodeling, removal of cellular debris, and maintenance of neural network stability. During neurodegenerative disease, this tightly regulated neuron–microglia communication becomes disrupted. Injured neurons release danger-associated signals including glutamate, nucleotides, and high-mobility group box protein-1 (HMGB1), which activate microglia and stimulate the release of pro-inflammatory cytokines, reactive oxygen species, and other neurotoxic mediators (Suzumura, 2013). Sustained activation of microglia amplifies neuroinflammation and accelerates neuronal injury, contributing to progressive neurodegeneration. Because microglial behavior is strongly shaped by neuronal activity, interventions that modulate neural activity offer a promising approach to regulating neuron–microglia signaling (Fig. 1).

Neuromodulation techniques offer a potential approach to influence these interactions by altering neuronal excitability, synaptic plasticity, and inflammatory signaling. Non-invasive brain stimulation methods such as

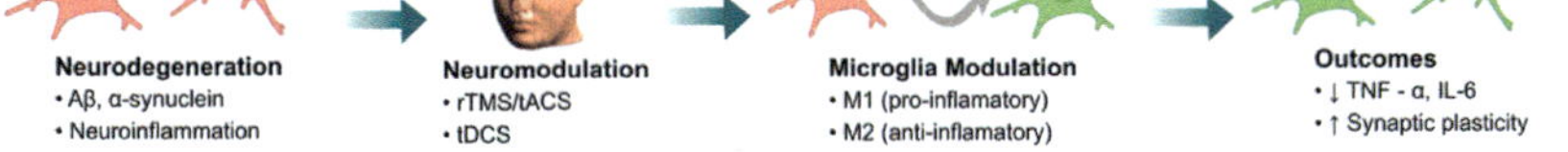
M1
M2
Neurodegeneration
• Aβ, α-synuclein
• Neuroinflammation
Neuromodulation
• rTMS/tACS
• tDCS
Microglia Modulation
• M1 (pro-inflamatory)
• M2 (anti-inflamatory)
Outcomes
• ↓ TNF - α, IL-6
• ↑ Synaptic plasticity

Fig. 1 Shifting the neuroimmune balance. Pathological proteins drive microglia into a harmful inflammatory state (M1). Neuromodulation redirects these cells toward a protective (M2) state, lowering toxic cytokines and helping synapses recover.

repetitive transcranial magnetic stimulation (rTMS) generate time-varying magnetic fields that induce electric currents in cortical tissue, thereby modulating neuronal firing patterns and network activity (Uzair et al., 2022). Depending on stimulation frequency and protocol, rTMS can induce long-term potentiation-like or long-term depression-like effects, leading to sustained changes in synaptic plasticity and circuit dynamics. These activity-dependent changes in neuronal signaling can subsequently influence glial cells, linking neuromodulation to neuroimmune regulation. Experimental studies indicate that neuromodulation can directly modify microglial activation states and inflammatory pathways. For example, rTMS has been shown to reduce glial activation and decrease the release of pro-inflammatory cytokines, suggesting that neuromodulation can attenuate neuroinflammatory responses. In animal models of Parkinson's disease, rTMS reduces neuroinflammation by suppressing the HMGB1/TLR4 signaling pathway and decreasing microglial activation in the substantia nigra and striatum (Han et al., 2023). Similarly, rTMS can influence microglial polarization by shifting microglia away from pro-inflammatory phenotypes and toward neuroprotective states through mechanisms involving the let-7b-5p/HMGA2/NF-κB signaling pathway (Hong et al., 2022). These changes are associated with reduced inflammatory cytokine production and improved neuronal survival.

Evidence from neurodegenerative disease models further supports the role of neuromodulation in regulating neuron–microglia interactions. In Alzheimer's disease models, rTMS has been shown to reduce amyloid-β deposition, decrease neuroinflammatory cytokines such as IL-6 and TNF-α, and suppress excessive microglial activation, ultimately improving synaptic plasticity and cognitive performance (Ji et al., 2025). These findings suggest that neuromodulation may influence disease progression not only by modifying neuronal activity but also by enhancing glial-mediated clearance of pathological proteins and restoring neuroimmune balance. Neuromodulation approaches also have relevance for other neurodegenerative disorders characterized by neuroinflammation and cortical network dysfunction. For example, rTMS and transcranial direct current stimulation (tDCS) have been investigated in ALS, where cortical hyperexcitability and microglial activation are important features of disease pathophysiology (Della Toffola et al., 2025). These interventions aim to modulate cortical excitability, regulate inflammatory pathways, and restore disrupted neural network dynamics, thereby potentially slowing disease progression. In addition, transcranial alternating current stimulation (tACS), particularly at gamma frequencies, has been proposed as a strategy to restore disrupted neural oscillations observed in Alzheimer's disease (De Paolis et al., 2024). Because neural oscillations coordinate neuronal communication across distributed brain networks, modulating these oscillatory dynamics may indirectly regulate microglial responses by altering activity-dependent signaling pathways within neural circuits.

Collectively, these findings highlight neuromodulation as a promising strategy for regulating neuron–microglia interactions in neurodegenerative diseases. By modulating neural circuit activity, inflammatory signaling, and microglial activation states, neuromodulatory interventions may attenuate chronic neuroinflammation while preserving the beneficial functions of microglia. A deeper understanding of how neuromodulation reshapes neuron–microglia communication will therefore be critical for developing targeted therapeutic strategies aimed at modifying disease progression across neurodegenerative disorders.

4. Insights from animal models and human translational studies

Animal models and human translational studies have been fundamental for understanding the roles of microglia in neurodegenerative diseases and for exploring potential therapeutic strategies targeting neuroimmune signaling. Experimental models allow controlled investigation of microglial dynamics, including changes in morphology, gene expression, and inflammatory signaling that occur during aging, neuronal injury, and neurodegeneration. These studies demonstrate that microglia respond rapidly to pathological stimuli, undergoing functional transitions that can either support neuronal repair or promote neuroinflammatory damage depending on disease stage and environmental context (Edler et al., 2021).

A major advantage of animal models is the ability to experimentally manipulate microglial populations. Techniques such as pharmacological depletion, genetic targeting, and irradiation have been used to transiently remove microglia and examine the consequences of their repopulation. Experimental evidence suggests that newly repopulated microglia can reshape inflammatory signaling, influence synaptic remodeling, and support tissue repair in several neurological disease models (Zhou et al., 2025). These findings highlight the plasticity of microglial populations and suggest that modifying microglial states may represent a viable strategy for altering disease trajectories. Recent studies have extended these concepts toward therapeutic approaches that directly modify microglial populations. One emerging strategy is microglial replacement, in which dysfunctional or pathogenic microglia are depleted and replaced with donor or genetically engineered cells capable of restoring homeostatic functions. Advances in depletion strategies and cell engraftment techniques have demonstrated the feasibility of widespread microglial replacement in preclinical models, and early translational efforts are beginning to explore its clinical potential (Rao et al., 2025).

Parallel progress in molecular and experimental tools has also improved the ability to study microglia in both animal models and human tissue. The identification of microglia-specific markers, such as TMEM119, has enabled more accurate discrimination of microglia from other brain macrophages, facilitating detailed characterization of microglial transcriptional programs and functional states across development and disease conditions (Bennett et al., 2016). These tools have significantly expanded our ability to investigate microglial heterogeneity and their interactions with neuronal circuits. Human translational studies complement experimental research by providing in vivo evidence of microglial activation in neurodegenerative diseases. Imaging approaches such as positron emission tomography (PET) using translocator protein (TSPO) ligands allow indirect measurement of neuroinflammatory activity associated with microglial activation. Increased TSPO binding has been observed in several neurodegenerative disorders, including Parkinson's disease, suggesting that microglial activation is closely linked to disease progression and clinical severity (Politis et al., 2012).

Despite these advances, translating mechanistic insights from animal models to human disease remains challenging due to differences in microglial biology across species, limitations of current imaging approaches, and the complex heterogeneity of human neurodegenerative disorders (Smith & Dragunow, 2014). Nevertheless, integrating findings from experimental models, molecular tools, and human imaging studies is progressively improving our understanding of microglial dynamics and their potential as therapeutic targets in neurodegenerative diseases.

5. Biomarkers, therapeutic opportunities and future directions

Advances in neuroimaging and molecular profiling are enhancing our ability to investigate microglial activity in neurodegenerative diseases.

Imaging techniques such as PET using TSPO ligands provide in vivo measures of neuroinflammation, although improved specificity remains an important goal. In parallel, transcriptomic approaches, including single-cell sequencing, are uncovering substantial heterogeneity within microglial populations and identifying disease-associated microglial states that may serve as potential biomarkers. Increasing understanding of neuron–microglia interactions has also opened new therapeutic possibilities. Strategies aimed at modulating microglial activity, including pharmacological approaches, cell-based therapies, and neuromodulation, are being explored as potential means to regulate neuroinflammation and protect neural circuits. Continued integration of molecular, imaging, and translational research will be essential for developing targeted interventions that leverage microglial biology to modify the progression of neurodegenerative diseases.

References

Adamu, A., Li, S., Gao, F., & Xue, G. (2024). The role of neuroinflammation in neurodegenerative diseases: Current understanding and future therapeutic targets. *Frontiers in Aging Neuroscience, 16*, 1347987.

Bennett, M. L., Bennett, F. C., Liddelow, S. A., Ajami, B., Zamanian, J. L., Fernhoff, N. B., et al. (2016). New tools for studying microglia in the mouse and human CNS. *Proceedings of the National Academy of Sciences of the United States of America, 113*(12), E1738–E1746.

Borst, K., Dumas, A. A., & Prinz, M. (2021). Microglia: Immune and non-immune functions. *Immunity, 54*(10), 2194–2208.

Chen, W. W., Zhang, X., & Huang, W. J. (2016). Role of neuroinflammation in neurodegenerative diseases (Review). *Molecular Medicine Reports, 13*(4), 3391–3396.

Chen, Y., Yin, P., Chen, Q., Zhang, Y., Tang, Y., Jin, W., et al. (2025). Neurodegenerative diseases and immune system: From pathogenic mechanism to therapy. *Neural Regeneration Research.*

De Marchi, F., Munitic, I., Vidatic, L., Papić, E., Rački, V., Nimac, J., et al. (2023). Overlapping neuroimmune mechanisms and therapeutic targets in neurodegenerative disorders. *Biomedicines, 11*(10).

De Paolis, M. L., Paoletti, I., Zaccone, C., Capone, F., D'Amelio, M., & Krashia, P. (2024). Transcranial alternating current stimulation (tACS) at gamma frequency: An up-and-coming tool to modify the progression of Alzheimer's disease. *Translational Neurodegeneration, 13*(1), 33.

De Schepper, S., Crowley, G., & Hong, S. (2021). Understanding microglial diversity and implications for neuronal function in health and disease. *Developmental Neurobiology, 81*(5), 507–523.

Della Toffola, J., Ricci, E., Quagliotto, M., Manganotti, P., & Benussi, A. (2025). Non-Invasive brain stimulation for amyotrophic lateral sclerosis: Current evidence and future perspectives. *Medicina (Kaunas, Lithuania), 61*(9).

Edler, M. K., Mhatre-Winters, I., & Richardson, J. R. (2021). Microglia in aging and Alzheimer's disease: A comparative species review. *Cells, 10*(5).

Femminella, G. D., Dani, M., Wood, M., Fan, Z., Calsolaro, V., Atkinson, R., et al. (2019). Microglial activation in early Alzheimer trajectory is associated with higher gray matter volume. *Neurology, 92*(12), e1331–e1343.

Fołta, J., Rzepka, Z., & Wrześniok, D. (2025). The role of inflammation in neurodegenerative diseases: Parkinson's disease, Alzheimer's disease, and multiple sclerosis. *International Journal of Molecular Sciences, 26*(11).

Gao, C., Jiang, J., Tan, Y., & Chen, S. (2023). Microglia in neurodegenerative diseases: Mechanism and potential therapeutic targets. *Signal Transduction and Targeted Therapy, 8*(1), 359.

Godeanu, S., & Cătălin, B. (2025). The complementary role of morphology in understanding microglial functional heterogeneity. *International Journal of Molecular Sciences, 26*(8).

Han, C., Zhang, X., Dou, K., Yao, W., Yao, M., Wan, Q., et al. (2023). Repetitive transcranial magnetic stimulation alleviates glial activation through suppressing HMGB1/TLR4 pathway in a rat model of Parkinson's disease. *Molecular Biology Reports, 50*(8), 6481–6492.

Hong, Y., Lyu, J., Zhu, L., Wang, X., Peng, M., Chen, X., et al. (2022). High-frequency repetitive transcranial magnetic stimulation (rTMS) protects against ischemic stroke by inhibiting M1 microglia polarization through let-7b-5p/HMGA2/NF-κB signaling pathway. *BMC Neuroscience, 23*(1), 49.

Ji, Y., Yang, C., Pang, X., Yan, Y., Wu, Y., Geng, Z., et al. (2025). Repetitive transcranial magnetic stimulation in Alzheimer's disease: Effects on neural and synaptic rehabilitation. *Neural Regeneration Research, 20*(2), 326–342.

Kempuraj, D., Thangavel, R., Natteru, P. A., Selvakumar, G. P., Saeed, D., Zahoor, H., et al. (2016). Neuroinflammation induces neurodegeneration. *Journal of Neurosurgery: Spine, 1*(1).

Mason, H. D., & McGavern, D. B. (2022). How the immune system shapes neurodegenerative diseases. *Trends in Neurosciences, 45*(10), 733–748.

Politis, M., Su, P., & Piccini, P. (2012). Imaging of microglia in patients with neurodegenerative disorders. *Frontiers in Pharmacology, 3*, 96.

Rao, Y., Bai, Y., Li, X., Du, B., & Peng, B. (2025). The evolution of microglia replacement: A new paradigm for CNS disease therapy. *Cell Stem Cell, 32*(12), 1807–1832.

Scheiblich, H., Trombly, M., Ramirez, A., & Heneka, M. T. (2020). Neuroimmune connections in aging and neurodegenerative diseases. *Trends in Immunology, 41*(4), 300–312.

Smith, A. M., & Dragunow, M. (2014). The human side of microglia. *Trends in Neurosciences, 37*(3), 125–135.

Sun, N., Victor, M. B., Park, Y. P., Xiong, X., Scannail, A. N., Leary, N., et al. (2023). Human microglial state dynamics in Alzheimer's disease progression. *Cell, 186*(20), 4386–4403.e29.

Suzumura, A. (2013). Neuron-microglia interaction in neuroinflammation. *Current Protein & Peptide Science, 14*(1), 16–20.

Tan, Y. L., Yuan, Y., & Tian, L. (2020). Microglial regional heterogeneity and its role in the brain. *Molecular Psychiatry, 25*(2), 351–367.

Uzair, M., Abualait, T., Arshad, M., Yoo, W. K., Mir, A., Bunyan, R. F., et al. (2022). Transcranial magnetic stimulation in animal models of neurodegeneration. *Neural Regeneration Research, 17*(2), 251–265.

Wang, H. (2021). Microglia heterogeneity in Alzheimer's disease: Insights from single-cell technologies. *Frontiers in Synaptic Neuroscience, 13*, 773590.

Zang, X., Chen, S., Zhu, J., Ma, J., & Zhai, Y. (2022). The emerging role of central and peripheral immune systems in neurodegenerative diseases. *Frontiers in Aging Neuroscience, 14*, 872134.

Zhou, K., Wang, Y., Xu, Y., Zhang, Y., & Zhu, C. (2025). Exploring microglial replacement: From disease models to clinical translation. *Brain, Behavior, and Immunity, 129*, 179–185.

CHAPTER EIGHT

Glial control of extracellular α-synuclein propagation in LRRK2 Parkinson's disease

Indrani Datta* **and Dibyam Debasish Sahu**
Department of Biophysics, National Institute of Mental Health and Neurosciences, Institute of National Importance, Bengaluru, Karnataka, India
*Corresponding author. e-mail address: indranidatta.nimhans@gmail.com

Contents

Advances in Immunology, Volume 171
ISSN 0065-2776, https://doi.org/10.1016/bs.ai.2026.04.005

Abstract

Parkinson's disease (PD) pathology extends well beyond dopaminergic neuronal loss, with glial cells—microglia and astrocytes—emerging as active architects of α-synuclein spread rather than passive bystanders. This review synthesises current evidence on how mutations in Leucine-Rich Repeat Kinase 2 (LRRK2), the most common genetic cause of familial PD, fundamentally corrupt glial handling of extracellular α-synuclein. We first outline the biology of extracellular α-synuclein—its cellular sources, conformational spectrum, prion-like propagation mechanisms, and principal glial clearance routes—before examining LRRK2 domain architecture, its downstream Rab GTPase signalling cascade, and the cellular processes it governs in glia. We then detail how LRRK2 mutations reconfigure microglial responses: driving constitutive NLRP3 inflammasome priming, impairing phagolysosomal degradation of α-synuclein aggregates, and redirecting phagocytosed cargo into pathogenic exosomal release via the LRRK2–Rab10–LYTL axis. In astrocytes, LRRK2 mutations disrupt annexin A2-mediated phagocytosis, impair chaperone-mediated autophagy and lysosomal acidification, deplete membrane cholesterol through Rab8A/Rab10 hyperphosphorylation, compromise glutamate transporter surface expression, and promote the secretion of phospho-α-synuclein-enriched extracellular vesicles that are neurotoxic to co-cultured dopaminergic neurons. Crucially, dysfunctional microglia and astrocytes do not operate independently—they form a self-amplifying feed-forward circuit in which microglial cytokines (IL-1α, TNF-α, C1q) drive A1 astrocyte conversion, tunnelling nanotube-mediated aggregate exchange propagates rather than resolves α-synuclein burden, and successive waves of neuronal death perpetuate the cycle. We highlight that these mechanisms are mutation-specific: the GTPase-domain variant I1371V, characterised through our group's patient-derived iPSC platform, drives qualitatively distinct membrane and metabolic dysfunction compared with the kinase-domain variant G2019S, underscoring the need for variant-tailored therapeutic strategies. We review human iPSC-based models—including microglia-like cells, midbrain-patterned astrocytes, and 3D midbrain organoids—that have proven indispensable for resolving cell-autonomous from non-cell-autonomous contributions of LRRK2 mutations. Finally, we evaluate emerging therapeutic strategies targeting LRRK2 kinase activity, NLRP3 inflammasome activation, extracellular α-synuclein immunotherapy, and glial lysosomal enhancement, including intranasal mesenchymal stromal cell-derived small extracellular vesicles. We conclude by identifying key unanswered questions regarding the relative dominance of microglial versus astrocytic clearance at different disease stages, the full pathogenic landscape of understudied LRRK2 variants, and the tractability of glial biomarkers as pharmacodynamic endpoints in clinical trials.

1. Introduction: Beyond the neuron-centric paradigm of Parkinson's disease

Parkinson's disease (PD) is traditionally described as the death of dopaminergic neurons in the substantia nigra pars compacta (SNpc), leading to the main motor symptoms of tremor, rigidity, and bradykinesia (Paisán-Ruíz et al., 2004). However, this neuron-focused perspective overlooks a growing body of evidence showing that glial cells—primarily microglia and astrocytes—are not just passive responders to neuronal damage but play a key role in shaping α-synuclein pathobiology from its earliest stages. Post-mortem studies, PET neuroimaging, and animal model research all indicate that microglial activation and reactive astrogliosis occur before noticeable neurodegeneration in vulnerable brain regions (Yun et al., 2018).

A core aspect of PD development is the abnormal buildup and spread of α-synuclein protein. Although it lacks a standard signal for extracellular release, both soluble and aggregated forms of α-synuclein have been found in tissue culture media and bodily fluids, including brain interstitial fluid, plasma, and cerebrospinal fluid (CSF) (El-Agnaf et al., 2003; El-Agnaf et al., 2006; Emmanouilidou et al., 2011; Hansson et al., 2014; Lee et al., 2005, 2014; Tokuda et al., 2010). Post-mortem brain analyses show that, through prion-like spread, α-synuclein monomers can form large aggregates in pathological states (Brás & Outeiro, 2021; De Boni et al., 2022; Stuendl et al., 2016). These aggregates, secreted by dopaminergic neurons into CSF, interact with astrocytes (Braak et al., 2007; Raj et al., 2023; Wakabayashi et al., 2000), and can trigger neuroinflammation (Lee et al., 2010).

PD was once seen as entirely idiopathic because its origins and mechanisms were unknown (Billingsley et al., 2018). However, family studies identified monogenic PD variants, where mutations in a single gene can cause the disease (Farrer, 2006). Specifically, autosomal-dominant mutations occur in LRRK2, SNCA, and VPS35, while autosomal-recessive mutations are found in PARK7, PRKN, and PINK1 (Billingsley et al., 2018; Farrer, 2006; Giasson et al., 2006; Trinh et al., 2014; Helley et al., 2017; Pang et al., 2019; Morais & Vos, 2022; Smith & Schapira, 2022).

The identification of LRRK2 mutations as the most common genetic factor in familial and some sporadic PD (Zimprich et al., 2004; Nalls et al., 2019) has broadened the understanding of glial PD biology. LRRK2 is highly expressed in glial cells, including the two primary types, astrocytes and microglia: microglia phagocytose extracellular α-synuclein aggregates, and astrocytes scavenge and attempt to degrade them (Rostami et al., 2017; Smethurst et al., 2022). When these clearance mechanisms fail, as seen in LRRK2-mutant glia, the balance shifts from containment to amplification of pathology. It is also found in peripheral immune cells, with levels increasing in response to inflammatory stimuli like interferon-γ (Schapansky et al., 2018; Panagiotakopoulou et al., 2020). This pattern indicates that LRRK2 may play a crucial role in linking immune activation to α-synuclein processing in glia

2. Biology of extracellular α-synuclein

2.1 Sources of extracellular α-synuclein

α-Synuclein is a 140-amino acid protein found in presynaptic terminals, encoded by the SNCA gene. It normally exists as a natively unfolded monomer, but in PD it misfolds, oligomerizes, and forms fibrillar aggregates rich in β-sheets that constitute the core of Lewy bodies. The protein has three main domains: an amphipathic N-terminal region (amino acids 1–61) with KTKEGV motifs that facilitate membrane binding, a hydrophobic non-amyloid β-component (NAC) region (amino acids 62–95) crucial for aggregation, and an acidic C-terminal region (amino acids 96–140) that interacts with ligands. Importantly, α-synuclein contains a VKKDQ/KFERQ-like motif that directs it to chaperone-mediated autophagy (CMA), a vital degradation pathway that is impaired in PD.

Extracellular α-synuclein comes from various cellular processes. Normally, neurons release small amounts of α-synuclein through unconventional secretory pathways that bypass the classical ER-Golgi route (Lee et al., 2013). Under disease conditions—such as lysosomal failure, oxidative stress, or proteasomal overload—this release increases markedly. Three main mechanisms have been identified: (i) exosomal release, where multivesicular bodies (MVBs) fuse with the plasma membrane to release exosome-bound α-synuclein; (ii) passive release from dying or permeabilised neurons; and (iii) an unconventional secretion pathway that completely avoids membrane-enclosed vesicles. Notably, lysosomal dysfunction—a hallmark of LRRK2-PD—significantly enhances exosomal α-synuclein release (Alvarez-Erviti et al., 2011; Abe et al., 2024). Abe et al. showed that lysosomal stress promotes the release of harmful α-synuclein from macrophage-lineage cells via the LRRK2-Rab10 pathway, linking LRRK2 kinase hyperactivity to higher extracellular α-synuclein levels (Alvarez-Erviti et al., 2011; Abe et al., 2024).

2.2 Structural forms and their differential glial handling

Extracellular α-synuclein exists as a conformational spectrum: natively unstructured monomers, prefibrillar oligomers, and mature fibrils (Danzer et al., 2007). This structural heterogeneity determines the glial cellular response. Monomeric α-synuclein preferentially activates microglial phagocytosis, whereas aggregated and fibrillar species tend to suppress clearance and instead promote inflammatory activation (Park et al., 2008). Higher-order oligomeric α-synuclein activates a proinflammatory microglial state by directly binding to the heterodimer TLR1/2 (Toll-like receptor 1 and 2) on the cell surface, which triggers the nuclear translocation of NF-κB (nuclear factor κB) and boosts the production of proinflammatory cytokines TNF-α and IL-1β through a MyD88-dependent pathway (Daniele et al., 2015). Fibrillar α-synuclein activates TLR4 and CD11b, triggering mitochondrial ROS generation, NLRP3 assembly, and caspase-1 activation, ultimately releasing mature IL-1β and IL-18 (Li et al., 2021). LRRK2 mutations amplify this downstream inflammatory response, as discussed in Section 4.

Exposure of astrocytes to extracellular WT α-synuclein triggers a form-dependent response: monomeric species are internalised mainly via clathrin-mediated endocytosis, whereas aggregated forms associate more strongly with plasma membrane lipid rafts (Raj et al., 2023, 2022). This interaction increases membrane rigidity, enhances store-operated calcium entry, and induces ER stress followed by mitochondrial membrane depolarization at 48 h (Raj et al., 2023, 2022). Functionally, WT aggregates impair antioxidant defences more than monomers, evidenced by greater reductions in Nrf2 nuclear localization and glutathione-related enzyme expression. Unexpectedly, glutamate uptake rises in astrocytes treated with aggregates due to upregulated GLAST1 expression, though glutamine synthase activity decreases and intracellular glutamate accumulates, disrupting the glutamate-glutamine cycle essential for neuronal neurotransmitter replenishment (Raj et al., 2022).

2.3 Prion-like propagation mechanisms

Braak and colleagues (Braak et al., 2003) and Luk et al. (Luk et al., 2012). demonstrated that α-synuclein spreads in a prion-like way: extracellular seeds are absorbed by recipient cells, guiding the misfolding of normal proteins. In addition to neuron-to-neuron transfer, microglia and astrocytes are now recognised as key intermediaries. Microglia can internalise α-synuclein aggregates, pass excess cargo to nearby microglia via tunnelling nanotubes (TNTs), and, when overwhelmed, release these aggregates via exosomes, which are then taken up by neurons (Li et al., 2021; Scheiblich et al., 2021, 2024). Astrocytes also transfer α-synuclein to microglia via TNTs (Rostami et al., 2021), and LRRK2-mutant astrocytes release phospho-α-synuclein-enriched EVs that are absorbed by and toxic to dopaminergic neurons in co-culture (Di Domenico et al., 2019). While the importance of cell–cell contact has been emphasized in prion diseases (Victoria et al., 2016), our study (Raj et al., 2024) highlights the role of the secretome of affected astrocytes in the presence of extracellular α-synuclein. Continuous exposure to extracellular α-synuclein induced astrocytic changes, including α-synuclein release, increased inflammatory cytokine levels, and reduced growth factor secretion. These changes lead to apoptosis and dysfunction in dopaminergic neurons, including neurite collapse, calcium responses, and impaired dopamine vesicle release (Raj et al., 2024).

2.4 Glial clearance mechanisms

Extracellular α-syn is cleared by three principal glial mechanisms: (i) microglial phagocytosis, driven by TLR2/4 and Fc receptor engagement, followed by lysosomal degradation; (ii) astrocytic uptake via clathrin-mediated endocytosis and lipid raft–mediated pathways, with degradation through the endolysosomal system and chaperone-mediated autophagy (CMA); and (iii) glymphatic clearance during sleep, mediated by AQP4-polarised astrocyte endfeet. In PD, each of these mechanisms is compromised—and LRRK2 mutations create additional, genotype-specific layers of clearance failure, as detailed in Sections 4 and 6.

3. LRRK2 signalling pathways relevant to glial function

3.1 Domain architecture and pathogenic mutations

LRRK2 is a large (~280 kDa), multidomain protein comprising an N-terminal armadillo-ankyrin-LRR scaffold, a central GTPase (ROC-COR)

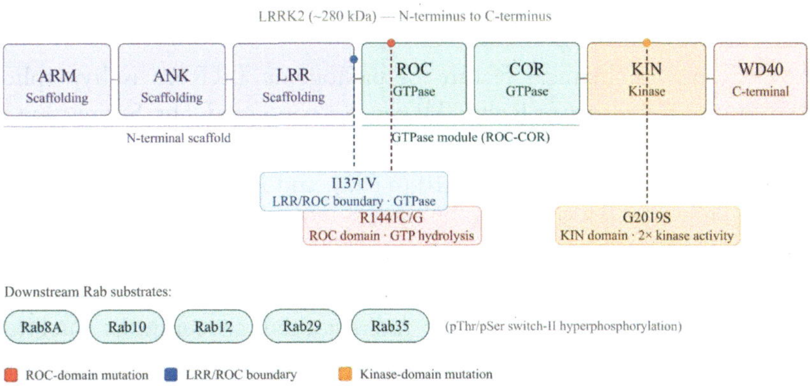

Fig. 1 LRRK2 domain architecture. The seven domains are shown in functional groupings: scaffolding (ARM-ANK-LRR), GTPase module (ROC-COR), kinase (KIN), and WD40. The three major PD mutations are pinned at their respective positions — R1441C/G in ROC, I1371V at the LRR/ROC boundary, and G2019S in KIN. Downstream Rab GTPase substrates are noted below.

domain, a serine/threonine kinase domain, and a C-terminal WD40 domain (Fig. 1) (Alessi & Pfeffer, 2024; Bosgraaf & Van Haastert, 2003; Gilsbach & Kortholt, 2014; Watanabe et al., 2020). The ROC domain binds and hydrolyses GTP, regulating LRRK2 membrane association, while the kinase domain phosphorylates downstream substrates. Pathogenic mutations cluster in the ROC-COR bi-lobe (e.g., R1441C/G, Y1699C, I1371V) and the kinase domain (G2019S). The G2019S substitution in the kinase activation loop increases kinase activity approximately 2-fold by altering the DFG-motif geometry (Liu et al., 2013; Nolen et al., 2004). ROC domain mutations, in contrast, impair GTPase activity and membrane cycling, and—as demonstrated by our group for I1371V—can drive markedly more severe downstream Rab hyperphosphorylation than kinase-domain mutations (Singh et al., 2026). I1371 resides in a deep hydrophobic pocket at the ROC–ROC dimer interface, where the Cδ methyl group of isoleucine completes van der Waals packing, creating a precisely tuned hydrophobic seal essential for proper GTPase cycling (Deng et al., 2008). Over 50 LRRK2 variants have been identified in PD patients, with G2019S predominating in European and North African populations and I1371V reported mainly in East Asian populations (Deng et al., 2008; Fernández-Pajarín et al., 2023; Janković et al., 2015; Lin et al., 2019; Paisán-Ruíz et al., 2005; Pankratz et al., 2006; Pirkevi et al., 2009; Sadhukhan et al., 2012; Seki et al., 2011).

3.2 Downstream signalling: The Rab GTPase cascade

The defining biochemical feature of pathogenic LRRK2 is hyperphosphorylation of a subset of Rab GTPases at a conserved Thr/Ser residue in their switch-II effector domain. The most extensively validated LRRK2 substrates are Rab8A (pT72), Rab10 (pT73), and Rab29 (pS71) (Liu et al., 2018; Pfeffer, 2018; Steger et al., 2016; Vieweg et al., 2020). Phosphorylated Rabs are functionally inactivated with respect to canonical effectors, instead acquiring new phospho-dependent binding partners (e.g., RILPL1, RILPL2, JIP3, JIP4) that redirect them to centriolar satellites, lysosomes, or tubular sorting compartments (Dhekne et al., 2018; Komori & Kuwahara, 2023). Rab29, which resides on the trans-Golgi network, acts as a master activator of LRRK2 by recruiting it to Golgi membranes where it further amplifies Rab8A and Rab10 phosphorylation (Kuwahara & Iwatsubo, 2020; Purlyte et al., 2018). More recently, Rab12 has been identified as a critical non-redundant activator of LRRK2 at damaged lysosomes, with loss of Rab12 reducing phospho-Rab10 levels by ~5-fold (Dhekne et al., 2023).

In glia, Rab phosphorylation events significantly influence vesicle trafficking, endolysosomal dynamics, and inflammatory signalling. Phosphorylated Rab10, through JIP4, promotes LYTL (LYsosomal Tubulation/sorting driven by LRRK2), a process where LAMP1-negative tubules bud off from stressed lysosomes, releasing membranous vesicles. This mechanism can divert α-syn cargo away from lysosomal degradation (Bonet-Ponce et al., 2020). Additionally, Rab8A phosphorylation mediated by LRRK2 disrupts endosomal recycling, leading to reduced surface localisation of dopamine and glutamate transporters, which strongly affects dopaminergic neurotransmission and astrocyte glutamate balance, respectively.

3.3 LRRK2-regulated cellular processes in glia

Beyond its role in Rab-dependent trafficking, LRRK2 influences various cellular functions directly related to glial management of α-synuclein. (i) Autophagy and mitophagy: The G2019S mutation in LRRK2 impair basal mitophagy in living organisms (Singh et al., 2021), and this defect can be reversed with LRRK2 kinase inhibitors (Singh et al., 2021). In astrocytes, G2019S decreases lysosome numbers and hinders CMA, resulting in α-synuclein buildup (Streubel-Gallasch et al., 2021). (ii) Membrane remodelling: Our research shows that I1371V causes targeted cholesterol depletion from membranes, disrupts lipid microdomains, lowers caveolin-1 levels, and changes membrane structure through Rab8A/Rab10 hyperphosphorylation, impairing sterol transport (Singh et al., 2026). These membrane alterations affect how signalling receptors are displayed on glial surfaces. (iii) Inflammatory signalling: LRRK2 phosphorylates substrates that enhance NF-κB–mediated cytokine production, and LRRK2 expression itself is increased by IFN-γ in microglia, creating a self-perpetuating inflammatory cycle (Panagiotakopoulou et al., 2020).

4. Microglial responses to extracellular α-synuclein in the LRRK2 context

4.1 Microglial sensing of α-synuclein

Microglia express a diverse array of receptors capable of recognising extracellular α synuclein. TLR2 recognises oligomeric α-synuclein and signals via MyD88-NF-κB to produce TNF-α, IL-6, and IL-1β (Li et al., 2021). TLR4 recognises fibrillar α-synuclein through the CD36 co-receptor system and activates both NF-κB (priming step) and NLRP3 inflammasome (activation step), leading to the maturation and release of pro-inflammatory cytokines like IL-1β (Li et al., 2021). Fc receptors mediate antibody-opsonised α-synuclein uptake and can drive microglial reactivity in the context of anti α synuclein immunotherapy. Scavenger receptors and CD11b contribute to non-specific phagocytosis. Importantly, LRRK2 is recruited to TLR-activated vesicles and modulates downstream signalling at multiple steps: it amplifies cytokine production, regulates the phagosomal-lysosomal trafficking of α-syn cargo, and influences antigen presentation (Ohtonen et al., 2023). In LRRK2-mutant microglia, IFN-γ further upregulates LRRK2 expression and kinase activity, creating a genotype-specific inflammatory amplification loop (Panagiotakopoulou et al., 2020).

4.2 Phagocytosis and lysosomal processing of α-syn

Microglial phagocytosis of α-syn aggregates is the most effective clearance mechanism among CNS cells in vitro (Choi & Chung, 2025; Harackiewicz & Grembecka, 2024; Sinha et al., 2021). Following receptor-mediated or bulk uptake, α-synuclein-containing phagosomes fuse with lysosomes for degradation via the autophagy-lysosome pathway (ALP). LRRK2 regulates this process through Rab-dependent control of phagosomal maturation and lysosomal function. In G2019S microglia, hyperphosphorylation of Rab8A and Rab10 impairs phagosomal-endosomal fusion, slowing α-syn delivery to lysosomes (Abe et al., 2024). Lysosomal stress—induced by accumulating α-syn aggregates—further activates LRRK2 via Rab12 recruitment to damaged lysosomal membranes (Dhekne et al., 2023) amplifying Rab10 phosphorylation and triggering LYTL-mediated exosomal release of α-syn cargo rather than degradation (Boecker et al., 2021). Thus, LRRK2 mutations redirect the fate of phagocytosed α-synuclein from lysosomal destruction to exosomal propagation—a critical shift that converts microglia from clearance cells into unwitting amplifiers of α-synuclein spread.

4.3 NLRP3 inflammasome activation in LRRK2-mutant microglia

The NLRP3 inflammasome is a central mediator of glial neuroinflammation in PD. α-Syn aggregates prime the NLRP3 inflammasome through TLR-NF-κB signalling and subsequently activate it through K^+ efflux, ROS generation, and lysosomal damage (Li et al., 2021). Activated NLRP3 recruits the adaptor ASC and cleaves procaspase-1, producing mature IL-1β and IL-18 and driving pyroptosis—an inflammatory mode of cell death that further amplifies the extracellular release of α-synuclein and damage-associated molecular patterns (Li et al., 2021; Hu et al., 2024). NLRP3 levels are significantly elevated in activated microglia in the substantia nigra of PD patients (Anderson et al., 2021). In G2019S LRRK2-mutant microglia, NLRP3 inflammasome activation is heightened: nuclear ASC speck formation—a hallmark of inflammasome priming—occurs constitutively under basal conditions in G2019S mouse microglia and in human monocyte-derived microglia-like cells from LRRK2-PD patients, in contrast to wild-type controls where it requires exogenous priming (Panagiotakopoulou et al., 2020). This suggests that LRRK2 mutations create a tonically primed inflammatory state in microglia that lowers the threshold for NLRP3 activation in response to α-syn (Fig. 2). IL-1β release is consistently elevated in immune cells harbouring G2019S mutations, and circulating IL-1β levels are elevated in PD patients (Hu et al., 2015; Kim et al., 2020).

4.4 Microglial exosomal release of α-synuclein

Beyond degradation failure, reactive microglia actively release α-synuclein-containing exosomes that seed pathology in adjacent neurons and glia. Guo et al. showed that microglial exosomes facilitate α-synuclein transmission in a PD mouse model and that reactive microglia release more exosomes with

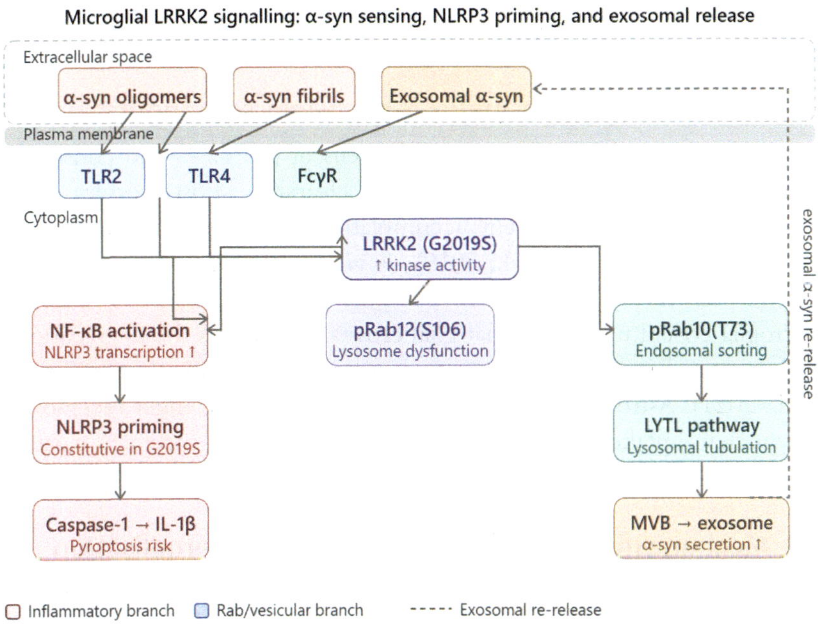

Fig. 2 Microglial LRRK2 signalling. Two parallel effector branches downstream of G2019S hyperactivation are shown: the left inflammatory arm (TLR2/4 → NF-κB → NLRP3 constitutive priming → caspase-1/IL-1β) and the right vesicular arm (pRab10-T73 → LYTL → MVB diversion → exosomal α-syn re-release). The dashed arc closing the loop back to extracellular space depicts the propagation cycle.

higher α-synuclein content than resting microglia (Guo et al., 2020). TLR2 activation on microglia enhances exosomal α-synuclein secretion via an autophagy-lysosome pathway impairment mechanism (Xia et al., 2021). In the specific context of LRRK2, Abe et al. demonstrated that lysosomal stress triggers LRRK2-Rab10 accumulation on lysosomal surfaces, with subsequent Rab10 phosphorylation by LRRK2 specifically driving exosomal release of pathogenic α-synuclein from macrophage lineage cells (Abe et al., 2024). iPSC-derived LRRK2-G2019S microglia from two PD patient lines showed elevated pro-inflammatory cytokines (TNF-α, IL-8) and altered phagocytic capacity, with transcriptomic profiling identifying significant upregulation of TLR2, TLR4, and innate immune activation pathways (Ohtonen et al., 2023; Kurniawan et al., 2025). Furthermore, LRRK2-G2019S microglia and neuromelanin synergise to drive dopaminergic neurodegeneration in iPSC-based neuron-microglia co-culture models, an effect reversible by immunomodulation (Blasco-Agell et al., 2025) (Fig. 2).

5. Astrocytic uptake and processing of extracellular α-synuclein

5.1 Astrocytes as major α-synuclein scavengers

Astrocytes are the most abundant glial cells of the CNS and constitute a major reservoir for extracellular α-syn clearance. Post-mortem studies reveal significant α-synuclein accumulation in SNpc astrocytes of PD patients (Di Domenico et al., 2019). *In vitro*, astrocytes internalise fibrillar α-synuclein more avidly than neurons, and iPSC-derived astrocyte-microglia co-cultures show that glial crosstalk enhances the degradation of both α-synuclein and Aβ aggregates compared to monocultures (Rostami et al., 2021). Astrocytes express TLR2, TLR4, and scavenger receptors for α-synuclein uptake, and also participate in glymphatic-mediated clearance via AQP4-polarised endfeet at the perivascular space.

5.2 Mechanisms of astrocytic α-synuclein internalisation

Astrocytic α-synuclein uptake occurs via clathrin-mediated endocytosis —implicated in the bulk internalisation of extracellular α-syn oligomers and fibrils—and via lipid raft–mediated, caveolin-dependent pathways, which are particularly relevant for monomeric α-syn and plasma membrane–associated species. Annexin A2 (AnxA2) plays a critical role in the actin-mediated internalisation of α-synuclein aggregates in astrocytes; in G2019S Lrrk2 astrocytes, AnxA2 delocalises from the plasma membrane and fails to correctly recruit to α-synuclein inclusions, directly impairing phagocytosis (Streubel-Gallasch et al., 2021). LRRK2 kinase inhibition with MLi-2 partially rescues this AnxA2 localisation defect (Streubel-Gallasch et al., 2021).

5.3 Lysosomal degradation pathways and their failure

Once internalised, α-synuclein follows the endolysosomal pathway: early endosome → late endosome/MVB → lysosome, with CMA providing an alternative route for monomeric α-synuclein tagged by KFERQ-like motifs. Lysosomal degradation requires sustained acidification (pH 4.5–5.0) and the activity of hydrolases including cathepsins B, D, and L. Streubel-Gallasch et al. demonstrated that G2019S LRRK2 astrocytes accumulate significantly more fibrillar α-synuclein than wild-type or Lrrk2-knockout astrocytes following identical α-synuclein pulse-chase experiments, attributable to a reduction in lysosomal-like structures and impaired endolysosomal maturation (Streubel-Gallasch et al., 2021). TLR2 activation—an upstream trigger of LRRK2-mediated signalling—acutely impairs CMA in both PD neurons and astrocytes, potentiating α-synuclein pathology seeded by pre-formed fibrils and inducing A1 neurotoxic astrocyte markers (Weiss et al., 2024). In A53T-α-synuclein iPSC-derived astrocytes, lysosomal malfunction and failure of both proteasomal and autophagic proteostasis produce cell-intrinsic α-synuclein accumulation that is transferred to co-cultured neurons (Di Domenico et al., 2019).

5.4 Consequences of astrocytic α-synuclein accumulation

Failed astrocytic α-synuclein degradation triggers reactive astrogliosis, characterised by morphological hypertrophy, upregulation of GFAP and vimentin, and a shift toward a pro-inflammatory secretome. Accumulating α-synuclein in astrocytes disrupts calcium homeostasis by impairing ER and mitochondrial functions, the ALP mechanism, and altering glutamate uptake capacity—effects directly demonstrated in our group's characterisation of astrocytes (Raj et al., 2023, 2022, 2024). LRRK2 I1371V iPSC-derived astrocytes intrinsically displayed significantly reduced expression of glutamate transporters SLC1A2 and SLC1A3, attributable to impaired Rab10-mediated trafficking from the Golgi to the plasma membrane (Banerjee et al., 2023). The resulting glutamate accumulation in the extracellular space poses an excitotoxic risk to neighbouring neurons. Simultaneously, deficient Nrf2-mediated glutathione synthesis and reduced ATP generation in I1371V astrocytes impair the overall antioxidant defence of the nigrostriatal niche (Banerjee et al., 2023). Further, in the presence of extracellular α-synuclein aggregates, the LRRK2 I1371V astrocytes showed a more pro-inflammatory signature and higher release of α-synuclein due to influx of higher Ca^{2+} through the formation of amyloid pores (Datta et al., 2026).

6. LRRK2-driven astrocyte dysfunction: Mechanisms and consequences

6.1 Altered vesicle trafficking and MVB biogenesis

Studies in human iPSC-derived G2019S astrocytes reveal profound alterations in MVB biogenesis and EV secretion. Di Domenico et al. demonstrated that G2019S astrocytes accumulate phospho-α-syn (pS129) within smaller, non-perinuclearly distributed MVBs compared to isogenic controls (Di Domenico et al., 2019). The ratio of phosphorylated to total α-synuclein in MVBs was markedly higher in mutant astrocytes, suggesting that the LRRK2 G2019S mutation specifically routes pathogenic α-synuclein species into the MVB-EV secretory pathway (De Rus Jacquet et al., 2021). EVs from G2019S astrocytes fail to provide neurotrophic support to co-cultured dopaminergic neurons and instead induce neurite atrophy (De Rus Jacquet et al., 2021). While total EV numbers were unchanged, the cargo composition—enriched in pathological α-synuclein—represents a qualitative shift from trophic to neurotoxic extracellular communication.

6.2 Lysosomal impairment and cholesterol metabolism

LRRK2 mutations impair lysosomal biogenesis, acidification, and hydrolase trafficking in astrocytes. G2019S astrocytes show reduced lysosomal number detectable by TEM, and altered localisation of lysosomal markers compared with isogenic controls (Streubel-Gallasch et al., 2021). Similarly, our data suggests that LRRK2 I1371V astrocytes showed impairment in lysosomal function through reduction in Cathepsin D activity (Banerjee et al., 2026), with accumulation of cargo in the lysosomes upon exposure to extracellular α-synuclein. Our group's analysis of I1371V cells revealed a uniquely severe disruption of membrane sterol metabolism: I1371V-expressing SH-SY5Y cells, U87 glia-like cells, and iPSC-derived floor-plate cells exhibited selective depletion of membrane cholesterol—without changes in total cellular cholesterol—due to impaired sterol vesicular transport downstream of Rab8A/Rab10 hyperphosphorylation (Singh et al., 2026). This membrane cholesterol depletion disrupted lipid microdomain (raft) organisation, reduced caveolin-1 expression, increased membrane fluidity, and altered membrane topology, collectively impairing the surface expression of the dopamine transporter (DAT) (Singh et al., 2026). That GW5074 (a non-selective LRRK2 modulator) rescued these I1371V phenotypes more effectively than the kinase-selective MLi-2 underscores the distinct GTPase-domain pathobiology of non-G2019S mutations (Singh et al., 2026).

6.3 Effects on receptor and transporter localisation

The membrane trafficking defects in LRRK2-mutant glia extend to functionally critical receptors and transporters. In I1371V astrocytes, reduced SLC1A2 (EAAT2) and SLC1A3 (EAAT1) surface expression leads to extracellular glutamate accumulation (Banerjee et al., 2023). In dopaminergic neurons and floor-plate cells, I1371V impairs DAT surface localisation, reduces dopamine uptake capacity, and affects the Sonic Hedgehog (SHH) signalling pathway by diminishing floor plate cell responsiveness to SHH (Potdar et al., 2024). These findings illuminate how a single GTPase-domain LRRK2 mutation, by disrupting cholesterol and Rab-dependent trafficking, creates a cascade of receptor mis-localisation with broad functional consequences for the nigrostriatal circuit. Multiple reports have reported impaired Trafficking of the glutamate transporter as well as increased glutamate levels for cells and animals harboring the LRRK2 G2019S mutation (Di Iacovo et al., 2025; Iovino et al., 2022; Mercatelli et al., 2025).

7. Microglia–astrocyte crosstalk in LRRK2 Parkinson's disease

The interaction between microglia and astrocytes in PD is not additive but synergistic, creating self-amplifying neurotoxic circuits that accelerate dopaminergic degeneration. In the LRRK2 context, this crosstalk acquires additional complexity because both cell types independently harbour LRRK2-driven dysfunction.

7.1 Cytokine-mediated glial state conversion

Activated microglia release a triad of cytokines—IL-1α, TNF-α, and complement component C1q—that together are necessary and sufficient to convert astrocytes to a neurotoxic A1 phenotype (Liddelow et al., 2017). A1 astrocytes lose their neurotrophic functions and instead release toxic lipids, complement proteins, and additional cytokines that kill neurons and oligodendrocytes (Yun et al., 2018; Liddelow et al., 2017) demonstrated that blocking A1 astrocyte conversion using the GLP-1R agonist NLY01 was neuroprotective in two mouse models of PD, positioning microglia-to-astrocyte cytokine signalling as a tractable therapeutic target. In LRRK2-PD, where G2019S microglia constitutively produce elevated IL-1β and TNF-α (Kim et al., 2020; Ho et al., 2017, 2018; Russo et al., 2018), the rate of A1 conversion is expected to be higher than in sporadic PD, creating a more rapidly progressing neurotoxic glial environment.

7.2 Tunnelling nanotubes and direct α-synuclein exchange

TNTs mediate direct inter-glial transfer of α-synuclein aggregates, lysosomal vesicles, and mitochondria between microglia, between astrocytes and microglia, and between glia and neurons. Scheiblich et al. (2021) showed that TNTs enable cooperative microglial degradation of fibrillar α-synuclein, with overloaded microglia distributing aggregate cargo to less-burdened neighbours via TNT-mediated lysosomal transfer. More recently, the same group confirmed that neurons transfer pathological α-synuclein into neighbouring microglia through TNTs, enabling a form of transcellular aggregate disposal (Scheiblich et al., 2021). In LRRK2-mutant glia, where lysosomal capacity is compromised, this TNT-mediated aggregate redistribution may paradoxically propagate

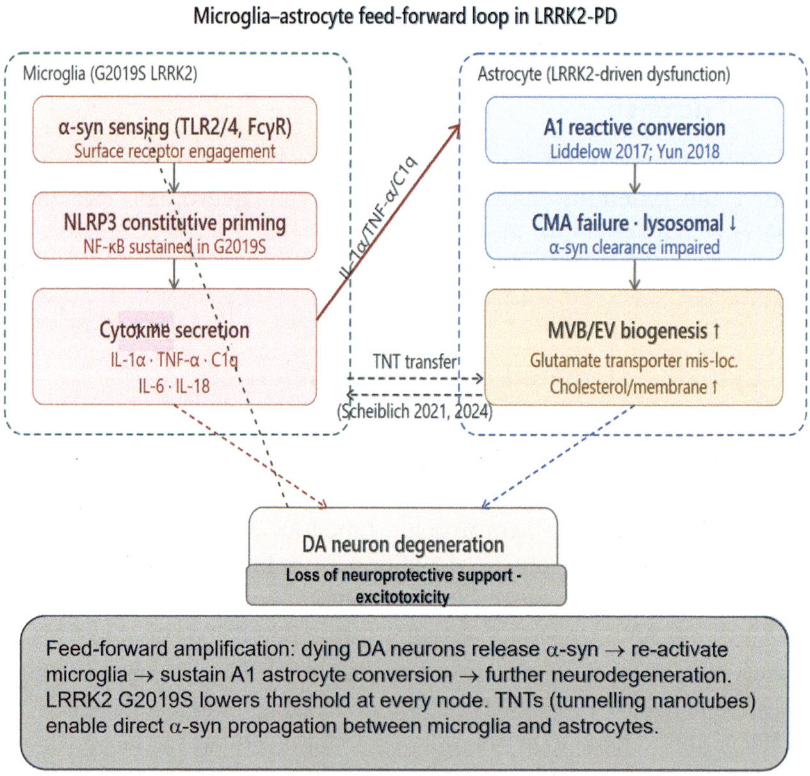

Fig. 3 Microglia–astrocyte feed-forward loop. The left compartment depicts G2019S microglial activation leading to constitutive NLRP3 priming and cytokine secretion (IL-1α, TNF-α, C1q). These signals drive A1 reactive conversion of astrocytes (right compartment), which in turn fail to clear α-syn and shed it via MVB/EV pathways. Dying dopaminergic neurons (bottom) release further α-syn, closing the amplification cycle. Bidirectional TNT-mediated transfer is shown as the dashed bridge.

rather than contain α-synuclein pathology, as cargo arriving in recipient cells with impaired lysosomal function is incompletely degraded and instead re-released (Rostami et al., 2017; Abounit et al., 2016; Chakraborty et al., 2023; Dilsizoglu Senol et al., 2021).

7.3 The feed-forward inflammatory loop and dopaminergic neurotoxicity

The neurotoxic feedback loop in LRRK2-PD can be summarised as follows: (i) LRRK2-hyperactivated microglia incompletely degrade α-synuclein aggregates and re-release them via exosomes; (ii) extracellular α-synuclein seeds neighbouring neurons and activates local microglia via TLR2/4 and NLRP3; (iii) activated microglia release IL-1α, TNF-α, and C1q, converting astrocytes to A1 state; (iv) A1 astrocytes fail to degrade their own α-synuclein burden (exacerbated by LRRK2-mutant lysosomal dysfunction) and becomes hub for spread of α-synuclein that are neurotoxic; (v) toxic glial-derived signals kill dopaminergic neurons, releasing more α-synuclein. LRRK2 mutations amplify each step of this cycle, both in microglia (via kinase-dependent inflammatory amplification) and astrocytes (via trafficking-mediated clearance failure) (Fig. 3).

8. Human iPSC models illuminate glial mechanisms in LRRK2-PD

The complexity of LRRK2-driven glial dysfunction—and its heterogeneity across mutations—demands human cellular platforms that transcend rodent models. LRRK2 ia a multidomain protein and the point mutations of LRRK2 reported in PD patients is often not present in small model organisms such as C. elegans, zebra fish and drosophila. Additionally, a study has demonstrated differences in stability, activity, and the effects of mutations between human and mouse LRRK2 (Langston et al., 2016). It is also revealed that inflammatory signaling differently alters chromatin accessibility and gene expression of the PD-associated kinase LRRK2 in humans and mice (Beilina et al., 2026). Thus, it is important to study LRRK2 mutational changes in human-origin cells, especially in iPSC-derived cell systems from PD patients carrying LRRK2 mutations. Human iPSC technology now enables the derivation of patient-specific dopaminergic neurons, astrocytes, and microglia-like cells, with isogenic gene-corrected controls providing rigorous experimental comparators.

8.1 iPSC-derived microglia in LRRK2-PD

Ohtonen et al. (2023) demonstrated that iPSC-derived microglial-like cells (iMGLs) from G2019S patients recapitulate the transcriptional signature of microglia in the human idiopathic PD midbrain, with spatial transcriptomics confirming a shared PD-microglial profile characterised by upregulation of neuroinflammation and cytokine activation pathways. Functionally, G2019S iMGLs showed elevated TNF-α and IL-8 secretion upon LPS + IFN-γ stimulation, and altered phagocytosis and mitochondrial respiration in a donor-dependent manner (Ohtonen et al., 2023). In 3D midbrain organoid models, LRRK2-G2019S microglia with metabolic dysregulation—including impaired serine biosynthesis and upregulated glycolysis—caused dopaminergic neurodegeneration that was not observed with wild-type microglia (Kurniawan et al., 2025). Importantly, LRRK2-mutant microglia and extracellular neuromelanin synergise in iPSC co-culture models to drive dopaminergic neuron loss, with immunomodulatory drugs reversing this effect (Blasco-Agell et al., 2025).

8.2 iPSC-derived astrocytes in LRRK2-PD: Contributions from our group

iPSC-Derived Midbrain patterned astrocytes harboring the LRRK2 G2019S mutation have impaired functioning of the ECM and associated signalling, leading to altered response to inflammatory stimuli (Booth et al., 2019). These mutation-carrying astrocytes showed increased expression of alpha-synuclein (Sonninen et al., 2020), aberrant mitochondrial morphology, decreased mitochondrial activity and ATP production along with an increase of glycolysis and increased production of reactive oxygen species (Ramos-Gonzalez et al., 2021), altered metabolism, disturbed Ca2 + homeostasis and increased release of cytokines upon inflammatory stimulation (Sonninen et al., 2020). They also exhibit increased accumulation of LRRK2 and Phospho-α-synuclein in the shedded Multivesicular bodies, pointing to impaired astrocyte-to-neuron trophic signaling (De Rus Jacquet et al., 2021; Reinhardt et al., 2013).

The diseased astrocytes when co-cultured with dopaminergic neurons, led to abnormal, astrocyte-derived α-synuclein accumulation in the neurons. Dysfunctional chaperone-mediated autophagy (CMA), impaired macroautophagy and impaired mitochondrial transfer to neurons are all contributing factors to the observed dopaminergic neurodegeneration (Di Domenico et al., 2019; Reinhardt et al., 2013; Ding et al., 2025).

Our group has systematically characterised the cellular biology of LRRK2 I1371V across the dopaminergic lineage using patient-derived iPSCs. We generated the first iPSC line (NIMHi001-A) from a PD patient of East Indian ethnicity carrying LRRK2 I1371V (Datta et al., 2020). Subsequent differentiation to dopaminergic neurons revealed reduced progenitor yield, impaired FOXA2/CLIC5 floor-plate marker expression, higher α-synuclein pathology, and reduced vesicular dopamine release (Jagtap et al., 2022). Floor-plate cell analysis demonstrated that I1371V specifically impairs SHH signalling responsiveness, explaining the ontogenic origin of reduced DA neuron yield (Potdar et al., 2024). In astrocytes differentiated from the same I1371V iPSC line—we demonstrated significant cell-intrinsic dysfunctions in glutamate uptake, Nrf2-mediated antioxidant defence, and ATP generation, attributable to impaired SLC1A2/SLC1A3 surface expression and dysregulated glutamate metabolism (Banerjee et al., 2023). Our most recent study of membrane biology in I1371V cells showed that these GTPase-domain cells exhibit more severe membrane cholesterol depletion and Rab8A/Rab10 hyperphosphorylation than G2019S kinase-domain cells, underscoring the pathogenic heterogeneity across LRRK2 variants (Singh et al., 2026).

8.3 Midbrain organoids and co-culture systems

Three-dimensional midbrain organoid models incorporating dopaminergic neurons, astrocytes, and microglia—derived from the same patient iPSC background—enable the simultaneous study of neuron-glia interactions in a spatially organised context that approximates the human midbrain.

Single-cell RNA-sequencing data of mBOs harboring the LRRK2 G2019S variant showed altered neurodevelopment, resulting in an untimely and incomplete differentiation with reduced cellular variability (Smits et al., 2019; Zagare et al., 2022). The mBOs showed elevated LRRK2 kinase activity and reduction of dopaminergic markers *TH* (Ha et al., 2020; Kim et al., 2019), *AADC, VMAT2,* and *DAT (*Kim et al., 2019*).* There was also a reduction in mature neuronal markers *NURR1, PITX3, EN1, TH, and MAPT.* The mutant organoids also showed localization of phospho-α-synuclein(Serine 129) positive vesicles with endosomes positive for EEA1 and LC3B as compared to healthy control organoids. These defects were rescued upon treatment with LRRK2 kinase inhibitor (Kim et al., 2019).

Kurniawan et al. (2025) showed that healthy midbrain organoids cocultured with LRRK2-G2019S microglia had significantly lower levels of tyrosine hydroxylase (TH) positive cells, linking the proinflammatory effect of the mutation on microglial activity in the midbrain (Kurniawan et al., 2025).

These co-culture and organoid platforms are the experimental systems of choice for probing cell-autonomous versus non-cell-autonomous contributions of LRRK2 mutations, and for testing therapies that must modulate glial biology in a human cellular context.

9. Therapeutic targeting of LRRK2-mediated glial dysfunction

9.1 LRRK2 kinase inhibitors

LRRK2 kinase inhibitors represent the most clinically advanced therapeutic strategy. MLi-2, BIIB122 (DNL201/DNL151), and GW5074 are the most studied compounds, with BIIB122/DNL151 now in Phase 2 trials (NCT05418673) evaluating disease modification in early LRRK2-PD (Fig. 4). Mechanistically, LRRK2 kinase inhibition reduces phospho-Rab10 levels, restores lysosomal function, rescues mitophagy, and reduces pS129-αSyn in various in vivo and in vitro models (Singh et al., 2021; Thirstrup et al., 2017; Ho et al., 2019; Ilieva et al., 2024; Gomez-Sequeda et al., 2025). In G2019S astrocytes, MLi-2 partially rescues AnxA2-mediated α-synuclein phagocytosis (Streubel-Gallasch et al., 2021). However, important cautions apply: (i) kinase-selective inhibitors may be insufficient for GTPase-domain mutations like I1371V, which require broader LRRK2 modulation (Singh et al., 2026); (ii) chronic systemic LRRK2 inhibition carries pulmonary and renal safety liabilities observed in preclinical species; and (iii) optimal therapeutic windows and dosing schedules for glial-specific effects remain undefined. Antisense oligonucleotides targeting LRRK2 mRNA (BIIB094) offer an alternative approach with CNS-selective activity and are in Phase 1 evaluation (Fig. 4).

9.2 NLRP3 inflammasome inhibitors

Targeting the NLRP3 inflammasome represents a promising glial-specific strategy, given the central role of microglial NLRP3 activation in PD neuroinflammation (Fig. 4). Gordon et al. demonstrated that the NLRP3 inhibitor MCC950 prevented α-syn pathology and dopaminergic neurodegeneration in a mouse PFF model (Gordon et al., 2018).

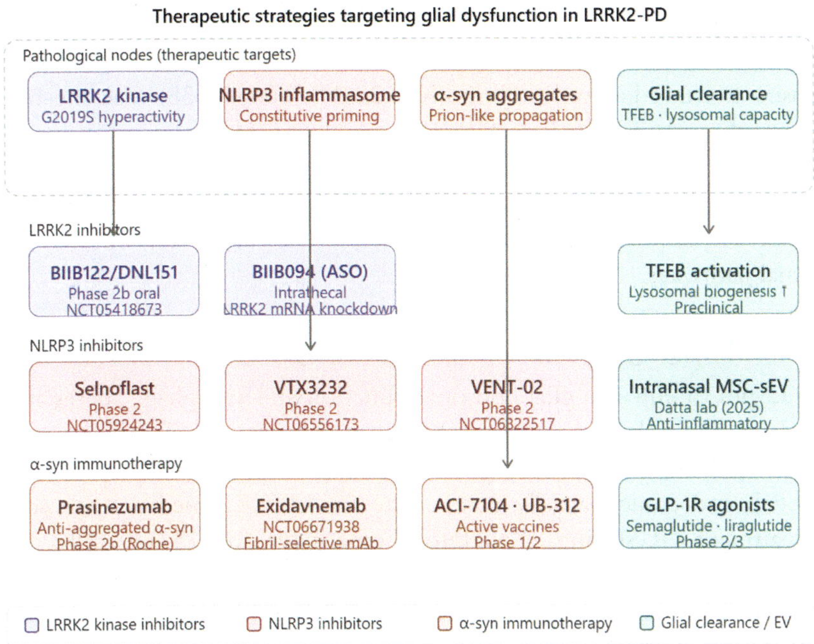

Fig. 4 Therapeutic landscape. Four target classes are organised in columns: LRRK2 kinase inhibitors (BIIB122/DNL151 Phase 2b, BIIB094 ASO), NLRP3 inflammasome inhibitors (selnoflast, VTX3232, VENT-02 — all Phase 2), α-syn immunotherapies (prasinezumab, exidavnemab, ACI-7104/UB-312), and glial clearance strategies (TFEB activation, intranasal MSC-sEV from the Datta lab, GLP-1R agonists).

In the clinical arena, selnoflast (RO-7486967) is in Phase 2 evaluation in early PD (NCT05924243), and VTX3232 is in Phase 2a trials (NCT06556173). VENT−02, another brain-penetrant NLRP3 inhibitor, completed Phase 1a showing significant IL-1β inhibition in blood (NCT06822517). In the LRRK2 context, NLRP3 inhibition may be particularly valuable given the constitutive inflammasome priming in G2019S microglia (Panagiotakopoulou et al., 2020). However, NLRP3 has homeostatic immune functions, and complete or prolonged inhibition may impair pathogen clearance.

9.3 Immunotherapies targeting extracellular α-synuclein

Passive and active immunisation strategies aim to reduce extracellular α-syn burden by antibody-mediated clearance. Prasinezumab (PRX002), targeting the C-terminal of aggregated α-syn, showed promising Phase 1b data but did not meet its Phase 2 primary endpoint, with post-hoc analyses suggesting motor-symptom slowing in specific subgroups. BAN0805 (exidavnemab), targeting aggregated forms, showed dose-dependent plasma α-syn reduction and is in Phase 2a (NCT06671938). Vaccine-based approaches (ACI-7104.056, UB-312) are also in early clinical evaluation. In LRRK2-PD, where glial α-syn handling is impaired, reducing extracellular α-synuclein load via immunotherapy may synergise with LRRK2 kinase inhibition—lowering the burden on already-compromised lysosomal pathways.

9.4 Enhancing glial clearance pathways

Strategies to enhance glial lysosomal function and autophagy represent an underexplored but mechanistically rational approach. TFEB activation—upregulating lysosomal biogenesis—has shown promise in preclinical PD models and could partially compensate for LRRK2-mediated lysosomal impairment. Restoring cholesterol homeostasis in I1371V cells using cyclodextrin-based cholesterol modulators is a potential approach informed by our group's finding of membrane cholesterol depletion as a central I1371V phenotype (Singh et al., 2026). GLP-1R agonists that block microglial A1 astrocyte conversion (Yun et al., 2018) and intranasal delivery of therapeutic extracellular vesicles from healthy MSCs—shown by our group to restore motor deficits and neurogenesis in PD rat models (Mondal et al., 2025) —represent additional avenues for glia-targeted neuroprotection. Our group's ongoing work with iMSC-derived small EVs as a cell-free, intranasal therapeutic platform aims to combine immunomodulation, neuroprotection, and anti-inflammatory effects in a scalable product (Mondal et al., 2025; Ghanty et al., 2026).

10. Future directions and unanswered questions

Despite significant progress, fundamental questions remain. Do microglia or astrocytes dominate α-synuclein clearance in the human LRRK2-PD brain, and does this balance shift with disease stage? Currently, in vitro data suggest microglial superiority for phagocytic clearance, while astrocytes may be more significant in early disease when neuronal α-syn loads are subthreshold for overt microglial activation. Longitudinal human iPSC organoid studies combining multimodal single-cell approaches will be needed. How does the I1371V mutation reshape glial biology relative to G2019S, and are there additional understudied variants with unique glial phenotypes? Our group's characterisation of I1371V astrocytes has established that GTPase-domain variants are not merely weaker versions of G2019S but drive qualitatively distinct cellular dysfunction (Banerjee et al., 2023; Singh et al., 2026). A systematic multi-variant glial comparison platform is needed. Can glial dysfunction be therapeutically reversed once established, or only prevented? The distinction between preventive and restorative glial targeting is critical for the design of clinical trials, which enrol patients with existing pathology. What is the contribution of peripheral LRRK2-expressing immune cells—monocytes, macrophages, T cells—to the CNS inflammatory milieu of LRRK2-PD ? LRRK2 is highly expressed in peripheral monocytes and its expression is induced by immune stimuli; pathological α-syn is known to recruit LRRK2-expressing monocytes to the brain. Elucidating the axis of peripheral–central immune crosstalk in LRRK2-PD may reveal accessible therapeutic targets.

11. Conclusions

The evidence reviewed here establishes that LRRK2 mutations fundamentally reshape how glial cells detect, internalise, degrade, and propagate extracellular α-synuclein. Microglia harbouring LRRK2 mutations are tonically primed for NLRP3-mediated inflammatory activation, exhibit impaired lysosomal clearance of α-syn, and redirect phagocytosed aggregates into pathogenic exosomal release pathways via the LRRK2-Rab10-LYTL axis. Astrocytes with LRRK2 mutations fail as α-syn scavengers, propagate phospho-α-syn-enriched EVs to neurons, impair glutamate homeostasis, and succumb to oxidative stress due to Nrf2-GSH pathway failure. Together, dysfunctional microglia and astrocytes form a bidirectional, amplifying circuit—each cell type's impairment exacerbating the other's—that accelerates the progression of dopaminergic neurodegeneration beyond what either cell type alone contributes. Critically, as our group's work on LRRK2 I1371V demonstrates, these mechanisms are mutation-specific: GTPase-domain and kinase-domain variants drive distinct glial pathobiology, necessitating variant-tailored therapeutic strategies. Future progress requires longitudinal human iPSC models, multi-variant comparative platforms, and clinical trial designs that incorporate glial biomarkers as pharmacodynamic endpoints. Targeting glial LRRK2 signalling—and its downstream inflammatory and trafficking consequences—represents one of the most mechanistically grounded and therapeutically promising frontiers in PD research.

References

Abe, T., Kuwahara, T., Suenaga, S., Sakurai, M., Takatori, S., & Iwatsubo, T. (2024). Lysosomal stress drives the release of pathogenic α-synuclein from macrophage lineage cells via the LRRK2-Rab10 pathway. *iScience, 27*, 108893. https://doi.org/10.1016/j.isci.2024.108893.

Abounit, S., Bousset, L., Loria, F., Zhu, S., de Chaumont, F., Pieri, L., et al. (2016). Tunneling nanotubes spread fibrillar α-synuclein by intercellular trafficking of lysosomes. *The EMBO Journal, 35*, 2120–2138. https://doi.org/10.15252/embj.201593411.

Alessi, D. R., & Pfeffer, S. R. (2024). Leucine-rich repeat kinases. *Annual Review of Biochemistry, 93*, 261–287. https://doi.org/10.1146/annurev-biochem-030122-051144.

Alvarez-Erviti, L., Seow, Y., Schapira, A. H., Gardiner, C., Sargent, I. L., Wood, M. J. A., et al. (2011). Lysosomal dysfunction increases exosome-mediated alpha-synuclein release and transmission. *Neurobiology of Disease, 42*, 360–367. https://doi.org/10.1016/j.nbd.2011.01.029.

Anderson, F. L., Von Herrmann, K. M., Andrew, A. S., Kuras, Y. I., Young, A. L., Scherzer, C. R., et al. (2021). Plasma-borne indicators of inflammasome activity in Parkinson's disease patients. *NPJ Parkinson's Disease, 7*, 2. https://doi.org/10.1038/s41531-020-00147-6.

Banerjee, R., Raj, A., Potdar, C., Pal, P., Yadav, R., Kamble, N., et al. (2023). Astrocytes differentiated from LRRK2-I1371V Parkinson's-disease-induced pluripotent stem cells exhibit similar yield but cell-intrinsic dysfunction in glutamate uptake and metabolism, ATP generation, and Nrf2-mediated glutathione machinery. *Cells, 12*, 1592. https://doi.org/10.3390/cells12121592.

Banerjee, R., Santhoshkumar, R., Holla, V., Kamble, N., Yadav, R., Pal, P. K., et al. (2026). LRRK2 I1371V impairs astrocytic glucose metabolism and triggers multi-organellar dysfunction in PD. *bioRxiv*. https://doi.org/10.64898/2026.01.19.700314.

Beilina, A., Park, J.-H., Landeck, N., Chia, R., Ding, J., Reed, X., et al. (2026). Inflammatory signaling differentially changes chromatin accessibility and gene expression of the PD- associated kinase LRRK2 between human and mice. *Molecular Neurodegeneration*. https://doi.org/10.1186/s13024-026-00938-0.

Billingsley, K. J., Bandres-Ciga, S., Saez-Atienzar, S., & Singleton, A. B. (2018). Genetic risk factors in Parkinson's disease. *Cell and Tissue Research, 373*, 9–20. https://doi.org/10.1007/s00441-018-2817-y.

Blasco-Agell, L., Pons-Espinal, M., Testa, V., Roch, G., Montero-Muñoz, J., Fernandez-Carasa, I., et al. (2025). LRRK2-mutant microglia and neuromelanin synergize to drive dopaminergic neurodegeneration in an iPSC-based Parkinson's disease model. *Communications Biology, 8*, 1203. https://doi.org/10.1038/s42003-025-08544-4.

Boecker, C. A., Goldsmith, J., Dou, D., Cajka, G. G., & Holzbaur, E. L. F. (2021). Increased LRRK2 kinase activity alters neuronal autophagy by disrupting the axonal transport of autophagosomes. *Current Biology: CB, 31*, 2140–2154.e6. https://doi.org/10.1016/j.cub.2021.02.061.

Bonet-Ponce, L., Beilina, A., Williamson, C. D., Lindberg, E., Kluss, J. H., Saez-Atienzar, S., et al. (2020). LRRK2 mediates tubulation and vesicle sorting from lysosomes. *Science Advances, 6*, eabb2454. https://doi.org/10.1126/sciadv.abb2454.

Booth, H. D. E., Wessely, F., Connor-Robson, N., Rinaldi, F., Vowles, J., Browne, C., et al. (2019). RNA sequencing reveals MMP2 and TGFB1 downregulation in LRRK2 G2019S Parkinson's iPSC-derived astrocytes. *Neurobiology of Disease, 129*, 56–66. https://doi.org/10.1016/j.nbd.2019.05.006.

Bosgraaf, L., & Van Haastert, P. J. M. (2003). Roc, a Ras/GTPase domain in complex proteins. *Biochimica et Biophysica Acta (BBA) - Molecular Cell Research, 1643*, 5–10. https://doi.org/10.1016/j.bbamcr.2003.08.008.

Braak, H., Sastre, M., & Del Tredici, K. (2007). Development of α-synuclein immunoreactive astrocytes in the forebrain parallels stages of intraneuronal pathology in sporadic Parkinson's disease. *Acta Neuropathologica (Berl), 114*, 231–241. https://doi.org/10.1007/s00401-007-0244-3.

Braak, H., Tredici, K. D., Rüb, U., De Vos, R. A. I., Jansen Steur, E. N. H., & Braak, E. (2003). Staging of brain pathology related to sporadic Parkinson's disease. *Neurobiology of Aging, 24*, 197–211. https://doi.org/10.1016/S0197-4580(02)00065-9.

Brás, I. C., & Outeiro, T. F. (2021). Alpha-synuclein: Mechanisms of release and pathology progression in synucleinopathies. *Cells, 10*, 375. https://doi.org/10.3390/cells10020375.

Chakraborty, R., Nonaka, T., Hasegawa, M., & Zurzolo, C. (2023). Tunnelling nanotubes between neuronal and microglial cells allow bi-directional transfer of α-synuclein and mitochondria. *Cell Death & Disease, 14*, 329. https://doi.org/10.1038/s41419-023-05835-8.

Choi, Y., & Chung, W.-S. (2025). Glial phagocytosis for synapse and toxic proteins in neurodegenerative diseases. *Molecular Neurodegeneration, 20*, 81. https://doi.org/10.1186/s13024-025-00870-9.

Daniele, S. G., Béraud, D., Davenport, C., Cheng, K., Yin, H., & Maguire-Zeiss, K. A. (2015). Activation of MyD88-dependent TLR1/2 signaling by misfolded α-synuclein, a protein linked to neurodegenerative disorders. *Science Signaling, 8*. https://doi.org/10.1126/scisignal.2005965.

Danzer, K. M., Haasen, D., Karow, A. R., Moussaud, S., Habeck, M., Giese, A., et al. (2007). Different species of α-synuclein oligomers induce calcium influx and seeding. *The Journal of Neuroscience, 27*, 9220–9232. https://doi.org/10.1523/JNEUROSCI.2617-07.2007.

Datta, I., Banerjee, R., Holla, V., Kamble, N., Yadav, R., & Pal, P. (2026). LRRK2-I1371V disrupts astrocyte membrane homeostasis and paradoxically enhances α-synuclein. *Toxicity Despite Impaired Clearance*. https://doi.org/10.21203/rs.3.rs-7255076/v1.

Datta, I., Sowmithra, Jagtap, S., Potdar, C., Yadav, R., & Pal, P. (2020). Generation of induced pluripotent stem cells (NIMHi001-A) from a Parkinson's disease patient of East Indian ethnicity carrying LRRK2 I1371V variant. *Stem Cell Research, 44*, 101768. https://doi.org/10.1016/j.scr.2020.101768.

De Boni, L., Watson, A. H., Zaccagnini, L., Wallis, A., Zhelcheska, K., Kim, N., et al. (2022). Brain region-specific susceptibility of lewy body pathology in synucleinopathies is governed by α-synuclein conformations. *Acta Neuropathologica (Berl), 143*, 453–469. https://doi.org/10.1007/s00401-022-02406-7.

De Rus Jacquet, A., Tancredi, J. L., Lemire, A. L., DeSantis, M. C., Li, W.-P., & O'Shea, E. K. (2021). The LRRK2 G2019S mutation alters astrocyte-to-neuron communication via extracellular vesicles and induces neuron atrophy in a human iPSC-derived model of Parkinson's disease. *eLife, 10*, e73062. https://doi.org/10.7554/eLife.73062.

Deng, J., Lewis, P. A., Greggio, E., Sluch, E., Beilina, A., & Cookson, M. R. (2008). Structure of the ROC domain from the Parkinson's disease-associated leucine-rich repeat kinase 2 reveals a dimeric GTPase. *Proceedings of the National Academy of Sciences, 105*, 1499–1504. https://doi.org/10.1073/pnas.0709098105.

Dhekne, H. S., Tonelli, F., Yeshaw, W. M., Chiang, C. Y., Limouse, C., Jaimon, E., et al. (2023). Genome-wide screen reveals Rab12 GTPase as a critical activator of Parkinson's disease-linked LRRK2 kinase. *eLife, 12*, e87098. https://doi.org/10.7554/eLife.87098.

Dhekne, H. S., Yanatori, I., Gomez, R. C., Tonelli, F., Diez, F., Schüle, B., et al. (2018). A pathway for Parkinson's disease LRRK2 kinase to block primary cilia and Sonic hedgehog signaling in the brain. *eLife, 7*, e40202. https://doi.org/10.7554/eLife.40202.

Di Domenico, A., Carola, G., Calatayud, C., Pons-Espinal, M., Muñoz, J. P., Richaud-Patin, Y., et al. (2019). Patient-specific iPSC-derived astrocytes contribute to non-cell-autonomous neurodegeneration in Parkinson's disease. *Stem Cell Reports, 12*, 213–229. https://doi.org/10.1016/j.stemcr.2018.12.011.

Di Iacovo, A., D'Agostino, C., Bhatt, M., Romanazzi, T., Giovannardi, S., Cinquetti, R., et al. (2025). The kinase LRRK2 is required for the physiological function and expression of the glial glutamate transporter EAAT2 (SLC1A2). *Journal of Neurochemistry, 169*, e16265. https://doi.org/10.1111/jnc.16265.

Dilsizoglu Senol, A., Samarani, M., Syan, S., Guardia, C. M., Nonaka, T., Liv, N., et al. (2021). α-Synuclein fibrils subvert lysosome structure and function for the propagation of protein misfolding between cells through tunneling nanotubes. *PLoS Biology, 19*, e3001287. https://doi.org/10.1371/journal.pbio.3001287.

Ding, M., Wang, F., Jiang, L.-L., Ma, C., Qi, Y.-W., Liu, J.-Y., et al. (2025). LRRK2 G2019S mutation contributes to mitochondrial transfer dysfunction in a Drp1-STX17-dependent manner. *Translational Neurodegeneration, 14*, 64. https://doi.org/10.1186/s40035-025-00525-1.

El-Agnaf, O. M. A., Salem, S. A., Paleologou, K. E., Cooper, L. J., Fullwood, N. J., Gibson, M. J., et al. (2003). α-Synuclein implicated in Parkinson's disease is present in extracellular biological fluids, including human plasma. *The FASEB Journal, 17*, 1–16. https://doi.org/10.1096/fj.03-0098fje.

El-Agnaf, O. M. A., Salem, S. A., Paleologou, K. E., Curran, M. D., Gibson, M. J., Court, J. A., et al. (2006). Detection of oligomeric forms of α-synuclein protein in human plasma as a potential biomarker for Parkinson's disease. *The FASEB Journal, 20*, 419–425. https://doi.org/10.1096/fj.03-1449com.

Emmanouilidou, E., Elenis, D., Papasilekas, T., Stranjalis, G., Gerozissis, K., Ioannou, P. C., et al. (2011). Assessment of α-synuclein secretion in mouse and human brain parenchyma. *PLoS One, 6*, e22225. https://doi.org/10.1371/journal.pone.0022225.

Farrer, M. J. (2006). Genetics of Parkinson disease: Paradigm shifts and future prospects. *Nature Reviews. Genetics, 7*, 306–318. https://doi.org/10.1038/nrg1831.

Fernández-Pajarín, G., Sesar, Á., Jiménez-Martín, I., Ares, B., & Castro, A. (2023). Progression and treatment of a series of patients with advanced LRRK2-associated Parkinson's disease. *Neurologia (Barcelona, Spain), 38*, 350–356. https://doi.org/10.1016/j.nrleng.2020.06.014.

Ghanty, R., Mondal, K., Kamble, N., Datta, I., & Pdf, S. (2026). Pre-motor mesenchymal stromal cell dysfunction drives immune dysregulation in Parkinson's Disease. *Implications for Allogeneic Cell Therapy*. https://doi.org/10.2139/ssrn.6034155.

Giasson, B. I., Covy, J. P., Bonini, N. M., Hurtig, H. I., Farrer, M. J., Trojanowski, J. Q., et al. (2006). Biochemical and pathological characterization of Lrrk2. *Annals of Neurology, 59*, 315–322. https://doi.org/10.1002/ana.20791.

Gilsbach, B. K., & Kortholt, A. (2014). Structural biology of the LRRK2 GTPase and kinase domains: Implications for regulation. *Frontiers in Molecular Neuroscience, 7*. https://doi.org/10.3389/fnmol.2014.00032.

Gomez-Sequeda, N., Jimenez-Del-Rio, M., Velez-Pardo, C. (2025). Inhibiting LRRK2 kinase activity protects against the pathology associated with the presenilin 1 Ile416Thr mutation in cholinergic neurons. https://doi.org/10.1101/2025.09.17.25336024.

Gordon, R., Albornoz, E. A., Christie, D. C., Langley, M. R., Kumar, V., Mantovani, S., et al. (2018). Inflammasome inhibition prevents α-synuclein pathology and dopaminergic neurodegeneration in mice. *Science Translational Medicine, 10*, eaah4066. https://doi.org/10.1126/scitranslmed.aah4066.

Guo, M., Wang, J., Zhao, Y., Feng, Y., Han, S., Dong, Q., et al. (2020). Microglial exosomes facilitate α-synuclein transmission in Parkinson's disease. *Brain, 143*, 1476–1497. https://doi.org/10.1093/brain/awaa090.

Ha, J., Kang, J. S., Lee, M., Baek, A., Kim, S., Chung, S.-K., et al. (2020). Simplified brain organoids for rapid and robust modeling of brain disease. *Frontiers in Cell and Developmental Biology, 8*, 594090. https://doi.org/10.3389/fcell.2020.594090.

Hansson, O., Hall, S., Öhrfelt, A., Zetterberg, H., Blennow, K., Minthon, L., et al. (2014). Levels of cerebrospinal fluid α-synuclein oligomers are increased in Parkinson's disease with dementia and dementia with Lewy bodies compared to Alzheimer's disease. *Alzheimer's Research & Therapy, 6*, 25. https://doi.org/10.1186/alzrt255.

Harackiewicz, O., & Grembecka, B. (2024). The role of microglia and astrocytes in the pathomechanism of neuroinflammation in Parkinson's disease—Focus on alpha-synuclein. *Journal of Integrative Neuroscience, 23*, 203. https://doi.org/10.31083/j.jin2311203.

Helley, M. P., Pinnell, J., Sportelli, C., & Tieu, K. (2017). Mitochondria: A common target for genetic mutations and environmental toxicants in Parkinson's disease. *Frontiers in Genetics, 8*, 177. https://doi.org/10.3389/fgene.2017.00177.

Ho, D. H., Je, A. R., Lee, H., Son, I., Kweon, H.-S., Kim, H.-G., et al. (2018). LRRK2 kinase activity induces mitochondrial fission in microglia via Drp1 and modulates neuroinflammation. *Experimental Neurobiology, 27*, 171–180. https://doi.org/10.5607/en.2018.27.3.171.

Ho, D. H., Nam, D., Seo, M. K., Park, S. W., Son, I., & Seol, W. (2019). Leucine-rich repeat kinase 2 (LRRK2) phosphorylates Rab10 in glia and neurons. *Biomedical Science Letters, 25*, 177–184. https://doi.org/10.15616/BSL.2019.25.2.177.

Ho, D. H., Seol, W., Eun, J. H., & Son, I. (2017). Phosphorylation of p53 by LRRK2 induces microglial tumor necrosis factor α-mediated neurotoxicity. *Biochemical and Biophysical Research Communications, 482*, 1088–1094. https://doi.org/10.1016/j.bbrc.2016.11.163.

Hu, B., Zhang, J., Huang, J., Luo, B., Zeng, X., & Jia, J. (2024). NLRP3/1-mediated pyroptosis: Beneficial clues for the development of novel therapies for Alzheimer's disease. *Neural Regeneration Research, 19*, 2400–2410. https://doi.org/10.4103/1673-5374.391311.

Hu, Y., Yu, S.-Y., Zuo, L.-J., Cao, C.-J., Wang, F., Chen, Z.-J., et al. (2015). Parkinson disease with REM sleep behavior disorder: Features, α-synuclein, and inflammation. *Neurology, 84*, 888–894. https://doi.org/10.1212/WNL.0000000000001308.

Ilieva, N. M., Hoffman, E. K., Ghalib, M. A., Greenamyre, J. T., & De Miranda, B. R. (2024). LRRK2 kinase inhibition protects against Parkinson's disease-associated environmental toxicants. *Neurobiology of Disease, 196*, 106522. https://doi.org/10.1016/j.nbd.2024.106522.

Iovino, L., Giusti, V., Pischedda, F., Giusto, E., Plotegher, N., Marte, A., et al. (2022). Trafficking of the glutamate transporter is impaired in LRRK2-related Parkinson's disease. *Acta Neuropathologica (Berl), 144*, 81–106. https://doi.org/10.1007/s00401-022-02437-0.

Jagtap, S., Potdar, C., Yadav, R., Pal, P. K., & Datta, I. (2022). Dopaminergic neurons differentiated from LRRK2 I1371V-induced pluripotent stem cells display a lower yield, α-synuclein pathology, and functional impairment. *ACS Chemical Neuroscience, 13*, 2632–2645. https://doi.org/10.1021/acschemneuro.2c00297.

Janković, M. Z., Kresojević, N. D., Dobričić, V. S., Marković, V. V., Petrović, I. N., Novaković, I. V., et al. (2015). Identification of novel variants in LRRK2 gene in patients with Parkinson's disease in Serbian population. *Journal of the Neurological Sciences, 353*, 59–62. https://doi.org/10.1016/j.jns.2015.04.002.

Kim, C., Beilina, A., Smith, N., Li, Y., Kim, M., Kumaran, R., et al. (2020). LRRK2 mediates microglial neurotoxicity via NFATc2 in rodent models of synucleinopathies. *Science Translational Medicine, 12*, eaay0399. https://doi.org/10.1126/scitranslmed.aay0399.

Kim, H., Park, H. J., Choi, H., Chang, Y., Park, H., Shin, J., et al. (2019). Modeling G2019S-LRRK2 sporadic Parkinson's disease in 3D midbrain organoids. *Stem Cell Reports, 12*, 518–531. https://doi.org/10.1016/j.stemcr.2019.01.020.

Komori, T., & Kuwahara, T. (2023). An update on the interplay between LRRK2, Rab GTPases and Parkinson's disease. *Biomolecules, 13*, 1645. https://doi.org/10.3390/biom13111645.

Kurniawan, H., Nickels, S. L., Zagare, A., Zuccoli, E., Rosety, I., Gomez-Giro, G., et al. (2025). The Parkinson's disease-associated LRRK2-G2019S variant restricts serine metabolism, leading to microglial inflammation and dopaminergic neuron degeneration. *Journal of Neuroinflammation, 22*, 244. https://doi.org/10.1186/s12974-025-03577-2.

Kuwahara, T., & Iwatsubo, T. (2020). The emerging functions of LRRK2 and Rab GTPases in the endolysosomal system. *Frontiers in Neuroscience, 14*, 227. https://doi.org/10.3389/fnins.2020.00227.

Langston, R. G., Rudenko, I. N., & Cookson, M. R. (2016). The function of orthologues of the human Parkinson's disease gene *LRRK2* across species: Implications for disease modelling in preclinical research. *The Biochemical Journal, 473*, 221–232. https://doi.org/10.1042/BJ20150985.

Lee, H.-J., Bae, E.-J., & Lee, S.-J. (2014). Extracellular α-synuclein—a novel and crucial factor in Lewy body diseases. *Nature Reviews Neurology, 10*, 92–98. https://doi.org/10.1038/nrneurol.2013.275.

Lee, H.-J., Cho, E.-D., Lee, K. W., Kim, J.-H., Cho, S.-G., & Lee, S.-J. (2013). Autophagic failure promotes the exocytosis and intercellular transfer of α-synuclein. *Experimental & Molecular Medicine, 45*, e22. https://doi.org/10.1038/emm.2013.45.

Lee, H.-J., Patel, S., & Lee, S.-J. (2005). Intravesicular localization and exocytosis of α-synuclein and its aggregates. *The Journal of Neuroscience, 25*, 6016–6024. https://doi.org/10.1523/JNEUROSCI.0692-05.2005.

Lee, H.-J., Suk, J.-E., Patrick, C., Bae, E.-J., Cho, J.-H., Rho, S., et al. (2010). Direct transfer of alpha-synuclein from neuron to astroglia causes inflammatory responses in synucleinopathies. *The Journal of Biological Chemistry, 285*, 9262–9272. https://doi.org/10.1074/jbc.M109.081125.

Li, Y., Xia, Y., Yin, S., Wan, F., Hu, J., Kou, L., et al. (2021). Targeting microglial α-synuclein/TLRs/NF-kappaB/NLRP3 inflammasome axis in Parkinson's disease. *Frontiers in Immunology, 12*, 719807. https://doi.org/10.3389/fimmu.2021.719807.

Liddelow, S. A., Guttenplan, K. A., Clarke, L. E., Bennett, F. C., Bohlen, C. J., Schirmer, L., et al. (2017). Neurotoxic reactive astrocytes are induced by activated microglia. *Nature, 541*, 481–487. https://doi.org/10.1038/nature21029.

Lin, H.-I., Cheng, Y.-C., Ko, H.-W., Wen, C.-H., Lu, H.-E., Huang, C.-Y., et al. (2019). Generation of induced pluripotent stem cells (IBMSi011-A) from a patient with Parkinson's disease carrying LRRK2 p.I1371V mutation. *Stem Cell Research, 37*, 101447. https://doi.org/10.1016/j.scr.2019.101447.

Liu, M., Bender, S. A., Cuny, G. D., Sherman, W., Glicksman, M., & Ray, S. S. (2013). Type II kinase inhibitors show an unexpected inhibition mode against Parkinson's disease-linked LRRK2 mutant G2019S. *Biochemistry, 52*, 1725–1736. https://doi.org/10.1021/bi3012077.

Liu, Z., Bryant, N., Kumaran, R., Beilina, A., Abeliovich, A., Cookson, M. R., et al. (2018). LRRK2 phosphorylates membrane-bound Rabs and is activated by GTP-bound Rab7L1 to promote recruitment to the trans-Golgi network. *Human Molecular Genetics, 27*, 385–395. https://doi.org/10.1093/hmg/ddx410.

Luk, K. C., Kehm, V., Carroll, J., Zhang, B., O'Brien, P., Trojanowski, J. Q., et al. (2012). Pathological α-synuclein transmission initiates parkinson-like neurodegeneration in nontransgenic mice. *Science (New York, N. Y.), 338*, 949–953. https://doi.org/10.1126/science.1227157.

Mercatelli, D., Brugnoli, A., Di Maio, A., Albanese, F., Shimshek, D. R., Usiello, A., et al. (2025). Enhancement of D1 dopaminergic responses in aged LRRK2 G2019S knock-in mice. *Neurobiology of Disease, 208*, 106881. https://doi.org/10.1016/j.nbd.2025.106881.

Mondal, K., Ghanty, R., Mahadevan, A., Waghmare, G., Santhoshkumar, R., Bn, N., et al. (2025). Intranasal delivery of DPSC-derived small extracellular vesicles-encased phloroglucinol attenuates non-motor and motor deficits and promotes neurogenesis in an in vivo rat model of Parkinson's disease. *Stem Cell Research & Therapy, 16*, 570. https://doi.org/10.1186/s13287-025-04573-2.

Morais, V. A., & Vos, M. (2022). Reduced penetrance of Parkinson's disease models. *Med Genetics, 34*, 117–124. https://doi.org/10.1515/medgen-2022-2138.

Nalls, M. A., Blauwendraat, C., Vallerga, C. L., Heilbron, K., Bandres-Ciga, S., Chang, D., et al. (2019). Identification of novel risk loci, causal insights, and heritable risk for Parkinson's disease: a meta-analysis of genome-wide association studies. *Lancet Neurology, 18*, 1091–1102. https://doi.org/10.1016/S1474-4422(19)30320-5.

Nolen, B., Taylor, S., & Ghosh, G. (2004). Regulation of protein kinases. *Molecular Cell, 15*, 661–675. https://doi.org/10.1016/j.molcel.2004.08.024.

Ohtonen, S., Giudice, L., Jäntti, H., Fazaludeen, M. F., Shakirzyanova, A., Gómez-Budia, M., et al. (2023). Human iPSC-derived microglia carrying the LRRK2-G2019S mutation show a Parkinson's disease related transcriptional profile and function. *Scientific Reports, 13*, 22118. https://doi.org/10.1038/s41598-023-49294-9.

Paisán-Ruíz, C., Jain, S., Evans, E. W., Gilks, W. P., Simón, J., Van Der Brug, M., et al. (2004). Cloning of the gene containing mutations that cause PARK8-linked Parkinson's disease. *Neuron, 44*, 595–600. https://doi.org/10.1016/j.neuron.2004.10.023.

Paisán-Ruíz, C., Lang, A. E., Kawarai, T., Sato, C., Salehi-Rad, S., Fisman, G. K., et al. (2005). LRRK2 gene in Parkinson disease: Mutation analysis and case control association study. *Neurology, 65*, 696–700. https://doi.org/10.1212/01.wnl.0000167552.79769.b3.

Panagiotakopoulou, V., Ivanyuk, D., De Cicco, S., Haq, W., Arsić, A., Yu, C., et al. (2020). Interferon-γ signaling synergizes with LRRK2 in neurons and microglia derived from human induced pluripotent stem cells. *Nature Communications, 11*, 5163. https://doi.org/10.1038/s41467-020-18755-4.

Pang, S. Y.-Y., Ho, P. W.-L., Liu, H.-F., Leung, C.-T., Li, L., Chang, E. E. S., et al. (2019). The interplay of aging, genetics and environmental factors in the pathogenesis of Parkinson's disease. *Translational Neurodegeneration, 8*, 23. https://doi.org/10.1186/s40035-019-0165-9.

Pankratz, N., Pauciulo, M. W., Elsaesser, V. E., Marek, D. K., Halter, C. A., Rudolph, A., et al. (2006). Mutations in LRRK2 other than G2019S are rare in a north American-based sample of familial Parkinson's disease. *Movement disorders : official journal of the Movement Disorder Society, 21*, 2257–2260. https://doi.org/10.1002/mds.21162.

Park, J., Paik, S. R., Jou, I., & Park, S. M. (2008). Microglial phagocytosis is enhanced by monomeric α-synuclein, not aggregated α-synuclein: Implications for Parkinson's disease. *Glia, 56*, 1215–1223. https://doi.org/10.1002/glia.20691.

Pfeffer, S. R. (2018). LRRK2 and Rab GTPases. *Biochemical Society Transactions, 46*, 1707–1712. https://doi.org/10.1042/BST20180470.

Pirkevi, C., Lesage, S., Condroyer, C., Tomiyama, H., Hattori, N., Ertan, S., et al. (2009). A LRRK2 G2019S mutation carrier from Turkey shares the Japanese haplotype. *Neurogenetics, 10*(3), 271. https://doi.org/10.1007/s10048-009-0173-5.

Potdar, C., Jagtap, S., Singh, K., Yadav, R., Pal, P. K., & Datta, I. (2024). Impaired sonic hedgehog responsiveness of induced pluripotent stem cell-derived floor plate cells carrying the LRRK2-I1371V mutation contributes to the ontogenic origin of lower dopaminergic neuron yield. *Stem Cells and Development, 33*, 306–320. https://doi.org/10.1089/scd.2023.0283.

Purlyte, E., Dhekne, H. S., Sarhan, A. R., Gomez, R., Lis, P., Wightman, M., et al. (2018). Rab29 activation of the Parkinson's disease-associated LRRK2 kinase. *The EMBO Journal, 37*, 1–18. https://doi.org/10.15252/embj.201798099.

Raj, A., Banerjee, R., Holla, V., Kamble, N., Yadav, R., Pal, P. K., et al. (2024). Dysregulation of protein degradation and alteration of secretome in α-synuclein-exposed astrocytes: Implications for dopaminergic neuronal dysfunction. *Cell Communication and Signaling: CCS, 22*, 574. https://doi.org/10.1186/s12964-024-01928-9.

Raj, A., Banerjee, R., Santhoshkumar, R., Sagar, C., & Datta, I. (2023). Presence of extracellular alpha-synuclein aggregates trigger astrocytic degeneration through enhanced membrane rigidity and deregulation of store-operated calcium entry (SOCE) into the endoplasmic reticulum. *Molecular Neurobiology, 60*, 5309–5329. https://doi.org/10.1007/s12035-023-03400-0.

Raj, A., Kaushal, A., & Datta, I. (2022). Impact of monomeric and aggregated wild-type and A30P/A53T double-mutant α-synuclein on antioxidant mechanism and glutamate metabolic profile of cultured astrocytes. *Journal of Neuroscience Research, 100*, 681–706. https://doi.org/10.1002/jnr.24994.

Ramos-Gonzalez, P., Mato, S., Chara, J. C., Verkhratsky, A., Matute, C., & Cavaliere, F. (2021). Astrocytic atrophy as a pathological feature of Parkinson's disease with LRRK2 mutation. *NPJ Parkinson's Disease, 7*, 31. https://doi.org/10.1038/s41531-021-00175-w.

Reinhardt, P., Schmid, B., Burbulla, L. F., Schöndorf, D. C., Wagner, L., Glatza, M., et al. (2013). Genetic correction of a LRRK2 mutation in human iPSCs links Parkinsonian neurodegeneration to ERK-dependent changes in gene expression. *Cell Stem Cell, 12*, 354–367. https://doi.org/10.1016/j.stem.2013.01.008.

Rostami, J., Holmqvist, S., Lindström, V., Sigvardson, J., Westermark, G. T., Ingelsson, M., et al. (2017). Human astrocytes transfer aggregated alpha-synuclein via tunneling nanotubes. *The Journal of Neuroscience, 37*, 11835–11853. https://doi.org/10.1523/JNEUROSCI.0983-17.2017.

Rostami, J., Mothes, T., Kolahdouzan, M., Eriksson, O., Moslem, M., Bergström, J., et al. (2021). Crosstalk between astrocytes and microglia results in increased degradation of α-synuclein and amyloid-β aggregates. *Journal of Neuroinflammation, 18*, 124. https://doi.org/10.1186/s12974-021-02158-3.

Russo, I., Di Benedetto, G., Kaganovich, A., Ding, J., Mercatelli, D., Morari, M., et al. (2018). Leucine-rich repeat kinase 2 controls protein kinase A activation state through phosphodiesterase 4. *Journal of Neuroinflammation, 15*, 297. https://doi.org/10.1186/s12974-018-1337-8.

Sadhukhan, T., Vishal, M., Das, G., Sharma, A., Mukhopadhyay, A., Das, S. K., et al. (2012). Evaluation of the role of LRRK2 gene in Parkinson's disease in an East Indian cohort. *Disease Markers, 32*, 355–362. https://doi.org/10.3233/DMA-2012-0898.

Schapansky, J., Khasnavis, S., DeAndrade, M. P., Nardozzi, J. D., Falkson, S. R., Boyd, J. D., et al. (2018). Familial knockin mutation of LRRK2 causes lysosomal dysfunction and accumulation of endogenous insoluble α-synuclein in neurons. *Neurobiology of Disease, 111*, 26–35. https://doi.org/10.1016/j.nbd.2017.12.005.

Scheiblich, H., Dansokho, C., Mercan, D., Schmidt, S. V., Bousset, L., Wischhof, L., et al. (2021). Microglia jointly degrade fibrillar alpha-synuclein cargo by distribution through tunneling nanotubes. *Cell, 184*, 5089–5106.e21. https://doi.org/10.1016/j.cell.2021.09.007.

Scheiblich, H., Eikens, F., Wischhof, L., Opitz, S., Jüngling, K., Cserép, C., et al. (2024). Microglia rescue neurons from aggregate-induced neuronal dysfunction and death through tunneling nanotubes. *Neuron, 112*, 3106–3125.e8. https://doi.org/10.1016/j.neuron.2024.06.029.

Seki, N., Takahashi, Y., Tomiyama, H., Rogaeva, E., Murayama, S., Mizuno, Y., et al. (2011). Comprehensive mutational analysis of LRRK2 reveals variants supporting association with autosomal dominant Parkinson's disease. *Journal of Human Genetics, 56*, 671–675. https://doi.org/10.1038/jhg.2011.79.

Singh, F., Prescott, A. R., Rosewell, P., Ball, G., Reith, A. D., & Ganley, I. G. (2021). Pharmacological rescue of impaired mitophagy in Parkinson's disease-related LRRK2 G2019S knock-in mice. *eLife, 10*, e67604. https://doi.org/10.7554/eLife.67604.

Singh, K., Banerjee, R., Potdar, C., Shaw, A., Rakshith, R., Kamble, N., et al. (2026). Membrane dysfunction as a central mechanism in LRRK2-associated Parkinson's disease: Comparative analysis of G2019S and I1371V variants. *Cells, 15*, 342. https://doi.org/10.3390/cells15040342.

Sinha, A., Kushwaha, R., Molesworth, K., Mychko, O., Makarava, N., & Baskakov, I. V. (2021). Phagocytic activities of reactive microglia and astrocytes associated with prion diseases are dysregulated in opposite directions. *Cells, 10*, 1728. https://doi.org/10.3390/cells10071728.

Smethurst, P., Franklin, H., Clarke, B. E., Sidle, K., & Patani, R. (2022). The role of astrocytes in prion-like mechanisms of neurodegeneration. *Brain, 145*, 17–26. https://doi.org/10.1093/brain/awab366.

Smith, L., & Schapira, A. H. V. (2022). GBA variants and Parkinson disease: Mechanisms and treatments. *Cells, 11*, 1261. https://doi.org/10.3390/cells11081261.

Smits, L. M., Reinhardt, L., Reinhardt, P., Glatza, M., Monzel, A. S., Stanslowsky, N., et al. (2019). Modeling Parkinson's disease in midbrain-like organoids. *NPJ Parkinson's Disease, 5*, 5. https://doi.org/10.1038/s41531-019-0078-4.

Sonninen, T.-M., Hämäläinen, R. H., Koskuvi, M., Oksanen, M., Shakirzyanova, A., Wojciechowski, S., et al. (2020). Metabolic alterations in Parkinson's disease astrocytes. *Scientific Reports, 10*, 14474. https://doi.org/10.1038/s41598-020-71329-8.

Steger, M., Tonelli, F., Ito, G., Davies, P., Trost, M., Vetter, M., et al. (2016). Phosphoproteomics reveals that Parkinson's disease kinase LRRK2 regulates a subset of Rab GTPases. *eLife, 5*, e12813. https://doi.org/10.7554/eLife.12813.

Streubel-Gallasch, L., Giusti, V., Sandre, M., Tessari, I., Plotegher, N., Giusto, E., et al. (2021). Parkinson's disease–Associated LRRK2 interferes with astrocyte-mediated alpha-synuclein clearance. *Molecular Neurobiology, 58*, 3119–3140. https://doi.org/10.1007/s12035-021-02327-8.

Stuendl, A., Kunadt, M., Kruse, N., Bartels, C., Moebius, W., Danzer, K. M., et al. (2016). Induction of α-synuclein aggregate formation by CSF exosomes from patients with Parkinson's disease and dementia with Lewy bodies. *Brain, 139*, 481–494. https://doi.org/10.1093/brain/awv346.

Thirstrup, K., Dächsel, J. C., Oppermann, F. S., Williamson, D. S., Smith, G. P., Fog, K., et al. (2017). Selective LRRK2 kinase inhibition reduces phosphorylation of endogenous Rab10 and Rab12 in human peripheral mononuclear blood cells. *Scientific Reports*, 7, 10300. https://doi.org/10.1038/s41598-017-10501-z.

Tokuda, T., Qureshi, M. M., Ardah, M. T., Varghese, S., Shehab, S. A. S., Kasai, T., et al. (2010). Detection of elevated levels of α-synuclein oligomers in CSF from patients with Parkinson disease. *Neurology, 75*, 1766–1770. https://doi.org/10.1212/WNL.0b013e3181fd613b.

Trinh, J., Amouri, R., Duda, J. E., Morley, J. F., Read, M., Donald, A., et al. (2014). A comparative study of Parkinson's disease and leucine-rich repeat kinase 2 p.G2019S parkinsonism. *Neurobiology of Aging, 35*, 1125–1131. https://doi.org/10.1016/j.neurobiolaging.2013.11.015.

Victoria, G. S., Arkhipenko, A., Zhu, S., Syan, S., & Zurzolo, C. (2016). Astrocyte-to-neuron intercellular prion transfer is mediated by cell-cell contact. *Scientific Reports, 6*, 20762. https://doi.org/10.1038/srep20762.

Vieweg, S., Mulholland, K., Bräuning, B., Kachariya, N., Lai, Y.-C., Toth, R., et al. (2020). PINK1-dependent phosphorylation of Serine111 within the SF3 motif of Rab GTPases impairs effector interactions and LRRK2-mediated phosphorylation at Threonine72. *The Biochemical Journal, 477*, 1651–1668. https://doi.org/10.1042/BCJ20190664.

Wakabayashi, K., Hayashi, S., Yoshimoto, M., Kudo, H., & Takahashi, H. (2000). NACP/α-synuclein-positive filamentous inclusions in astrocytes and oligodendrocytes of Parkinson's disease brains. *Acta Neuropathologica (Berl), 99*, 14–20. https://doi.org/10.1007/PL00007400.

Watanabe, R., Buschauer, R., Böhning, J., Audagnotto, M., Lasker, K., Lu, T.-W., et al. (2020). The in situ structure of Parkinson's disease-linked LRRK2. *Cell, 182*, 1508–1518.e16. https://doi.org/10.1016/j.cell.2020.08.004.

Weiss, F., Hughes, L., Fu, Y., Bardy, C., Halliday, G. M., & Dzamko, N. (2024). Astrocytes contribute to toll-like receptor 2-mediated neurodegeneration and alpha-synuclein pathology in a human midbrain Parkinson's model. *Translational Neurodegeneration, 13*, 62. https://doi.org/10.1186/s40035-024-00448-3.

Xia, Y., Zhang, G., Kou, L., Yin, S., Han, C., Hu, J., et al. (2021). Reactive microglia enhance the transmission of exosomal α-synuclein via toll-like receptor 2. *Brain, 144*, 2024–2037. https://doi.org/10.1093/brain/awab122.

Yun, S. P., Kam, T.-I., Panicker, N., Kim, S., Oh, Y., Park, J.-S., et al. (2018). Block of A1 astrocyte conversion by microglia is neuroprotective in models of Parkinson's disease. *Nature Medicine, 24*, 931–938. https://doi.org/10.1038/s41591-018-0051-5.

Zagare, A., Barmpa, K., Smajic, S., Smits, L. M., Grzyb, K., Grünewald, A., et al. (2022). Midbrain organoids mimic early embryonic neurodevelopment and recapitulate LRRK2-p.Gly2019Ser-associated gene expression. *American Journal of Human Genetics, 109*, 311–327. https://doi.org/10.1016/j.ajhg.2021.12.009.

Zimprich, A., Biskup, S., Leitner, P., Lichtner, P., Farrer, M., Lincoln, S., et al. (2004). Mutations in LRRK2 cause autosomal-dominant Parkinsonism with pleomorphic pathology. *Neuron, 44*, 601–607. https://doi.org/10.1016/j.neuron.2004.11.005.

CHAPTER NINE

Microglial advances in Parkinson's disease

Manuel Debasa-Mouce[a], Alberto Ouro[a,b], Joshua De Leon[c], Shelly Gulkarov[d], Allison B. Reiss[c,d], and Anastasia Bougea[e,*]

[a]NeuroAging Group (NEURAL), Clinical Neurosciences Research Laboratory (LINC), Health Research Institute of Santiago de Compostela (IDIS), Santiago de Compostela, Spain
[b]de Investigación Biomédica en Red en Enfermedades Neurodegenerativas (CIBERNED), Instituto de Salud Carlos III, Madrid, Spain
[c]Department of Foundations of Medicine, NYU Grossman Long Island School of Medicine, Mineola, NY, United States
[d]Department of Medicine, NYU Grossman Long Island School of Medicine, Mineola, NY, United States
[e]Department of Neurology, Medical School National and Kapodistrian University of Athens, Athens, Greece
*Corresponding author. e-mail address: abougea@med.uoa.gr

Contents

Abstract

Microglia perform the function of CNS macrophages and act as the primary immune cells in the brain. They surveil the environment, phagocytose cellular debris, maintain homeostasis and respond to tissue damage. While under physiological conditions they

Advances in Immunology, Volume 171
ISSN 0065-2776, https://doi.org/10.1016/bs.ai.2026.06.003

play a role in supporting neurons, activated microglia participate directly in the degeneration of neurons in the substantia nigra, as the hallmark of the Parkinsons disease (PD). Their detrimental effects result from direct phagocytosis of dopaminergic neurons as well as via neuroinflammation and release of toxic reactive oxygen and nitrogen species. This pathological shift is driven by a complex interplay of genetic predispositions, such as LRRK2 and GBA mutations, and environmental triggers like toxins and gut dysbiosis.A central mechanism of this neurodegeneration involves extracellular α-synuclein acting as a danger signal (DAMP), which activates microglial Toll-like receptors (e.g., TLR2) to initiate a severe inflammatory cascade. Furthermore, the extreme biophysical stability of aggregated α-synuclein overwhelms the microglial endolysosomal network, leading to lysosomal failure, "frustrated phagocytosis," and the active propagation of the disease via exosomal shedding. Relieving this maladaptive chronic neuroinflammation is a primary therapeutic goal. Modern strategies aim to break this vicious cycle through precise interventions like NLRP3 inflammasome inhibition and autophagy enhancement. Concurrently, advanced fluid biomarkers, such as seed amplification assays (SAA), alongside multidimensional neuroimaging techniques (PET, SPECT, MRI), are proving crucial for detecting these early microglial and pathological changes to guide personalized, disease-modifying therapies of PD.

1. Dual nature of microglial function

Microglia perform the function of CNS macrophages and act as the primary immune cells in the brain (Jurga et al., 2020). They surveil the environment, phagocytose cellular debris, maintain homeostasis and respond to tissue damage. They are capable of migration and chemotaxis. Microglia share CD11b and CD68 markers with macrophages (Brandenburg et al., 2020). Microglia originate in the yolk sac from cells of the mesoderm lineage and account for approximately 10 % of the total cells in the adult brain (Prinz et al., 2019; Thion et al., 2018). Although there are a relatively large number of markers that characterize microglia, the most selective for this cell type are the transmembrane protein 119 (TMEM119) and purinergic receptor P2Y12R (Banerjee et al., 2021). In the adult brain, it is estimated that microglia renew themselves at a rate of 28 % per year (Réu et al., 2017).

Microglia can interact with neurons in both a protective and destructive fashion. Microglia may take on a range of phenotypes that express different surface marker molecules. These phenotypes span the gamut from an M1 pro-inflammatory state to an M2 anti-inflammatory state with M1 microglia exerting toxic effects on neurons while M2 microglia foster tissue maintenance and repair (Rim et al., 2024; Song & Suk, 2017). Under physiological conditions, they play a role in supporting neurons throughout the adult brain (Augusto-Oliveira et al., 2019). However, activated microglia participate directly in the degeneration of neurons in the substantia nigra (Martin et al., 2025). Their detrimental effects result from direct phagocytosis of dopaminergic neurons as well as via neuroinflammation and release of toxic reactive oxygen and nitrogen species (Casanova et al., 2026; Isik et al., 2023).

Activated microglia provoke neuroinflammation through NF-κB signaling, which leads to transcription of pro-inflammatory mediators such as TNF-α, IL-1β, and TGF-β (Zhang et al., 2026). Oligomeric β-sheet–enriched alpha-synuclein and dysfunctional mitochondria provoke an inflammatory response from microglia (Deyell et al., 2023; Marchi et al., 2023). Both alpha-synuclein and metabolic products of dysfunctional mitochondria incite this response by acting as damage-associated molecular patterns (DAMPs). alpha-Synuclein interacts with the TLR2 receptor on the microglial surface to bring on an inflammatory response (Bisht et al., 2026; Leandrou et al., 2024; Xia et al., 2021) and can cause a transition from the M2 to the M1 phenotype (Guo et al., 2022). In the brain of the person with PD, damaged dopaminergic neurons release neuromelanins, formed during catecholamine metabolism, into the extracellular space where they are phagocytosed by microglia, inducing activation and a neuroinflammatory response (Zucca et al., 2023). In an LPS-induced murine PD model, Cai et al. found that microglia drove synapse elimination in the early stages of neurodegeneration and this microglial effect required complement receptor 3 (CR3) since knockdown of microglial CR3 was synapse-sparing (Cai et al., 2026). Relieving the maladaptive chronic neuroinflammation driven by microglia is one of the main approaches pursued by investigators for the treatment of PD (Zhang et al., 2025).

2. Specific genetic and environmental factors that trigger microglial activation

The etiopathogenesis of Parkinson's Disease (PD) is now viewed by the modern scientific community not as a simple and one-dimensional degeneration of neurons, but as an exceptionally complex interplay between genetic predisposition and environmental insults (Tan et al., 2020). In this dynamic environment, microglial cells, which constitute the primary line of defense and immunity of the Central Nervous System, act as the ultimate convergence point for these heterogeneous factors (Hickman et al., 2018). Under physiological conditions, the architecture and function of microglial cells are strictly regulated to maintain brain homeostasis, support neuroplasticity, and clear metabolic debris. However, specific genetic mutations and prolonged exposure to environmental toxins can skew these cells toward a chronic, maladaptive, and highly aggressive phenotype. This state quickly ceases to be protective and transforms into one of the main driving forces of neurodegeneration, creating a toxic, dead-end microenvironment for the vulnerable dopaminergic neurons.

2.1 Genetic drivers of microglial dysfunction

Modern genome-wide association studies (GWAS) have radically changed the way we perceive the disease, revealing numerous genetic risk loci that are expressed at much higher levels in microglial cells than in the neurons themselves (Colonna & Butovsky, 2017). This pivotal finding demonstrates that, in a very large percentage of patients, the immune system does not merely react passively to the cell death that is already occurring, but is genetically programmed to malfunction from the start, undermining brain health.

One of the most characteristic examples of this genetic predisposition involves mutations in the LRRK2 gene, with the G2019S mutation standing out as the most frequent cause of the familial form of the disease and as a significant risk factor for sporadic cases. The LRRK2 protein is produced in massive quantities within microglial cells, where it functions as an orchestrator of critical processes, controlling cytoskeletal dynamics, the process of autophagy, and the intensity of the inflammatory response (Wallings & Tansey, 2019). As long as it functions normally, it maintains cellular balance. However, when it carries pathogenic mutations, the enzymatic activity of the kinase increases uncontrollably, trapping the microglia in a state of permanent hyperarousal (Blasco-Agell et al., 2024). These mutated cells lose their ability to contain inflammation, exhibit defects in the mechanics of autophagy, and react violently to normal environmental stimuli, massively secreting cytokines such as TNF-α (Wallings & Tansey, 2019).

In a parallel research path, the decisive influence of the GBA gene, which encodes the enzyme glucocerebrosidase, is identified. Heterozygous mutations in this gene represent the most widespread genetic risk factor for the development of the disease (Sidransky et al., 2009). Although the scientific community historically focused on the effects of these mutations within neurons, their destructive action on microglial cells is equally critical. The reason is simple: microglia rely absolutely on the flawless operation of their lysosomes to function as the "cleaners" of the brain. Glucocerebrosidase deficiency paralyzes this ability, making the cells incapable of breaking down the toxic α-synuclein (Schöndorf et al., 2014).

This inability creates the phenomenon of frustrated phagocytosis, which triggers intracellular alarms leading to the release of inflammatory factors, while simultaneously radically altering the structure of lipids in the cell membrane. Finally, the role of the SNCA gene itself, which encodes alpha-synuclein, is crucial. While mutations in this gene primarily destroy neuronal function, the overproduction or incorrect spatial folding of the protein also puts microglial cells in a state of exhaustion, which, unable to remove the constantly increasing volume of extracellular aggregates, gradually collapse (Tan et al., 2020).

2.2 Environmental triggers and the "Double Hit" hypothesis

Shifting the focus from the genetic background to the external environment, a multitude of epidemiological data confirm that the development of the disease is strongly linked to long-term exposure to specific toxins, which act as direct triggers of the microglial response. Characteristic examples are agricultural pesticides, such as rotenone and paraquat, which have been extensively incriminated. Rotenone acts by violently inhibiting mitochondrial complex I, causing a dramatic drop in cellular energy levels and a sharp increase in oxidative stress. Because microglial cells are extremely sensitive to any change in oxygen levels, they react immediately by activating the NADPH oxidase enzyme (NOX2) and releasing toxic superoxide radicals into the environment, which exterminate the dopaminergic neurons (Gao et al., 2003). Similarly, paraquat traps the microglia in a chronic inflammatory state through exhausting redox reactions.

One of the most innovative approaches in recent years concerns the investigation of the gut-brain axis, with the gastrointestinal system emerging as the possible true starting point of the pathology. Any disturbance in the balance of the intestinal flora (dysbiosis) destroys the integrity of the intestinal barrier, allowing bacterial toxins to enter the systemic circulation (Sampson et al., 2016). The resulting inflammation penetrates the blood-brain barrier and puts the microglia on alert. The now prevailing theory argues that pathological α-synuclein is initially formed in the gut and uses the vagus nerve as a transport pathway to the brain, resulting in microglial cells in the brainstem being activated decades before any motor disturbance is observed (Sampson et al., 2016). Furthermore, head traumas are recognized as an extremely aggravating factor, as they cause micro-ruptures in the blood-brain barrier, allowing the peripheral immune system to invade the brain tissue. This inflammatory reaction often does not subside, with the microglia remaining in a state of prolonged, low-grade excitation, performing a cumulative destruction that manifests clinically much later (Braak et al., 2003).

3. Targeting the alpha-synuclein-microglia axis

The interaction between microglia and α-synuclein is the central engine of neuroinflammation in PD. This relationship is not unidirectional; rather, it forms a feed-forward loop often described as the "vicious cycle" of neurodegeneration (Tan et al., 2020) (Fig. 1). Breaking this axis is a primary goal of current therapeutic development.

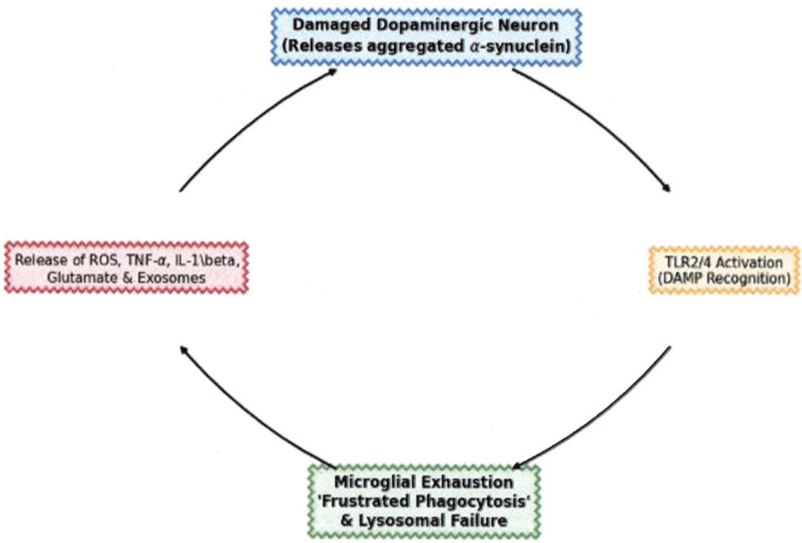

Fig. 1 The vicious cycle of microglial activation and neurodegeneration in Parkinson's disease. Pathological, aggregated alpha-synuclein released from damaged dopaminergic neurons acts as a Damage-Associated Molecular Pattern (DAMP). It binds to microglial pattern recognition receptors (such as TLR2 and TLR4), initiating an intracellular signaling cascade via NF-κB. The extreme biophysical stability of these aggregates overwhelms the lysosomal machinery, leading to lysosomal membrane permeabilization and "frustrated phagocytosis". Consequently, microglia shift to a neurotoxic state, releasing pro-inflammatory cytokines, reactive oxygen species (ROS), and glutamate. This toxic microenvironment exacerbates dopaminergic neuron death, which in turn releases more alpha-synuclein, perpetuating a relentless cycle of neurodegeneration. Microglia further propagate the pathology via exosomes.

3.1 The mechanism of recognition

The destructive, continuous interaction between pathological alpha-synuclein and microglial cells constitutes the central core that fuels neuroinflammation in PD (Tan et al., 2020). The zero point of this cycle is recognition. In their physiological function, microglial cells do not arbitrarily attack neurons, but are exclusively stimulated by specific danger signals. The problematic, aggregated forms of alpha-synuclein are perceived by the immune system exactly as such signals (DAMPs). As soon as the suffering neurons shed these protein remnants, the microglia detect them instantly utilizing receptors on their surface. A leading role is played by Toll-like receptors, especially TLR2 and TLR4 (Fellner et al., 2013; Kim et al., 2013). The physical connection of these receptors with the pathological fibrils directly triggers the NF-κB intracellular signaling pathway, which commands the production of potent pro-inflammatory cytokines (Kim et al., 2013).

3.2 Failure of clearance and "Frustrated Phagocytosis"

In a healthy brain, microglia act as highly efficient scavengers, successfully phagocytosing and degrading extracellular proteins through an intricate endolysosomal network. In PD, however, this vital clearance process is catastrophically overwhelmed. The underlying issue is not just the sheer volume of extracellular alpha-synuclein, but the extreme biophysical stability of the protein's aggregated forms. Pathological alpha-synuclein folds into dense, β-sheet-rich fibrillar structures that are highly resistant to proteolytic cleavage. When microglia internalize these aggregates via endocytosis, the cargo is delivered to the lysosomes for destruction. However, the structural integrity of the fibrils overwhelms local hydrolases, including vital enzymes like Cathepsin D and glucocerebrosidase. As the lysosomal lumen fills with this indigestible material, the organelle swells, leading to severe lysosomal membrane permeabilization (LMP). This leakage of acidic contents and digestive enzymes into the cytosol triggers profound cellular stress, culminating in a state known as "frustrated phagocytosis."

Under these conditions, the microglial cell becomes metabolically exhausted, often forced to shift from efficient oxidative phosphorylation to rapid but unsustainable glycolysis (Hickman et al., 2018). Consequently, these exhausted microglia completely abandon their homeostatic and neurosupportive roles. The synthesis of crucial neurotrophic factors, such as Brain-Derived Neurotrophic Factor (BDNF) and Insulin-like Growth Factor 1 (IGF-1), sharply declines. Instead, the stressed microglia perpetually discharge reactive oxygen species

(ROS) and excitatory amino acids like glutamate into the extracellular space. This accumulation of glutamate hyperactivates NMDA receptors on neighboring dopaminergic neurons, causing massive calcium influx and subsequent excitotoxic death. This neuronal death inevitably releases even more monomeric and aggregated α-synuclein into the extracellular matrix, definitively closing the loop of the neurodegenerative vicious cycle.

3.3 Microglia as vectors of disease propagation

A particularly concerning aspect of the alpha-synuclein-microglia axis is the potential role of these immune cells in actively spreading the disease throughout the brain. The propagation of PD pathology follows a predictable anatomical trajectory, classically described by Braak staging. While direct trans-synaptic spread between neurons is a primary focus of the "prion-like" hypothesis, the "Trojan horse" role of microglia is gaining significant traction. Microglia are highly motile surveyors of the brain parenchyma. When they engulf α-synuclein in a highly affected region, they may physically migrate to adjacent, unaffected tissues before their metabolic collapse. Because their lysosomal machinery is impaired, the internalized α-synuclein is not destroyed. Ironically, the acidic, highly oxidative environment of the failing lysosome may actually accelerate the structural cross-linking and aggregation of the protein, rendering it even more toxic. If these exhausted microglia ultimately undergo necrosis or apoptosis, they burst and release this heavily compacted, highly nucleating form of alpha-synuclein into the new environment. Alternatively, living but dysfunctional microglia actively expel these toxic aggregates via the secretion of exosomes. These nanovesicles, derived from multivesicular bodies, protect the enclosed alpha-synuclein from extracellular proteases and facilitate its highly efficient uptake by neighboring healthy neurons. Through this exosomal shedding, microglia effectively seed Lewy body pathology in pristine brain regions (Braak et al., 2003). Furthermore, emerging evidence suggests these immune cells might also physically transfer aggregates directly to adjacent cells through fragile actin bridges known as tunneling nanotubes, further cementing their role as vectors of disease propagation (Braak et al., 2003).

4. Therapeutic interventions targeting the axis

Parkinson's disease treatments are currently limited in their efficacy; they can lessen motor symptoms but do not slow the progression of the

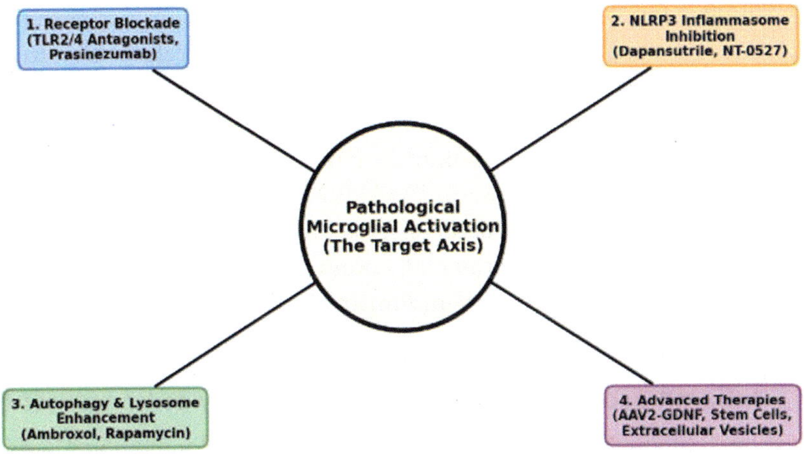

Fig. 2 Emerging therapeutic interventions targeting the alpha-synuclein-microglia axis. Current disease-modifying strategies aim to break the neurodegenerative cycle at multiple critical nodes: (1) Receptor Blockade (e.g., TLR2/4 antagonists, monoclonal antibodies) to prevent initial recognition; (2) Inflammasome Inhibition (e.g., NLRP3 inhibitors) to decouple protein uptake from inflammatory bursts; (3) Autophagy & Lysosomal Enhancement (e.g., GCase chaperones like Ambroxol) to alleviate frustrated phagocytosis; and (4) Advanced Therapies (Gene and Stem Cell therapies) to restore neurotrophic support and replace lost populations.

disease (Balestrino & Schapira, 2020). The complex pathophysiology of PD makes it very challenging to develop disease-modifying therapies despite the many possible molecular targets and the huge resources devoted to this goal (Mari & Mestre, 2022). However, the elucidation of the α-synuclein-microglial axis presents multiple highly specific, druggable targets aimed at halting disease progression (Fig. 2).

4.1 Pharmacological interventions: Receptor blockade and monoclonal antibodies

The first major line of pharmacological intervention focuses on Receptor Blockade at the microglial membrane. By utilizing targeted small molecules to antagonize Pattern Recognition Receptors, specifically TLR2 and TLR4, researchers aim to essentially "blind" the microglia to extracellular alpha-synuclein. This blockade intercepts the neuroinflammatory signaling cascade at its very inception, preventing the activation of the downstream MyD88 and NF-κB pathways, thereby completely halting the transcription and release of pro-inflammatory cytokines (Fellner et al., 2013; Kim et al., 2013).

Simultaneously, monoclonal antibody therapy has gained extensive traction as a method to clear extracellular aggregates before they trigger microglia. Prasinezumab, an investigational humanized monoclonal antibody targeting aggregated alpha-synuclein, has entered several clinical trials after showing good efficacy in animal models (Pagano et al., 2024; Teil & Huot, 2026). While the Phase 2 PASADENA study did not meet its primary endpoint, post hoc analyses suggested it slowed the deterioration of motor signs in a subgroup with rapidly progressing symptoms (Taylor et al., 2025; Xiao & Tan, 2025). Prasinezumab has since moved into Phase III clinical trials.

4.2 Inflammasome inhibition and autophagy enhancement

A second highly promising avenue is inflammasome inhibition. Because blocking surface receptors might indiscriminately suppress necessary immune surveillance against actual pathogens, targeting downstream cytosolic complexes offers a more refined approach. The NLRP3 inflammasome is highly expressed in microglia and its transcription is triggered by alpha-synuclein (Haque et al., 2020; Pike et al., 2021; Xu et al., 2025). Small molecule inhibitors of the NLRP3 inflammasome work by sterically hindering the assembly of the complex, effectively decoupling protein uptake from the catastrophic release of IL-1β and IL-18 (Singh et al., 2023). Several compounds are currently under investigation. For instance, NT-0527 is a brain-penetrant, orally bioavailable inhibitor showing anti-inflammatory effects in animal models (Harrison et al., 2025). Its successor, NT-0796, showed reduced neuroinflammation in a Phase 1b/2a trial over 4 weeks with good safety, despite some debate on the inflammasome's exact role in PD (Clarke et al., 2025; Senkevich et al., 2024). Furthermore, VTX3232 showed a good safety profile, reducing plasma and CSF inflammatory markers in a 28-day Phase 2a study (Bultinck et al., 2026), while Usnoflast (ZYIL1) induced positive changes in locomotor and neurogenesis genes in PD murine models (More et al., 2025; Yeole et al., 2025). Finally, dapansutrile (OLT1177), which has been safely evaluated in humans for various diseases (Klück et al., 2020; Lonnemann et al., 2020; Sánchez-Fernández et al., 2019), crosses the BBB in PD mouse models to reduce alpha-synuclein aggregation and improve dopaminergic survival (Amo-Aparicio et al., 2023; Luque et al., 2026), with a Phase 2 trial currently underway.

Conversely, enhancing autophagy and restoring lysosomal competence (often through drug repurposing) addresses the root cause of frustrated phagocytosis. Ambroxol hydrochloride, a mucolytic drug, is being repurposed as a pharmacological chaperone for the lysosomal enzyme glucocerebrosidase (GCase). Reduced GCase activity correlates with alpha-synuclein accumulation (Richter et al., 2014). Ambroxol stabilizes GCase, aiding its transport to the lysosome and upregulating its activity both in vitro and in vivo (Baden et al., 2023; Colucci et al., 2023; Istaiti et al., 2021; Mullin et al., 2020; Siemeling et al., 2024). The Phase 3 ASPro-PD trial in the UK is currently recruiting. Concurrently, drugs like Rapamycin inhibit the mTOR pathway to artificially upregulate macroautophagy, helping microglia digest the backlog of internalized alpha-synuclein (Schöndorf et al., 2014).

4.3 Advanced therapeutics: Gene, cell, and extracellular vesicle therapies

Advanced therapeutic strategies encompass gene therapy, stem cell transplantation, and the use of extracellular vesicles. Regarding gene therapy, viral vectors and plasmids are being used to deliver disease-modifying therapies directly to brain cells (Haggerty et al., 2020). For example, polymeric nanoparticles delivering the human *GBA1* gene improved motor deficits and neuroprotection in PD mouse models (Huh et al., 2023; Kwatra et al., 2026). Additionally, AAV-GAD delivers the glutamic acid decarboxylase gene to the subthalamic nucleus to increase inhibitory GABA, modulating pathologic excitatory activity with significant improvements noted in Phase 2 trials (LeWitt et al., 2011; Ngo & Vo, 2019; Tai, 2022; Tian et al., 2024). Another approach, AAV2-GDNF (AB-1005), delivers glial cell line-derived neurotrophic factor into the putamen to foster dopaminergic survival (Chmielarz & Saarma, 2020; Elsworth et al., 2008), showing stability and motor improvement in early human trials (Van Laar et al., 2025).

In the realm of stem cells, replacing midbrain dopaminergic neurons is a rapidly growing area. Phase I/II trials have transplanted iPS cell-derived dopaminergic progenitors directly into the putamen, showing graft survival, dopamine production, and motor stability without tumor formation over 24 months (Fričová et al., 2020; Kayhanian & Barker, 2026; Sawamoto et al., 2025; Takahashi et al., 2025). Similarly, bemdaneprocel (cryopreserved midbrain dopaminergic progenitors) was safely tolerated and yielded functional improvements (Tabar et al., 2025).

Lastly, extracellular vesicles **(EVs)** can transfer therapeutic cargo (like miRNA) across the blood-brain barrier (Zafarjonovna et al., 2026; Zhao et al., 2022). In mouse models, mesenchymal stem cell-derived EVs delivering miRNA-181a-2–3p knocked down the inflammatory EGR1 transcription factor, protecting dopaminergic neurons (Ma et al., 2022; Yu et al., 2018). Furthermore, intravenously administered colostrum-derived EVs, enriched in neuroregulatory components, reduced microglial activation and preserved neurons in MPTP-treated mice (Hollingsworth et al., 2026; Mustapha & Taib, 2021). However, standardizing and purifying EVs for human trials remains a major hurdle (Primorac et al., 2026).

5. Diagnostic, progression, and imaging biomarkers

Although PD is primarily defined by the accumulation of alpha-synuclein in Lewy bodies, several patients also exhibit additional pathological features, such as β-amyloid deposits and tau aggregates (Irwin et al., 2017). A key difficulty in PD research lies in its marked clinical heterogeneity. Quantitative biomarkers play a crucial role by enabling earlier diagnosis, longitudinal monitoring, and patient stratification based on distinct underlying pathologies (Höglinger et al., 2024; Simuni et al., 2024; Vijiaratnam et al., 2021). Historically, neuroimaging and fluid biomarkers have had limitations (Hall et al., 2016; Mollenhauer et al., 2016, 2017; Simuni et al., 2018), but recent advances in seed amplification assays (SAA) and novel imaging techniques are demonstrating increasing potential (Cho et al., 2021; del Campo et al., 2023; Grossauer et al., 2023; Paslawski et al., 2023; Pereira et al., 2023).

5.1 Fluid and genetic biomarkers

A defining feature of PD is the accumulation of intracellular alpha-synuclein aggregates. While total alpha-synuclein levels can be quantified in biological fluids, results are highly variable (Mollenhauer, 2014). Thus, the field is moving toward more specific species and accessible biofluids.

Regarding serum biomarkers, the ultimate goal is to identify blood-based candidates for a more accessible, non-invasive alternative (Tönges et al., 2022). Total alpha-synuclein in serum has yielded inconsistent results due to erythrocyte abundance (Ganguly et al., 2021; Tönges et al., 2022; Zubelzu et al., 2022). However, specific species, like phosphorylated (PS129) and neuron-derived extracellular vesicle alpha-synuclein, show improved specificity (Agliardi et al., 2021; Stuendl et al., 2021; Tian et al., 2019). Most importantly, alpha-synuclein seed amplification assays (SAA) have emerged as a major advance. These methods accurately distinguish PD patients from controls and identify prodromal stages, with positivity rates varying by genetic background (e.g., highest in *GBA* mutations) (Bargar et al., 2021; Brockmann et al., 2021; Groveman et al., 2018; Iranzo et al., 2021; Kang et al., 2019; Kluge et al., 2022; Rossi et al., 2020; Siderowf et al., 2023; Zarkali, Thomas, et al., 2024). Other prominent candidates include Neurofilament light chain (NfL) and GFAP, which are structural proteins reflecting axonal and astrocytic damage, respectively. While NfL consistently predicts cognitive impairment (Buhmann et al., 2022; Tönges et al., 2022), combining it with GFAP enhances prognostic value for Parkinson's disease dementia (PDD) (Batzu et al., 2022; Tang et al., 2023; Teng et al., 2023). Amyloid and tau (particularly p-tau) in plasma show some promise when combined with alpha-synuclein to improve diagnostic accuracy (Ren et al., 2022; Tönges et al., 2022). Finally, inflammatory biomarkers (such as IL-6, IL-1β, TNF-α, CRP) and miRNAs (like hsa-miR-144–3p) are being explored, though high heterogeneity currently limits their standalone applicability (Chan et al., 2021; Huh et al., 2021; Qu et al., 2023; Shen et al., 2022; Tönges et al., 2022; Zago et al., 2022; Zhang et al., 2024).

Cerebrospinal Fluid (CSF) Biomarkers directly reflect brain pathology (Kwon et al., 2022). Total alpha-synuclein levels in CSF are typically reduced in PD, but SAA in CSF has proven highly accurate, especially in prodromal stages (Berg & Klein, 2023; Schneider & Alcalay, 2017; Siderowf et al., 2023; Stewart et al., 2015). GFAP and YKL-40 in CSF are elevated during neurodegeneration and neuroinflammation but lack disease specificity (Llorens et al., 2017; Lotankar et al., 2017; McGrowder et al., 2021; Morenas-Rodríguez et al., 2019). Furthermore, beta-amyloid 1–42, total tau, and p-tau in CSF are crucial for differential diagnosis; an Alzheimer-like CSF profile strongly suggests dementia with Lewy bodies (DLB) rather than PD (Kang et al., 2013; Schade & Mollenhauer, 2014; Spies et al., 2010; Walker et al., 2019).

Finally, genetic biomarkers complement clinical diagnosis. Mutations in LRRK2 (PARK8) and SNCA (PARK1/4) directly drive α-synuclein pathology (Kouli et al., 2018; Liu et al., 2016; Ramirez et al., 2006; Rideout et al., 2020), while GBA1 mutations impair lysosomal function, associating with earlier onset and cognitive decline (Nichols et al., 2009). Other loci, such as *MAPT*, *DJ-1* (PARK7), *BIN1*, and *TMEM175*, highlight shared mechanisms across neurodegenerative diseases (Chia et al., 2021; Lotankar et al., 2017; Schellenberg & Montine, 2012; Shi et al., 2011). (Table 1).

Table 1 Fluid and genetic biomarkers in PD.

Biomarker	Type/source	Biological sample	Main utility	Key findings/ performance	Limitations	References
alpha-synuclein (total)	Protein aggregation	Serum/CSF	Diagnosis	downarrow CSF levels in PD; inconsistent serum results	High variability, low specificity	Førland et al. (2020), Schneider and Alcalay (2017)
alpha-synuclein (oligomeric/ PS129)	Pathological species	Blood (erythrocytes)	Diagnosis/ progression	Associated with severity and motor progression	Methodological variability	Tian et al. (2019)
alpha-synuclein (EV-derived)	Neuron-derived vesicles	Plasma	Differential diagnosis	Distinguishes PD vs DLB/PSP	Limited standardization	Agliardi et al. (2021), Stuendl et al. (2021),
alpha-synuclein SAA	Seeding assay	Plasma, CSF, saliva, skin, gland	Early diagnosis/ prodromal	Sensitivity ~88–95 %, specificity ~92–98 %; detects prodromal PD	Variable across genetic subtypes	Zarkali, Thomas, et al. (2024)
NfL	Axonal damage marker	Plasma/CSF	Progression/ differential diagnosis	Predicts cognitive decline; distinguishes PD vs atypical syndromes (~90 %)	Not disease-specific; age-dependent	Tönges et al. (2022)

GFAP	Astrocytic injury marker	Plasma/CSF	Cognitive decline/ progression	Predicts conversion to PDD; improves models with NfL	Low specificity	Batzu et al. (2022), Tang et al. (2023), Teng et al. (2023)
Amyloid-β (Aβ42)	AD-related protein	Plasma/CSF	Cognitive decline	downarrow levels correlate with cognitive impairment	Inconsistent in serum	Kang et al. (2013)
Tau/p-tau	AD-related proteins	Plasma/CSF	Cognitive decline/ diagnosis	uparrow p-tau in PD; better when combined with alpha-synuclein (AUC ~0.8)	Variable results	Schade and Mollenhauer (2014)
Inflammatory markers	Neuroinflammat-ion	Serum/EVs	Severity/ progression	Elevated cytokines; panels reach AUC >0.8	High heterogeneity, low specificity	Chan et al. (2021), Qu et al. (2023), Shen et al. (2022)
Multi-protein panels	Proteomic panels	Serum	Cognitive decline prediction	Moderate accuracy (AUC ~0.8)	Limited validation	Chan et al. (2021), Qu et al. (2023), Shen et al. (2022)
miRNAs	Non-coding RNAs	Plasma/ exosomes	Diagnosis	Panels show good accuracy (AUC ~0.87)	Lack of standardization	Tönges et al. (2022), Zago et al. (2022), Zhang et al. (2024)

(continued)

Table 1 Fluid and genetic biomarkers in PD. *(cont'd)*

Biomarker	Type/source	Biological sample	Main utility	Key findings/performance	Limitations	References
YKL-40	Neuroinflammation	CSF	Progression/co-pathology	Elevated in neurodegeneration	Low specificity	Llorens et al. (2017), Morenas-Rodríguez et al. (2019)
GBA1 mutations	Genetic	DNA	Risk/stratification	Earlier onset, more cognitive decline	Not diagnostic alone	Nichols et al. (2009)
LRRK2 mutations	Genetic	DNA	Risk/subtype identification	Common familial PD cause	Variable phenotype	Liu et al. (2016), Rideout et al. (2020)
SNCA (PARK1/4)	Genetic	DNA	Pathogenesis	Linked to alpha-synuclein aggregation	Rare mutations	Ramirez et al. (2006)
MAPT	Genetic	DNA	Risk/tau pathology	Associated with neurodegeneration	Non-specific	Schellenberg and Montine (2012)

DJ-1 (PARK7)	Genetic/protein	DNA/serum	Pathogenesis	Reduced levels lead to uparrow alpha-syn aggregation	Not specific	Lotankar et al. (2017), Shi et al. (2011)
BIN1/ TMEM175	Genetic loci	DNA	Risk/ differential diagnosis	Shared pathways with DLB/AD	Emerging evidence	Chia et al. (2021)

Aβ42: Amyloid beta 42; **AD:** Alzheimer's disease; **APOE:** Apolipoprotein E; **AUC:** Area under the curve; **BIN1:** Bridging integrator 1; **CRP:** C-reactive protein; **CSF:** Cerebrospinal fluid; **DLB:** Dementia with Lewy bodies; **DNA:** Deoxyribonucleic acid; **EVs:** Extracellular vesicles; **GBA1:** Glucosylceramidase beta 1; **GFAP:** Glial fibrillary acidic protein; **IL-1β:** Interleukin-1 beta, **IL-6:** Interleukin-6; **LRRK2:** Leucine-rich repeat kinase 2; **MAPT:** Microtubule-associated protein tau; **MIA:** Melanoma inhibitory activity; **miRNAs:** MicroRNAs; **NfL:** Neurofilament light chain; **PD:** Parkinson's disease; **PDD:** Parkinson's disease dementia; **PSP:** Progressive supranuclear palsy; **p-tau:** Phosphorylated tau; **SAA:** Seed amplification assay; **SNCA:** Synuclein alpha; **TMEM175:** Transmembrane protein 175; **TNF-α:** Tumor necrosis factor-alpha.

5.2 Neuroimaging insights

Neuroimaging combines molecular, structural, and functional readouts that dissect PD pathology beyond classical nigrostriatal degeneration (Bidesi et al., 2021; Cilia et al., 2026; Saeed et al., 2020; Schröter et al., 2025; Weingarten et al., 2015). Since no single modality fulfills all roles (diagnosis, prognosis, treatment monitoring), multimodal approaches are favored.

5.2.1 Dopaminergic, metabolic, and perfusion imaging (PET & SPECT)

Dopaminergic imaging remains the most clinically validated approach. DAT SPECT and DAT PET are gold standards for visualizing presynaptic transporter loss, distinguishing PD from essential tremor and prodromal conditions like REM sleep behavior disorder (Akdemir et al., 2021; Cilia et al., 2026; De Feo et al., 2023; Palermo et al., 2021; Tinaz et al., 2018; Treglia et al., 2012). Similarly, cardiac MIBG scintigraphy assesses sympathetic denervation and often outperforms DAT-SPECT in early diagnosis (De Feo et al., 2023; Horsager et al., 2020; McKeith et al., 2017; Orimo et al., 1999; Treglia et al., 2012; Yoshita et al., 1998). [18 F]DOPA PET measures dopamine precursor uptake but can underestimate terminal loss due to early compensatory AADC activity (Ibrahim et al., 2016; Kaasinen & Vahlberg, 2017; Stormezand et al., 2020). Unlike presynaptic imaging, metabolic and perfusion imaging (FDG-PET) captures systems-level functional consequences, revealing reproducible networks of hypometabolism (e.g., parietal cortices) and hypermetabolism (e.g., pallidal-thalamic regions) that excel at differentiating atypical parkinsonian disorders (González-Redondo et al., 2014; Zarkali, Thomas, et al., 2024). In comparing modalities, PET offers higher sensitivity and quantification, while SPECT is more accessible and cost-effective (Beer et al., 2011; Davis et al., 2020; Khalil et al., 2011).

5.2.2 Structural and microstructural magnetic resonance imaging (MRI)

MRI has shifted from being relatively uninformative to a dynamic biomarker domain, particularly through techniques interrogating the substantia nigra (Hwang et al., 2023; Zucca et al., 2017). Neuromelanin-sensitive MRI (NM-MRI) visualizes signal loss in the substantia nigra and locus coeruleus (Cho et al., 2021; Sulzer et al., 2018), while the loss of the swallow-tail sign on susceptibility-sensitive sequences offers high diagnostic sensitivity. Furthermore, iron-sensitive MRI (using QSM or R2*) detects in vivo iron accumulation, which promotes α-synuclein aggregation; baseline QSM strongly predicts longitudinal motor and cognitive decline (Barbosa et al., 2015; Cao et al., 2023; Lancione et al., 2022; Langkammer et al., 2012; Li et al., 2020; Ostrerova-Golts et al., 2000; Sun et al., 2020; Thomas et al., 2020). Free water imaging estimates extracellular expansion due to neuronal loss, distinguishing early PD effectively (Arnaldi et al., 2021; Ohtsuka et al., 2014). Finally, while conventional structural MRI and cortical atrophy show high inter-individual heterogeneity (Filippi et al., 2020; Laansma et al., 2021; Mak et al., 2015; Pyatigorskaya et al., 2014; Torres-Parga et al., 2025), white matter imaging and connectivity metrics (using advanced diffusion models like fixel-based analysis and fMRI) are emerging as robust prognostic markers for cognitive impairment and dementia conversion (Caspell-Garcia et al., 2017; Duncan et al., 2016; Pietracupa et al., 2023; Pysz et al., 2010; Volpicelli-Daley et al., 2011; Zarkali et al., 2021; Zarkali, Hannaway, et al., 2024).

6. Future directions

As we move beyond the simplistic view of neuroinflammation as merely a secondary, reactive event in PD, the field is undergoing a paradigm shift toward a highly nuanced understanding of immune modulation. The future of PD therapeutics lies not in broadly suppressing the immune system—an approach that carries significant risks including opportunistic infections and the impairment of essential cellular clearance mechanisms—but rather in the targeted "reprogramming" of microglia to restore their innate protective functions (Colonna & Butovsky, 2017). The next decade of translational research will likely focus heavily on three interconnected pillars: high-resolution cellular phenotyping, the development of precision biomarkers, and the deployment of personalized immunotherapies. This transition represents a vital shift away from the traditional "one-size-fits-all" pharmacological approach toward a sophisticated precision medicine model, recognizing that PD is a heterogeneous syndrome with highly variable neuroinflammatory drivers.

6.1 Defining specific cellular pathways

The historical classification of microglia into binary M1 (neurotoxic) and M2 (neuroprotective) states is now universally considered obsolete within the context of chronic neurodegeneration (Smajic et al., 2022). The advent of single-cell resolution technologies, such as single-cell RNA sequencing (scRNA-seq) and spatial transcriptomics, is currently revolutionizing our understanding of microglial heterogeneity. In models of Alzheimer's and ALS, researchers have successfully identified distinct "Disease-Associated Microglia" (DAM) (Keren-Shaul et al., 2017). In PD, the microglial landscape is likely even more complex due to the interplay with dopamine metabolism, iron accumulation, and neuromelanin. Recent studies utilizing post-mortem human midbrain tissue have begun to reveal specific glial activation states that appear distinct to PD pathology (Kamath et al., 2022; Smajic et al., 2022). Future research must precisely define the transcriptional signature of PD-associated microglia in the substantia nigra compared to those in the cortex or striatum (Roy et al., 2025).

A rapidly emerging frontier is the field of immunometabolism. We now recognize that the functional phenotype of a microglial cell is inextricably linked to its primary metabolic fuel. Pro-inflammatory microglia rely heavily on aerobic glycolysis, which allows for the rapid production of ATP necessary to fuel massive oxidative bursts (Wallings & Tansey, 2019). Conversely, resting and reparative microglia rely predominantly on oxidative phosphorylation (OXPHOS). Defining specific metabolic switches, such as mTOR or HIF-1$ \alpha$ pathways, offers a highly novel therapeutic avenue. By utilizing small molecules to force a metabolic shift back toward OXPHOS, clinicians might successfully dampen chronic inflammation without bluntly blocking essential cytokine receptors (Gao et al., 2023). Furthermore, aberrant reactivation of synaptic pruning mechanisms via the complement cascade may contribute to early loss of striatal dopaminergic connectivity long before overt neuronal cell death occurs (Gao et al., 2023).

6.2 Developing personalized therapies

The failure of many broad-spectrum anti-inflammatory clinical trials in the past likely stems from a profound lack of patient stratification. For a specific subset of patients, robust neuroinflammation may be a primary, driving force of the pathology; for others, it may merely be a late-stage secondary response (Tan et al., 2020). To successfully implement personalized therapy, the field urgently requires sophisticated tools to monitor neuroinflammation in vivo. While TSPO-PET imaging has been successfully used to visualize broad neuroinflammatory activity (Gerhard et al., 2006), current ligands cannot distinguish between destructive and protective microglial phenotypes. Next-generation radiotracers designed to target specific markers, such as the active NLRP3 inflammasome, could soon allow clinicians to visualize "hotspots" of pathogenic inflammation (Alonge et al., 2025).

Alongside advanced imaging, the high-throughput analysis of CSF and serum for specific cytokine expression profiles, soluble TREM2 levels, or LRRK2 kinase activity within exosomes will be essential to accurately identify "inflammatory subtypes" (Alonge et al., 2025). The most immediate application of this framework lies within genetically defined cohorts. For patients harboring *LRRK2* mutations, highly specific kinase inhibitors (such as DNL201) have advanced into clinical trials, aiming to normalize altered lysosomal pH and autophagic flux directly in individuals predisposed to LRRK2 overactivity (Jennings et al., 2022). Similarly, for *GBA* mutation carriers, pharmacological chaperones like Ambroxol are being utilized to correct misfolding of the mutant glucocerebrosidase enzyme, enhancing intrinsic microglial capacity to process complex lipids and clear toxic aggregates (Schöndorf et al., 2014).

In conclusion, the future of PD treatment fundamentally relies upon dissecting and understanding the profound heterogeneity of the microglial response. By defining highly specific cellular and metabolic pathways through high-throughput sequencing, and meticulously matching these inflammatory signatures to individual patient biomarker profiles, the scientific community moves ever closer to a reality where the brain's immune system is effectively transformed from a relentless driver of pathology into a powerful, precisely controlled ally in neural repair and neuroprotection.

References

Agliardi, C., Meloni, M., Guerini, F. R., Zanzottera, M., Bolognesi, E., Baglio, F., & Clerici, M. (2021). Oligomeric α-Syn and SNARE complex proteins in peripheral extracellular vesicles of neural origin are biomarkers for Parkinson's disease. *Neurobiology of Disease, 148*, 105185. https://doi.org/10.1016/J.NBD.2020.105185.

Akdemır, Ü.Ö., Bora, H. A. T., Atay, L.Ö., Akdemİr, Ü.Ö., Bora, H. A. T., & Atay, L.Ö. (2021). Dopamine transporter SPECT imaging in Parkinson's disease and parkinsoniandisorders. *Turkish Journal of Medical Sciences, 51*(2), 400–410. https://doi.org/10.3906/sag-2008-253.

Alonge, P., Balistreri, C. R., Torrente, A., Magro, D., Rubino, E., & Monastero, R. (2025). TREM 2 in Parkinson's disease: A promising candidate gene for disease susceptibility and progression. *Brain Sciences, 15*(4), https://doi.org/10.3390/BRAINSCI15040379.

Amo-Aparicio, J., Daly, J., Højen, J. F., & Dinarello, C. A. (2023). Pharmacologic inhibition of NLRP3 reduces the levels of α-synuclein and protects dopaminergic neurons in a model of Parkinson's disease. *Journal of Neuroinflammation, 20*(1), https://doi.org/10.1186/S12974-023-02830-W.

Arnaldi, D., Chincarini, A., Hu, M. T., Sonka, K., Boeve, B., Miyamoto, T., ... Nobili, F. (2021). Dopaminergic imaging and clinical predictors for phenoconversion of REM sleep behaviour disorder. *Brain: A Journal of Neurology, 144*(1), 278–287. https://doi.org/10.1093/BRAIN/AWAA365.

Augusto-Oliveira, M., Arrifano, G. P., Lopes-Araújo, A., Santos-Sacramento, L., Takeda, P. Y., Anthony, D. C., ... Crespo-Lopez, M. E. (2019). What do microglia really do in healthy adult brain? *Cells 2019, 8*(10), *8*. https://doi.org/10.3390/CELLS8101293.

Baden, P., Perez, M. J., Raji, H., Bertoli, F., Kalb, S., Illescas, M., ... Deleidi, M. (2023). Glucocerebrosidase is imported into mitochondria and preserves complex I integrity and energy metabolism. *Nature Communications, 14*(1), 1930. https://doi.org/10.1038/S41467-023-37454-4.

Balestrino, R., & Schapira, A. H. V. (2020). Parkinson disease. *European Journal of Neurology, 27*(1), 27–42. https://doi.org/10.1111/ENE.14108.

Banerjee, A., Lu, Y., Do, K., Mize, T., Wu, X., Chen, X., & Chen, J. (2021). Validation of induced microglia-like cells (iMG cells) for future studies of brain diseases. *Frontiers in Cellular Neuroscience, 15*. https://doi.org/10.3389/FNCEL.2021.629279.

Barbosa, J. H. O., Santos, A. C., Tumas, V., Liu, M., Zheng, W., Haacke, E. M., & Salmon, C. E. G. (2015). Quantifying brain iron deposition in patients with Parkinson's disease using quantitative susceptibility mapping, R2 and R2*. *Magnetic Resonance Imaging, 33*(5), 559–565. https://doi.org/10.1016/j.mri.2015.02.021.

Bargar, C., Wang, W., Gunzler, S. A., LeFevre, A., Wang, Z., Lerner, A. J., ... Chen, S. G. (2021). Streamlined alpha-synuclein RT-QuIC assay for various biospecimens in Parkinson's disease and dementia with Lewy bodies. *Acta Neuropathologica Communications, 9*(1), https://doi.org/10.1186/S40478-021-01175-W.

Batzu, L., Rota, S., Hye, A., Heslegrave, A., Trivedi, D., Gibson, L. L., ... Aarsland, D. (2022). Plasma p-tau181, neurofilament light chain and association with cognition in Parkinson's disease. *Npj Parkinson's Disease, 8*(1), 154. https://doi.org/10.1038/s41531-022-00384-x.

Beer, A. J., Kessler, H., Wester, H.-J., & Schwaiger, M. (2011). PET imaging of integrin αVβ3 expression. *Theranostics, 1*, 48–57. https://doi.org/10.7150/thno/v01p0048.

Berg, D., & Klein, C. (2023). α-Synuclein seed amplification and its uses in Parkinson's disease. *The Lancet Neurology, 22*(5), 369–371. https://doi.org/10.1016/S1474-4422(23)00124-2.

Bidesi, N. S. R., Vang Andersen, I., Windhorst, A. D., Shalgunov, V., & Herth, M. M. (2021). The role of neuroimaging in Parkinson's disease. *Journal of Neurochemistry, 159*(4), 660–689. https://doi.org/10.1111/jnc.15516.

Bisht, K. S., Kumari, M., & Maiti, T. K. (2026). N-terminal KTKEGV motif lysine residues of α-Synuclein are critical for TLR2 interaction and activation. *Archives of Biochemistry and Biophysics, 776*. https://doi.org/10.1016/j.abb.2025.110701.

Blasco-Agell, L., Pons-Espinal, M., Testa, V., Roch, G., Montero-Muñoz, J., Fernandez-Carasa, I., ... Consiglio, A. (2024). LRRK2-mutant microglia trigger dopaminergic neurodegeneration when activated by neuromelanin. *BioRxiv*. https://doi.org/10.1101/2024.10.07.616997.

Braak, H., Del Tredici, K., Rüb, U., De Vos, R. A. I., Jansen Steur, E. N. H., & Braak, E. (2003). Staging of brain pathology related to sporadic Parkinson's disease. *Neurobiology of Aging, 24*(2), 197–211. https://doi.org/10.1016/S0197-4580(02)00065-9.

Brandenburg, S., Blank, A., Bungert, A. D., & Vajkoczy, P. (2020). Distinction of microglia and macrophages in glioblastoma: Close relatives, different tasks? *International Journal of Molecular Sciences, 22*(1), 194. https://doi.org/10.3390/IJMS22010194.

Brockmann, K., Quadalti, C., Lerche, S., Rossi, M., Wurster, I., Baiardi, S., ... Parchi, P. (2021). Association between CSF alpha-synuclein seeding activity and genetic status in Parkinson's disease and dementia with Lewy bodies. *Acta Neuropathologica Communications, 9*(1), https://doi.org/10.1186/S40478-021-01276-6.

Buhmann, C., Lezius, S., Pötter-Nerger, M., Gerloff, C., Kuhle, J., & Choe, C. (2022). Age-adjusted serum neurofilament predicts cognitive decline in Parkinson's disease (MARK-PD). *Movement Disorders, 37*(2), 435–436. https://doi.org/10.1002/MDS.28909;WEBSITE:WEBSITE:MOVEMENTDISORDERS;JOURNAL:JOURNAL:15318257;REQUESTEDJOURNAL:JOURNAL:15318257;WGROUP:STRING:PUBLICATION.

Bultinck, J., Yuan, S., Cantuti-Castelvetri, L., Brosens, L., Bracke, D., Collins, J., ... Ogilvie, K. (2026). NLRP3 inhibition by VTX3232 tempers inflammation resulting in reduced body weight, hyperglycemia, and hepatic steatosis in obese male mice. *Molecular Metabolism, 103*. https://doi.org/10.1016/j.molmet.2025.102282.

Cai, L., Zhang, Y., Li, J., Hu, L., Meng, Q., Shao, J., ... Hu, G. (2026). Complement receptor 3 (CR3)-dependent microglial synapse elimination drives Parkinson's disease pathogenesis in systemic inflammation. *Cell Death & Disease, 17*(1), https://doi.org/10.1038/S41419-026-08557-9.

Cao, Q., Han, X., Tang, D., Qian, H., Yan, K., Shi, X., ... Zhang, J. (2023). Diagnostic value of combined magnetic resonance imaging techniques in the evaluation of Parkinson disease. *Quantitative Imaging in Medicine and Surgery, 13*(10), 6503–6516. https://doi.org/10.21037/QIMS-23-87/COIF).

Casanova, P. V., Freitag-Berenguel, I., Saavedra-López, E., Usandizaga-Estarloa, M., Ríos-Cuadrado, C., Martínez-Remedios, P., ... Barcia, C. (2026). Microglial low-affinity FcγR mediates the phagocytic elimination of dopaminergic neurons in Parkinson's disease degeneration. *Npj Parkinson's Disease, 12*(1), 35. https://doi.org/10.1038/s41531-025-01249-9.

Caspell-Garcia, C., Simuni, T., Tosun-Turgut, D., Wu, I. W., Zhang, Y., Nalls, M., ... Weintraub, D. (2017). Multiple modality biomarker prediction of cognitive impairment in prospectively followed de novo Parkinson disease. *PLoS One, 12*(5), e0175674. https://doi.org/10.1371/JOURNAL.PONE.0175674.

Chan, L., Chung, C. C., Chen, J. H., Yu, R. C., & Hong, C. T. (2021). Cytokine profile in plasma extracellular vesicles of Parkinson's disease and the association with cognitive function. *Cells, 10*(3), 1–9. https://doi.org/10.3390/CELLS10030604.

Chia, R., Sabir, M. S., Bandres-Ciga, S., Saez-Atienzar, S., Reynolds, R. H., Gustavsson, E., ... Scholz, S. W. (2021). Genome sequencing analysis identifies new loci associated with Lewy body dementia and provides insights into its genetic architecture. *Nature Genetics, 53*(3), 294–303. https://doi.org/10.1038/s41588-021-00785-3.

Chmielarz, P., & Saarma, M. (2020). Neurotrophic factors for disease-modifying treatments of Parkinson's disease: Gaps between basic science and clinical studies. *Pharmacological Reports: PR, 72*(5), 1195–1217. https://doi.org/10.1007/S43440-020-00120-3.

Cho, S. J., Bae, Y. J., Kim, J. M., Kim, D., Baik, S. H., Sunwoo, L., ... Kim, J. H. (2021). Diagnostic performance of neuromelanin-sensitive magnetic resonance imaging for patients with Parkinson's disease and factor analysis for its heterogeneity: A systematic review and meta-analysis. *European Radiology, 31*(3), 1268–1280. https://doi.org/10.1007/S00330-020-07240-7.

Cilia, R., Arnaldi, D., Ballanger, B., Ceravolo, R., Micco, R. D., Sole, A. D., ... Eimeren, T. van. (2026). Neuroimaging and pathology biomarkers in Parkinson's disease and Parkinsonism. *Brain Sciences, 16*(1), 110. https://doi.org/10.3390/brainsci16010110.

Clarke, N., Thornton, P., Reader, V., Lindsay, N., Digby, Z., Mullen, B., ... Watt, A. P. (2025). Anti-neuroinflammatory and anti-inflammatory effects of the NLRP3 inhibitor NT-0796 in subjects with Parkinson's disease. *Movement Disorders: Official Journal of the Movement Disorder Society, 40*(10), 2199–2208. https://doi.org/10.1002/MDS.30307.

Colonna, M., & Butovsky, O. (2017). Microglia function in the central nervous system during health and neurodegeneration. *Annual Review of Immunology, 35*, 441–468. https://doi.org/10.1146/ANNUREV-IMMUNOL-051116-052358.

Colucci, F., Avenali, M., De Micco, R., Fusar Poli, M., Cerri, S., Stanziano, M., ... Cilia, R. (2023). Ambroxol as a disease-modifying treatment to reduce the risk of cognitive impairment in GBA-associated Parkinson's disease: A multicentre, randomised, double-blind, placebo-controlled, phase II trial. The AMBITIOUS study protocol. *BMJ Neurology Open, 5*(2), https://doi.org/10.1136/BMJNO-2023-000535.

Davis, K. M., Ryan, J. L., Aaron, V. D., & Sims, J. B. (2020). PET and SPECT imaging of the brain: History, technical considerations, applications, and radiotracers. *Seminars in Ultrasound, CT and MRI, 41*(6), 521–529. https://doi.org/10.1053/j.sult.2020.08.006.

De Feo, M. S., Frantellizzi, V., Locuratolo, N., Di Rocco, A., Farcomeni, A., Pauletti, C., ... Spanu, A. (2023). Role of functional neuroimaging with 123I-MIBG and 123I-FP-CIT in De Novo Parkinson's disease: A multicenter study. *Life (Chicago, Ill.: 1978), 13*(8), 1786. https://doi.org/10.3390/LIFE13081786.

del Campo, M., Vermunt, L., Peeters, C. F. W., Sieben, A., Hok-A-Hin, Y. S., Lleó, A., ... Teunissen, C. E. (2023). CSF proteome profiling reveals biomarkers to discriminate dementia with Lewy bodies from Alzheimer's disease. *Nature Communications, 14*(1), https://doi.org/10.1038/S41467-023-41122-Y.

Deyell, J. S., Sriparna, M., Ying, M., & Mao, X. (2023). The Interplay between α-synuclein and microglia in α-synucleinopathies. *International Journal of Molecular Sciences, 24*(3), https://doi.org/10.3390/IJMS24032477.

Duncan, G. W., Firbank, M. J., Yarnall, A. J., Khoo, T. K., Brooks, D. J., Barker, R. A., ... O'Brien, J. T. (2016). Gray and white matter imaging: A biomarker for cognitive impairment in early Parkinson's disease? *Movement Disorders: Official Journal of the Movement Disorder Society, 31*(1), 103–110. https://doi.org/10.1002/MDS.26312.

Elsworth, J. D., Redmond, D. E., Leranth, C., Bjugstad, K. B., Sladek, J. R., Collier, T. J., ... Roth, R. H. (2008). AAV2-mediated gene transfer of GDNF to the striatum of MPTP monkeys enhances the survival and outgrowth of co-implanted fetal dopamine neurons. *Experimental Neurology, 211*(1), 252–258. https://doi.org/10.1016/j.expneurol.2008.01.026.

Fellner, L., Irschick, R., Schanda, K., Reindl, M., Klimaschewski, L., Poewe, W., ... Stefanova, N. (2013). Toll-like receptor 4 is required for α-synuclein dependent activation of microglia and astroglia. *Glia, 61*(3), 349. https://doi.org/10.1002/GLIA.22437.

Filippi, M., Sarasso, E., Piramide, N., Stojkovic, T., Stankovic, I., Basaia, S., ... Agosta, F. (2020). Progressive brain atrophy and clinical evolution in Parkinson's disease. *NeuroImage: Clinical, 28*. https://doi.org/10.1016/j.nicl.2020.102374.

Førland, M. G., Tysnes, O. B., Aarsland, D., Maple-Grødem, J., Pedersen, K. F., Alves, G., & Lange, J. (2020). The value of cerebrospinal fluid α-synuclein and the tau/α-synuclein ratio for diagnosis of neurodegenerative disorders with Lewy pathology. *European Journal of Neurology, 27*(1), 43–50. https://doi.org/10.1111/ENE.14032;REQUESTEDJOURNAL:JOURNAL:14681331;WGROUP:STRING:PUBLICATION.

Fričová, D., Korchak, J. A., & Zubair, A. C. (2020). Challenges and translational considerations of mesenchymal stem/stromal cell therapy for Parkinson's disease. *Npj Regenerative Medicine, 5*(1), 20. https://doi.org/10.1038/s41536-020-00106-y.

Ganguly, U., Singh, S., Pal, S., Prasad, S., Agrawal, B. K., Saini, R. V., & Chakrabarti, S. (2021). Alpha-synuclein as a biomarker of Parkinson's disease: Good, but not good enough. *Frontiers in Aging Neuroscience, 13*, 702639. https://doi.org/10.3389/FNAGI.2021.702639/FULL.

Gao, C., Jiang, J., Tan, Y., & Chen, S. (2023). Microglia in neurodegenerative diseases: Mechanism and potential therapeutic targets. *Signal Transduction and Targeted Therapy, 8*(1), 359. https://doi.org/10.1038/s41392-023-01588-0.

Gao, H. M., Liu, B., & Hong, J. S. (2003). Critical role for microglial NADPH oxidase in rotenone-induced degeneration of dopaminergic neurons. *The Journal of Neuroscience: The Official Journal of the Society for Neuroscience, 23*(15), 6181–6187. https://doi.org/10.1523/JNEUROSCI.23-15-06181.2003.

Gerhard, A., Pavese, N., Hotton, G., Turkheimer, F., Es, M., Hammers, A., ... Brooks, D. J. (2006). In vivo imaging of microglial activation with [11C](R)-PK11195 PET in idiopathic Parkinson's disease. *Neurobiology of Disease, 21*(2), 404–412. https://doi.org/10.1016/j.nbd.2005.08.002.

González-Redondo, R., García-García, D., Clavero, P., Gasca-Salas, C., García-Eulate, R., Zubieta, J. L., ... Rodríguez-Oroz, M. C. (2014). Grey matter hypometabolism and atrophy in Parkinson's disease with cognitive impairment: A two-step process. *Brain, 137*(8), 2356–2367. https://doi.org/10.1093/BRAIN/AWU159.

Grossauer, A., Hemicker, G., Krismer, F., Peball, M., Djamshidian, A., Poewe, W., ... Heim, B. (2023). α-Synuclein seed amplification assays in the diagnosis of synucleinopathies using cerebrospinal fluid-a systematic review and meta-analysis. *Movement Disorders Clinical Practice, 10*(5), 737–747. https://doi.org/10.1002/MDC3.13710.

Groveman, B. R., Orrù, C. D., Hughson, A. G., Raymond, L. D., Zanusso, G., Ghetti, B., ... Caughey, B. (2018). Rapid and ultra-sensitive quantitation of disease-associated jα-synuclein seeds in brain and cerebrospinal fluid by αSyn RT-QuIC. *Acta Neuropathologica Communications, 6*(1), https://doi.org/10.1186/S40478-018-0508-2.

Guo, S., Wang, H., & Yin, Y. (2022). Microglia polarization from M1 to M2 in neurodegenerative diseases. *Frontiers in Aging Neuroscience, 14.* https://doi.org/10.3389/FNAGI.2022.815347.

Haggerty, D. L., Grecco, G. G., Reeves, K. C., & Atwood, B. (2020). Adeno-associated viral vectors in neuroscience research. *Molecular Therapy Methods and Clinical Development, 17,* 69–82. https://doi.org/10.1016/j.omtm.2019.11.012.

Hall, S., Surova, Y., Öhrfelt, A., Blennow, K., Zetterberg, H., & Hansson, O. (2016). Longitudinal measurements of cerebrospinal fluid biomarkers in Parkinson's disease. *Movement Disorders: Official Journal of the Movement Disorder Society, 31*(6), 898–905. https://doi.org/10.1002/MDS.26578.

Haque, M. E., Akther, M., Jakaria, M., Kim, I. S., Azam, S., & Choi, D. K. (2020). Targeting the microglial NLRP3 inflammasome and its role in Parkinson's disease. *Movement Disorders: Official Journal of the Movement Disorder Society, 35*(1), 20–33. https://doi.org/10.1002/MDS.27874.

Harrison, D., Billinton, A., Bock, M. G., Clarke, N. P., Digby, Z., Gabel, C. A., ... Watt, A. P. (2025). Profile of NT-0527, a brain penetrant NLRP3 Inflammasome inhibitor suitable as an in vivo tool compound for neuroinflammatory disorders. *RSC Medicinal Chemistry, 16*(11), 5318–5332. https://doi.org/10.1039/D5MD00639B.

Hickman, S., Izzy, S., Sen, P., Morsett, L., & El Khoury, J. (2018). Microglia in neurodegeneration. *Nature Neuroscience, 21*(10), 1359. https://doi.org/10.1038/S41593-018-0242-X.

Höglinger, G. U., Adler, C. H., Berg, D., Klein, C., Outeiro, T. F., Poewe, W., ... Lang, A. E. (2024). A biological classification of Parkinson's disease: The SynNeurGe research diagnostic criteria. *The Lancet Neurology, 23*(2), 191–204. https://doi.org/10.1016/S1474-4422(23)00404-0.

Hollingsworth, D., Srivastava, S., Akter, S., Kumar, M., Dey, S. S., Panja, S., ... Sil, S. (2026). Colostrum extracellular vesicles are neuroprotective in models of Parkinson's disease. *Theranostics, 16*(8), 4190. https://doi.org/10.7150/THNO.128257.

Horsager, J., Andersen, K. B., Knudsen, K., Skjærbæk, C., Fedorova, T. D., Okkels, N., ... Borghammer, P. (2020). Brain-first versus body-first Parkinson's disease: A multimodal imaging case-control study. *Brain: A Journal of Neurology, 143*(10), 3077–3088. https://doi.org/10.1093/BRAIN/AWAA238.

Huh, Y. E., Park, H., Chiang, M. S. R., Tuncali, I., Liu, G., Locascio, J. J., ... Scherzer, C. R. (2021). Glucosylceramide in cerebrospinal fluid of patients with GBA-associated and idiopathic Parkinson's disease enrolled in PPMI. *NPJ Parkinson's Disease,* 7(1), https://doi.org/10.1038/S41531-021-00241-3.

Huh, Y. E., Usnich, T., Scherzer, C. R., Klein, C., & Chung, S. J. (2023). GBA1 variants and Parkinson's disease: Paving the way for targeted therapy. *Journal of Movement Disorders, 16*(3), 261–278. https://doi.org/10.14802/JMD.23023.

Hwang, K. S., Langley, J., Tripathi, R., Hu, X. P., & Huddleston, D. E. (2023). In vivo detection of substantia nigra and locus coeruleus volume loss in Parkinson's disease using neuromelanin-sensitive MRI: Replication in two cohorts. *PLoS One, 18*(4), https://doi.org/10.1371/JOURNAL.PONE.0282684.

Ibrahim, N., Kusmirek, J., Struck, A. F., Floberg, J. M., Perlman, S. B., Gallagher, C., & Hall, L. T. (2016). The sensitivity and specificity of F-DOPA PET in a movement disorder clinic. *American Journal of Nuclear Medicine and Molecular Imaging, 6*(1), 102. https://pmc.ncbi.nlm.nih.gov/articles/PMC4749509/.

Iranzo, A., Fairfoul, G., Ayudhaya, A. C. N., Serradell, M., Gelpi, E., Vilaseca, I., ... Green, A. J. E. (2021). Detection of α-synuclein in CSF by RT-QuIC in patients with isolated rapid-eye-movement sleep behaviour disorder: a longitudinal observational study. *The Lancet Neurology, 20*(3), 203–212. https://doi.org/10.1016/S1474-4422(20)30449-X.

Irwin, D. J., Grossman, M., Weintraub, D., Hurtig, H. I., Duda, J. E., Xie, S. X., ... Trojanowski, J. Q. (2017). Neuropathological and genetic correlates of survival and dementia onset in synucleinopathies: A retrospective analysis. *The Lancet Neurology, 16*(1), 55. https://doi.org/10.1016/S1474-4422(16)30291-5.

Isik, S., Yeman Kiyak, B., Akbayir, R., Seyhali, R., & Arpaci, T. (2023). Microglia mediated neuroinflammation in Parkinson's disease. *Cells, 12*(7), https://doi.org/10.3390/CELLS12071012.

Istaiti, M., Revel-Vilk, S., Becker-Cohen, M., Dinur, T., Ramaswami, U., Castillo-Garcia, D., ... Zimran, A. (2021). Upgrading the evidence for the use of ambroxol in Gaucher disease and GBA related Parkinson: Investigator initiated registry based on real life data. *American Journal of Hematology, 96*(5), 545–551. https://doi.org/10.1002/AJH.26131.

Jennings, D., Huntwork-Rodriguez, S., Henry, A. G., Sasaki, J. C., Meisner, R., Diaz, D., ... Troyer, M. D. (2022). Preclinical and clinical evaluation of the LRRK2 inhibitor DNL201 for Parkinson's disease. *Science Translational Medicine, 14*(648), https://doi.org/10.1126/SCITRANSLMED.ABJ2658;WEBSITE:WEBSITE:AAAS-SITE;WGROUP:STRING:PUBLICATION.

Jurga, A. M., Paleczna, M., & Kuter, K. Z. (2020). Overview of general and discriminating markers of differential microglia phenotypes. *Frontiers in Cellular Neuroscience, 14*. https://doi.org/10.3389/FNCEL.2020.00198.

Kaasinen, V., & Vahlberg, T. (2017). Striatal dopamine in Parkinson disease: A meta-analysis of imaging studies. *Annals of Neurology, 82*(6), 873–882. https://doi.org/10.1002/ANA.25103.

Kamath, T., Abdulraouf, A., Burris, S. J., Langlieb, J., Gazestani, V., Nadaf, N. M., ... Macosko, E. Z. (2022). Single-cell genomic profiling of human dopamine neurons identifies a population that selectively degenerates in Parkinson's disease. *Nature Neuroscience, 25*(5), 588–595. https://doi.org/10.1038/s41593-022-01061-1.

Kang, J.-H., Irwin, D. J., Chen-Plotkin, A. S., Siderowf, A., Caspell, C., Coffey, C. S., ... Ranola, M. (2013). Association of cerebrospinal fluid β-amyloid 1-42, T-tau, P-tau181, and α-synuclein levels with clinical features of drug-naive patients with early Parkinson disease. *JAMA Neurology, 70*(10), 1277–1287. https://doi.org/10.1001/JAMANEUROL.2013.3861.

Kang, U. J., Boehme, A. K., Fairfoul, G., Shahnawaz, M., Ma, T. C., Hutten, S. J., ... Soto, C. (2019). Comparative study of cerebrospinal fluid α-synuclein seeding aggregation assays for diagnosis of Parkinson's disease. *Movement Disorders: Official Journal of the Movement Disorder Society, 34*(4), 536–544. https://doi.org/10.1002/MDS.27646.

Kayhanian, S., & Barker, R. A. (2026). Clinical trial highlights: Dopamine cell-replacement therapies. *Journal of Parkinson's Disease, 16*(1), https://doi.org/10.1177/1877718X251397277.

Keren-Shaul, H., Spinrad, A., Weiner, A., Matcovitch-Natan, O., Dvir-Szternfeld, R., Ulland, T. K., ... Amit, I. (2017). A unique microglia type associated with restricting development of Alzheimer's disease. *Cell, 169*(7), 1276–1290.e17. https://doi.org/10.1016/j.cell.2017.05.018.

Khalil, M. M., Tremoleda, J. L., Bayomy, T. B., & Gsell, W. (2011). Molecular SPECT imaging: An overview. *International Journal of Molecular Imaging, 2011*, 1–15. https://doi.org/10.1155/2011/796025.

Kim, C., Ho, D. H., Suk, J. E., You, S., Michael, S., Kang, J., ... Lee, S. J. (2013). Neuron-released oligomeric α-synuclein is an endogenous agonist of TLR2 for paracrine activation of microglia. *Nature Communications, 4*. https://doi.org/10.1038/NCOMMS2534.

Klück, V., Jansen, T. L. T. A., Janssen, M., Comarniceanu, A., Efdé, M., Tengesdal, I. W., ... Joosten, L. A. B. (2020). Dapansutrile, an oral selective NLRP3 inflammasome inhibitor, for treatment of gout flares: An open-label, dose-adaptive, proof-of-concept, phase 2a trial. *The Lancet. Rheumatology, 2*(5), e270–e280. https://doi.org/10.1016/S2665-9913(20)30065-5.

Kluge, A., Bunk, J., Schaeffer, E., Drobny, A., Xiang, W., Knacke, H., ... Zunke, F. (2022). Detection of neuron-derived pathological α-synuclein in blood. *Brain, 145*(9), 3058–3071. https://doi.org/10.1093/BRAIN/AWAC115.

Kouli, A., Torsney, K. M., & Kuan, W. L. (2018). Parkinson's disease: Etiology, neuropathology, and pathogenesis. *Exon Publications,* 3–26. https://doi.org/10.15586/CODONPUBLICATIONS.PARKINSONSDISEASE.2018.CH1.

Kwatra, M., Kwak, G., Li, H., Suk, J. S., & Ko, H. S. (2026). Polymeric nanoparticle-mediated GBA1 gene therapy is neuroprotective in a preclinical model of Parkinson's disease. *Drug Delivery and Translational Research, 16*(3), https://doi.org/10.1007/S13346-025-01944-3.

Kwon, E. H., Tennagels, S., Gold, R., Gerwert, K., Beyer, L., & Tönges, L. (2022). Update on CSF Biomarkers in Parkinson's disease. *Biomolecules 2022, 12*(2), *12.* https://doi.org/10.3390/BIOM12020329.

Laansma, M. A., Bright, J. K., Al-Bachari, S., Anderson, T. J., Ard, T., Assogna, F., ... van der Werf, Y. D. (2021). International multicenter analysis of brain structure across clinical stages of Parkinson's disease. *Movement Disorders: Official Journal of the Movement Disorder Society, 36*(11), 2583–2594. https://doi.org/10.1002/MDS.28706.

Lancione, M., Donatelli, G., Del Prete, E., Campese, N., Frosini, D., Cencini, M., ... Cosottini, M. (2022). Evaluation of iron overload in nigrosome 1 via quantitative susceptibility mapping as a progression biomarker in prodromal stages of synucleinopathies. *Neuroimage, 260.* https://doi.org/10.1016/j.neuroimage.2022.119454.

Langkammer, C., Schweser, F., Krebs, N., Deistung, A., Goessler, W., Scheurer, E., ... Reichenbach, J. R. (2012). Quantitative susceptibility mapping (QSM) as a means to measure brain iron? A post mortem validation study. *Neuroimage, 62*(3), 1593–1599. https://doi.org/10.1016/j.neuroimage.2012.05.049.

Leandrou, E., Chalatsa, I., Anagnostou, D., Machalia, C., Semitekolou, M., Filippa, V., ... Emmanouilidou, E. (2024). α-Synuclein oligomers potentiate neuroinflammatory NF-κB activity and induce Cav3.2 calcium signaling in astrocytes. *Translational Neurodegeneration, 13*(1), https://doi.org/10.1186/S40035-024-00401-4.

LeWitt, P. A., Rezai, A. R., Leehey, M. A., Ojemann, S. G., Flaherty, A. W., Eskandar, E. N., ... Feigin, A. (2011). AAV2-GAD gene therapy for advanced Parkinson's disease: A double-blind, sham-surgery controlled, randomised trial. *The Lancet Neurology, 10*(4), 309–319. https://doi.org/10.1016/S1474-4422(11)70039-4.

Li, J., Cao, F., Yin, H. L., Huang, Z. J., Lin, Z. T., Mao, N., ... Wang, G. (2020). Ferroptosis: Past, present and future. *Cell Death & Disease, 11*(2), https://doi.org/10.1038/S41419-020-2298-2.

Liu, G., Boot, B., Locascio, J. J., Jansen, I. E., Winder-Rhodes, S., Eberly, S., ... Nalls, M. A. (2016). Specifically neuropathic Gaucher's mutations accelerate cognitive decline in Parkinson's. *Annals of Neurology, 80*(5), 674–685. https://doi.org/10.1002/ANA.24781;WGROUP:STRING:PUBLICATION.

Llorens, F., Thüne, K., Tahir, W., Kanata, E., Diaz-Lucena, D., Xanthopoulos, K., ... Zerr, I. (2017). YKL-40 in the brain and cerebrospinal fluid of neurodegenerative dementias. *Molecular Neurodegeneration, 12*(1), 83. https://doi.org/10.1186/S13024-017-0226-4.

Lonnemann, N., Hosseini, S., Marchetti, C., Skouras, D. B., Stefanoni, D., D'Alessandro, A., ... Korte, M. (2020). The NLRP3 inflammasome inhibitor OLT1177 rescues cognitive impairment in a mouse model of Alzheimer's disease. *Proceedings of the National Academy of Sciences of the United States of America, 117*(50), 32145–32154. https://doi.org/10.1073/PNAS.2009680117.

Lotankar, S., Prabhavalkar, K. S., & Bhatt, L. K. (2017). Biomarkers for Parkinson's disease: Recent advancement. *Neuroscience Bulletin, 33*(5), 585–597. https://doi.org/10.1007/S12264-017-0183-5.

Luque, M., Matic, M., Heras-Garvin, A., Amo-Aparicio, J., Luk, K. C., Haindl, M. T., ... Stefanova, N. (2026). Clinically advanced NLRP3 inhibitor modulates microglial transcriptome and alleviates α-synuclein-induced progression of parkinsonism. *Journal of Neuroinflammation, 23*(1), 76. https://doi.org/10.1186/S12974-026-03716-3.

Ma, J., Shi, X., Li, M., Chen, S., Gu, Q., Zheng, J., ... Li, X. (2022). MicroRNA-181a-2-3p shuttled by mesenchymal stem cell-secreted extracellular vesicles inhibits oxidative stress in Parkinson's disease by inhibiting EGR1 and NOX4. *Cell Death Discovery, 8*(1), https://doi.org/10.1038/S41420-022-00823-X.

Mak, E., Su, L., Williams, G. B., Firbank, M. J., Lawson, R. A., Yarnall, A. J., ... O'Brien, J. T. (2015). Baseline and longitudinal grey matter changes in newly diagnosed Parkinson's disease: ICICLE-PD study. *Brain: A Journal of Neurology, 138*(Pt 10), 2974–2986. https://doi.org/10.1093/BRAIN/AWV211.

Marchi, S., Guilbaud, E., Tait, S. W. G., Yamazaki, T., & Galluzzi, L. (2023). Mitochondrial control of inflammation. *Nature Reviews. Immunology, 23*(3), 159–173. https://doi.org/10.1038/S41577-022-00760-X.

Mari, Z., & Mestre, T. A. (2022). The disease modification conundrum in Parkinson's disease: Failures and hopes. *Frontiers in Aging Neuroscience, 14*. https://doi.org/10.3389/FNAGI.2022.810860.

Martin, J., Lai, G. J., Park, C. Y., West, C., Van Brunt, T., Ahmed, S., ... Riessland, M. (2025). Age-related nigral downregulation of the Parkinson's risk factor FAM49B primes human microglia for inflammaging. *Npj Aging, 12*(1), 1. https://doi.org/10.1038/s41514-025-00296-z.

McGrowder, D. A., Miller, F., Vaz, K., Nwokocha, C., Wilson-Clarke, C., Anderson-Cross, M., ... Alexander-Lindo, R. (2021). Cerebrospinal fluid biomarkers of Alzheimer's disease: Current evidence and future perspectives. *Brain Sciences, 11*(2), 1–56. https://doi.org/10.3390/BRAINSCI11020215.

McKeith, I. G., Boeve, B. F., Dickson, D. W., Halliday, G., Taylor, J. P., Weintraub, D., ... Kosaka, K. (2017). Diagnosis and management of dementia with Lewy bodies: Fourth consensus report of the DLB Consortium. *Neurology, 89*(1), 88–100. https://doi.org/10.1212/WNL.0000000000004058.

Mollenhauer, B. (2014). Quantification of α-synuclein in cerebrospinal fluid: How ideal is this biomarker for Parkinson's disease? *Parkinsonism & Related Disorders, 20*(.1), S76–S79. https://doi.org/10.1016/S1353-8020(13)70020-8.

Mollenhauer, B., Caspell-Garcia, C. J., Coffey, C. S., Taylor, P., Shaw, L. M., Trojanowski, J. Q., ... Galasko, D. (2017). Longitudinal CSF biomarkers in patients with early Parkinson disease and healthy controls. *Neurology, 89*(19), 1959–1969. https://doi.org/10.1212/WNL.0000000000004609.

Mollenhauer, B., Zimmermann, J., Sixel-Döring, F., Focke, N. K., Wicke, T., Ebentheuer, J., ... Trenkwalder, C. (2016). Monitoring of 30 marker candidates in early Parkinson disease as progression markers. *Neurology, 87*(2), 168. https://doi.org/10.1212/WNL.0000000000002651.

More, S. A., Ghosh, A., Kulkarni, O. P., & Ramesh Mulay, S. (2025). Role of persistent necroinflammation in chronic tissue remodeling and organ fibrosis. *American Journal of Physiology. Cell Physiology, 330*(1), C40–C55. https://doi.org/10.1152/AJPCELL.00416.2025.

Morenas-Rodríguez, E., Alcolea, D., Suárez-Calvet, M., Muñoz-Llahuna, L., Vilaplana, E., Sala, I., ... Lleó, A. (2019). Different pattern of CSF glial markers between dementia with Lewy bodies and Alzheimer's disease. *Scientific Reports, 9*(1), 7803. https://doi.org/10.1038/s41598-019-44173-8.

Mullin, S., Smith, L., Lee, K., D'Souza, G., Woodgate, P., Elflein, J., ... Schapira, A. H. V. (2020). Ambroxol for the treatment of patients with Parkinson disease with and without glucocerebrosidase gene mutations: A nonrandomized, noncontrolled trial. *JAMA Neurology, 77*(4), 427–434. https://doi.org/10.1001/JAMANEUROL.2019.4611.

Mustapha, M., & Taib, C. N. M. (2021). MPTP-induced mouse model of Parkinson's disease: A promising direction of therapeutic strategies. *Bosnian Journal of Basic Medical Sciences, 21*(4), 422–433. https://doi.org/10.17305/BJBMS.2020.5181.

Ngo, D. H., & Vo, T. S. (2019). An updated review on pharmaceutical properties of gamma-aminobutyric acid. *Molecules 2019, 24*(15), *24*. https://doi.org/10.3390/MOLECULES24152678.

Nichols, W. C., Pankratz, N., Marek, D. K., Pauciulo, M. W., Elsaesser, V. E., Halter, C. A., ... Foroud, T. (2009). Mutations in GBA are associated with familial Parkinson disease susceptibility and age at onset. *Neurology, 72*(4), 310–316. https://doi.org/10.1212/01.WNL.0000327823.81237.D1;REQUESTEDJOURNAL:JOURNAL:WNL;JOURNAL:JOURNAL:WNL;ISSUE:ISSUE:.

Ohtsuka, C., Sasaki, M., Konno, K., Kato, K., Takahashi, J., Yamashita, F., & Terayama, Y. (2014). Differentiation of early-stage parkinsonisms using neuromelanin-sensitive magnetic resonance imaging. *Parkinsonism and Related Disorders, 20*(7), 755–760. https://doi.org/10.1016/j.parkreldis.2014.04.005.

Orimo, S., Ozawa, E., Nakade, S., Sugimoto, T., & Mizusawa, H. (1999). (123)I-metaiodobenzylguanidine myocardial scintigraphy in Parkinson's disease. *Journal of Neurology, Neurosurgery, and Psychiatry, 67*(2), 189–194. https://doi.org/10.1136/JNNP.67.2.189.

Ostrerova-Golts, N., Petrucelli, L., Hardy, J., Lee, J. M., Farer, M., & Wolozin, B. (2000). The A53T alpha-synuclein mutation increases iron-dependent aggregation and toxicity. *The Journal of Neuroscience: The Official Journal of the Society for Neuroscience, 20*(16), 6048–6054. https://doi.org/10.1523/JNEUROSCI.20-16-06048.2000.

Pagano, G., Taylor, K. I., Anzures Cabrera, J., Simuni, T., Marek, K., Postuma, R. B., ... Bonni, A. (2024). Prasinezumab slows motor progression in rapidly progressing early-stage Parkinson's disease. *Nature Medicine, 30*(4), 1096–1103. https://doi.org/10.1038/s41591-024-02886-y.

Palermo, G., Giannoni, S., Bellini, G., Siciliano, G., & Ceravolo, R. (2021). Dopamine transporter imaging, current status of a potential biomarker: A comprehensive review. *International Journal of Molecular Sciences, 22*(20), https://doi.org/10.3390/IJMS222011234.

Paslawski, W., Khosousi, S., Hertz, E., Markaki, I., Boxer, A., & Svenningsson, P. (2023). Large-scale proximity extension assay reveals CSF midkine and DOPA decarboxylase as supportive diagnostic biomarkers for Parkinson's disease. *Translational Neurodegeneration, 12*(1), https://doi.org/10.1186/S40035-023-00374-W.

Pereira, J. B., Kumar, A., Hall, S., Palmqvist, S., Stomrud, E., Bali, D., ... Hansson, O. (2023). DOPA decarboxylase is an emerging biomarker for Parkinsonian disorders including preclinical Lewy body disease. *Nature Aging, 3*(10), 1201–1209. https://doi.org/10.1038/S43587-023-00478-Y.

Pietracupa, S., Belvisi, D., Piervincenzi, C., Tommasin, S., Pasqua, G., Petsas, N., ... Pantano, P. (2023). White and gray matter alterations in de novo PD patients: Which matter most? *Journal of Neurology, 270*(5), 2734–2742. https://doi.org/10.1007/S00415-023-11607-3.

Pike, A. F., Varanita, T., Herrebout, M. A. C., Plug, B. C., Kole, J., Musters, R. J. P., ... Veerhuis, R. (2021). α-Synuclein evokes NLRP3 inflammasome-mediated IL-1β secretion from primary human microglia. *Glia, 69*(6), 1413–1428. https://doi.org/10.1002/GLIA.23970.

Primorac, D., Brlek, P., Bulić, L., Hrvatin, N., Škaro, V., Projić, P., ... Mobasheri, A. (2026). Clinical applications of extracellular vesicles: Promises and pitfalls. *International Journal of Molecular Sciences, 27*(3), https://doi.org/10.3390/IJMS27031509.

Prinz, M., Jung, S., & Priller, J. (2019). Microglia biology: One century of evolving concepts. *Cell, 179*(2), 292–311. https://doi.org/10.1016/j.cell.2019.08.053.

Pyatigorskaya, N., Gallea, C., Garcia-Lorenzo, D., Vidailhet, M., & Lehericy, S. (2014). A review of the use of magnetic resonance imaging in Parkinson's disease. *Therapeutic Advances in Neurological Disorders, 7*(4), 206–220. https://doi.org/10.1177/1756285613511507; WEBSITE:WEBSITE:SAGE;ISSUE:ISSUE:.

Pysz, M. A., Gambhir, S. S., & Willmann, J. K. (2010). Molecular imaging: Current status and emerging strategies. *Clinical Radiology, 65*(7), 500–516. https://doi.org/10.1016/j.crad.2010.03.011.

Qu, Y., Li, J., Qin, Q., Wang, D., Zhao, J., An, K., ... Xue, Z. (2023). A systematic review and meta-analysis of inflammatory biomarkers in Parkinson's disease. *Npj Parkinson's Disease, 9*(1), 18. https://doi.org/10.1038/s41531-023-00449-5.

Ramirez, A., Heimbach, A., Gründemann, J., Stiller, B., Hampshire, D., Cid, L. P., ... Kubisch, C. (2006). Hereditary parkinsonism with dementia is caused by mutations in ATP13A2, encoding a lysosomal type 5 P-type ATPase. *Nature Genetics, 38*(10), 1184–1191. https://doi.org/10.1038/ng1884.

Ren, J., Pan, C., Wang, Y., Xue, C., Lin, H., Xu, J., ... Liu, W. (2022). Plasma α-synuclein and phosphorylated tau 181 as a diagnostic biomarker panel for de novo Parkinson's disease. *Journal of Neurochemistry, 161*(6), 506–515. https://doi.org/10.1111/JNC.15601;SUBPAGE:STRING:FULL.

Réu, P., Khosravi, A., Bernard, S., Mold, J. E., Salehpour, M., Alkass, K., ... Frisén, J. (2017). The lifespan and turnover of microglia in the human brain. *Cell Reports, 20*(4), 779–784. https://doi.org/10.1016/j.celrep.2017.07.004.

Richter, F., Fleming, S. M., Watson, M., Lemesre, V., Pellegrino, L., Ranes, B., ... Chesselet, M. F. (2014). A GCase chaperone improves motor function in a mouse model of synucleinopathy. *Neurotherapeutics: the Journal of the American Society for Experimental NeuroTherapeutics, 11*(4), 840. https://doi.org/10.1007/S13311-014-0294-X.

Rideout, H. J., Chartier-Harlin, M. C., Fell, M. J., Hirst, W. D., Huntwork-Rodriguez, S., Leyns, C. E. G., ... Taymans, J. M. (2020). The current state-of-the art of LRRK2-based biomarker assay development in Parkinson's disease. *Frontiers in Neuroscience, 14*, 566602. https://doi.org/10.3389/FNINS.2020.00865/TEXT.

Rim, C., You, M. J., Nahm, M., & Kwon, M. S. (2024). Emerging role of senescent microglia in brain aging-related neurodegenerative diseases. *Translational Neurodegeneration, 13*(1), https://doi.org/10.1186/S40035-024-00402-3.

Rossi, M., Candelise, N., Baiardi, S., Capellari, S., Giannini, G., Orrù, C. D., ... Parchi, P. (2020). Ultrasensitive RT-QuIC assay with high sensitivity and specificity for Lewy body-associated synucleinopathies. *Acta Neuropathologica, 140*(1), 49–62. https://doi.org/10.1007/S00401-020-02160-8.

Roy, I., Thomas, R. A., Ambriz, G. J., Farhan, S., Piscopo, V. E. C., & Durcan, T. M. (2025). Single nuclear RNA sequencing shows altered microglial and astrocytic functions in post-mortem Parkinson's disease tissue. *BioRxiv*. https://doi.org/10.1101/2025.11.13.687853.

Saeed, U., Lang, A. E., & Masellis, M. (2020). Neuroimaging advances in Parkinson's disease and atypical Parkinsonian syndromes. *Frontiers in Neurology, 11*. https://doi.org/10.3389/FNEUR.2020.572976.

Sampson, T. R., Debelius, J. W., Thron, T., Janssen, S., Shastri, G. G., Ilhan, Z. E., ... Mazmanian, S. K. (2016). Gut microbiota regulate motor deficits and neuroinflammation in a model of Parkinson's disease. *Cell, 167*(6), 1469–1480.e12. https://doi.org/10.1016/j.cell.2016.11.018.

Sánchez-Fernández, A., Skouras, D. B., Dinarello, C. A., & López-Vales, R. (2019). OLT1177 (Dapansutrile), a selective NLRP3 inflammasome inhibitor, ameliorates experimental autoimmune encephalomyelitis pathogenesis. *Frontiers in Immunology, 10*. https://doi.org/10.3389/FIMMU.2019.02578.

Sawamoto, N., Doi, D., Nakanishi, E., Sawamura, M., Kikuchi, T., Yamakado, H., ... Takahashi, J. (2025). Phase I/II trial of iPS-cell-derived dopaminergic cells for Parkinson's disease. *Nature, 641*(8064), 971–977. https://doi.org/10.1038/S41586-025-08700-0.

Schade, S., & Mollenhauer, B. (2014). Biomarkers in biological fluids for dementia with Lewy bodies. *Alzheimer's Research & Therapy, 6*(5), 72. https://doi.org/10.1186/S13195-014-0072-3.

Schellenberg, G. D., & Montine, T. J. (2012). The genetics and neuropathology of Alzheimer's disease. *Acta Neuropathologica, 124*(3), 305–323. https://doi.org/10.1007/S00401-012-0996-2.

Schneider, S. A., & Alcalay, R. N. (2017). Neuropathology of genetic synucleinopathies with parkinsonism: Review of the literature. *Movement Disorders, 32*(11), 1504–1523. https://doi.org/10.1002/MDS.27193,CTYPE.STRING.JOURNAL.

Schöndorf, D. C., Aureli, M., McAllister, F. E., Hindley, C. J., Mayer, F., Schmid, B., ... Deleidi, M. (2014). iPSC-derived neurons from GBA1-associated Parkinson's disease patients show autophagic defects and impaired calcium homeostasis. *Nature Communications, 5*(1), 4028. https://doi.org/10.1038/ncomms5028.

Schröter, N., Groppa, S., Rijntjes, M., Gonzalez-Escamilla, G., Urbach, H., Jost, W. H., & Rau, A. (2025). Neuroimaging in advanced Parkinson's disease: Insights into pathophysiology, biomarkers, and personalized therapies. *Journal of Neural Transmission (Vienna, Austria: 1996), 132*(11), 1655–1664. https://doi.org/10.1007/s00702-025-02942-y.

Senkevich, K., Liu, L., Alvarado, C. X., Leonard, H. L., Nalls, M. A., & Gan-Or, Z. (2024). Lack of genetic evidence for NLRP3 inflammasome involvement in Parkinson's disease pathogenesis. *Npj Parkinson's Disease, 10*(1), 145. https://doi.org/10.1038/s41531-024-00744-9.

Shen, J., Amari, N., Zack, R., Skrinak, R. T., Unger, T. L., Posavi, M., ... Chen-Plotkin, A. S. (2022). Plasma MIA, CRP, and albumin predict cognitive decline in Parkinson's disease. *Annals of Neurology, 92*(2), 255–269. https://doi.org/10.1002/ANA.26410;WGROUP:STRING:PUBLICATION.

Shi, M., Bradner, J., Hancock, A. M., Chung, K. A., Quinn, J. F., Peskind, E. R., ... Zhang, J. (2011). Cerebrospinal fluid biomarkers for Parkinson disease diagnosis and progression. *Annals of Neurology, 69*(3), 570–580. https://doi.org/10.1002/ANA.22311;PAGE:STRING:ARTICLE/CHAPTER.

Siderowf, A., Concha-Marambio, L., Lafontant, D. E., Farris, C. M., Ma, Y., Urenia, P. A., ... Soto, C. (2023). Assessment of heterogeneity among participants in the Parkinson's progression markers initiative cohort using α-synuclein seed amplification: A cross-sectional study. *The Lancet Neurology, 22*(5), 407–417. https://doi.org/10.1016/S1474-4422(23)00109-6.

Sidransky, E., Nalls, M. A., Aasly, J. O., Aharon-Peretz, J., Annesi, G., Barbosa, E. R., ... Ziegler, S. G. (2009). Multicenter analysis of glucocerebrosidase mutations in Parkinson's disease. *The New England Journal of Medicine, 361*(17), 1651–1661. https://doi.org/10.1056/NEJMOA0901281.

Siemeling, O., Slingerland, S., van der Zee, S., & van Laar, T. (2024). Study protocol of the GRoningen early-PD Ambroxol treatment (GREAT) trial: a randomized, double-blind, placebo-controlled, single center trial with ambroxol in Parkinson patients with a GBA mutation. *BMC Neurology, 24*(1), https://doi.org/10.1186/S12883-024-03629-9.

Simuni, T., Chahine, L. M., Poston, K., Brumm, M., Buracchio, T., Campbell, M., ... Marek, K. (2024). A biological definition of neuronal α-synuclein disease: towards an integrated staging system for research. *The Lancet Neurology, 23*(2), 178–190. https://doi.org/10.1016/S1474-4422(23)00405-2.

Simuni, T., Siderowf, A., Lasch, S., Coffey, C. S., Caspell-Garcia, C., Jennings, D., ... Marek, K. (2018). Longitudinal change of clinical and biological measures in early Parkinson's disease: Parkinson's progression markers initiative cohort. *Movement Disorders: Official Journal of the Movement Disorder Society, 33*(5), 771–782. https://doi.org/10.1002/MDS.27361.

Singh, J., Habean, M. L., & Panicker, N. (2023). Inflammasome assembly in neurodegenerative diseases. *Trends in Neurosciences, 46*(10), 814–831. https://doi.org/10.1016/J.TINS.2023.07.009.

Smajic, S., Prada-Medina, C. A., Landoulsi, Z., Ghelfi, J., Delcambre, S., Dietrich, C., ... Spielmann, M. (2022). Single-cell sequencing of human midbrain reveals glial activation and a Parkinson-specific neuronal state. *Brain: A Journal of Neurology, 145*(3), 964–978. https://doi.org/10.1093/BRAIN/AWAB446.

Song, G. J., & Suk, K. (2017). Pharmacological modulation of functional phenotypes of microglia in neurodegenerative diseases. *Frontiers in Aging Neuroscience, 9*(MAY), https://doi.org/10.3389/FNAGI.2017.00139.

Spies, P. E., Slats, D., Sjogren, J. M. C., Kremer, B. P. H., Verhey, F. R. J., Rikkert, M. G. M. O., & Verbeek, M. M. (2010). The cerebrospinal fluid amyloid β42/40 ratio in the differentiation of Alzheimers disease from non-Alzheimers dementia. *Current Alzheimer Research,* 7(5), 470–476. https://doi.org/10.2174/156720510791383796.

Stewart, T., Sossi, V., Aasly, J. O., Wszolek, Z. K., Uitti, R. J., Hasegawa, K., ... Zhang, J. (2015). Phosphorylated α-synuclein in Parkinson's disease: Correlation depends on disease severity. *Acta Neuropathologica Communications, 3*(1), 7. https://doi.org/10.1186/S40478-015-0185-3.

Stormezand, G. N., Chaves, L. T., Vállez García, D., Doorduin, J., De Jong, B. M., Leenders, K. L., ... Dierckx, R. A. J. O. (2020). Intrastriatal gradient analyses of 18F-FDOPA PET scans for differentiation of Parkinsonian disorders. *NeuroImage: Clinical, 25*, 102161. https://doi.org/10.1016/J.NICL.2019.102161.

Stuendl, A., Kraus, T., Chatterjee, M., Zapke, B., Sadowski, B., Moebius, W., ... Schneider, A. (2021). α-Synuclein in plasma-derived extracellular vesicles is a potential biomarker of Parkinson's disease. *Movement Disorders, 36*(11), 2508–2518. https://doi.org/10.1002/MDS.28639;CTYPE:STRING:JOURNAL.

Sulzer, D., Cassidy, C., Horga, G., Kang, U. J., Fahn, S., Casella, L., ... Zecca, L. (2018). Neuromelanin detection by magnetic resonance imaging (MRI) and its promise as a biomarker for Parkinson's disease. *Npj Parkinson's Disease, 4*(1), 11. https://doi.org/10.1038/s41531-018-0047-3.

Sun, J., Lai, Z., Ma, J., Gao, L., Chen, M., Chen, J., ... Ma, T. (2020). Quantitative evaluation of iron content in idiopathic rapid eye movement sleep behavior disorder. *Movement Disorders: Official Journal of the Movement Disorder Society, 35*(3), 478–485. https://doi.org/10.1002/MDS.27929.

Tabar, V., Sarva, H., Lozano, A. M., Fasano, A., Kalia, S. K., Yu, K. K. H., ... Henchcliffe, C. (2025). Phase I trial of hES cell-derived dopaminergic neurons for Parkinson's disease. *Nature, 641*(8064), 978–983. https://doi.org/10.1038/s41586-025-08845-y.

Tai, C. H. (2022). Subthalamic burst firing: A pathophysiological target in Parkinson's disease. *Neuroscience and Biobehavioral Reviews, 132*, 410–419. https://doi.org/10.1016/J.NEUBIOREV.2021.11.044.

Takahashi, R., Nakanishi, E., Yamakado, H., Sawamoto, N., & Takahashi, J. (2025). Allogenic transplantation therapy of iPS cell-derived dopamine progenitors for Parkinson's disease –Current status of the Kyoto trial and future perspectives. *Parkinsonism and Related Disorders, 135*. https://doi.org/10.1016/j.parkreldis.2025.107833.

Tan, E. K., Chao, Y. X., West, A., Chan, L. L., Poewe, W., & Jankovic, J. (2020). Parkinson disease and the immune system - associations, mechanisms and therapeutics. *Nature Reviews. Neurology, 16*(6), 303–318. https://doi.org/10.1038/S41582-020-0344-4.

Tang, Y., Han, L., Li, S., Hu, T., Xu, Z., Fan, Y., ... Wang, J. (2023). Plasma GFAP in Parkinson's disease with cognitive impairment and its potential to predict conversion to dementia. *Npj Parkinson's Disease, 9*(1), 23. https://doi.org/10.1038/s41531-023-00447-7.

Taylor, K. I., Lipsmeier, F., Scelsi, M. A., Volkova-Volkmar, E., Rukina, D., Popp, W., ... Bamdadian, A. (2025). Exploratory digital outcome measures of motor sign progression in Parkinson's disease patients treated with prasinezumab. *Npj Digital Medicine, 8*(1), 365. https://doi.org/10.1038/s41746-025-01572-8.

Teil, M., & Huot, P. (2026). The challenges of experimental pharmacology in identifying novel treatments for Parkinson's disease. *Current Opinion in Neurobiology, 97*, 103164. https://doi.org/10.1016/J.CONB.2025.103164.

Teng, X., Mao, S., Wu, H., Shao, Q., Zu, J., Zhang, W., ... Xu, C. (2023). The relationship between serum neurofilament light chain and glial fibrillary acidic protein with the REM sleep behavior disorder subtype of Parkinson's disease. *Journal of Neurochemistry, 165*(2), 268–276. https://doi.org/10.1111/JNC.15780;REQUESTEDJOURNAL:JOURNAL:14714159;ISSUE:ISSUE:.

Thion, M. S., Ginhoux, F., & Garel, S. (2018). Microglia and early brain development: An intimate journey. *Science (New York, N. Y.), 362*(6411), 185–189. https://doi.org/10.1126/SCIENCE.AAT0474.

Thomas, G. E. C., Leyland, L. A., Schrag, A. E., Lees, A. J., Acosta-Cabronero, J., & Weil, R. S. (2020). Brain iron deposition is linked with cognitive severity in Parkinson's disease. *Journal of Neurology, Neurosurgery, and Psychiatry, 91*(4), 418–425. https://doi.org/10.1136/JNNP-2019-322042.

Tian, C., Liu, G., Gao, L., Soltys, D., Pan, C., Stewart, T., ... Zhang, J. (2019). Erythrocytic α-synuclein as a potential biomarker for Parkinson's disease. *Translational Neurodegeneration, 8*(1), 15. https://doi.org/10.1186/S40035-019-0155-Y.

Tian, Y., Geng, S., Liu, T., Wang, Q., Lian, J., Lin, L., ... Liu, P. (2024). Unveiling MRI markers for Parkinson's disease: GABAergic dysfunction and cortical changes. *NeuroImage: Clinical, 43*. https://doi.org/10.1016/j.nicl.2024.103661.

Tinaz, S., Chow, C., Kuo, P. H., Krupinski, E. A., Blumenfeld, H., Louis, E. D., & Zubal, G. (2018). Semiquantitative analysis of dopamine transporter scans in patients with Parkinson disease. *Clinical Nuclear Medicine, 43*(1), e1–e7. https://doi.org/10.1097/RLU.0000000000001885.

Tönges, L., Buhmann, C., Klebe, S., Klucken, J., Kwon, E. H., Müller, T., ... Lingor, P. (2022). Blood-based biomarker in Parkinson's disease: Potential for future applications in clinical research and practice. *Journal of Neural Transmission, 129*(9), 1201–1217. https://doi.org/10.1007/S00702-022-02498-1.

Torres-Parga, A., Gershanik, O., Cardona, S., Guerrero, J., Gonzalez-Ojeda, L. M., & Cardona, J. F. (2025). Diagnostic performance of T1-Weighted MRI gray matter biomarkers in Parkinson's disease: A systematic review and meta-analysis. *Parkinsonism and Related Disorders, 140*. https://doi.org/10.1016/j.parkreldis.2025.108009.

Treglia, G., Cason, E., Stefanelli, A., Cocciolillo, F., Di Giuda, D., Fagioli, G., & Giordano, A. (2012). MIBG scintigraphy in differential diagnosis of Parkinsonism: A meta-analysis. *Clinical Autonomic Research: Official Journal of the Clinical Autonomic Research Society, 22*(1), 43–55. https://doi.org/10.1007/S10286-011-0135-5.

Van Laar, A. D., Christine, C. W., Phielipp, N., Larson, P. S., Elder, J. B., Merola, A., ... Bankiewicz, K. S. (2025). Intraputaminal delivery of adeno-associated virus serotype 2-Glial cell line-derived neurotrophic factor in mild or moderate Parkinson's disease. *Movement Disorders: Official Journal of the Movement Disorder Society, 40*(7), 1297–1306. https://doi.org/10.1002/MDS.30193.

Vijiaratnam, N., Simuni, T., Bandmann, O., Morris, H. R., & Foltynie, T. (2021). Progress towards therapies for disease modification in Parkinson's disease. *The Lancet Neurology, 20*(7), 559–572. https://doi.org/10.1016/S1474-4422(21)00061-2.

Volpicelli-Daley, L. A., Luk, K. C., Patel, T. P., Tanik, S. A., Riddle, D. M., Stieber, A., ... Lee, V. M. Y. (2011). Exogenous α-synuclein fibrils induce lewy body pathology leading to synaptic dysfunction and neuron death. *Neuron, 72*(1), 57–71. https://doi.org/10.1016/j.neuron.2011.08.033.

Walker, L., Stefanis, L., & Attems, J. (2019). Clinical and neuropathological differences between Parkinson's disease, Parkinson's disease dementia and dementia with Lewy bodies – current issues and future directions. *Journal of Neurochemistry, 150*(5), 467–474. https://doi.org/10.1111/JNC.14698;CSUBTYPE:STRING:SPECIAL;PAGE:STRING:ARTICLE/CHAPTER.

Wallings, R. L., & Tansey, M. G. (2019). LRRK2 regulation of immune-pathways and inflammatory disease. *Biochemical Society Transactions, 47*(6), 1581–1595. https://doi.org/10.1042/BST20180463.

Weingarten, C. P., Sundman, M. H., Hickey, P., & Chen, N. kuei (2015). Neuroimaging of Parkinson's disease: Expanding views. *Neuroscience and Biobehavioral Reviews, 59*, 16–52. https://doi.org/10.1016/j.neubiorev.2015.09.007.

Xia, Y., Zhang, G., Kou, L., Yin, S., Han, C., Hu, J., ... Wang, T. (2021). Reactive microglia enhance the transmission of exosomal α-synuclein via toll-like receptor 2. *Brain: A Journal of Neurology, 144*(7), 2024–2037. https://doi.org/10.1093/BRAIN/AWAB122.

Xiao, B., & Tan, E. K. (2025). Prasinezumab slows motor progression in Parkinsons disease: Beyond the clinical data. *Npj Parkinson's Disease, 11*(1), 31. https://doi.org/10.1038/s41531-025-00886-4.

Xu, W., Huang, Y., & Zhou, R. (2025). NLRP3 inflammasome in neuroinflammation and central nervous system diseases. *Cellular & Molecular Immunology, 22*(4), 341–355. https://doi.org/10.1038/s41423-025-01275-w.

Yeole, A., Khanna, L., Doshi, M., Sharma, A., Uttarwar, P., Doshi, S., ... Parmar, D. (2025). A phase 2, proof-of-concept, placebo-controlled, randomized, multicenter, double-blind study to evaluate the efficacy, safety, tolerability, pharmacokinetics, and pharmacodynamics of Usnoflast (ZYIL1) in patients with amyotrophic lateral sclerosis. *Amyotrophic Lateral Sclerosis & Frontotemporal Degeneration, 26*(7–8), 794–801. https://doi.org/10.1080/21678421.2025.2515900.

Yoshita, M., Hayashi, M., & Hirai, S. (1998). Decreased myocardial accumulation of 123I-meta-iodobenzyl guanidine in Parkinson's disease. *Nuclear Medicine Communications, 19*(2), 137–142. https://doi.org/10.1097/00006231-199802000-00007.

Yu, Q., Huang, Q., Du, X., Xu, S., Li, M., & Ma, S. (2018). Early activation of Egr-1 promotes neuroinflammation and dopaminergic neurodegeneration in an experimental model of Parkinson's disease. *Experimental Neurology, 302*, 145–154. https://doi.org/10.1016/J.EXPNEUROL.2018.01.009.

Zafarjonovna, A. Z., Aysulu, E., Matlyuba, S., Rashid, H., Azamatovich, J. B., Ahmadjon, A., ... Ishankulov, A. (2026). Small extracellular vesicles as emerging biomarkers and therapeutic targets in neurodegenerative diseases. *Clinica Chimica Acta, 587*. https://doi.org/10.1016/j.cca.2026.120932.

Zago, E., Dal Molin, A., Dimitri, G. M., Xumerle, L., Pirazzini, C., Bacalini, M. G., ... Zago, E. (2022). Early downregulation of hsa-miR-144-3p in serum from drug-naïve Parkinson's disease patients. *Scientific Reports, 12*(1), 1330. https://doi.org/10.1038/s41598-022-05227-6.

Zarkali, A., Hannaway, N., Mccolgan, P., Heslegrave, A. J., Veleva, E., Laban, R., ... Weil, R. S. (2024). Neuroimaging and plasma evidence of early white matter loss in Parkinson's disease with poor outcomes. *Brain Communications, 6*(3), https://doi.org/10.1093/BRAINCOMMS/FCAE130.

Zarkali, A., McColgan, P., Leyland, L. A., Lees, A. J., & Weil, R. S. (2021). Visual dysfunction predicts cognitive impairment and white matter degeneration in Parkinson's disease. *Movement Disorders: Official Journal of the Movement Disorder Society, 36*(5), 1191–1202. https://doi.org/10.1002/MDS.28477.

Zarkali, A., Thomas, G. E. C., Zetterberg, H., & Weil, R. S. (2024). Neuroimaging and fluid biomarkers in Parkinson's disease in an era of targeted interventions. *Nature Communications, 15*(1), 5661. https://doi.org/10.1038/s41467-024-49949-9.

Zhang, F., Yang, W., Sun, R., Duan, X., Yang, Y., Wang, A., & Tian, Y. (2026). Cytokine-microglia interactions in neuroinflammation: Mechanisms, disease dynamics, and therapeutic strategies. *Antioxidants & Redox Signaling, 44*(7–9), https://doi.org/10.1177/15230864251401591.

Zhang, W. T., Wang, Y. J., Yao, Y. F., Zhang, G. X., Zhang, Y. N., & Gao, S. S. (2024). Circulating microRNAs as potential biomarkers for the diagnosis of Parkinson's disease: A meta-analysis. *Neurología, 39*(7), 573–583. https://doi.org/10.1016/J.NRL.2022.03.002.

Zhang, Z., Niu, K., Huang, T., Guo, J., Xarbat, G., Gong, X., ... Zhang, T. (2025). Microglia depletion reduces neurodegeneration and remodels extracellular matrix in a mouse Parkinson's disease model triggered by α-synuclein overexpression. *Npj Parkinson's Disease, 11*(1), 15. https://doi.org/10.1038/s41531-024-00846-4.

Zhao, Y., Haney, M. J., Fallon, J. K., Rodriguez, M., Swain, C. J., Arzt, C. J., ... Batrakova, E. V. (2022). Using extracellular vesicles released by GDNF-transfected macrophages for therapy of Parkinson disease. *Cells, 11*(12), https://doi.org/10.3390/CELLS11121933.

Zubelzu, M., Morera-Herreras, T., Irastorza, G., Gómez-Esteban, J. C., & Murueta-Goyena, A. (2022). Plasma and serum alpha-synuclein as a biomarker in Parkinson's disease: A meta-analysis. *Parkinsonism and Related Disorders, 99*, 107–115. https://doi.org/10.1016/j.parkreldis.2022.06.001.

Zucca, F. A., Capucciati, A., Bellei, C., Sarna, M., Sarna, T., Monzani, E., ... Zecca, L. (2023). Neuromelanins in brain aging and Parkinson's disease: Synthesis, structure, neuroinflammatory, and neurodegenerative role. *IUBMB Life, 75*(1), 55–65. https://doi.org/10.1002/IUB.2654.

Zucca, F. A., Segura-Aguilar, J., Ferrari, E., Muñoz, P., Paris, I., Sulzer, D., ... Zecca, L. (2017). Interactions of iron, dopamine and neuromelanin pathways in brain aging and Parkinson's disease. *Progress in Neurobiology, 155*, 96–119. https://doi.org/10.1016/j.pneurobio.2015.09.012.

CHAPTER TEN

Microglia in Alzheimer's disease: Insights into disease progression and therapy

Vaishali Saini, Srija Mukherjee[1], Chaitali Vora[1], Himanshi Jindal[1], and Hem Chandra Jha*
Mehta Family School of Biosciences and Biomedical Engineering, Indian Institute of Technology, Indore, Madhya Pradesh, India
*Corresponding author. e-mail address: hemcjha@iiti.ac.in

Contents

Abstract

The role of microglia, once seen as bystanders, has recently shifted to that of central regulators in disease pathology. The shift has been observed in M1/M2-polarized microglia to multiple configurations, including disease-associated microglia (DAM), lipid-droplet-accumulating microglia (LDAM), senescent microglia, and interferon-responsive microglia. This chapter provides a comprehensive synthesis of microglial biology across multiple interfaces, including transcriptomic, lipid-associated metabolic, cell senescence, and metabolic reprogramming. Metabolic disharmony in microglia occurs when lipid dysregulation and inflammasome activation occurs, leading to chronic inflammation beyond the basic phagocytic repair function of microglia. The TREM2-associated therapeutic

[1] These authors contributed equally.

Advances in Immunology, Volume 171
ISSN 0065-2776, https://doi.org/10.1016/bs.ai.2026.06.004

trajectory also shows a translational gap with mechanistic and clinical benefits. We also identify the need for critical disease-associated microglial biomarkers and intervention strategies. Moreover, advanced iPSC-derived microglia and chimeric models often yield specialized organoid co-cultures, accelerating microglia-mediated therapeutic studies. Collectively, this chapter entails microglia as a central player in AD. This positions microglia biology as a metabolically plastic, spatially organized immune-regulated microenvironment that can efficiently aid in reprogramming and AD therapeutics.

1. Introduction

Neurological disorders have been narrated as a neuron-centered catastrophe, such as Alzheimer's disease (AD), characterized by the accumulation of amyloid beta, tau hyperphosphorylation, malfunctioned synapses, and neuron death. The brain-resident immune cells, or microglia, have been cast as reactive bystanders, suggesting a role at damage sites as they become activated and contribute to inflammation. Interestingly, over the last few decades, microglia have emerged as central players in genetic and molecular modulation of AD progression. The primary microglia roles include debris clearance, synaptic maintenance, and communication among themselves and between neurons and astrocytes (Badimon et al., 2020). Microglial activation states are categorized into homeostatic and reactive states. Reactive microglia act as inflammatory mediators and exhibit a fluid-like nature, which is classified into M1 and M2 phenotypes based on their pro- and anti-inflammatory properties, respectively (Scheld et al., 2026). Of note, this dichotomy requires a comprehensive exploration of states of intermediate and disease-associated microglia (DAM). During the early stages of AD, the reactive microglia are involved in reduced Aβ deposition via phagocytosis (Wu et al., 2025). Although functionally advantageous, the overactivation of microglia via an inflammatory feedback loop might trigger neuronal damage and plaque deposition (Wang et al., 2025).

Genome-wide association studies (GWAS) led to the crucial identification of microglia as central players in AD progression, with Shade *et al.* identifying new risk loci in multiple neuropathologies. Interestingly, PIK3R5, which is highly expressed in microglia, was shown to be associated with neurofibrillary tangles (NFT) (Shade et al., 2024). Moreover, another study identified numerous risk factors associated with AD that are primarily expressed in microglia. The study identified 9 unique microglial clusters, including MS4A6A, EED, INPP5D, and RABEP1 (Cardona et al., 2025).

This implies the role of microglia in the development of neurological disorders. Beyond GWAS, several functional studies, such as the role of TREM2 as a lipid-sensing receptor, have elucidated the crucial role of microglial clustering around amyloid plaques (Wang et al., 2015). Using the 5XFAD mouse model, microglia-specific TFEB overexpression restored autophagy-lysosomal pathway (ALP) function, a pathway increasingly recognized as a key driver of AD progression. TFEB-mediated targeted activation in microglia can thus help reprogram degradative immune pathways and enhance Aβ clearance, thereby improving cognitive outcomes in AD (Kim et al., 2026). Yet another study showed that the mitigation of cognitive decline using induced pluripotent stem cell-generated microglia (iMGL) in the same mouse model. Of note, extracellular vesicles (EVs) derived from iMGL reduced Aβ plaques and microglial activation. This highlights neuroprotective signature of such microglia in AD mouse model (Krattli et al., 2026). Such repositioning of microglia as central drivers also led to the identification of distinct microglial phenotypes, including DAM, interferon-responsive, lipid-droplet-accumulating, and senescence-like (Toda Robert et al., 2026). More importantly, microglia are not just static; they incur dynamic transitions. In the early stages of AD, microglia reprogram to a protective state, while as pathology accumulates, they shift toward a chronic inflammatory, metabolically impaired state. This heterogeneity explains the failure of anti-inflammatory interventions as a part of improving AD symptoms. Transcriptomics identified different transcriptional trajectories in AD mice with genes associated with late-onset AD (Grubman et al., 2021). Such advances converge with microglial metabolism to identify microglial functions, such as lipid droplet accumulation, as targets for therapeutic intervention. Ideally, reprogramming microglia rather than suppressing them would limit maladaptive inflammatory cascades while retaining their beneficial phagocytic states. TREM2 agonism, inflammasome inhibition, complement pathway modulation, and metabolic interventions thus aim at restoring microglial fitness (Sprenger et al., 2025).

This chapter explores the comprehensive examination of emerging literature and the current role of microglia in AD progression. The identification of whether microglia are beneficial or detrimental in AD remains elusive; thus, we also aim to address the dichotomy of microglial states. We also discuss how these insights are being translated into therapeutic strategies that harness microglial function to ameliorate AD pathology.

2. New microglial taxonomies: Single-cell and spatial atlases

Microglia are now recognized as transcriptionally diverse and spatially dynamic innate immune cells, whose activation states are more precisely defined by single-cell and spatial omics approaches rather than by the binary M1/M2 polarization framework (Paolicelli et al., 2022; Gao et al., 2023). Comprehensive transcriptomic and proteomic analyses spanning development, aging, and disease have uncovered a continuum of phenotypes defined by coordinated gene expression modules and anatomical context. Within this complex and multidimensional framework, an expanding family of disease-associated microglial states has been delineated in neurodegenerative and inflammatory conditions, including disease-associated microglia (DAM), the microglial neurodegenerative phenotype (MGnD), and lipid-droplet–accumulating microglia (LDAM), among others (Sunna et al., 2023; Wei & Li, 2022). DAM and MGnD are characterized by downregulation of homeostatic "sensome" genes such as *P2RY12, CX3CR1* and *TMEM119*, coupled to upregulation of phagocytic, lysosomal and lipid metabolism programs centered on *APOE, TREM2, LPL, CST7* and related risk genes, and have been implicated in amyloid, tau and α-synuclein pathologies (Casali & Reed-Geaghan, 2021; Javanmehr et al., 2022; Krasemann et al., 2017). LDAM is predominantly identified in aging and chronic injury and is characterized by intracellular lipid droplet accumulation, oxidative stress signatures and impaired phagocytic capacity, thereby connecting disrupted immunometabolic processes with persistent neuroinflammation (Sung et al., 2025).

DAM were initially identified in AD mouse models as a TREM2-APOE-driven transcriptional program marked by downregulation of homeostatic genes (e.g. *P2ry12, Cx3cr1, Tmem119*) and upregulation of phagocytosis and lipid metabolism genes such as *Apoe, Lpl, Cst7, Trem2* (Deczkowska et al., 2018; Xu et al., 2022). Functionally, DAM clusters around amyloid plaques and other protein aggregates show enhanced phagocytic and lysosomal activity along with expression of inflammatory mediators. This suggests both neuroprotective and neurotoxic potential depending on various stages of microglia. The MGnD (neurodegenerative microglia) phenotype features *APOE*-dependent suppression of homeostatic genes and induction of complement, phagocytic, and metabolic programs, partly overlapping with DAM but distinct from classical "M1" signatures (Gao et al., 2023). Additional disease-associated states include interferon-responsive, proliferative, and border-associated programs, as well as disease-associated border macrophages (DaBAMs) in perivascular niches (Sun & Jiang, 2024; Vara-Pérez & Movahedi, 2025).

Comparative human-mouse studies converge on the idea that microglial activation is organized into conserved regulatory modules such as TREM2-APOE-driven lipid-phagocytic programs whose deployment, composition and spatial restriction diverge substantially between species (Cantoni et al., 2015). In both mouse AD models and human AD tissue, TREM2 loss-of-function attenuates the full acquisition of amyloid-responsive or DAM-like signatures (Zhao et al., 2022). This indicates a shared reliance on TREM2-dependent signaling with differential downstream transcriptional responses. At baseline, purified human cortical microglia show broad overlap with mouse core microglial genes such as *CX3CR1, P2RY12, ITGAM* but display preferential enrichment of innate immune receptors, including multiple TLRs, Fcγ receptors and SIGLEC family members that are not uniformly part of the mouse "signature" (Galatro et al., 2017). These human-enriched receptors, such as SIGLEC-11 and related inhibitory SIGLECs, modulate phagocytosis and oxidative burst, suggesting that human microglia are tuned toward stronger, yet more tightly checkpointed, sensing of tissue damage and immune complexes than their murine counterparts (Galatro et al., 2017). Age-associated shifts have been observed in longitudinal and cross-sectional profiling of the human microglia wherein the lipid and carbohydrate metabolism, interferon pathways, and APOE-related modules have been described (Lee et al., 2023). Moreover, certain AD-associated risk factors are critical while modeling in wild-type and single-transgene mouse lines when compared to human AD cortex. Large human microglial atlases such as HuMicA reveal multiple disease-associated subclasses (inflammatory and lipid-rich DAM, stress-related and border-associated states) across diverse brain disorders (Martins-Ferreira et al., 2025). Many only partially resemble mouse DAM or MGnD and show human-specific markers and pathways, indicating that "DAM-like" states are not one-to-one orthologues. Xenotransplantation of human microglia into mouse brains confirms human-specific, AD risk gene-enriched trajectories in response to Aβ, emphasizing the need for human tissue-based references.

High-resolution spatial transcriptomics in AD mouse models using platforms such as CosMx and Stereo-seq shows that amyloid plaques are embedded within discrete microglial niches characterized by dense accumulations of DAM-like cells and plaque-induced gene (PIG) modules (Mallach et al., 2024). Across hippocampus and cortex, microglia exhibit a relatively stereotyped transcriptional response to plaques, whereas astrocytic states vary markedly between regions, indicating that astrocytes provide a key axis of spatial heterogeneity. Within these niches, increasing microglial density and activation are tightly coupled to astrocyte acquisition of neurotoxic, complement- and cytokine-enriched signatures and to a shift in nearby neurons toward increased GABAergic and reduced glutamatergic signaling, linking plaque-proximal microglial states to local synaptic imbalance and circuit dysfunction. Human spatial transcriptomic studies of AD cortex similarly reveal plaque-glia niches that can be stratified by Aβ load and glial content, where GFAP/IBA1-enriched spots show coordinated upregulation of DAM, human AD-associated microglial, plaque-induced, and disease-associated astrocyte signatures (Avey et al., 2025). These glial-rich niches display downregulation of synaptic and axonal genes and enrichment of immune and stress pathways, supporting the view that reactive microglia-astrocyte networks create toxic inflammatory microenvironments around dense-core plaques (Hasel et al., 2023). Layer-resolved maps further assign glial and neuronal clusters to cortical laminae (L1-L6), white matter and meningeal regions, revealing that particular microglial states preferentially localize to plaque-rich deep layers, juxtacortical white matter or perivascular territories, thereby establishing spatially circumscribed immune microdomains with distinct effector programs and degrees of synaptic compromise (Bayraktar et al., 2018) (Fig. 1).

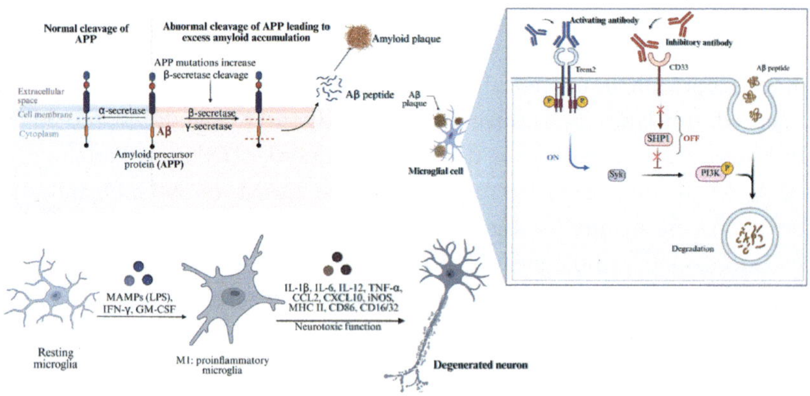

Fig. 1 Transition of resting to proinflammatory microglia leads to neurodegeneration. Microglial polarization occurs when multiple cytokines are induced to transition microglia from M0 to M1 (proinflammatory) state. This M1 microglia in turn release cytokines such as IL-6 that leads to degeneration of neurons. This also causes abnormal plaque clearance and hence higher deposition.

3. Lipid biology & lipid-laden microglia (LDAM)

Lipid-laden microglia, also known as lipid droplet-accumulating microglia (LDAM) are a dysfunctional microglial state characterized by the accumulation of triglyceride-rich lipid droplets (Marschallinger et al., 2020). These cells show impaired phagocytic capacity, increased pro-inflammatory signaling, and metabolic shifts away from oxidative phosphorylation toward glycolysis. LDAM were first described in aged mice as a distinct microglial state with abundant lipid droplets, defective phagocytosis, high ROS, and a pro-inflammatory transcriptome compared with homeostatic or classical DAM microglia (Sung et al., 2025). Triglyceride synthesis and lipid droplet formation involving enzymes such as ACSL1 and PLIN2 are involved in metabolic programming and act as innate immune triggers to bacterial products of amyloid fibrils (Kandpal et al., 2026; Singh et al., 2025a). Lipid droplets in LDAM constitute triglycerides and cholesterol esters. The abundance of such droplets is associated with downregulation of oxidative phosphorylation pathways and a subsequent shift towards glycolysis. Such changes interact to the TREM2-APOE associated signaling which ultimately leads to loss of microglia homeostatic markers and an enhanced inflammation. Beyond a risk factor in AD, APOE4 also acts as a genetic driver of LDAM which leads to impairment of lipid clearance. This was observed in both human iPSC derived microglia (iMG) and AD brain tissues (Haney et al., 2024). Higher LD accumulation occurs in APOE4/4 cells when compared to APOE3/3 which might be attributed to involvement of triglyceride synthesis via ACSL1 and DGAT1/2. APOE4-mediated remodeling of microglia LD proteome leads to entrapment of cholesterol esters in foam-cell-like state with defective reverse cholesterol transport (Stephenson et al., 2024). This eventually leads to lysosomal overload, impaired lipophagy, and neurotoxic extracellular lipid export via APOE4. Transcriptomics of LD-high microglia revealed an over-expression of NF-κB-associated cytokines (e.g., TNF, IL-1β) and chemokines with suppressed homeostatic genes (Wang et al., 2022). This marks a persistently inflamed LDAM state that gets intensified through NF-κB1/STAT4 activation. The APOE4-LDAM axis displays a conserved immunometabolic dysfunction which is elevated by genetic risks thus offering therapeutic benefits through ACSL1 blockade or lipophagy activation of microglial homeostasis (Table 1).

Table 1 Reported abundance of lipid-laden microglia (LDAM) across model systems and human cohorts.

Model system	Condition	Reported LDAM
Mouse aging	Aged mouse brain	Striking buildup of LDAM in aging mouse cortex; LDAM are a distinct microglial state enriched in old vs young brains (Marschallinger et al., 2020)
Human aging (AD)	Aged-matched controls and AD temporal cortex	LDAM clusters are enriched in AD brain sections (Marschallinger et al., 2020)
Human scRNA-seq (AD)	Postmortem AD with APOE4/4, APOE3/3	APOE4/4 AD brain has the highest percentage of LDAM; APOE3/3 AD has intermediate; aged-matched controls show the least LDAM (Haney et al., 2024).
Mouse AD (5xFAD)	Aβ-plaque-rich cortex	65 % of LDAM localized within plaque-associated regions (Marschallinger et al., 2020)
Human iPSC-microglia	APOE4/4 vs APOE3/3 iMG exposed to fAβ	APOE4/4 iMG show significantly higher LDAM fractions after fAβ compared with APOE3/3 isogenic controls, linking APOE4 genotype to LDAM predisposition (Haney et al., 2024; Mao et al., 2025)

4. Microglial senescence and aging phenotypes in Alzheimer's disease

Microglial senescence has been observed as a distinctive cellular phenotype in AD and can be segregated from classical and DAM microglial states. The convergence of aging and chronic Aβ exposure accelerates genomic, proteomic, and organellar damage that leads to oxidative stress with involvement of double-strand breaks, telomere dysfunction, and epigenetic erosion (Anderton et al., 2024). Persistent stress activates ATMATR kinase signaling and stabilizes p53 with p21-CIP1-mediated CDK2 inhibition (Hu et al., 2012). Parallel oxidative and mitogenic stress derepresses CDKN2A locus which further induces p16^INK4a and p15^INK4b ultimately maintaining retinoblastoma through CDK4/6 suppression (Kumari & Jat, 2021). Such checkpoints enable irreversible cell-cycle exit coupled with DNA damage response (DDR) and inflammatory signaling via NF-κB and C/EBPβ activation (Solier et al., 2012).

Senescent microglia exhibit dystrophic features, including fragmented processes alongside reduced arborization and impaired actin polymerization with reduced Rac1/cdc42 signaling. Such a phenotype is an outcome mitochondrial dysfunction (Davies et al., 2017). Chronic ROS exposure amplifies oxidative DNA damage and lipid peroxidation, reinforcing a self-propagating redox–DDR loop (Chen et al., 2025). Simultaneously, sustained PARP1 activation during base excision repair consumes intracellular NAD^+, constraining sirtuin (SIRT1/SIRT3) activity and suppressing mitochondrial biogenesis, antioxidant defenses, and metabolic flexibility (Cantó & Auwerx, 2011). Reduced NAMPT-dependent NAD^+ salvage and impaired AMPK signaling further entrench metabolic rigidity, biasing senescent microglia toward aerobic glycolysis and persistent inflammatory output (Nishida et al., 2022).

At the chromatin level, senescence is stabilized by large-scale epigenetic remodeling. Accessibility is lost at homeostatic loci such as P2RY12, TMEM119, and CX3CR1, disrupting surveillance and chemotactic gene networks, while inflammatory super-enhancers acquire H3K27ac and remain constitutively active (Zhang et al., 2023). Formation of senescence-associated heterochromatin foci, enrichment of H3K9me3, and stochastic DNA methylation drift lock microglia into a low-plasticity transcriptional state that partially overlaps with DAM signatures but lacks adaptive reparative or Aβ-compacting capacity. Functionally, senescent microglia are defined by acquisition of a senescence-associated secretory phenotype (SASP) that generates a chronic neurotoxic microenvironment. Constitutive NF-κB signaling-sustained by unresolved DDR cues, cytosolic DNA leakage activating cGAS-STING pathways, and loss of IL-10/SOCS-mediated negative feedback-drives long-term secretion of IL-1β, IL-6, TNF-α, CCL2, CXCL10, and complement components (C1q, C3) (Ng et al., 2023). Matrix metalloproteinases, prostaglandins, and reactive oxygen and nitrogen species further degrade extracellular structure and sensitize synapses to injury. Unlike transient immune activation, SASP signaling persists locally around Aβ deposits, impairing synaptic plasticity, suppressing long-term potentiation, and lowering the threshold for tau hyperphosphorylation and trans-synaptic spread (Muneer et al., 2016).

Concurrently, senescence-associated lysosomal and autophagic collapse exacerbates sterile inflammation. Defective v-ATPase–dependent acidification, cathepsin inactivation, and impaired autophagosome–lysosome fusion prevent degradation of engulfed material, leading to accumulation of lipofuscin, oxidized lipids, and cholesterol esters that act as damage-associated molecular patterns (Colacurcio & Nixon, 2016). These signals chronically activate the NLRP3 inflammasome, promoting caspase-1-dependent IL-1β maturation and perpetuating inflammation independent of new Aβ deposition. Collectively, senescent microglia become metabolically and transcriptionally locked-optimized for cytokine production but deficient in clearance and repair-thereby converting molecular aging into sustained synaptic dysfunction and network-level neurodegeneration (Saini et al., 2023; Xu & Núñez, 2023).

5. Metabolic reprogramming and functional trade-offs

Metabolic remodeling provides the energetic substrate linking microglial senescence to neurodegenerative cascades. Senescent microglia display impaired mitochondrial electron transport, elevated mitochondrial DNA lesions, defective mitophagy, and chronic NAD^+ depletion secondary to sustained PARP-driven repair activity (Li et al., 2022). NAD^+ loss restricts sirtuin-dependent transcriptional control and mitochondrial biogenesis, diverting metabolism toward aerobic glycolysis. This configuration supports cytokine synthesis but fails to meet ATP-intensive requirements for cytoskeletal remodeling, chemotaxis, and phagocytic cup formation (Bonkowski & Sinclair, 2016). Concurrently, disrupted cholesterol homeostasis and APOE-regulated lipid flux drive lipid droplet accumulation, compromising lysosomal acidification and suppressing TREM2-mediated reparative signaling. These senescent microglia also act as mediators of chronic synaptic and network dysfunction (Li et al., 2025). This framework justifies both senolytic approaches that ablate irreversibly senescent microglia and senomorphic strategies aimed at repressing SASP transmission or reconstituting mitochondrial and lysosomal fitness, underscoring the importance of interventions distinguishing reversible dysfunction from terminal senescence (Tripathi et al., 2026).

Microglial identity is defined metabolically by enforcing phagocytic efficacy that defines aging and neurodegenerative burden. In homeostatic states, microglia preferentially engage mitochondrial oxidative phosphorylation (OXPHOS) to sustain high-yield ATP generation, redox equilibrium, and anabolic flexibility (Leng & Zhang, 2023). Such energetics enables actin turnover, vesicular trafficking, chemotaxis, and debris clearance. Chronic Aβ-induced mitochondrial impairment shows aerobic glycolysis instead of Warburg effect which stems from persistent DNA damage and NF-κB-mediated inflammatory signalling. This shows that metabolic potential is constrained due to damaged microglia leading to reduced functional diversity (Cameron et al., 2019). The OXPHOS-glycolysis ratio, displaying balanced phagocytic and cytokine mechanisms is efficiently maintained via mitochondrial membrane potential and ATP buffering (Grubelnik et al., 2025). Glycolytic by-products hinder with nucleotide and lipid precursor availability which also supports inflammasome activation (Kierans & Taylor, 2024).

Monocarboxylate Transporters (MCT1, MCT4) regulate lactate shuttling and maintain intracellular NAD^+/NADH ratios. Mislocalization due to aging might lead to lactate retention and cytoplasmic acidification ultimately suppressing mitochondrial respiration (Ammar et al., 2023). Lactate mediates histone lactylation and induces proinflammatory transcripts which alter chromatin structure. Parallel to this, reduced pyruvate imports lower α-ketoglutarate levels which causes demethylation and anti-inflammatory programming (Wang et al., 2026). Loss of purinergic receptor, P2RY12, from healthy microglia causes reduced chemotaxis mediated by mitochondria. Chronic inflammation and DNA damage along with P2RY12 down-regulation causes impaired mitochondrial potential and calcium-mediated signaling. Such a transition shifts surveillant microglia to a pro-inflammatory state leading to critical pathways such as PARP activation and defective NAD + regeneration (Lou et al., 2016). Such an entrapment of microglia selectively leads to NF-κB-driven cytokine production and impairs efficient clearing mechanisms (Yusri et al., 2025). This leads to chronic neuroinflammation coexisting with inefficient Aβ removal which reduces microglial competence (Lopez-Ortiz et al., 2025). Therefore, there is a need for central therapeutic targets which would be able to restore microglia functioning for efficient clearing mechanisms.

Microglia have also been implicated in cortical circuit formation with divergent expression among different species. Of note, neural cells diverged rapidly on the human lineage and have 328 differentially expressed genes (DEGs) when compared to chimpanzee (175) and gorilla (164). These DEGs were disease-associated genes such as SNCA. Interestingly, the proportion of DEGs near human accelerated regions (HARs) were highest among microglia which could be attributed to intronic and flanking regions

(Jorstad et al., 2023). This indicates faster divergence in non-neuronal cell types. Converging literature shows a plausible connection between HARs within microbiota-microglia axis. This could become regulatory through microglial function and maturation via immune and metabolic signaling (He et al., 2024). Parallel to this, HARs control neurodevelopment and immune gene networks by acting as human-specific enhancers (Singh et al., 2025b).

6. Inflammasomes, NLRP3 and neuroinflammation: Translational potential through immunotherapy

Alzheimer diseases is chronic, widespread progressive neurodegenerative diseases, initially presenting with cognitive disorders, memory impairment which significantly leads to challenges in activities and early onset of psychiatric symptoms. The pathology of AD patients has been linked to accumulation of β-amyloid (Aβ) plaques, formation of neurofibrils tangles and hyperphosphorylation of tau proteins (Li & Gong, 2025).

Inflammasomes are cellular protein complexes that regulate inflammation in brain and other tissues. They plays a crucial role in neuroinflammation and present in neurons, microglia and astrocytes where they detect the signals from damaged cells. NLRP3 are most extensively studied inflammasomes in brain cells and it is linked to several neurological disorders such as Alzheimer diseases. In transgenic models' suppression of NLRP3 has been shown to decrease the accumulation of Aβ, mitochondrial dysfunctioning, synaptic deterioration and cognitive impairment. Due to the activation of NLRP3, transition of microglial states towards inflammation, adaptor protein ASC and procaspase-1, which collectively activate caspase-1, leads to production of inflammatory molecules such as IL-1β and IL-18 and facilitates aggregation of Aβ. Peripheral blood mononuclear cells from AD patients shows hyperactivation of NLRP3 link to central nervous system pathology (Han et al., 2024) (Fig. 2).

MCC950 is a diarylsulphonylurea-containing small molecule inhibitor of NLRP3 by inhibiting the ATPase activity of NACHT domain and preventing oligomerization, ASC recruitment and inflammasome assembly. This small molecule inhibits microglial NLRP3 activation in mice model as well and reduces release of pro-inflammatory cytokines induced activation of γδ T cells also it decreases the aggregation of Aβ plaques in APP/PS1 brains and improves neurobehavior and amyloid accumulation (Dempsey et al., 2017).

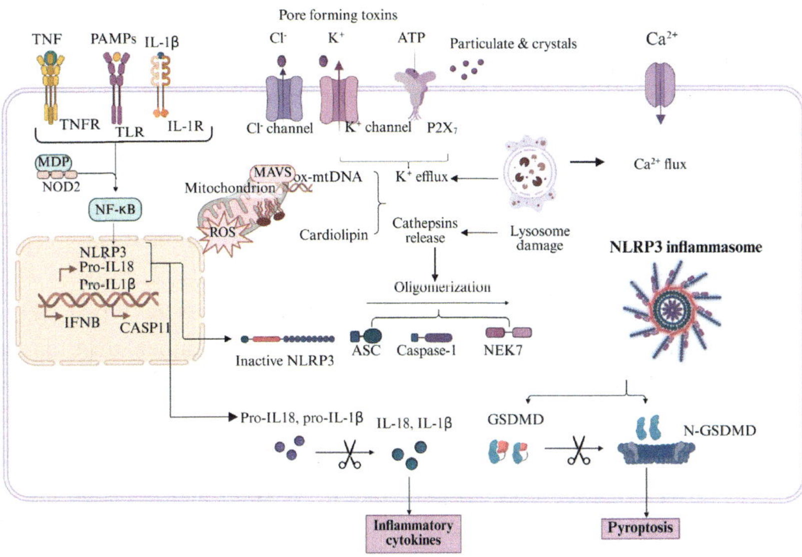

Fig. 2 Mitochondria and NLRP3 inflammasome mediated microglial activation. Several receptors such as including TNFR, TLR, IL-1R, and Chloride/potassium channels are involved in activation of downstream signalling molecules such as NF-kB and NLRP3. These release pro-inflammatory pathways to further induce neuroinflammation.

MCC950 not only reduces the activation of NLRP3 but also modulates the autophagy pathways by reducing the autophagic flux and induces transcriptional & functional changes to improve the neuron activity and BDNF expression in sporadic AD models. This inhibitor reduces the activation of inflammasome by these markers such as CD11b & CD68 which reflects the alteration in immune system (He et al., 2020). Some other inhibitors such as BAL-0028 and BAL-0598 which potentially inhibit gain of function mutation in nucleotide binding domain/helical domain 2 through human NLRP3-AID PBMCs and cellular models. Mutations include severe neonatal-onset multisystem inflammatory diseases (NOMID) variants (D303H, K568N, Y570C) and somatic mutations (D303H, K565E, E567G, K568N, Y570C) that causes hyperactivation of NLRP3 in AD person which elevates neuroinflammation (Wilhelmsen et al., 2025).

Some immunotherapies, either active or passive anti-amyloid antibodies, mediates beneficial effects during microglial activation. The potential of anti-Aβ monoclonal antibodies to suppress the progression of Alzheimer's disease progression which depend on the solubility of Aβ antibodies in the brain which also effects on neuropathological mechanisms and reduces the cerebral Aβ (Loeffler, 2023). Anti- Aβ monoclonal antibodies (mAbs) bind at specific site includes protofibrils & fibrillar plaques which facilitates clearance through microglial Fcγ receptor engagement. Further, the IgG1 Fc region first interacts with FcγIIa & FcγIIIa, activates the immunoreceptor tyrosine-based activation motif signaling pathways that includes IP3-mediated Ca2+ mobilization, Syk/PLCγ2 phosphorylation & Rac1-Arp2/3 nucleation complex-driven cytoskeletal remodeling which further facilitates the upregulation of phagocytosis machinery of Aβ-antibody immune complexes, complement receptors & lipid metabolism genes such as (C1qa, C3b, Apoe & LpI) leads to elimination of synapsis (Elamin et al., 2025; Yadollahikhales & Rojas, 2023). NLRP3 interacts with TLR4/complement primarily rather than directly regulating FcγR phagocytosis. Excessive NLRP3 reduces risks of attenuating phagocytosis during early phases of treatment. NLRP3 inhibitors when pairs with anti- Aβ monoclonal antibodies, people are segregated by APOE geneotype, amyloid & tau levels, markers such as IL-1β which is responsible for inflammation (De Weerd et al., 2025).

7. Therapeutic targeting: The TREM2 story and Imaging biomarkers to monitor microglial biology in patients

Triggering receptor expressed on myeloid cells 2 (TREM2) functions as a lipid- and damage-sensing receptor that orchestrates microglial immunometabolism adaptation in neurodegenerative contexts. Structurally, TREM2 is a single-pass transmembrane receptor that associates with the ITAM-containing adaptor DAP12 (TYROBP), enabling phosphorylation-dependent recruitment of SYK kinase and activation of downstream PI3K–AKT–mTOR and ERK signaling cascades (Deming et al., 2018). This signaling axis regulates actin remodeling, survival, proliferation, and metabolic reprogramming. Importantly, TREM2 binds an array of lipid ligands, including phosphatidylserine, sulfatides, apolipoproteins (notably ApoE), and lipoprotein particles, thereby positioning it as a central node in microglial lipid sensing (Li et al., 2022). In AD, TREM2 signaling is required for the transition of homeostatic microglia into DAM, a transcriptional state characterized by upregulation of genes involved in lipid metabolism (LPL, APOE), phagocytosis (CTSD), and lysosomal function (Nugent et al., 2020). Loss-of-function variants such as R47H impair ligand binding and downstream signaling, resulting in defective microglial clustering around amyloid plaques, reduced plaque compaction, and increased axonal dystrophy (Cheng-Hathaway et al., 2018). TREM2 deficiency disrupts cholesterol efflux and mitochondrial fitness, promoting lipid accumulation and contributing to LDAM. Thus, TREM2 integrates extracellular lipid cues with intracellular metabolic programs, and its dysfunction drives a failure of microglial containment responses in AD (Ishikawa et al., 2025).

These mechanistic insights provided the rationale for therapeutic agonism of TREM2, exemplified by the monoclonal antibody AL002, designed to stabilize receptor conformation and enhance downstream signaling (Long et al., 2024). In preclinical models, including 5xFAD and APP knock-in mice, TREM2 agonist antibodies increased microglial proliferation, enhanced plaque-associated microglial clustering, and promoted compaction of amyloid fibrils into less neurotoxic conformations (Wang et al., 2020). Transcriptomic analyses demonstrated upregulation of DAM-associated gene programs and partial restoration of lipid metabolic pathways, including increased expression of cholesterol transporters and lysosomal enzymes. Furthermore, TREM2 activation improved mitochondrial bioenergetics, reducing reactive oxygen species (ROS) accumulation and enhancing phagocytic capacity. Translation into human systems, including iPSC-derived microglia and chimeric xenotransplantation models, confirmed that AL002 induces conserved signaling responses, including SYK phosphorylation and increased soluble TREM2 (sTREM2) shedding, a biomarker of receptor engagement (Long et al., 2024). Favorable pharmacokinetics and pharmacodynamics have been shown in clinical studies which modulate inflammatory cytokines by dose-dependent increment of CSF sTREM2. A phase 2 clinical trial could not show improved cognitive function even with clear biological activity (Wu et al., 2025). This could be due to difference in clinical outcomes which is perceived through certain considerations including the time of intervention as TREM2 is involved in early plaque deposition and thus becomes less efficient in latter stages of the disease (Yu et al., 2025). Moreover, sustained activation could also cause maladaptive states including LDAM formation via persistent lipid update and partial catabolism. Additionally, the variability among the population is due to difference in APOE genotype and microglia activation. Collectively, such differences suggest TREM2-targeted therapies would require time-dependent dosing and temporal stratification, and combinatorial approaches to achieve maximum clinical benefit (Wu et al., 2026).

The development of imaging biomarkers becomes essential for in vivo characterization of microglial dynamics and for therapeutic purposes. Positron emission tomography (PET) imaging utilized to target translocator protein (TSPO) remains the most common approach to assess neuroinflammation (Tronel et al., 2017). TSPO is upregulated in microglia and astrocytes that are activated because of neuroinflammation which is detected by certain radioligands including [^{11}C]-PBR28, [^{18}F]-DPA-714. TSPO-PET remains limited as it lacks cellular specificity and sensitivity to genetic polymorphisms such as rs6971 that affect the binding affinity and complicates quantitative interpretation (Zheng et al., 2016). Multiple emerging strategies aim to overcome such limitations that target microglia-specific markers including TREM2, CSF1R, and P2RY12 and integrates advanced MRI techniques to assess structural and metabolic modalities (Bobotis et al., 2024). Multimodal biomarker frameworks involving lipidomic and single transcriptomic profiling offer comprehensive approach to elucidate different microglial states and transitions. Spatial and temporal mapping of microglial activation can also be correlated to amyloid or tau pathology to enable assessment of various therapeutic interventions as means to restore microglial functioning.

8. Human models & platform technologies accelerating discovery and conceptual reframing through open questions

Translating microglia biology has been a critical limitation, leading to reliance on rodent models. Rodent models rely on labeling depleting microglia in addition to altering gene expression, such as CX3CR1+/GFP transgenic, CSF1R-deficient, or CD11b-Cre transgenic mice. To recapitulate the functional and genetic architecture of human microglia, human induced pluripotent stem cell-derived microglia (iMGL) have emerged to enable patient-specific microglial behavior in vitro (Dolan et al., 2023). The iMGLs have transcriptomic signatures similar to those of primary human microglia from both adult and fetus (Abud et al., 2017). The authors of this study noted that, in addition to their functional similarity, iMGLs can also be used to study AD. The two characteristics that make iMGLs beneficial are their ability to internalize Aβ or tau (Abud et al., 2017). This finding is crucial as iMGLs can be utilized to identify therapeutic targets against amyloid aggregates via high-throughput drug-screening assays to promote clearance or degradation.

Beyond in vitro, numerous chimeric mouse models have been extended to iMGLs in *vivo*. Such models use iPSC-derived progenitor cells for transplantation into the postnatal brains of humanized immunodeficient mice, enabling them to study human microglia in a surrogate brain environment (Hasselmann et al., 2019). Interestingly, the transplanted microglia responded to Aβ plaques, providing a powerful tool for demonstrating a chimeric model with genetically modified microglia. Another study by Mancuso et al. generated expression profiles of human stem cell-derived microglia xenotransplanted in the APP mouse model (Mancuso et al., 2024). This aids in identifying a multipronged response to AD pathology and, in turn, supports translational research.

Recent advancements in this area have also been made in treatment of certain disorders. (Chen et al., 2025) showed that the microglial transplantation strategy without conditioning, known as tricyclic microglial depletion for transplantation (TCMDT), is crucial for the engraftment of exogenous microglia (Chen et al., 2025). The transplantation could efficiently rescue microglial dysfunction and also mitigate AD pathology. This is also complemented in vitro by utilizing human iPSC-derived brain organoids. A multifactorial disease such as AD would benefit from such advanced models, as brain organoids (BOs) have recently been incorporated or co-cultured with microglia. This is shown by Wenzel *et al.*, who demonstrated that Aβ oligomerization is promoted in BO co-cultures, coinciding with a significant increase in IBA1 levels (Wenzel et al., 2024). This overcomes the initial stages of the Aβ challenge and can also help develop effective therapies for AD and provide improved diagnostic tools to identify its various subtypes.

9. Conclusion

This chapter collectively explains the dynamics of microglial biology with their involvement as state-dependent regulators in AD pathogenesis rather than simply acting as inflammatory mediators. The convergence of single-cell transcriptomics, spatial omics, metabolomics, and consequential integration with iPSCs has revealed an unprecedented solution for understanding microglial heterogeneity along with both protective and pathological functions. This also differs in context-specific interactions such as genetic background, disease stages and cerebral microenvironment.

Several critical gaps still exist as the causal and consequential nature of senescent, dysfunctional microglia remain unresolved. Interestingly, the consequences of microglia polarization or senescence are largely unknown in non-amyloid AD plaques. Furthermore, future research shall involve multi-omic profiling of human microglia across disease stages alongside efficient CNS-selective delivery mechanisms of modulating microglia in AD therapeutics. Ultimately, such selective reprogramming of microglia towards restorative states would preserve immune competence while also resolving chronic inflammation.

Acknowledgments

We thank Centre for Rural Development and Technology, IIT Indore, grant no. IITI/CRDT/2022–23/05, Anusandhan National Research Foundation, ANRF/PAIR/2025/000018/PAIR-A(G), and PMRF grant ID: 2103365. We thank the Ministry of Human Resource Development (MHRD), Govt. of India for providing financial support in the form of a fellowship to Vaishali Saini, Srija Mukherjee, and Chaitali Vora. The funding bodies do not have a role in study design and manuscript preparation. We acknowledge the Indian Institute of Technology Indore for providing support in the form of facilities.

Authors' contribution

Hem Chandra Jha: Conceptualization; Vaishali Saini: Conceptualization, content writing, draft preparation; Himanshi Jindal, Srija Mukherjee, Chaitali Vora: Content writing and editing; Figure preparation: Himanshi Jindal; Table preparation: Srija Mukherjee; Dr. Hem Chandra Jha: Conceptualization, review, editing, fund acquisition and project administration.

All authors read and approved the manuscript and declare no conflict of interest.

References

Abud, E. M., Ramirez, R. N., Martinez, E. S., Healy, L. M., Nguyen, C. H. H., Newman, S. A., ... Blurton-Jones, M. (2017). iPSC-derived human microglia-like cells to study neurological diseases. *Neuron, 94*, 278–293.e9. https://doi.org/10.1016/j.neuron.2017.03.042.

Ammar, N., Hildebrandt, M., Geismann, C., Röder, C., Gemoll, T., Sebens, S., ... Schäfer, H. (2023). Monocarboxylate transporter-1 (MCT1)-mediated lactate uptake protects pancreatic adenocarcinoma cells from oxidative stress during glutamine scarcity thereby promoting resistance against inhibitors of glutamine metabolism. *Antioxidants, 12*, 1818. https://doi.org/10.3390/antiox12101818.

Anderton, E., Chamoli, M., Bhaumik, D., King, C. D., Xie, X., Foulger, A., ... Lithgow, G. J. (2024). Amyloid β accelerates age-related proteome-wide protein insolubility. *GeroScience, 46*, 4585–4602. https://doi.org/10.1007/s11357-024-01169-1.

Avey, D. R., Ng, B., Vialle, R. A., Kearns, N. A., De Paiva Lopes, K., Iatrou, A., ... Wang, Y. (2025). Uncovering plaque-glia niches in human Alzheimer's disease brains using spatial transcriptomics. *Molecular Neurodegeneration Advances, 1*, 2. https://doi.org/10.1186/s44477-025-00002-z.

Badimon, A., Strasburger, H. J., Ayata, P., Chen, X., Nair, A., Ikegami, A., ... Schaefer, A. (2020). Negative feedback control of neuronal activity by microglia. *Nature, 586*, 417–423. https://doi.org/10.1038/s41586-020-2777-8.

Bayraktar, O.A., Bartels, T., Polioudakis, D., Holmqvist, S., Haim, L.B. , Young, A.M.H., ... Prakash, K. (2018). Single-cell in situ transcriptomic map of astrocyte cortical layer diversity. https://doi.org/10.1101/432104.

Bobotis, B. C., Halvorson, T., Carrier, M., & Tremblay, M.-È. (2024). Established and emerging techniques for the study of microglia: Visualization, depletion, and fate mapping. *Frontiers in Cellular Neuroscience, 18*, 1317125. https://doi.org/10.3389/fncel.2024.1317125.

Bonkowski, M. S., & Sinclair, D. A. (2016). Slowing ageing by design: The rise of NAD+ and sirtuin-activating compounds. *Nature Reviews. Molecular Cell Biology, 17*, 679–690. https://doi.org/10.1038/nrm.2016.93.

Cameron, A. M., Castoldi, A., Sanin, D. E., Flachsmann, L. J., Field, C. S., Puleston, D. J., ... Pearce, E. J. (2019). Inflammatory macrophage dependence on NAD+ salvage is a consequence of reactive oxygen species–mediated DNA damage. *Nature Immunology, 20*, 420–432. https://doi.org/10.1038/s41590-019-0336-y.

Cantó, C., & Auwerx, J. (2011). Interference between PARPs and SIRT1: A novel approach to healthy ageing? *Aging, 3*, 543–547. https://doi.org/10.18632/aging.100326.

Cantoni, C., Bollman, B., Licastro, D., Xie, M., Mikesell, R., Schmidt, R., ... Piccio, L. (2015). TREM2 regulates microglial cell activation in response to demyelination in vivo. *Acta Neuropathologica (Berl.), 129*, 429–447. https://doi.org/10.1007/s00401-015-1388-1.

Cardona, C. L., Wei, L., Kim, J., Angeles, E., Singh, G., Chen, S., ... Sproul, A. A. (2025). High throughput identification of genetic regulators of microglial inflammatory processes in Alzheimer's disease. *Journal of Neuroinflammation, 22*, 294. https://doi.org/10.1186/s12974-025-03562-9.

Casali, B. T., & Reed-Geaghan, E. G. (2021). Microglial function and regulation during development, homeostasis and Alzheimer's disease. *Cells, 10*, 957. https://doi.org/10.3390/cells10040957.

Chen, D., Wang, C., Chen, X., Li, J., Chen, S., Li, Y., ... Zhong, L. (2025). Brain-wide microglia replacement using a nonconditioning strategy ameliorates pathology in mouse models of neurological disorders. *Science Translational Medicine, 17*, eads6111. https://doi.org/10.1126/scitranslmed.ads6111.

Chen, Y.-S., Tian, H.-X., Rong, D.-C., Wang, L., Chen, S., Zeng, J., ... Zhou, H.-H. (2025). ROS homeostasis in cell fate, pathophysiology, and therapeutic interventions. *Molecular Biomedicine, 6*, 89. https://doi.org/10.1186/s43556-025-00338-8.

Cheng-Hathaway, P. J., Reed-Geaghan, E. G., Jay, T. R., Casali, B. T., Bemiller, S. M., Puntambekar, S. S., ... Landreth, G. E. (2018). The Trem2 R47H variant confers loss-of-function-like phenotypes in Alzheimer's disease. *Molecular Neurodegeneration, 13*, 29. https://doi.org/10.1186/s13024-018-0262-8.

Colacurcio, D. J., & Nixon, R. A. (2016). Disorders of lysosomal acidification—The emerging role of v-ATPase in aging and neurodegenerative disease. *Ageing Research Reviews, 32*, 75–88. https://doi.org/10.1016/j.arr.2016.05.004.

Davies, D. S., Ma, J., Jegathees, T., & Goldsbury, C. (2017). Microglia show altered morphology and reduced arborization in human brain during aging and Alzheimer's disease. *Brain Pathology (Zurich, Switzerland), 27*, 795–808. https://doi.org/10.1111/bpa.12456.

De Weerd, L., Hummel, S., Müller, S. A., Paris, I., Sandmann, T., Eichholtz, M., ... Haass, C. (2025). Early intervention anti-Aβ immunotherapy attenuates microglial activation without inducing exhaustion at residual plaques. *Molecular Neurodegeneration, 20*, 92. https://doi.org/10.1186/s13024-025-00878-1.

Deczkowska, A., Keren-Shaul, H., Weiner, A., Colonna, M., Schwartz, M., & Amit, I. (2018). Disease-associated microglia: A universal immune sensor of neurodegeneration. *Cell, 173*, 1073–1081. https://doi.org/10.1016/j.cell.2018.05.003.

Deming, Y., Li, Z., Benitez, B. A., & Cruchaga, C. (2018). Triggering receptor expressed on myeloid cells 2 (TREM2): A potential therapeutic target for Alzheimer disease? *Expert Opinion on Therapeutic Targets, 22*, 587–598. https://doi.org/10.1080/14728222.2018.1486823.

Dempsey, C., Rubio Araiz, A., Bryson, K. J., Finucane, O., Larkin, C., Mills, E. L., ... Lynch, M. A. (2017). Inhibiting the NLRP3 inflammasome with MCC950 promotes non-phlogistic clearance of amyloid-β and cognitive function in APP/PS1 mice. *Brain, Behavior, and Immunity, 61*, 306–316. https://doi.org/10.1016/j.bbi.2016.12.014.

Dolan, M.-J., Therrien, M., Jereb, S., Kamath, T., Gazestani, V., Atkeson, T., ... Stevens, B. (2023). Exposure of iPSC-derived human microglia to brain substrates enables the generation and manipulation of diverse transcriptional states in vitro. *Nature Immunology, 24*, 1382–1390. https://doi.org/10.1038/s41590-023-01558-2.

Elamin, S. A., Al Shibli, A. N., Shaito, A., Al-Maadhadi, M. J. M. B., Zolezzi, M., & Pedersen, S. (2025). Anti-amyloid monoclonal antibody therapies in Alzheimer's disease – a scoping review. *Neuroscience, 589*, 50–61. https://doi.org/10.1016/j.neuroscience.2025.10.011.

Galatro, T. F., Holtman, I. R., Lerario, A. M., Vainchtein, I. D., Brouwer, N., Sola, P. R., ... Eggen, B. J. L. (2017). Transcriptomic analysis of purified human cortical microglia reveals age-associated changes. *Nature Neuroscience, 20*, 1162–1171. https://doi.org/10.1038/nn.4597.

Gao, C., Jiang, J., Tan, Y., & Chen, S. (2023). Microglia in neurodegenerative diseases: Mechanism and potential therapeutic targets. *Signal Transduction and Targeted Therapy, 8*, 359. https://doi.org/10.1038/s41392-023-01588-0.

Grubelnik, V., Zmazek, J., & Marhl, M. (2025). The synergistic impact of glycolysis, mitochondrial OxPhos, and PEP cycling on ATP production in beta cells. *International Journal of Molecular Sciences, 26*, 1454. https://doi.org/10.3390/ijms26041454.

Grubman, A., Choo, X. Y., Chew, G., Ouyang, J. F., Sun, G., Croft, N. P., ... Polo, J. M. (2021). Transcriptional signature in microglia associated with Aβ plaque phagocytosis. *Nature Communications, 12*, 3015. https://doi.org/10.1038/s41467-021-23111-1.

Han, Q., Li, W., Chen, P., Wang, L., Bao, X., Huang, R., ... Chen, X. (2024). Microglial NLRP3 inflammasome-mediated neuroinflammation and therapeutic strategies in depression. *Neural Regen. Res. 19*, 1890–1898. https://doi.org/10.4103/1673-5374.390964.

Haney, M. S., Pálovics, R., Munson, C. N., Long, C., Johansson, P. K., Yip, O., ... Wyss-Coray, T. (2024). APOE4/4 is linked to damaging lipid droplets in Alzheimer's disease microglia. *Nature, 628*, 154–161. https://doi.org/10.1038/s41586-024-07185-7.

Hasel, P., Aisenberg, W. H., Bennett, F. C., & Liddelow, S. A. (2023). Molecular and metabolic heterogeneity of astrocytes and microglia. *Cell Metabolism, 35*, 555–570. https://doi.org/10.1016/j.cmet.2023.03.006.

Hasselmann, J., Coburn, M. A., England, W., Figueroa Velez, D. X., Kiani Shabestari, S., Tu, C. H., ... Blurton-Jones, M. (2019). Development of a chimeric model to study and manipulate human microglia in vivo. *Neuron, 103*, 1016–1033.e10. https://doi.org/10.1016/j.neuron.2019.07.002.

He, H., He, H., Mo, L., Yuan, Q., Xiao, C., Ma, Q., ... Zhang, J. (2024). Gut microbiota regulate stress resistance by influencing microglia-neuron interactions in the hippocampus. *Brain, Behavior, and Immunity - Health, 36*, 100729. https://doi.org/10.1016/j.bbih.2024.100729.

He, X., Xu, J., Li, G., Li, M., Li, L., Pei, Z., ... Hu, X. (2020). NLRP3-dependent microglial training impaired the clearance of amyloid-beta and aggravated the cognitive decline in Alzheimer's disease. *Cell Death & Disease, 11*, 849. https://doi.org/10.1038/s41419-020-03072-x.

Hu, W., Feng, Z., & Levine, A. J. (2012). The regulation of multiple p53 stress responses is mediated through MDM2. *Genes Cancer, 3*, 199–208. https://doi.org/10.1177/1947601912454734.

Ishikawa, K., Fujikawa, R., Okita, K., Kimura, F., Watanabe, T., Katsurabayashi, S., & Iwasaki, K. (2025). Microglia in brain aging and age-related diseases: Friends or foes? *International Journal of Molecular Sciences, 26*, 11494. https://doi.org/10.3390/ijms262311494.

Javanmehr, N., Saleki, K., Alijanizadeh, P., & Rezaei, N. (2022). Microglia dynamics in aging-related neurobehavioral and neuroinflammatory diseases. *Journal of Neuroinflammation, 19*, 273. https://doi.org/10.1186/s12974-022-02637-1.

Jorstad, N. L., Song, J. H. T., Exposito-Alonso, D., Suresh, H., Castro-Pacheco, N., Krienen, F. M., ... Bakken, T. E. (2023). Comparative transcriptomics reveals human-specific cortical features. *Science (New York, N. Y.), 382*, eade9516. https://doi.org/10.1126/science.ade9516.

Kandpal, M., Verma, T. P., Singh, S., Parmar, H., & Jha, H. C. (2026). Metabolomic and lipidomic signatures of *Helicobacter pylori* infection: Unveiling biochemical pathways associated with neurodegeneration. *iMetaOmics*, e70088. https://doi.org/10.1002/imo2.70088.

Kierans, S. J., & Taylor, C. T. (2024). Glycolysis: A multifaceted metabolic pathway and signaling hub. *The Journal of Biological Chemistry, 300*, 107906. https://doi.org/10.1016/j.jbc.2024.107906.

Kim, Y., Ha, T.-Y., Kondaurova, O., Lee, M.-S., & Chang, K.-A. (2026). Microglia TFEB activation attenuates Alzheimer's disease pathology by enhancing autophagy-lysosomal function. *Journal of Neuroinflammation, 23*, 88. https://doi.org/10.1186/s12974-026-03728-z.

Krasemann, S., Madore, C., Cialic, R., Baufeld, C., Calcagno, N., El Fatimy, R., ... Butovsky, O. (2017). The TREM2-APOE pathway drives the transcriptional phenotype of dysfunctional microglia in neurodegenerative diseases. *Immunity, 47*, 566–581.e9. https://doi.org/10.1016/j.immuni.2017.08.008.

Krattli, R. P., Markarian, M., Madan, S., Swami, D., McQuade, A., Baulch, J. E., ... Acharya, M. M. (2026). Comparing functional consequences of human IPSC -microglia and neural stem cell-derived extracellular vesicles in mitigating cognitive decline in Alzheimer's disease. *Aging Cell, 25*, e70341. https://doi.org/10.1111/acel.70341.

Kumari, R., & Jat, P. (2021). Mechanisms of cellular senescence: Cell cycle arrest and senescence associated secretory phenotype. *Frontiers in Cell and Developmental Biology, 9*, 645593. https://doi.org/10.3389/fcell.2021.645593.

Lee, S., Devanney, N. A., Golden, L. R., Smith, C. T., Schwartz, J. L., Walsh, A. E., ... Johnson, L. A. (2023). APOE modulates microglial immunometabolism in response to age, amyloid pathology, and inflammatory challenge. *Cell Reports, 42*, 112196. https://doi.org/10.1016/j.celrep.2023.112196.

Leng, L., & Zhang, J. (2023). Microglial metabolic reconfiguration provides a new strategy for the treatment of Alzheimer's disease. *Neural Regeneration Research*. https://doi.org/10.4103/1673-5374.367842.

Li, R.-Y., Qin, Q., Yang, H.-C., Wang, Y.-Y., Mi, Y.-X., Yin, Y.-S., ... Tang, Y. (2022). TREM2 in the pathogenesis of AD: A lipid metabolism regulator and potential metabolic therapeutic target. *Molecular Neurodegeneration, 17*, 40. https://doi.org/10.1186/s13024-022-00542-y.

Li, Y., Xia, X., Wang, Y., & Zheng, J. C. (2022). Mitochondrial dysfunction in microglia: A novel perspective for pathogenesis of Alzheimer's disease. *Journal of Neuroinflammation, 19*, 248. https://doi.org/10.1186/s12974-022-02613-9.

Li, Y., Zhao, Q., Wang, Y., Du, W., Yang, R., Wu, J., & Li, Y. (2025). Lipid droplet accumulation in microglia and their potential roles. *Lipids in Health and Disease, 24*, 215. https://doi.org/10.1186/s12944-025-02633-3.

Li, Z., & Gong, C. (2025). NLRP3 inflammasome in Alzheimer's disease: Molecular mechanisms and emerging therapies. *Frontiers in Immunology, 16*, 1583886. https://doi.org/10.3389/fimmu.2025.1583886.

Loeffler, D. A. (2023). Antibody-mediated clearance of brain amyloid-β: Mechanisms of action, effects of natural and monoclonal anti-Aβ antibodies, and downstream effects. *Journal of Alzheimer's Disease Reports, 7*, 873–899. https://doi.org/10.3233/ADR-230025.

Long, H., Simmons, A., Mayorga, A., Burgess, B., Nguyen, T., Budda, B., ... Rosenthal, A. (2024). Preclinical and first-in-human evaluation of AL002, a novel TREM2 agonistic antibody for Alzheimer's disease. *Alzheimer's Research & Therapy, 16*, 235. https://doi.org/10.1186/s13195-024-01599-1.

Lopez-Ortiz, A. O., Doceti, M., Thomas, J., Duffy, A., Coburn, M., K. Okojie, A., ... Eyo, U. B. (2025). Transcriptional regulation of microglial metabolic and activation states by P2RY12. *Glia, 73*, 2464–2482. https://doi.org/10.1002/glia.70078.

Lou, N., Takano, T., Pei, Y., Xavier, A. L., Goldman, S. A., & Nedergaard, M. (2016). Purinergic receptor P2RY12-dependent microglial closure of the injured blood–brain barrier. *Proceedings of the National Academy of Sciences of the United States of America, 113*, 1074–1079. https://doi.org/10.1073/pnas.1520398113.

Mallach, A., Zielonka, M., Van Lieshout, V., An, Y., Khoo, J. H., Vanheusden, M., ... De Strooper, B. (2024). Microglia-astrocyte crosstalk in the amyloid plaque niche of an Alzheimer's disease mouse model, as revealed by spatial transcriptomics. *Cell Reports, 43*, 114216. https://doi.org/10.1016/j.celrep.2024.114216.

Mancuso, R., Fattorelli, N., Martinez-Muriana, A., Davis, E., Wolfs, L., Van Den Daele, J., ... De Strooper, B. (2024). Xenografted human microglia display diverse transcriptomic states in response to Alzheimer's disease-related amyloid-β pathology. *Nature Neuroscience, 27*, 886–900. https://doi.org/10.1038/s41593-024-01600-y.

Mao, M., Ma, X., Wang, X., & Ye, J. (2025). Microglial APOE4 promotes neuron degeneration in Alzheimer's disease through inhibition of lipid droplet autophagy. *Acta Pharmaceutica Sinica B, 15*, 657–660. https://doi.org/10.1016/j.apsb.2024.10.009.

Marschallinger, J., Iram, T., Zardeneta, M., Lee, S. E., Lehallier, B., Haney, M. S., ... Wyss-Coray, T. (2020). Lipid-droplet-accumulating microglia represent a dysfunctional and proinflammatory state in the aging brain. *Nature Neuroscience, 23*, 194–208. https://doi.org/10.1038/s41593-019-0566-1.

Martins-Ferreira, R., Calafell-Segura, J., Leal, B., Rodríguez-Ubreva, J., Martínez-Saez, E., Mereu, E., ... Ballestar, E. (2025). The human microglia atlas (HuMicA) unravels changes in disease-associated microglia subsets across neurodegenerative conditions. *Nature Communications, 16*, 739. https://doi.org/10.1038/s41467-025-56124-1.

Muneer, P. M. A., Pfister, B. J., Haorah, J., & Chandra, N. (2016). Role of matrix metalloproteinases in the pathogenesis of traumatic brain injury. *Molecular Neurobiology, 53*, 6106–6123. https://doi.org/10.1007/s12035-015-9520-8.

Ng, P. Y., Zhang, C., Li, H., & Baker, D. J. (2023). Senescent microglia represent a subset of disease-associated microglia in P301S mice. *Journal of Alzheimer's Disease, 95*, 493–507. https://doi.org/10.3233/JAD-230109.

Nishida, T., Naguro, I., & Ichijo, H. (2022). NAMPT-dependent NAD+ salvage is crucial for the decision between apoptotic and necrotic cell death under oxidative stress. *Cell Death Discovery, 8*, 195. https://doi.org/10.1038/s41420-022-01007-3.

Nugent, A. A., Lin, K., Van Lengerich, B., Lianoglou, S., Przybyla, L., Davis, S. S., ... Di Paolo, G. (2020). TREM2 regulates microglial cholesterol metabolism upon chronic phagocytic challenge. *Neuron, 105*, 837–854.e9. https://doi.org/10.1016/j.neuron.2019.12.007.

Saini, V., Rani, A., Kumar, A., Jha, K., Karnati, S., & Jha, H. C. (2023). Altered synaptic plasticity: Plausible mechanisms associated with viral infections. *Future Virology, 18*, 733–752. https://doi.org/10.2217/fvl-2023-0105.

Scheld, M., Jülich, N., Vöhringer, K., Zendedel, A., Beyer, C., Kant, S., ... Sanadgol, N. (2026). Activated microglia-derived extracellular vesicles elicit a pro-inflammatory astrocytic response via cargo-dependent mechanisms. *Biomolecules, 16*, 224. https://doi.org/10.3390/biom16020224.

Shade, L. M. P., Katsumata, Y., Abner, E. L., Aung, K. Z., Claas, S. A., Qiao, Q., ... Fardo, D. W. (2024). GWAS of multiple neuropathology endophenotypes identifies new risk loci and provides insights into the genetic risk of dementia. *Nature Genetics, 56*, 2407–2421. https://doi.org/10.1038/s41588-024-01939-9.

Singh, S., Saini, V., & Jha, H. C. (2025a). The role of secondary genomes in neurodevelopment and co-evolutionary dynamics. *International review of neurobiology*. Elsevier. 245–297. https://doi.org/10.1016/bs.irn.2025.03.008.

Singh, S., Saini, V., Kandpal, M., Waghmare, T.S., Prusty, B.K., & Jha, H.C. (2025b). Coevolution of the human brain and microbiome: roles of accelerated regions and maternal microbiota in neurodevelopment. https://doi.org/10.31234/osf.io/k3ebh_v1.

Solier, S.-W., Zhang, Y., Ballestrero, A., Pommier, Y., & Zoppoli, G. (2012). DNA damage response pathways and cell cycle checkpoints in colorectal cancer: Current concepts and future perspectives for targeted treatment. *Current Cancer Drug Targets, 12*, 356–371. https://doi.org/10.2174/156800912800190901.

Sprenger, K. G., Lietzke, E. E., Melchior, J. T., & Bruce, K. D. (2025). Lipid and lipoprotein metabolism in microglia: Alzheimer's disease mechanisms and interventions. *Journal of Lipid Research, 66*, 100872. https://doi.org/10.1016/j.jlr.2025.100872.

Stephenson, R.A., Johnson, K.R., Cheng, L., Yang, L.G., Root, J.T., Gopalakrishnan, J., ... Narayan, P.S. (2024). Triglyceride metabolism controls inflammation and APOE4 -associated disease states in microglia. https://doi.org/10.1101/2024.04.11.589145.

Sun, R., & Jiang, H. (2024). Border-associated macrophages in the central nervous system. *Journal of Neuroinflammation, 21*, 67. https://doi.org/10.1186/s12974-024-03059-x.

Sung, S., Kim, H.-J., Cha, S. J., Nahm, M., Kim, S. H., & Kwon, M.-S. (2025). Microglial lipid droplets as therapeutic targets in age-related neurodegenerative diseases. *Npj Aging, 12*, 2. https://doi.org/10.1038/s41514-025-00295-0.

Sunna, S., Bowen, C. A., Ramelow, C. C., Santiago, J. V., Kumar, P., & Rangaraju, S. (2023). Advances in proteomic phenotyping of microglia in neurodegeneration. *Proteomics, 23*, 2200183. https://doi.org/10.1002/pmic.202200183.

Toda Robert, A., McQuade, A., Koppes-den Hertog, S. J., Erlebach, L., Kronenberg-Versteeg, D., Kampmann, M., ... Van Der Kant, R. (2026). Comparative lipidomics of iPSC-derived microglia protocols reveal lipid droplet and immune differences mediated by media composition. *Stem Cell Reports, 21*, 102779. https://doi.org/10.1016/j.stemcr.2025.102779.

Tripathi, U., Suda, M., Kulshreshtha, V., Piatkowski, B. T., Palmer, A. K., Giorgadze, N., ... Kirkland, J. L. (2026). Senolytic-resistant senescent cells have a distinct SASP profile and functional impact: The path to developing senosensitizers. *Aging Cell, 25*, e70358. https://doi.org/10.1111/acel.70358.

Tronel, C., Largeau, B., Santiago Ribeiro, M., Guilloteau, D., Dupont, A.-C., & Arlicot, N. (2017). Molecular targets for PET imaging of activated microglia: The current situation and future expectations. *International Journal of Molecular Sciences, 18*, 802. https://doi.org/10.3390/ijms18040802.

Vara-Pérez, M., & Movahedi, K. (2025). Border-associated macrophages as gatekeepers of brain homeostasis and immunity. *Immunity, 58*, 1085–1100. https://doi.org/10.1016/j.immuni.2025.04.005.

Wang, C., Fan, L., Khawaja, R. R., Liu, B., Zhan, L., Kodama, L., ... Gan, L. (2022). Microglial NF-κB drives tau spreading and toxicity in a mouse model of tauopathy. *Nature Communications, 13*, 1969. https://doi.org/10.1038/s41467-022-29552-6.

Wang, J., Wu, J., Ma, X., Wu, Y., Xiao, Z., Zhou, X., ... Zhao, Q. (2025). A double-edged sword: Exploring the neuroprotective/damaging mechanisms of complement activation in Alzheimer's disease. *Aging and Health Research, 5*, 100267. https://doi.org/10.1016/j.ahr.2025.100267.

Wang, S., Mustafa, M., Yuede, C. M., Salazar, S. V., Kong, P., Long, H., ... Colonna, M. (2020). Anti-human TREM2 induces microglia proliferation and reduces pathology in an Alzheimer's disease model. *The Journal of Experimental Medicine, 217*, e20200785. https://doi.org/10.1084/jem.20200785.

Wang, X., Luo, X., Xiao, R., Liu, X., Zhou, F., Jiang, D., ... Xiao, Y. (2026). Targeting metabolic-epigenetic-immune axis in cancer: Molecular mechanisms and therapeutic implications. *Signal Transduction-Targeted Therapy, 11*, 28. https://doi.org/10.1038/s41392-025-02334-4.

Wang, Y., Cella, M., Mallinson, K., Ulrich, J. D., Young, K. L., Robinette, M. L., ... Colonna, M. (2015). TREM2 lipid sensing sustains the microglial response in an Alzheimer's disease model. *Cell, 160*, 1061–1071. https://doi.org/10.1016/j.cell.2015.01.049.

Wei, Y., & Li, X. (2022). Different phenotypes of microglia in animal models of Alzheimer disease. *Immunity & Ageing: I & A, 19*, 44. https://doi.org/10.1186/s12979-022-00300-0.

Wenzel, T. J., Desjarlais, J. D., & Mousseau, D. D. (2024). Human brain organoids containing microglia that have arisen innately adapt to a β-amyloid challenge better than those in which microglia are integrated by co-culture. *Stem Cell Research & Therapy, 15*, 258. https://doi.org/10.1186/s13287-024-03876-0.

Wilhelmsen, K., Deshpande, A., Tronnes, S., Mahanta, M., Banicki, M., Cochran, M., ... Coll, R. C. (2025). Discovery of potent and selective inhibitors of human NLRP3 with a novel mechanism of action. *The Journal of Experimental Medicine, 222*, e20242403. https://doi.org/10.1084/jem.20242403.

Wu, J., Geng, C., Liu, L., & Tang, Y. (2025). Advancement of disease-modifying therapy of Alzheimer's disease: From the perspective of new revised criteria for diagnosis and staging of Alzheimer's disease. *MedPlus, 2*, 100112. https://doi.org/10.1016/j.medp.2025.100112.

Wu, X., Miller, J. A., Lee, B. T. K., Wang, Y., & Ruedl, C. (2025). Reducing microglial lipid load enhances β amyloid phagocytosis in an Alzheimer's disease mouse model. *Science Advances, 11*, eadq6038. https://doi.org/10.1126/sciadv.adq6038.

Wu, Z., Yu, S., Hu, Y., Hu, X., Yang, L., Jiang, Y., ... Cheng, L. (2026). TREM2 facilitates myelin debris clearance but exacerbates chronic inflammation and fibrosis after spinal cord injury. *CNS Neuroscience & Therapeutics, 32*, e70777. https://doi.org/10.1002/cns.70777.

Xu, J., & Núñez, G. (2023). The NLRP3 inflammasome: Activation and regulation. *Trends in Biochemical Sciences, 48*, 331–344. https://doi.org/10.1016/j.tibs.2022.10.002.

Xu, Y.-J., Au, N. P. B., & Ma, C. H. E. (2022). Functional and phenotypic diversity of microglia: Implication for microglia-based therapies for Alzheimer's disease. *Frontiers in Aging Neuroscience, 14*, 896852. https://doi.org/10.3389/fnagi.2022.896852.

Yadollahikhales, G., & Rojas, J. C. (2023). Anti-Amyloid immunotherapies for Alzheimer's disease: A 2023 clinical update. *Neurotherapeutics: the Journal of the American Society for Experimental NeuroTherapeutics, 20*, 914–931. https://doi.org/10.1007/s13311-023-01405-0.

Yu, H., Zhang, L., Song, B., Ren, K., Chen, X., Dai, Y., ... Wei, Z. (2025). TREM2-mediated regulation of microglial activity: A promising target for the treatment of ischemic stroke. *Journal of Translational Medicine, 23*, 782. https://doi.org/10.1186/s12967-025-06799-3.

Yusri, K., Jose, S., Vermeulen, K. S., Tan, T. C. M., & Sorrentino, V. (2025). The role of NAD+ metabolism and its modulation of mitochondria in aging and disease. *npj Metabolic Health and Disease, 3*, 26. https://doi.org/10.1038/s44324-025-00067-0.

Zhang, D., Zhu, Y., Ju, Y., Zhang, H., Zou, X., She, S., ... Guan, Y. (2023). TEAD4 antagonizes cellular senescence by remodeling chromatin accessibility at enhancer regions. *Cellular and Molecular Life Sciences: CMLS, 80*, 330. https://doi.org/10.1007/s00018-023-04980-9.

Zhao, N., Qiao, W., Li, F., Ren, Y., Zheng, J., Martens, Y. A., ... Bu, G. (2022). Elevating microglia TREM2 reduces amyloid seeding and suppresses disease-associated microglia. *The Journal of Experimental Medicine, 219*, e20212479. https://doi.org/10.1084/jem.20212479.

Zheng, J., Winkeler, A., Peyronneau, M.-A., Dollé, F., & Boisgard, R. (2016). Evaluation of PET imaging performance of the TSPO radioligand [18F]DPA-714 in mouse and rat models of cancer and inflammation. *Molecular Imaging and Biology: MIB: the Official Publication of the Academy of Molecular Imaging, 18*, 127–134. https://doi.org/10.1007/s11307-015-0877-x.

CHAPTER ELEVEN

Microglia extracellular traps (MiETs) in Neurodegeneration: Mechanisms, Evidence Gaps, and Untapped Therapeutic Promise

Lipika Sha and Sushmita Jha*
Department of Bioscience and Bioengineering, Indian Institute of Technology, Jodhpur, India
*Corresponding author. e-mail address: sushmitajha@iitj.ac.in

Contents

Abstract

Microglia are the resident myeloid cells of the central nervous system, they play essential roles in neural tissue homeostasis, including synaptic pruning, clearance of debris and protein aggregates, and regulation of neuroinflammatory processes. In neurodegenerative diseases such as Alzheimer's disease, Parkinson's disease, and amyotrophic lateral

Advances in Immunology, Volume 171
ISSN 0065-2776, https://doi.org/10.1016/bs.ai.2026.04.008

sclerosis, microglial activation and chronic glial-driven inflammation contribute substantially to neuronal dysfunction and loss. Beyond these well-characterised functions, recent evidence indicates that microglia can release chromatin-based extracellular traps (microglia extracellular traps, or MiETs), similar to the neutrophil extracellular traps (NETs) observed in peripheral immunity. Microglia ETs are induced by stimuli such as dopamine and microbial infection, dependent or independent of NADPH oxidase/ROS pathways and histone citrullination. This chapter provides a detailed examination of MiET formation, triggers, intracellular signalling, and structural components, as well as contribution to neurodegenerative pathology. Potential mechanisms include amplification of neuroinflammation via extracellular histones and proteases, disruption of the blood-brain barrier and extracellular matrix, synaptic damage, and possible facilitation of spread of misfolded protein aggregates. We situate MiET formation within the broader microglial functional repertoire (phagocytosis, cytokine production, synaptic stripping) and focus on how ET-dominant responses may compromise homeostatic or neuroprotective roles. The chapter reviews evidence from disease models, highlights key gaps and discusses translational implications. Targeting MiET formation or promoting the clearance of MiETs represents promising, yet unexplored, therapeutic avenues in neurodegenerative disease. By focusing on MiETs, this work expands the conceptual framework for microglial pathogenicity and invites future mechanistic and translational research.

1. Introduction

Microglia are the resident immune cells of the central nervous system (CNS). In addition to being the major immune cell of the CNS, microglia are also dynamic regulators of CNS homeostasis. They originate from mesoderm-derived hematopoietic progenitors that migrate into the brain during development. Through continuous surveillance of the neural microenvironment, they respond to subtle changes in neuronal activity, synaptic remodeling, and tissue damage, positioning them as key intermediaries between physiological maintenance, pathological inflammation, and neurodegenerative diseases.

Neurodegenerative diseases (NDs) are a heterogeneous group of disorders characterized by the progressive degeneration of the structure and function of the central or peripheral nervous system. It constitutes a diverse group of neurological conditions that collectively affect millions of individuals worldwide. These disorders are characterized by progressive dysfunction and neuronal loss in the central nervous system (CNS) or the peripheral nervous system (PNS), leading to a gradual decline in cognitive, motor, and functional abilities (Dugger & Dickson, 2017). This group encompasses several primary neuropsychiatric and neurological conditions, including Alzheimer's disease (AD), Parkinson's disease (PD), Multiple Sclerosis (MS), Amyotrophic Lateral Sclerosis (ALS), and Huntington's disease (HD), among others.

Globally, the impact and burden of NDs are significant, and dementia is one of the most common clinical outcomes of many neurodegenerative diseases, along with brain injuries (Matej et al., 2019; Ziukelis et al., 2022). According to the World Health Organization (WHO), an estimated 57 million people were living with dementia in 2021, with nearly 10 million new cases each year. Notably, Alzheimer's disease accounts for approximately 60–70 % of these cases, underscoring its dominant contribution to the global dementia burden. In addition, the WHO reports 3 million people living with neurological disorders worldwide. This growing burden has underscored the need to understand the factors driving neurodegeneration. Despite extensive epidemiological and clinical characterization of neurodegenerative disorders, the precise mechanisms driving progressive neuronal loss remain incompletely understood. Various factors contribute to progressive neuronal dysfunction and loss, including genetic, molecular, environmental, and cellular factors. While genetic, molecular, and environmental risk factors contribute to disease susceptibility, it is the downstream cellular responses within the CNS that ultimately determine disease onset, progression, and severity (Kline et al., 2021; Waubant et al., 2019). Cellular responses, such as impaired protein clearance, mitochondrial dysfunction, chronic neuroinflammation, and microglial dysregulation, represent common pathways through which various risk factors converge to drive neurodegeneration (Boland et al., 2018; Zhang, 2023). Among these responses, chronic neuroinflammation has emerged as a central driver of neurodegeneration, with dysregulated microglial activation playing a pivotal role in shaping neuronal survival, synaptic integrity, and disease progression across multiple neurodegenerative conditions (Kempuraj et al., 2016; Zhang et al., 2023). Hence, elucidating these cellular processes, particularly microglial responses, is critical for understanding disease progression and identifying effective therapeutic targets. This chapter provides an overview of microglial biology in neurodegenerative disorders, summarizes current knowledge of extracellular trap formation in the CNS, and neurodegenerative disorder while discussing the potential implications of MiETs in neuroinflammation and neurodegeneration, highlighting potential avenues for future research and therapeutic intervention.

2. Microglia biology

Microglia are resident innate immune cells of the brain. Microglia constitute approximately 5–20 % of all glial cells and serve as the principal resident immune cells of the brain (Frost & Schafer, 2016; Lawson et al., 1992, 1990). Microglia primarily function for CNS immune surveillance and homeostasis. In CNS injury, microglia help phagocytose and eliminate microbes, dead cells, protein aggregates, and other soluble antigens that may endanger the CNS. Emerging evidence suggest microglia plays a central role in CNS pathologies, including Alzheimer's disease (AD), Parkinson's disease (PD), schizophrenia, autism, and multiple sclerosis (MS) (Prinz et al., 2019). Hence, it is important to study the role of microglia in the CNS and neurodegenerative diseases.

2.1 Origin and development of microglia

Microglia originate from the yolk sac myeloid progenitors. These progenitor cells migrate from the embryo into the neural tube, where they proliferate and colonize the parenchyma (Ginhoux et al., 2010; Schulz et al., 2012). It shares several markers with macrophages of the same lineage, e.g., Toll-like receptors (TLRs) (Bsibsi et al., 2002; Olson & Miller, 2004), CD11b (Akiyama & McGeer, 1990), and F4/80 (Perry et al., 1985) while exhibiting comparatively lower expression of the leukocyte common antigen CD45 (Becher & Antel, 1996; Dick et al., n.d). For microglia to persist throughout an organism's lifetime, their development and maintenance require continuous engagement of the colony-stimulating factor 1 receptor (CSF1R) (Elmore et al., 2014). This tyrosine kinase receptor transmits intracellular signals, including activation of protein kinase B (also known as AKT) and extracellular signal-regulated kinases (ERK), which are necessary for microglial proliferation and survival. (Dai et al., 2002). CSF1R transmits these signals via two ligands, CSF1 and IL-34, released by neurons and glial cells (Ma et al., 2012); defects in either ligand can result in a partial reduction in microglial count (Lawson et al., 1992).

2.2 Morphology and dynamic behavior of microglia

Microglia are highly dynamic in morphology and function, as shown by two-photon imaging (Hierro-Bujalance et al., 2018; Nimmerjahn et al., 2005). Microglia display three morphological variants: resting ramified, activated, and amoeboid phagocytic (Ling & Wong, 1993). Under normal conditions, microglia are ramified, with branches and processes terminating in bulbous endings (Colonna & Butovsky, 2017). While in response to diverse stimuli such as injury, infection, or neurodegenerative processes, ramified microglia rapidly transition into an activated or amoeboid phagocytic state (Kreutzberg, 1996; Kawabori & Yenari, 2015). As injuries or inflammation induce changes in morphology, microglia cell bodies enlarge, cell processes shorten, and are directed toward the injury site to phagocytose damaged tissue, covering a smaller area (Colonna & Butovsky, 2017). The amoeboid morphology reflects a highly activated state associated with phagocytosis and proinflammatory function. While bipolar rod-shaped microglia that form strings of cells aligned end-to-end at the damaged site have also been observed after brain injury (Tam & Ma, 2014). Thus, microglia shape and movement reflect microglial responses to a wide variety of stimuli, including normal neuronal activity, physical, chemical, and microbial insults, as well as aggravated neuronal hyperactivity.

2.3 Microglial activation and phenotypic diversity

Changes in microglial shape can also reflect their functional state. The microglial activation states were historically categorized into two opposite phenotypes; the classical (M1) and the alternative (M2) (Tang & Le, 2016). Recent research reflects a continuum of phenotypes between M1 and M2 (Wes et al., 2016). While conventional M1 microglia were thought to produce proinflammatory cytokines and chemokines, conventional M2 activation was accepted to promote an anti-inflammatory response (Colonna & Butovsky, 2017). M1 activation of microglia is widely accepted as a neurotoxic state, typically induced by simultaneous activation of the toll-like receptor (TLR) and interferon gamma (IFN-γ) signaling pathways (Martínez-Hernández et al., 2023). These microglia produce proinflammatory cytokines and chemokines, such as tumor necrosis factor alpha (TNF-α), interleukin (IL)-6, IL-1β, IL-12, and CCL2 (Smith et al., 2012; Colonna & Butovsky, 2017). M1 microglia express NADPH oxidase, which generates superoxide and reactive oxygen species (ROS) (Bordt & Polster, 2014; Haslund-Vinding et al., 2017; Geng et al., 2020). Another important inflammatory mediator produced is matrix metalloproteinase 12 (MMP12), which also expresses high levels of MHC class II, costimulatory molecules, Fc receptors, and integrins (Jurga et al., 2020). Hence, M1 microglia themselves can induce inflammation and neurotoxicity. M2 activation corresponds to the anti-inflammatory and healing activities of microglia; it can be induced by IL-4, IL-13, IL-10, Fc receptor ligation by immunocomplexes, and detection of apoptotic cells (Cherry et al., 2014). M2 activation can occur through transcription factor activation, such as peroxisome proliferator-activated receptor gamma (PPARγ), liver X receptor (LXR), and retinoic acid receptor (RXR), by fatty acids, oxysterols, and 9-*cis*-retinoic acid, respectively (Saijo et al., 2013). Activated M2 microglia promote the secretion of anti-inflammatory cytokines, notably a variety of growth and neurotrophic factors, such as transforming growth factor-β (TGF-β), insulin-like growth factor I (IGF-I), fibroblast growth factor (FGF), colony-stimulating factor 1 (CSF1), nerve growth factor (NGF), brain-derived neurotrophic factor (BDNF), neurotrophin-4/5 (NT-4/5), and glial cell–derived neurotrophic factor (GDNF) (Colonna & Butovsky, 2017; Guo et al., 2022). These factors signal through tyrosine kinase receptors, which play key roles in regulating synaptic plasticity and strength. This versatility enables microglia to perform essential roles in repair, synaptic pruning, trophic support, debris clearance, and immune surveillance (Paolicelli et al., 2011; Neumann et al., 2009; Yang et al., 2010). However, the M1/M2 paradigm does not fully capture the diversity of microglial states observed in neurodegenerative conditions, as microglia can adopt complex phenotypes that do not conform strictly to these categories (Ransohoff, 2016). And the phenotypic diversity suggests that microglia response extends beyond classical cytokine-driven inflammation. And despite the usefulness of the M1/M2 framework in conceptualizing microglial responses in vitro, accumulating evidence indicates that this binary classification does not adequately reflect microglial activation states in vivo (Nahrendorf & Swirski, 2016). Instead, microglial phenotypes exist along a dynamic continuum, with cells rarely exhibiting a strictly polarized M1 or M2 profile.

2.4 Microglial receptors and signalling

Microglia play an essential role in the immune system and express a variety of pattern recognition receptors (PRRs), including TLRs (Toll-like Receptors), NLRs (nucleotide-binding leucine-rich repeat receptors), and CLRs (C-type lectin receptors) that aid the detection of pathogen-associated molecular patterns (PAMPs) and damage-associated molecular patterns (DAMPs) (Kigerl et al., 2014). Microglia can also phagocytose or endocytose apoptotic cells, protein aggregates, and lipoprotein particles, aided by surface recognition of these molecules by scavenger receptors such as CD36, SR1, and MARCO; LDL receptor family members, such as LDLR, ApoER2, and VLDL; and three receptor tyrosine kinases, namely, Tyro3, Axl, and Mertk (TAM) (Rebeck et al., 2006; Lemke, 2013; Areschoug & Gordon, 2009). In the innate immune system, microglia can also capture and endocytose immune complexes; for opsonized protein complexes, this is complemented by Fc receptors and complement receptors. Microglia also express chemokine receptors and integrins, such as CX3CR1, CXCR4, CD11b, and CD11c (Mizutani et al., 2012; Colonna & Butovsky, 2017). Microglia function is also regulated by receptors for proinflammatory and anti-inflammatory cytokines such as IFN-α/β, IFN-γ, TNF-α, IL-1β, IL-10, and TGF-β, which are produced in the CNS by glial cells or that reach the CNS via the circulation (Veroni et al., 2010; Prins et al., 2013; Kann et al., 2022; Colonna & Butovsky, 2017).

In addition to immune receptors, microglia also express neurotransmitter receptors. These receptors help microglia monitor neuronal activity, guide them towards neuronal synapses, regulate synaptic plasticity, and influence dendritic spine density (Cserép et al., 2019; Nebeling et al., n.d.; Cornell et al., 2021). This also helps detect damaged neurons and support neuronal regeneration. Neurotransmitters that help microglia perform these functions include glutamate ionotropic receptors, such as α-amino-3-hydroxy-5-methyl-4-isoxazolepropionic acid (AMPA) and N-methyl-D-aspartate (NMDA) receptors, as well as glutamate metabotropic receptors, such as mGluR2 (Hagino et al., 2004; Taylor et al., 2005). Microglia also express purinergic receptors for ATP, including P2Y12 and P2X7 (Eyo et al., 2014; Crabbé et al., 2019; Gómez Morillas et al., 2021). In resting microglia, P2Y12 is active but downregulated upon activation; it drives migration and phagocytosis (Koizumi et al., 2013). P2X7 promotes TNF-α release from microglia in response to ATP (1 mM) (Damani et al., 2011; Shieh et al., 2014). Adenosine receptors (e.g., A2a) promote secretion of inflammatory mediators and phagocytosis (Franco et al., 2021). And gamma-aminobutyric acid (GABA), as well as adrenergic, dopaminergic, and cholinergic receptors, modulate microglial inflammatory responses (Czapski & Strosznajder, 2021).

2.5 Microglia and CNS immunity

Microglia share several functional similarities with peripheral macrophages in innate and adaptive immune responses. Microglia are the first line of innate immunity in the CNS. In a variety of CNS pathologies microglia are activated in the presence of lipopolysaccharide (LPS), beta-amyloid (Aβ), thrombin, IFN-γ, and other proinflammatory cytokines (Dheen et al., n.d.). Activated microglia release cytokines and chemokines to recruit lymphocytes (Suzumura et al., 1996; Takami et al., 1997; Hartlage-Rübsamen et al., 1999; Si et al., 2002; Babcock et al., 2003; Chen et al., 2004; Floden et al., 2005).

In the adaptive immune context, when microglia are activated, MHC expression and costimulatory molecules (e.g., CD80 and CD60) are elevated, further stimulating T cells (Slavik et al., 1999; Van Kooten & Banchereau, 2000). Additionally, microglia play a role in phagocytosis and cytotoxicity during brain injury. Upon activation, microglial opsonic receptors, such as complement receptors (CR1, CR3, CR4) and Fc gamma receptors (I, II, III), are upregulated, enhancing phagocytosis (Peress et al., 1993; Barnum, 1999). In addition, in response to pathogens and cytokine stimulation, microglia release superoxide radicals and nitric oxide (NO) (Yang et al., 2010). Recently, microglia have also been reported to release extracellular traps as an immune response against pathogens and dopamine (Agrawal et al., 2021; Wang et al., 2019). Given the role of microglia in the immune system and CNS pathologies, it is important to understand their role in neurodegenerative diseases.

3. Role of microglia in neurodegenerative disease

Microglia constantly survey and interact with other cells in the CNS, including neurons, astrocytes, oligodendrocytes, and infiltrating immune cells. Microglia play roles in synapse pruning, maintenance of homeostasis, phagocytosis, and support of other glial cells. Microglia are activated in response to CNS, infection, injury and disease. Microglial activation is a consistent feature across neurodegenerative disorders; however, its functional consequences depend on the disease in context, as it can result in either neuroprotective or neurotoxic outcomes (Fig. 1).

3.1 Alzheimer's disease

Alzheimer's disease (AD) is one of the most common neurodegenerative diseases, as it accounts for 60–70 % of senile dementia (Association, 2018). In AD, extra-neuronal amyloid plaques are formed because of β-amyloid (Aβ) deposition and intracellular neurofibrillary tangles (NFTs) caused by abnormal aggregation of tau protein (Braak & Braak, 1991; Hardy & Selkoe, 2002). In AD brains, microglial activation was observed along with Aβ plaques, and these were correlated with tau and amyloid proteins (Hayes et al., 2002). Microglial activation has been correlated with translocator protein (TSPO), a PET-imaging biomarker for neuroinflammation, earlier known as the peripheral benzodiazepine receptor (PBR), expressed in mitochondria of activated glial cells, which has an elevated expression in

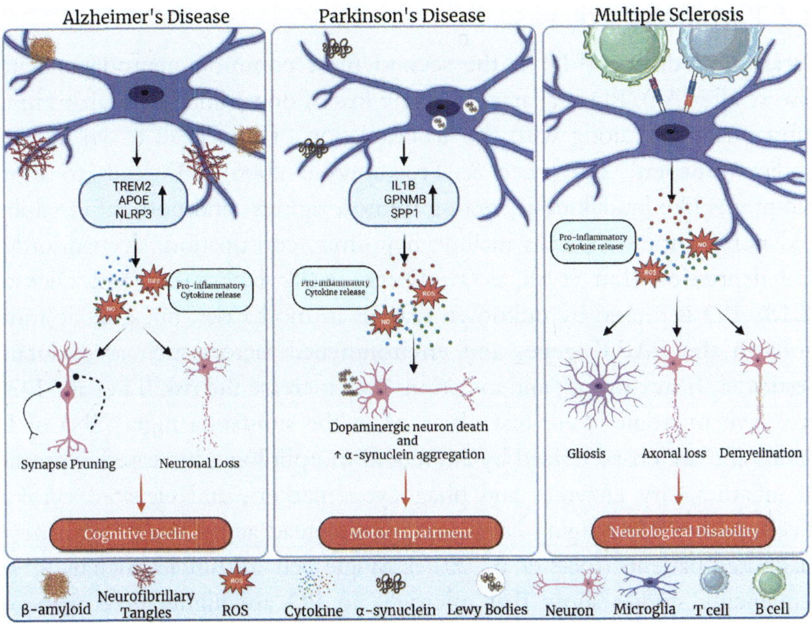

Fig. 1 During neurodegenerative disease, microglia activation leads to cytokine release and ROS production, resulting in disease progression as there is neuronal loss, while the microglia reside in a chronic activation state. *Created with Biorender.com.*

AD (Leng & Edison, 2021, Nutma et al., 2023, Fairley et al., 2024). Activated microglia are present in AD in various states. Keren-Shaul et al. first identified microglia in AD and termed them as disease-associated microglia (DAM), which participated in the clearance of Aβ (Keren-Shaul et al., 2017; Deczkowska et al., 2018). Additionally, single-cell RNA sequencing has revealed multiple microglial states in AD, including plaque-associated and disease-associated subtypes (Olah et al., 2020). These microglial subtypes have been reported to cluster near Aβ plaques, express genes related to phagocytosis, lipid handling, and migration, and may help clear Aβ, suggesting a protective role early in disease (Hsieh et al., 2009; Mazaheri et al., 2017). While some subtypes with possible neurotrophic or amyloid-responsive functions have also been described, they are involved in the TREM2 and APOE pathways (Hansen et al., 2017). Overall, microglial activation correlates strongly with Aβ and phosphorylated tau burden. And chronic exposure to growing pathology can drive them into dysfunctional states, contributing to disease progression.

3.2 Parkinson's disease

Parkinson's disease (PD) is the second most common neurodegenerative disease after AD. PD is characterized by loss of dopaminergic neurons in the substantia nigra, along with the accumulation of misfolded α-syn in Lewy bodies (Goedert, 2001; Lee & Trojanowski, 2006). PD leads to motor symptoms like bradykinesia, resting tremor, rigidity, and postural instability, and non-motor symptoms include hyposmia, constipation, sleep disorders, and depression (Liu et al., 2004; Davie, 2008; Jankovic, 2008; Dickson, 2018). PD is caused by unknown reasons in most cases, but genetic mutations in the PARK genes and environmental factors such as pollutants, pesticides, heavy metals, and infections may increase the risk (Li et al., 2021). Reactive microglia were first observed in the substantia nigra (SN) of PD brains and are characterized by amoeboid morphology, increased expression of inflammatory enzymes and phagocytic markers, and elevated cytokine levels, with PET imaging confirming widespread activation even in newly diagnosed patients (Joers et al., 2017). Single-cell and single-nucleus RNA-sequencing studies show that microglia in PD are highly heterogeneous, forming multiple subpopulations with distinct gene signatures and activation trajectories, rather than the M1/M2 phenotype. Some subsets show immune-activated profiles, including populations linked to α-synuclein pathology, and midbrain microglia appear more tolerogenic than striatal microglia. The reactive microglia migrate to injury sites, secrete pro- and anti-inflammatory factors, and clear debris, but are also associated with cytokine release, stress-response pathways, and inflammasome activation that may promote neurodegeneration. Additionally, peripheral immune signals can further influence brain inflammation and support infiltration of monocytes/macrophages (CCR2 + and CD163 + cells), which likely contribute to PD pathology, although the link between peripheral inflammation and central microglial activation is complex and not always direct. Overall, these findings highlight substantial microglial diversity and an important, context-dependent role in PD progression.

3.3 Multiple sclerosis

Multiple sclerosis (MS) is an autoimmune disease resulting in neurodegeneration, characterized by focal lesions of inflammation, axonal loss, gliosis, and demyelination (De Groot et al., 2001; Lassmann et al., 2007). In MS patients, myelin is disrupted, which is associated with activated microglia and macrophages (Prineas et al., 2001; Lassmann et al., 2007).

Brain biopsies also show that, in the early stages of MS, demyelination occurs in cortical and subcortical regions (Lucchinetti et al., 2011). Furthermore, in demyelinating diseases such as MS, oxidative injury plays an important role (Haider et al., 2011). Oxidative injury can occur via an oxidative burst in activated microglia and macrophages, which release reactive oxygen species (ROS) (Miller & Wachowicz n.d.). Along with ROS, (Nitric oxide) NO radicals can result in lesions, suggesting their role in the demyelination and neurodegeneration (Liu et al., 2001; Gray et al., 2008; Fischer et al., 2012). Together, these pieces of evidence indicate that activated microglia in MS promote demyelination. Microglia can also help in the remyelination process, i.e., myelin regeneration around axons, because they clear myelin debris and shape a local environment that supports repair via releasing factors like TNF-α, IGF-1, and FGF-2 (Albert et al., 2007; Lampron et al., 2015; Domingues et al., 2016). Overall, effective microglial responses are crucial for creating conditions that enable remyelination.

Among these unconventional responses, the formation of extracellular traps has recently gained attention as a potential amplifier of chronic neuroinflammation in the CNS. As various cells can form extracellular traps composed of RNA, DNA and histones in response to diverse stimuli, it is important to understand microglia extracellular traps (MiETs), as they may represent an overlooked mechanism of neuroinflammation in neurodegenerative diseases.

4. Extracellular traps

Extracellular traps (ETs) are webs of decondensed chromatin decorated with histones and antimicrobial proteins released by immune cells that can immobilize pathogens and modulate inflammation. ETs were first observed in neutrophils and considered a host defense response to present pathogens (Brinkmann et al., 2004). Neutrophil Extracellular Traps (NETs) are composed of DNA with cytoplasmic and granular proteins decorated on a scaffold of decondensed chromatin (Brinkmann et al., 2004). Subsequent research has demonstrated that multiple leukocyte populations, such as mast cells, basophils, eosinophils, macrophages, and microglia, can also release extracellular traps (Möllerherm et al., 2016; Von Köckritz-Blickwede et al., 2008; Morshed et al., 2014; Schorn et al., 2012; Yousefi et al., 2008; Agrawal et al., 2021).

4.1 Molecular composition of extracellular traps

Extracellular traps are composed of a decondensed chromatin backbone decorated with histones and antimicrobial proteins. ETs are composed of DNA, originating from the nucleus and/or mitochondria; they also contain histones, e.g., H2A, H2B, H4, along with modified histone citrullinated histone 3 (CitH3) (Yang et al., 2020; Karkowska-Kuleta et al., 2021; Papayannopoulos, 2018). Neutrophil extracellular traps (NETs) contain mitochondrial DNA during vital NETosis and nuclear DNA during lytic NETosis, although, in the presence of certain stimulants, the released NETs can contain both nuclear and mitochondrial DNA (Papayannopoulos, 2018). ET associated proteins vary depending on the cellular origin. Eosinophils, basophils, and macrophages release extracellular traps of mitochondrial origin (Yousefi et al., 2008; Aulik et al., 2012; Morshed et al., 2014). ET associated proteins may include neutrophil elastase (NE), myeloperoxidase (MPO), cathepsin G, calprotectin, azurocidin, proteinase 3 (PR3), α-defensisns, Heat shock protein 72, MMP1, MMP9, HMGB1, and LL-37 (Urban et al., 2009; Papayannopoulos et al., 2010; Dwyer et al., 2014; Metzler et al., 2014; Herster et al., 2020; Wang et al., 2024). These nucleic acids and proteins confer ETs with innate antimicrobial properties; play important roles in host defense, regulate cancer progression, and contribute to autoimmune diseases.

4.2 Mechanism of extracellular trap release

Extracellular traps (ETs) are released in response to stress and stimuli; this process is called ETosis. ETs are released mainly in two ways: lytic (suicidal) and non-lytic (vital). In lytic ETosis, cell death occurs simultaneously with the release of extracellular traps, whereas in non-lytic ETosis, cells remain viable even after nucleic acids are extruded as extracellular traps. In neutrophils, lytic ETosis is driven by reactive oxygen species (ROS). Various stimuli, such as Phorbol-12-myristate-13-acetate (PMA), IL-8, and calcium ionophore, activate protein kinase C, leading to NADPH oxidase-dependent ROS production (Hakkim et al., 2011), while ROS production can also occur independently of NADPH oxidase, such as in calcium ionophore-induced NETosis, where ROS production is dependent upon mitochondria (Douda et al., 2015). This increase in intracellular ROS ruptures azurophilic granules, releasing MPO and NE, which then further translocate to the nucleus (Branzk et al., 2014; Metzler et al., 2014; Papayannopoulos et al., 2010). Within the nucleus, NE cleaves histone and decondenses chromatin, which can also be mediated by peptidylargenine deiminase 4 (PAD4) via histone citrullination

(Papayannopoulos, 2018). Later, studies show that the interaction between neutrophils and platelets can lead to NETosis without causing cell death, as even after NET release, the plasma membrane remained intact (Clark et al., 2007). And this process was called non-lytic, or vital, NETosis. In vital NETosis, the cellular membrane remains intact, host defense mechanisms, such as phagocytosis, remain functional, and the process occurs faster than in lytic NETosis (Yipp et al., 2012). Non-lytic NETosis has been reported to be induced by platelets via the LPS-TLR4 axis, but the molecular mechanism still remains unclear (Clark et al., 2007; Pieterse et al., 2016). Study shows that in S. aureus-induced NETosis, inhibition of NADPH oxidase failed to exhibit formation of extracellular traps, suggesting that vital NETosis is independent of NADPH oxidase (Pilsczek et al., 2010). While signalling pathways for some stimulants have been studied, due to the diversity of upstream signalling pathways, the type of NETosis that results may vary. For example, lipopolysaccharide (LPS) from *P. aeruginosa* and *E. coli* O128:B12 can trigger ROS-dependent lytic NETosis, whereas when neutrophils are cocultured with platelets, LPS released by P. aeruginosa and E. coli O111:B4 induces vital NETosis. NETosis can also vary over time; it has been reported that neutrophils, when exposed to S. aureus, can undergo non-lytic NETosis in the early phase, then switch to lytic NETosis in later stages.

The mechanism of ET formation can also vary from cell to cell. In eosinophils, ETs are released as the cells lose nuclear integrity, and DNA-based extracellular traps are released in a lytic manner, with or without ROS, when exposed to *Aspergillus fumigatus*, PMA, or the calcium ionophore A23187, respectively (Barroso et al., 2021; Tomizawa et al., 2025). These eosinophil extracellular traps (EETs) can form through various molecular pathways, depending on the stimulus; aspergillus-induced ETosis requires PI3K and Akt signaling (Tomizawa et al., 2025). Additionally, LPS from gram-negative bacteria activates IL-5- or IFN-γ-primed eosinophils, resulting in the release of mitochondrial DNA in a ROS-dependent, non-lytic manner (Yousefi et al., 2008). Similarly, basophil extracellular traps (BETs) are released upon priming with IL-3, followed by activation of the complement factor 5a (C5a) receptor or FcεRI (Yousefi et al., 2015). BETs are composed of mitochondrial DNA, granule proteins basogranulin and mouse mast cell protease 8, and are formed in a ROS-dependent and NADPH oxidase-independent manner (Morshed et al., 2014; Yousefi et al., 2015).

Besides eosinophils, mast cells can release extracellular traps when stimulated with LPS, PMA, the M1 Protein-Fibrinogen complex, hydrogen peroxide (H_2O_2), glucose oxide, IL-23, and IL-1β (Von Köckritz-Blickwede et al., 2008; Lauth et al., 2009; Lin et al., 2011; Campillo-Navarro et al., 2017). Mast cells release extracellular traps in a ROS-dependent manner. Similarly, monocytes/macrophages can release ETs, and macrophages do so when stimulated by statins via inhibition of the sterol pathway, in a general mechanism involving NADPH oxidase and oxidative stress (Aulik et al., 2012; Chow et al., 2010). Additionally, microglia release extracellular traps in response to *Listeria monocytogenes,* ionomycin, PMA, and dopamine (DA) (Wang et al., 2019; Agrawal et al., 2021). *Listeria-* or PMA-induced microglia extracellular traps (MiETs) occur in a ROS- and NOX-dependent manner, whereas ionomycin induces ROS- and NOX-independent ETosis, involving ERK signalling (Wang et al., 2019). In case of DA-induced MiETs occurs in a non-lytic manner and are independent of ROS (Agrawal et al., 2021). Newer reports suggest that microglia can produce ETs when stimulated with SiO_2 nanoparticles (Fang et al., n.d; Liu et al., 2025).

4.3 Functional role of extracellular traps

Extracellular traps play a crucial role in immobilizing and killing bacteria, fungi, viruses, and parasites (Hirsch, 1958; Urban et al., 2006; Von Köckritz-Blickwede et al., 2008; Halverson et al., 2015). It is now widely accepted that the role of ETs is not only to prevent microbial invasion but also to contribute to host defense and to regulate various diseases (Abdallah et al., 2012; Branzk et al., 2014; Saitoh et al., 2012; Brinkmann et al., 2004). In ETs, NETs have been vastly studied for their role in various diseases (Papayannopoulos, 2018). NETs can damage tissues by killing epithelial and endothelial cells (Villanueva et al., 2011; Saffarzadeh et al., 2012). In sepsis and acute injury, NETs play a detrimental role, as free-circulating histones are cytotoxic (Villanueva et al., 2011; Yipp et al., 2012; Abrams et al., 2013). In this regard, NETs have a detrimental effect, and PAD4 plays a role, as its inhibition can reduce histone citrullination, minimize immune cell recruitment, and reduce liver damage in ischemia–reperfusion injury (Savchenko et al., 2014; Huang et al., 2015; Martinod et al., 2017). NETs also promote vascular occlusion, leading to deep vein thrombosis in patients with obesity and cancer (Fuchs et al., 2010; Martinod et al., 2013). Additionally, NETs can modulate sterile inflammation by regulating inflammatory cytokines directly or indirectly. NETs elevate genes encoding IL-6 and pro-IL-1β in macrophages (Warnatsch et al., 2015). Other components of NETs, such as neutrophil serine proteases, process pro-IL1β to its active form, and MPO promotes atherosclerosis via low-density lipoprotein (LDL) oxidation

(Karmakar et al., 2012; Milligan et al., 2016). NETs can also lead to an anti-inflammatory effect as NET aggregates degrade pro-inflammatory cytokines and chemokines (Schauer et al., 2014). As NETs are present in autoimmune disease conditions, they have been proposed to be the source of self-antigen that can also modulate these conditions (Garcia-Romo et al., 2011; Campbell et al., 2012; Lood et al., 2016). NETs also play a role in various cancers, such as pancreatic carcinoma, lung carcinoma, and adenocarcinoma, where NETs can result in tumor growth and promote metastasis (Boone et al., 2015; Coffelt et al., 2015; Wculek & Malanchi, 2015; Demers et al., 2016). Similarly, eosinophil extracellular traps (EETs) are also seen in multiple infectious, allergic, and autoimmune eosinophilic diseases (Yousefi et al., 2008; Dworski et al., 2011; Simon et al., 2011). Basophil extracellular traps (BETs) exhibit antibacterial activity, but they have not been further studied for their role in disease (Yousefi et al., 2015). Additionally, Microglia extracellular traps (MiETs) are present in the glioblastoma microenvironment, but their role remains to be elucidated (Agrawal et al., 2021). On the one hand, they protect the body against pathogen invasion; on the other hand, excessive or dysregulated ET release can promote tissue injury, autoimmunity, and tumor progression. Hence, maintaining a balance between protective and pathological ET activity is critical.

5. Extracellular traps in neurodegenerative disease

Recently, a significant role of ETs in the CNS has been recognized, making it essential to understand their release and signalling within the CNS. The cells that release extracellular traps, such as neutrophils, basophils, eosinophils, macrophages, and mast cells, except microglia, play a crucial role in innate immunity but are rarely found in the CNS in normal physiological conditions because of the presence of the blood-brain barrier (BBB). However, when the BBB is impaired or disrupted, as in trauma or disease, it allows immune cells, such as neutrophils, to infiltrate the brain. Neutrophil entry into the CNS is frequently accompanied by NETs release, which has been associated with BBB breakdown and secondary tissue damage. NETs components, such as histones, proteases, and matrix metalloproteinases, can degrade tight junction proteins, including occludin and claudin, thereby amplifying BBB dysfunction (Liu et al., 2012; Yang et al., 2007). While microglia involvement in neurodegenerative diseases is well established. The formation of microglial extracellular traps (MiETs), which are composed of components similar to those of NETs, remains poorly understood, underscoring the need for further investigation (Fig. 2).

5.1 Extracellular traps in Alzheimer's disease

Neuroinflammation and dementia are the hallmarks of Alzheimer's disease (AD). Recent studies suggest that neutrophils play an interesting role, as CD11b and ROS production are elevated in AD, suggesting neutrophil activation (Scali et al., 2002). Neutrophil presence in the brains of AD patients correlates with neurofibrillary tangles and amyloid-β (Aβ) burden, while gene expression signatures of neutrophils from AD patients suggest that neutrophils contribute to neuroinflammation (Song et al., 2022). Further studies show that not only neutrophils, but also neutrophil extracellular traps (NETs) may play a role in the pathogenesis of AD, as granule proteins of NETs play a role in neuroinflammation and AD (Pietronigro et al., 2017). Studies show that platelet activation in the intravascular space can occur upon exposure to Aβ, leading to increased Aβ production, ROS formation, and NET formation. Intravascular NETs are also produced when activated platelets release HMGB1 (Maugeri et al., 2014), which interacts with neutrophils via TLR-4/RAGE (Tadie et al., 2013; Huebener et al., 2015); this interaction induces the production of pro-inflammatory cytokines and upregulation of endothelial cell inflammatory markers (e.g., VCAM-1 and selectins).

Additionally, it has also been reported that in primary amyloidosis patients, amyloid fibrils can lead to neutrophil recruitment and NET formation via NADPH oxidase, while their components can fragment Aβ to oligomers, exerting neurotoxicity or neuroinflammation (Azevedo et al., 2012; Munir et al., 2021). In AD, reports show elevated neutrophil levels in the brain vasculature of mouse models, along with neutrophil adhesion and NET formation; additionally, extracellular myeloperoxidase (MPO) from NETs induces oxidative stress (Smyth et al., 2022). NETs can also damage the endothelial wall and the blood-brain barrier by releasing a mixture of nuclear proteins, proteases, NE, cathepsin G, MPO, and metalloproteinases (MMPs) (Stock et al., 2018). Further, a comprehensive bioinformatic analysis for Alzheimer's disease identifies five NET-related hub genes, NFKBIA, SOCS3, CCL2, TIMP1, and ACTB, that may act as biomarkers or therapeutic targets (Qiao & Shao, 2026).

5.2 Extracellular traps in multiple sclerosis

In Multiple Sclerosis (MS) patients, NET-associated proteins such as NE, MPO, and DNA-MPO complexes are elevated in plasma, which correlates

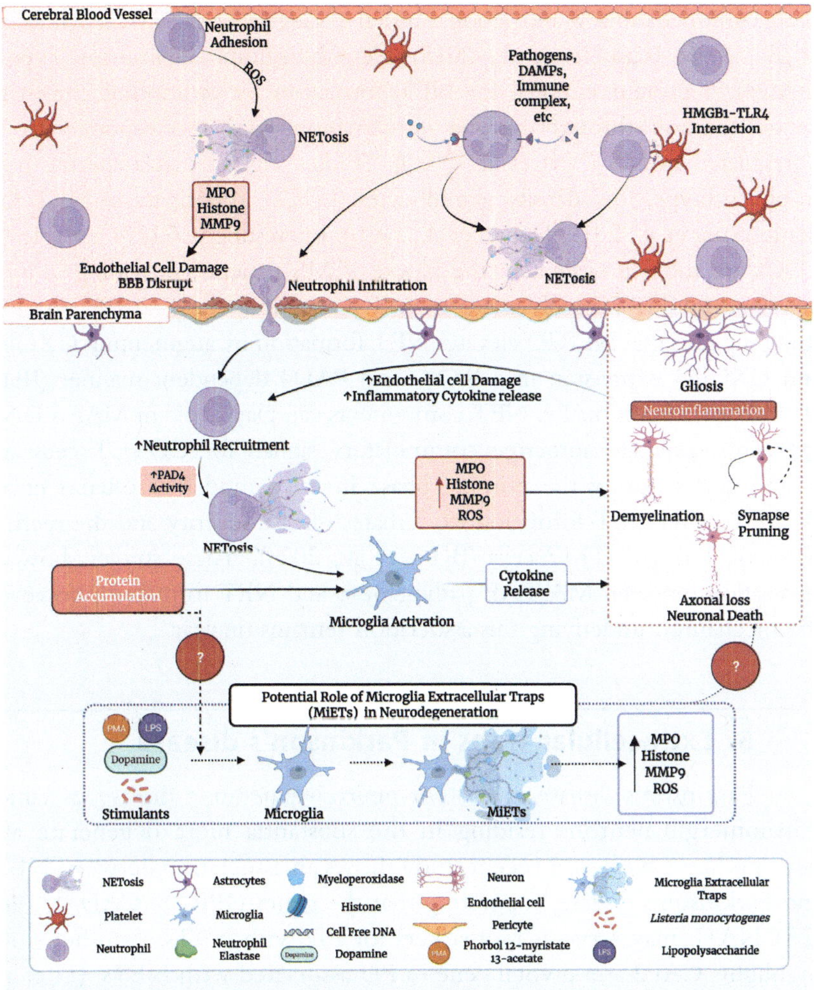

Fig. 2 Brain injuries lead to neutrophil adhesion to the brain microvascular endothelial cells (BMECs). Adhesion to BMECs and exposure to platelet-derived high-mobility group box-1 (HMGB1) via toll-like receptor-4 (TLR4) activate neutrophils and induce intravascular neutrophil extracellular trap (NET) production. NETs comprise neutrophil elastase, citrullinated histone H3, matrix metalloproteinases (MMPs), and cell-free DNA, which increase blood-brain barrier (BBB) permeability. Activated neutrophils can infiltrate the CNS through the BBB, and intraparenchymal neutrophils also undergo NETosis, resulting in neuronal damage and microglial activation, amplifying neuroinflammation and leading to neuronal loss. Further accumulation of protein in neurodegenerative disease can activate microglia, exacerbating the condition. While the role of microglia extracellular traps (MiETs) released in the CNS in response to various stimuli is not known in neurodegenerative disease. *Created with Biorender.com.*

with clinical disability and lesion burden (Naegele et al., 2012; Minohara et al., 2006; Rumble et al., 2015). Peptidylarginine Deiminase Type 4 (PAD4), a protein essential for NET formation by promoting chromatin decondensation through histone citrullination, was also reported to be upregulated in MS (Nali et al., 2020). Studies suggest that a specific neutrophil subtype, low-density granulocytes (LDGs), participate in NET formation (Ng et al., 2019; Denny et al., 2010). Interestingly, $CD14^{-}/CD15^{high}$ LDGs are more prevalent in the blood of MS patients, providing indirect evidence for NET involvement in MS (Ostendorf et al., 2019). Another study suggests that NLRP3 elevates NET formation by augmenting CXCR2 and CXCR4 expression in a ROS- and PAD4-dependent manner (Byun et al., 2024). Additionally, NET components can play a role in MA, as DNA extrusions generate autocrine costimulatory signals for CD4+ T cells and lymph nodes during the priming phase in mice models (Costanza et al., 2019). Finally, NET formation exacerbates disease severity and the recruitment of Th1 and Th17 cells (Byun et al., 2024). These studies show an association between MA/EAE pathogenesis and NET formation; however, the mechanism underlying this association remains unclear.

6. Extracellular traps in Parkinson's disease

Parkinson's disease is another neurodegenerative disease in which dopaminergic neurons residing in the substantia nigra degenerate and develop Lewy bodies. A recent study shows an association between NETs and Parkinson's disease, suggesting that the genes GPR78, CADM3, and CACNA1E may serve as biomarkers for PD with NETs. Another study highlights CAP2 as a pivotal gene in PD associated with NETs. (Li et al., 2024). Additionally, the disease exhibits elevated expression of neuronal nitric oxide synthase in circulating neutrophils, leading to enhanced nitric oxide synthesis and exacerbating inflammation by triggering the release of extracellular traps from dissociated neutrophils (Gatto et al., 2000; Manda-Handzlik et al., 2020).

Similarly, NETs have also been linked to pathological processes of neurological disorders, including stroke, amyotrophic lateral sclerosis, traumatic brain injury, brain tumors, and Huntington's disease, where peripheral immune dysregulation and chronic inflammation are increasingly recognized contributors to disease progression (Beers & Appel, 2019). Therapeutically, targeting ETs represents a promising yet complex strategy. Approaches include

DNase I to degrade extracellular DNA scaffolds, peptidylarginine deiminase 4 (PAD4) inhibitors to block NETosis, MPO inhibitors to reduce oxidative damage, and modulation of neutrophil recruitment (Papayannopoulos, 2018; Knight et al., 2015).

Beyond peripheral immune cells, microglia have been reported to release ET-like structures under non-sterile and sterile conditions. Previous studies have reported that microglia can release extracellular traps in response to *Listeria* infection and dopamine (Wang et al., 2019; Agrawal et al., 2021). These microglia ETs (MiETs) differ from the classical NETs in every aspect including their triggers, composition, and functional outputs. MiETs present in the glioblastoma (GBM) microenvironment. Although the mechanism of MiETs formation remains incompletely understood, the established role of microglia in neuroinflammation and neurodegenerative disease, where they exhibit both neuroprotective and neurotoxic roles, suggests that MiETs may play a role in these contexts.

7. Microglia extracellular traps in neurodegenerative disease

Microglia extracellular traps (MiETs) are web-like structures released by microglia in response to pathogenic and chemical stimuli, such as *Listeria monocytogenes*, *Weissella cibaria*, ionomycin, PMA, and dopamine (DA) (Agrawal et al., 2021; Eto et al., 2021; Wang et al., 2019). Mechanistically, MiET formation appears to involve chromatin decondensation driven by reactive oxygen species (ROS), PAD2-mediated histone citrullination, and the release of nuclear or mitochondrial DNA; it also consist of matrix metallopeptidases (MMP9 and MMP12), citrullinated histones (H3), and peptidyl arginine deiminase 2 (PAD2) that can act as damage-associated molecular patterns, promoting sustained microglial activation, extracellular matrix degradation, and blood–brain barrier disruption, processes closely associated with neurodegenerative pathology (Wang et al., 2019). Recent studies show that MiETs are released in response to silicon dioxide (SiO2) nanoparticles, which disrupt the blood-brain barrier, leading to neuronal pyroptosis via M1 polarization of microglia and ROS/NLRP3 axis as ROS can promote the assembly of NLRP3, Caspase1, and ASC to form inflammasomes, cleave downstream GSDMD, release the N-terminal domain, and ultimately resulting in the formation of pores on the cell membrane surface and releasing IL-1β and IL-18 (Abais et al., 2015; Liu et al., 2025). These overlaps significantly with molecular processes already implicated in neurodegenerative diseases, including oxidative stress, mitochondrial dysfunction, and dysregulated innate immune signaling.

Given microglia's role and protective function in the CNS, the inflammatory shift and dysfunctional phenotypes of microglia can serve as a central focus for target selection and interventions. In neurodegenerative disease, microglia exhibit impaired phagocytosis and pro-inflammatory activity, leading to Aβ and tau deposition and damaged synapses and neurons. Targeting microglia can enhance microglial phagocytic ability and mitigate neuroinflammation (Sun et al., 2024). Similarly, microglia can drive pathological progression and neurodegeneration via extracellular vesicles. Thus, targeting microglia by inhibiting microglial exosome synthesis and secretion can enhance phagocytosis and neuroinflammation, and promote microglial conversion to a protective phenotype (Gao et al., 2023). Along with microglia and microglial exosomes, microglia extracellular traps (MiETs) can also contribute to neurodegenerative diseases. As MiETs formation appears primarily as a stimulus and a pathological response, this suggests that inhibiting MiETs might not compromise normal microglial function.

Similar to NETs, excessive MiETs can be cleared or degraded by DNase I. Matrix Metalloproteases (MMPs) can potentially disrupt the BBB and damage tissues, as ETs consist of MMPs; MMP inhibitors can help in neurodegenerative disease. Further ROS and NOX released during MiETs can also contribute to the development of neurodegenerative diseases (Haider et al., 2011; Chen et al., 2012; Fischer et al., 2012). Similarly, other components of ET, such as myeloperoxidase (MPO) and citrullinated histones, have been associated with neurodegenerative disease; thus, inhibiting elevated MPO and histone citrullination is a potential target (Gray et al., 2008; Mastronardi et al., 2006; Petrozziello et al., 2020). Microglia extracellular traps also release extracellular nucleic acids, which can act as DAMPs and contribute to neurodegenerative disorders; these can be targeted as a potential therapeutic (Kunze et al., 2023). More strategies can be explored to target MiETs, but they also require understanding the role of MiETs in neurodegenerative disease beforehand.

8. Conclusion

Microglia are the primary resident immune cells of the CNS and help maintain constant immune surveillance by eliminating pathogens, cellular debris, and redundant synapses. They are also essential in neurodevelopment, CNS homeostasis, and neuroinflammation, with significant implications in neurodegenerative disease. Initially, to understand the role of microglia in the CNS and neurodegenerative disease, studies focused on their M1 and M2 phenotypes and their detrimental and supportive roles, as microglial function in neurodegenerative disease can be a double-edged sword. It can facilitate the clearance of misfolded proteins while also contributing to synapse loss, making microglia a therapeutic target.

Another aspect of microglia is the release of extracellular traps, as an innate immune response to pathogens and damage-associated signals. In parallel, neutrophils have been reported to infiltrate the CNS and to form neutrophil extracellular traps (NETs), which contribute to the disruption of the BBB and neuroinflammation, ultimately contributing to neurodegenerative disease via components such as metalloproteinases, proteases, cytokines, extracellular histones, DNA, and ROS. Similar to neutrophils, microglia release extracellular DNA containing citrullinated histone (CitH3), myeloperoxidase (MPO), peptidylarginine deiminase 2 (PAD2), MMP-9, and MMP-12. Microglia extracellular traps (MiETs) released are cytosolic reactive oxygen species (ROS) and NADPH-oxidase dependent or independent. As is well known, MMP-9 and histones associated with NETs disrupt BBB integrity, while ROS accumulation in AD patients can lead to mitochondrial dysfunction via aggravating Aβ aggregation, contributing to neuroinflammation and neurodegeneration. Additionally, MiETs also lead to neuronal loss, which can exacerbate the condition of neurodegeneration. As MiETs are composed of similar components to NETs, they can exert similar effects, suggesting that MiETs release may contribute to chronic neuroinflammation and neurodegeneration. Hence, making extracellular traps an important aspect to study as a therapeutic biomarker. Because NETs can exacerbate disease, many pharmacological inhibitors of NET formation have been reported, including DNase I, Cl-amidine, cyclosporine A, and ascomycin. Further pathway-specific inhibitors can also be used that inhibit upstream or downstream pathways of NETosis. There are also clinical trials that measure NETs as biomarkers rather than therapeutic targets, suggesting that ETs can be a potential therapeutic target. And given the role of microglia in CNS homeostasis and neurodegenerative disease, understanding the mechanisms, functional consequences, and pathological relevance of MiETs is essential.

References

Abais, J. M., Xia, M., Zhang, Y., Boini, K. M., & Li, P.-L. (2015). Redox regulation of NLRP3 inflammasomes: ROS as trigger or effector? *Antioxidants & Redox Signaling, 22*, 1111–1129. https://doi.org/10.1089/ars.2014.5994.

Abdallah, D. S. A., Lin, C., Ball, C. J., King, M. R., Duhamel, G. E., & Denkers, E. Y. (2012). Toxoplasma gondii triggers release of human and mouse neutrophil extracellular traps. *Infection and Immunity, 80*, 768. https://doi.org/10.1128/IAI.05730-11.

Abrams, S. T., Zhang, N., Manson, J., Liu, T., Dart, C., Baluwa, F., ... Toh, C.-H. (2013). Circulating histones are mediators of trauma-associated lung injury. *American Journal of Respiratory and Critical Care Medicine, 187*, 160–169. https://doi.org/10.1164/rccm.201206-1037OC.

Agrawal, I., Sharma, N., Saxena, S., Arvind, S., Chakraborty, D., Chakraborty, D. B., ... Jha, S. (2021). Dopamine induces functional extracellular traps in microglia. *iScience, 24*. https://doi.org/10.1016/j.isci.2020.101968.

Akiyama, H., & McGeer, P. L. (1990). Brain microglia constitutively express beta-2 integrins. *Journal of Neuroimmunology, 30*, 81–93. https://doi.org/10.1016/0165-5728(90)90055-r.

Albert, M., Antel, J., Brück, W., & Stadelmann, C. (2007). Extensive cortical remyelination in patients with chronic multiple sclerosis. *Brain Pathology (Zurich, Switzerland), 17*, 129–138. https://doi.org/10.1111/j.1750-3639.2006.00043.x.

Areschoug, T., & Gordon, S. (2009). Scavenger receptors: Role in innate immunity and microbial pathogenesis. *Cellular Microbiology, 11*, 1160–1169. https://doi.org/10.1111/j.1462-5822.2009.01326.x.

Association, A. (2018). 2018 Alzheimer's disease facts and figures. *Alzheimer's & Dementia: the Journal of the Alzheimer's Association, 14*, 367–429. https://doi.org/10.1016/j.jalz.2018.02.001.

Aulik, N. A., Hellenbrand, K. M., & Czuprynski, C. J. (2012). Mannheimia haemolytica and its leukotoxin cause macrophage extracellular trap formation by bovine macrophages. *Infection and Immunity, 80*, 1923–1933. https://doi.org/10.1128/IAI.06120-11.

Azevedo, E. P. C., Guimarães-Costa, A. B., Torezani, G. S., Braga, C. A., Palhano, F. L., Kelly, J. W., ... Foguel, D. (2012). Amyloid fibrils trigger the release of neutrophil extracellular traps (NETs), causing fibril fragmentation by NET-associated elastase. *The Journal of Biological Chemistry, 287*, 37206–37218. https://doi.org/10.1074/jbc.M112.369942.

Babcock, A. A., Kuziel, W. A., Rivest, S., & Owens, T. (2003). Chemokine expression by glial cells directs leukocytes to sites of axonal injury in the CNS. *The Journal of Neuroscience: the Official Journal of the Society for Neuroscience, 23*, 7922–7930. https://doi.org/10.1523/JNEUROSCI.23-21-07922.2003.

Barnum, S. R. (1999). Inhibition of complement as a therapeutic approach in inflammatory central nervous system (CNS) disease. *Molecular Medicine (Cambridge, Mass.), 5*, 569–582.

Barroso, M. V., Gropillo, I., Detoni, M. A. A., Thompson-Souza, G. A., Muniz, V. S., Vasconcelos, C. R. I., ... Neves, J. S. (2021). Structural and signaling events driving aspergillus fumigatus-induced human eosinophil extracellular trap release. *Frontiers in Microbiology, 12*. https://doi.org/10.3389/fmicb.2021.633696.

Becher, B., & Antel, J. P. (1996). Comparison of phenotypic and functional properties of immediately ex vivo and cultured human adult microglia. *Glia, 18*, 1–10. https://doi.org/10.1002/(SICI)1098-1136(199609)18:1%253C1::AID-GLIA1%253E3.0.CO;2-6.

Beers, D. R., & Appel, S. H. (2019 Feb). Immune dysregulation in amyotrophic lateral sclerosis: mechanisms and emerging therapies. *Lancet Neurol. 18*(2), 211–220. https://doi.org/10.1016/S1474-4422(18)30394-6. PMID: 30663610.

Boland, B., Yu, W. H., Corti, O., Mollereau, B., Henriques, A., Bezard, E., ... Millan, M. J. (2018). Promoting the clearance of neurotoxic proteins in neurodegenerative disorders of ageing. *Nature Reviews. Drug Discovery, 17*, 660–688. https://doi.org/10.1038/nrd.2018.109.

Boone, B. A., Orlichenko, L., Schapiro, N. E., Loughran, P., Gianfrate, G. C., Ellis, J. T., ... Zeh, H. J. (2015). The receptor for advanced glycation end products (RAGE) enhances autophagy and neutrophil extracellular traps in pancreatic cancer. *Cancer Gene Therapy, 22*, 326–334. https://doi.org/10.1038/cgt.2015.21.

Bordt, E. A., & Polster, B. M. (2014). NADPH oxidase- and mitochondria-derived reactive oxygen species in proinflammatory microglial activation: A bipartisan affair? *Free Radical Biology & Medicine, 76*, 34–46. https://doi.org/10.1016/j.freeradbiomed.2014.07.033.

Braak, H., & Braak, E. (1991). Neuropathological stageing of Alzheimer-related changes. *Acta Neuropathologica (Berl.), 82*, 239–259. https://doi.org/10.1007/BF00308809.

Branzk, N., Lubojemska, A., Hardison, S. E., Wang, Q., Gutierrez, M. G., Brown, G. D., & Papayannopoulos, V. (2014). Neutrophils sense microbe size and selectively release neutrophil extracellular traps in response to large pathogens. *Nature Immunology*, 2014 1511 15, 1017–1025. https://doi.org/10.1038/ni.2987.

Brinkmann, V., Reichard, U., Goosmann, C., Fauler, B., Uhlemann, Y., Weiss, D. S., Weinrauch, Y., & Zychlinsky, A. (2004). Neutrophil extracellular traps kill bacteria. *Science, 303*(5663), 1532–1535. https://doi.org/10.1126/science.1092385. PMID: 15001782.

Bsibsi, M., Ravid, R., Gveric, D., & van Noort, J. M. (2002). Broad expression of toll-like receptors in the human central nervous system. *Journal of Neuropathology and Experimental Neurology, 61*, 1013–1021. https://doi.org/10.1093/jnen/61.11.1013.

Byun, D. J., Lee, J., Ko, K., & Hyun, Y.-M. (2024). NLRP3 exacerbates EAE severity through ROS-dependent NET formation in the mouse brain. *Cell Commun. Signal. CCS, 22*, 96. https://doi.org/10.1186/s12964-023-01447-z.

Campbell, A. M., Kashgarian, M., & Shlomchik, M. J. (2012). NADPH oxidase inhibits the pathogenesis of systemic lupus erythematosus. *Science Translational Medicine, 4*, 157ra141. https://doi.org/10.1126/scitranslmed.3004801.

Campillo-Navarro, M., Leyva-Paredes, K., Donis-Maturano, L., González-Jiménez, M., Paredes-Vivas, Y., Cerbulo-Vázquez, A., ... Chacón-Salinas, R. (2017). Listeria monocytogenes induces mast cell extracellular traps. *Immunobiology, 222*, 432–439. https://doi.org/10.1016/J.IMBIO.2016.08.006.

Chen, C.-J., Chen, J.-H., Chen, S.-Y., Liao, S.-L., & Raung, S.-L. (2004). Upregulation of RANTES gene expression in neuroglia by Japanese encephalitis virus infection. *Journal of Virology, 78*, 12107–12119. https://doi.org/10.1128/JVI.78.22.12107-12119.2004.

Chen, X., Guo, C., & Kong, J. (2012). Oxidative stress in neurodegenerative diseases. *Neural Regeneration Research, 7*, 376–385. https://doi.org/10.3969/j.issn.1673-5374.2012.05.009.

Cherry, J. D., Olschowka, J. A., & O'Banion, M. K. (2014). Neuroinflammation and M2 microglia: The good, the bad, and the inflamed. *Journal of Neuroinflammation, 11*, 98. https://doi.org/10.1186/1742-2094-11-98.

Chow, O. A., Von Köckritz-Blickwede, M., Bright, A. T., Hensler, M. E., Zinkernagel, A. S., Cogen, A. L., ... Nizet, V. (2010). Statins enhance formation of phagocyte extracellular traps. *Cell Host & Microbe, 8*, 445–454. https://doi.org/10.1016/J.CHOM.2010.10.005.

Clark, S. R., Ma, A. C., Tavener, S. A., McDonald, B., Goodarzi, Z., Kelly, M. M., ... Kubes, P. (2007). Platelet TLR4 activates neutrophil extracellular traps to ensnare bacteria in septic blood. *Nature Medicine, 13*, 463–469. https://doi.org/10.1038/nm1565.

Coffelt, S. B., Kersten, K., Doornebal, C. W., Weiden, J., Vrijland, K., Hau, C.-S., ... de Visser, K. E. (2015). IL-17-producing γδ T cells and neutrophils conspire to promote breast cancer metastasis. *Nature, 522*, 345–348. https://doi.org/10.1038/nature14282.

Colonna, M., & Butovsky, O. (2017). Microglia function in the central nervous system during health and neurodegeneration. *Annual Review of Immunology, 35*, 441–468. https://doi.org/10.1146/annurev-immunol-051116-052358.

Cornell, J., Salinas, S., Huang, H.-Y., & Zhou, M. (2021). Microglia regulation of synaptic plasticity and learning and memory. *Neural Regeneration Research, 17*, 705–716. https://doi.org/10.4103/1673-5374.322423.

Costanza, M., Poliani, P. L., Portararo, P., Cappetti, B., Musio, S., Pagani, F., ... Sangaletti, S. (2019). DNA threads released by activated CD4+ T lymphocytes provide autocrine costimulation. *Proceedings of the National Academy of Sciences, 116*, 8985–8994. https://doi.org/10.1073/pnas.1822013116.

Crabbé, M., Van der Perren, A., Bollaerts, I., Kounelis, S., Baekelandt, V., Bormans, G., ... Van Laere, K. (2019). Increased P2X7 receptor binding is associated with neuroinflammation in acute but not chronic rodent models for Parkinson's disease. *Frontiers in Neuroscience, 13*, 799. https://doi.org/10.3389/fnins.2019.00799.

Cserép, C., Pósfai, B., Orsolits, B., Molnár, G., Heindl, S., Lénárt, N., ... Dénes, Á. (2019). Microglia monitor and protect neuronal function via specialized somatic purinergic junctions. *Cardiovascular Sciences*. https://doi.org/10.1101/606079.

Czapski, G. A., & Strosznajder, J. B. (2021). Glutamate and GABA in microglia-neuron cross-talk in Alzheimer's disease. *International Journal of Molecular Sciences, 22*, 11677. https://doi.org/10.3390/ijms222111677.

Dai, X.-M., Ryan, G. R., Hapel, A. J., Dominguez, M. G., Russell, R. G., Kapp, S., ... Stanley, E. R. (2002). Targeted disruption of the mouse colony-stimulating factor 1 receptor gene results in osteopetrosis, mononuclear phagocyte deficiency, increased primitive progenitor cell frequencies, and reproductive defects. *Blood, 99*, 111–120. https://doi.org/10.1182/blood.V99.1.111.

Damani, M. R., Zhao, L., Fontainhas, A. M., Amaral, J., Fariss, R. N., & Wong, W. T. (2011). Age-related alterations in the dynamic behavior of microglia. *Aging Cell, 10*, 263–276. https://doi.org/10.1111/j.1474-9726.2010.00660.x.

Davie, C. A. (2008). A review of Parkinson's disease. *British Medical Bulletin, 86*, 109–127. https://doi.org/10.1093/bmb/ldn013.

De Groot, C. J., Bergers, E., Kamphorst, W., Ravid, R., Polman, C. H., Barkhof, F., & van der Valk, P. (2001). Post-mortem MRI-guided sampling of multiple sclerosis brain lesions: Increased yield of active demyelinating and (p)reactive lesions. *Brain: A Journal of Neurology, 124*, 1635–1645. https://doi.org/10.1093/brain/124.8.1635.

Deczkowska, A., Keren-Shaul, H., Weiner, A., Colonna, M., Schwartz, M., & Amit, I. (2018). Disease-associated microglia: A universal immune sensor of neurodegeneration. *Cell, 173*, 1073–1081. https://doi.org/10.1016/j.cell.2018.05.003.

Demers, M., Wong, S. L., Martinod, K., Gallant, M., Cabral, J. E., Wang, Y., & Wagner, D. D. (2016). Priming of neutrophils toward NETosis promotes tumor growth. *Oncoimmunology, 5*, e1134073. https://doi.org/10.1080/2162402X.2015.1134073.

Denny, M. F., Yalavarthi, S., Zhao, W., Thacker, S. G., Anderson, M., Sandy, A. R., ... Kaplan, M. J. (2010). A distinct subset of proinflammatory neutrophils isolated from patients with systemic lupus erythematosus induces vascular damage and synthesizes type I IFNs. *Journal of Immunology Baltimore, MD 1950, 184*, 3284–3297. https://doi.org/10.4049/JIMMUNOL.0902199.

Dheen, S. T., Kaur, C., & Ling, E.-A., (n.d.) Microglial activation and its implications in the brain diseases. http://www.eurekaselect.com.

Dick, A. D., Ford, A. L., Forrester, J. V., & Sedgwick, J. D. (n.d.). Flow cytometric identification of a minority population of MHC class II positive cells in the normal rat retina distinct from CD45lowCD1 lb/c+CD4low parenchymal microglia. British Journal of Ophthalmology.

Dickson, D. W. (2018). Neuropathology of Parkinson disease. *Parkinsonism & Related Disorders, 46*(1), S30–S33. https://doi.org/10.1016/j.parkreldis.2017.07.033.

Domingues, H. S., Portugal, C. C., Socodato, R., & Relvas, J. B. (2016). Oligodendrocyte, astrocyte, and microglia crosstalk in myelin development, damage, and repair. *Frontiers in Cell and Developmental Biology, 4*, 71. https://doi.org/10.3389/fcell.2016.00071.

Douda, D. N., Khan, M. A., Grasemann, H., & Palaniyar, N. (2015). SK3 channel and mitochondrial ROS mediate NADPH oxidase-independent NETosis induced by calcium influx. *Proceedings of the National Academy of Sciences of the United States of America, 112*, 2817–2822. https://doi.org/10.1073/PNAS.1414055112.

Dugger, B. N., & Dickson, D. W. (2017). Pathology of neurodegenerative diseases. *Cold Spring Harbor Perspectives in Biology, 9*, a028035. https://doi.org/10.1101/cshperspect.a028035.

Dworski, R., Simon, H.-U., Hoskins, A., & Yousefi, S. (2011). Eosinophil and neutrophil extracellular DNA traps in human allergic asthmatic airways. *The Journal of Allergy and Clinical Immunology, 127*, 1260–1266. https://doi.org/10.1016/j.jaci.2010.12.1103.

Dwyer, M., Shan, Q., D'Ortona, S., Maurer, R., Mitchell, R., Olesen, H., ... Gadjeva, M. (2014). Cystic fibrosis sputum DNA has NETosis characteristics and neutrophil extracellular trap release is regulated by macrophage migration-inhibitory factor. *Journal of Innate Immunity, 6*, 765–779. https://doi.org/10.1159/000363242.

Elmore, M. R. P., Najafi, A. R., Koike, M. A., Dagher, N. N., Spangenberg, E. E., Rice, R. A., ... Green, K. N. (2014). Colony-stimulating factor 1 receptor signaling is necessary for microglia viability, unmasking a microglia progenitor cell in the adult brain. *Neuron, 82*, 380–397. https://doi.org/10.1016/j.neuron.2014.02.040.

Eto, S. F., Fernandes, D. C., Funnicelli, M. I. G., Alecrim, J. V. C., Souza, P. G., Carvalho, F. C. A., ... Pizauro, J. M. (2021). Microglia extracellular traps in Oreochromis niloticus infected with Weissella cibaria. *Fish & Shellfish Immunology, 113*, 148–153. https://doi.org/10.1016/J.FSI.2021.03.020.

Eyo, U. B., Peng, J., Swiatkowski, P., Mukherjee, A., Bispo, A., & Wu, L.-J. (2014). Neuronal hyperactivity recruits microglial processes via neuronal NMDA receptors and microglial P2Y12 receptors after status epilepticus. *The Journal of Neuroscience : the Official Journal of the Society for Neuroscience, 34*, 10528–10540. https://doi.org/10.1523/JNEUROSCI.0416-14.2014.

Fairley, L. H., Lai, K. O., Grimm, A., Eckert, A., & Barron, A. M. (2024). The mitochondrial translocator protein (TSPO) in Alzheimer's disease: Therapeutic and immunomodulatory functions. *Biochimie, 224*, 120–131. https://doi.org/10.1016/j.biochi.2024.07.003.

Fang, N., Chen, Y., Yikang, W., Yongli, W., Xu, J., Xiao, J., ... Yang, L. (n.d.) Targeting microglia extracellular traps via an "Internal-External" synergistic strategy to reshape the dysregulated microglia-neuron axis for spinal cord injury recovery. Advanced Functional Materials. n/a, e19846. https://doi.org/10.1002/adfm.202519846.

Fischer, M. T., Sharma, R., Lim, J. L., Haider, L., Frischer, J. M., Drexhage, J., ... Lassmann, H. (2012). NADPH oxidase expression in active multiple sclerosis lesions in relation to oxidative tissue damage and mitochondrial injury. *Brain, 135*, 886–899. https://doi.org/10.1093/brain/aws012.

Floden, A. M., Li, S., & Combs, C. K. (2005). Beta-amyloid-stimulated microglia induce neuron death via synergistic stimulation of tumor necrosis factor alpha and NMDA receptors. *The Journal of Neuroscience : the Official Journal of the Society for Neuroscience, 25*, 2566–2575. https://doi.org/10.1523/JNEUROSCI.4998-04.2005.

Franco, R., Lillo, A., Rivas-Santisteban, R., Reyes-Resina, I., & Navarro, G. (2021). Microglial adenosine receptors: From preconditioning to modulating the M1/M2 balance in activated cells. *Cells, 10*, 1124. https://doi.org/10.3390/cells10051124.

Frost, J. L., & Schafer, D. P. (2016). Microglia: Architects of the developing nervous system. *Trends in Cell Biology, 26*, 587–597. https://doi.org/10.1016/j.tcb.2016.02.006.

Fuchs, T. A., Brill, A., Duerschmied, D., Schatzberg, D., Monestier, M., Myers, D. D., ... Wagner, D. D. (2010). Extracellular DNA traps promote thrombosis. *Proceedings of the National Academy of Sciences of the United States of America, 107*, 15880–15885. https://doi.org/10.1073/PNAS.1005743107.

Gao, C., Jiang, J., Tan, Y., & Chen, S. (2023). Microglia in neurodegenerative diseases: Mechanism and potential therapeutic targets. *Signal Transduction and Targeted Therapy, 8*, 359. https://doi.org/10.1038/s41392-023-01588-0.

Garcia-Romo, G. S., Caielli, S., Vega, B., Connolly, J., Allantaz, F., Xu, Z., ... Pascual, V. (2011). Netting neutrophils are major inducers of type I IFN production in pediatric systemic lupus erythematosus. *Science Translational Medicine, 3*. https://doi.org/10.1126/SCITRANSLMED.3001201.

Gatto, E. M., Riobó, N. A., Carreras, M. C., Cherñavsky, A., Rubio, A., Satz, M. L., & Poderoso, J. J. (2000). Overexpression of neutrophil neuronal nitric oxide synthase in Parkinson's disease. *Nitric Oxide Biology & Chemistry, 4*, 534–539. https://doi.org/10.1006/niox.2000.0288.

Geng, L., Fan, L. M., Liu, F., Smith, C., & Li, J.-M. (2020). Nox2 dependent redox-regulation of microglial response to amyloid-β stimulation and microgliosis in aging. *Scientific Reports, 10*, 1582. https://doi.org/10.1038/s41598-020-58422-8.

Ginhoux, F., Greter, M., Leboeuf, M., Nandi, S., See, P., Gokhan, S., ... Merad, M. (2010). Fate mapping analysis reveals that adult microglia derive from primitive macrophages. *Science (New York, N. Y.), 330*, 841–845. https://doi.org/10.1126/science.1194637.

Goedert, M. (2001). Alpha-synuclein and neurodegenerative diseases. *Nature Reviews. Neuroscience, 2*, 492–501. https://doi.org/10.1038/35081564.

Gómez Morillas, A., Besson, V. C., & Lerouet, D. (2021). Microglia and neuroinflammation: What place for P2RY12? *International Journal of Molecular Sciences, 22*, 1636. https://doi.org/10.3390/ijms22041636.

Gray, E., Thomas, T. L., Betmouni, S., Scolding, N., & Love, S. (2008). Elevated myeloperoxidase activity in white matter in multiple sclerosis. *Neuroscience Letters, 444*, 195–198. https://doi.org/10.1016/j.neulet.2008.08.035.

Guo, S., Wang, H., & Yin, Y. (2022). Microglia polarization from M1 to M2 in neurodegenerative diseases. *Frontiers in Aging Neuroscience, 14*, 815347. https://doi.org/10.3389/fnagi.2022.815347.

Hagino, Y., Kariura, Y., Manago, Y., Amano, T., Wang, B., Sekiguchi, M., ... Noda, M. (2004). Heterogeneity and potentiation of AMPA type of glutamate receptors in rat cultured microglia. *Glia, 47*, 68–77. https://doi.org/10.1002/glia.20034.

Haider, L., Fischer, M. T., Frischer, J. M., Bauer, J., Höftberger, R., Botond, G., ... Lassmann, H. (2011). Oxidative damage in multiple sclerosis lesions. *Brain: A Journal of Neurology, 134*, 1914–1924. https://doi.org/10.1093/brain/awr128.

Hakkim, A., Fuchs, T. A., Martinez, N. E., Hess, S., Prinz, H., Zychlinsky, A., & Waldmann, H. (2011). Activation of the Raf-MEK-ERK pathway is required for neutrophil extracellular trap formation. *Nature Chemical Biology, 7*, 75–77. https://doi.org/10.1038/NCHEMBIO.496.

Halverson, T. W. R., Wilton, M., Poon, K. K. H., Petri, B., & Lewenza, S. (2015). DNA is an antimicrobial component of neutrophil extracellular traps. *PLoS Pathogens, 11*, e1004593. https://doi.org/10.1371/journal.ppat.1004593.

Hansen, D. V., Hanson, J. E., & Sheng, M. (2017). Microglia in Alzheimer's disease. *The Journal of Cell Biology, 217*, 459–472. https://doi.org/10.1083/jcb.201709069.

Hardy, J., & Selkoe, D. J. (2002). The amyloid hypothesis of Alzheimer's disease: Progress and problems on the road to therapeutics. *Science (New York, N. Y.), 297*, 353–356. https://doi.org/10.1126/science.1072994.

Hartlage-Rübsamen, M., Lemke, R., & Schliebs, R. (1999). Interleukin-1beta, inducible nitric oxide synthase, and nuclear factor-kappaB are induced in morphologically distinct microglia after rat hippocampal lipopolysaccharide/interferon-gamma injection. *Journal of Neuroscience Research, 57*, 388–398.

Haslund-Vinding, J., McBean, G., Jaquet, V., & Vilhardt, F. (2017). NADPH oxidases in oxidant production by microglia: activating receptors, pharmacology and association with disease. *British Journal of Pharmacology, 174*, 1733–1749. https://doi.org/10.1111/bph.13425.

Hayes, A., Thaker, U., Iwatsubo, T., Pickering-Brown, S. M., & Mann, D. M. A. (2002). Pathological relationships between microglial cell activity and tau and amyloid beta protein in patients with Alzheimer's disease. *Neuroscience Letters, 331*, 171–174. https://doi.org/10.1016/s0304-3940(02)00888-1.

Herster, F., Bittner, Z., Archer, N. K., Dickhöfer, S., Eisel, D., Eigenbrod, T., ... Weber, A. N. R. (2020). Neutrophil extracellular trap-associated RNA and LL37 enable self-amplifying inflammation in psoriasis. *Nature Communications, 11*. https://doi.org/10.1038/s41467-019-13756-4.

Hierro-Bujalance, C., Bacskai, B. J., & Garcia-Alloza, M. (2018). Vivo imaging of microglia with multiphoton microscopy. *Frontiers in Aging Neuroscience, 10*, 218. https://doi.org/10.3389/fnagi.2018.00218.

Hirsch, J. G. (1958). Bactericidal action of histone. *The Journal of Experimental Medicine, 108*, 925–944. https://doi.org/10.1084/jem.108.6.925.

Hsieh, C. L., Koike, M., Spusta, S. C., Niemi, E. C., Yenari, M., Nakamura, M. C., & Seaman, W. E. (2009). A role for TREM2 ligands in the phagocytosis of apoptotic neuronal cells by microglia. *Journal of Neurochemistry, 109*, 1144–1156. https://doi.org/10.1111/j.1471-4159.2009.06042.x.

Huang, H., Tohme, S., Al-Khafaji, A. B., Tai, S., Loughran, P., Chen, L., ... Tsung, A. (2015). Damage-associated molecular pattern-activated neutrophil extracellular trap exacerbates sterile inflammatory liver injury. *Hepatology (Baltimore, Md.), 62*, 600–614. https://doi.org/10.1002/hep.27841.

Huebener, P., Pradere, J.-P., Hernandez, C., Gwak, G.-Y., Caviglia, J. M., Mu, X., ... Schwabe, R. F. (2015). The HMGB1/RAGE axis triggers neutrophil-mediated injury amplification following necrosis. *The Journal of Clinical Investigation, 125*, 539–550. https://doi.org/10.1172/JCI76887.

Jankovic, J. (2008). Parkinson's disease: Clinical features and diagnosis. *Journal of Neurology, Neurosurgery, and Psychiatry, 79*, 368–376. https://doi.org/10.1136/jnnp.2007.131045.

Joers, V., Tansey, M. G., Mulas, G., & Carta, A. R. (2017). Microglial phenotypes in Parkinson's disease and animal models of the disease. *Progress in Neurobiology Multiple Mechanisms of Neurodegeneration and Progression, 155*, 57–75. https://doi.org/10.1016/j.pneurobio.2016.04.006.

Jurga, A. M., Paleczna, M., & Kuter, K. Z. (2020). Overview of general and discriminating markers of differential microglia phenotypes. *Frontiers in Cellular Neuroscience, 14*. https://doi.org/10.3389/fncel.2020.00198.

Kann, O., Almouhanna, F., & Chausse, B. (2022). Interferon γ: A master cytokine in microglia-mediated neural network dysfunction and neurodegeneration. *Trends in Neurosciences, 45*, 913–927. https://doi.org/10.1016/j.tins.2022.10.007.

Karkowska-Kuleta, J., Smolarz, M., Seweryn-Ozog, K., Satala, D., Zawrotniak, M., Wronowska, E., ... Rapala-Kozik, M. (2021). Proteinous components of neutrophil extracellular traps are arrested by the cell wall proteins of Candida albicans during fungal infection, and can be used in the host invasion. *Cells, 10*, 2736. https://doi.org/10.3390/cells10102736.

Karmakar, M., Sun, Y., Hise, A. G., Rietsch, A., & Pearlman, E. (2012). Cutting edge: IL-1β processing during Pseudomonas aeruginosa infection is mediated by neutrophil serine proteases and is independent of NLRC4 and caspase-1. *Journal of Immunology, 189*, 4231–4235. https://doi.org/10.4049/jimmunol.1201447.

Kawabori, M., & Yenari, M. A. (2015). The role of the microglia in acute CNS injury. *Metabolic Brain Disease, 30*, 381. https://doi.org/10.1007/S11011-014-9531-6.

Kempuraj, D., Thangavel, R., Natteru, P., Selvakumar, G., Saeed, D., Zahoor, H., ... Zaheer, A. (2016). Neuroinflammation Induces Neurodegeneration. *Journal of Neurology, Neurosurgery and Spine, 1*, 1003.

Keren-Shaul, H., Spinrad, A., Weiner, A., Matcovitch-Natan, O., Dvir-Szternfeld, R., Ulland, T. K., ... Amit, I. (2017). A unique microglia type associated with restricting development of Alzheimer's disease. *Cell, 169*, 1276–1290.e17. https://doi.org/10.1016/j.cell.2017.05.018.

Kigerl, K. A., de Rivero Vaccari, J. P., Dietrich, W. D., Popovich, P. G., & Keane, R. W. (2014). Pattern recognition receptors and central nervous system repair. *Experimental Neurology, 258*, 5–16. https://doi.org/10.1016/j.expneurol.2014.01.001.

Kline, E. M., Houser, M. C., Herrick, M. K., Seibler, P., Klein, C., West, A., & Tansey, M. G. (2021). Genetic and environmental factors in Parkinson's disease converge on immune function and inflammation. *Movement Disorders: Official Journal of the Movement Disorder Society, 36*, 25–36. https://doi.org/10.1002/mds.28411.

Knight, J. S., Subramanian, V., O'Dell, A. A., Yalavarthi, S., Zhao, W., Smith, C. K., Hodgin, J. B., Thompson, P. R., & Kaplan, M. J. (2015). Peptidylarginine deiminase inhibition disrupts NET formation and protects against kidney, skin and vascular disease in lupus-prone MRL/lpr mice. *Ann Rheum Dis*. *74*(12), 2199–2206. https://doi.org/10.1136/annrheumdis-2014-205365 Epub 2014 Aug 7. PMID: 25104775; PMCID: PMC4320672.

Koizumi, S., Ohsawa, K., Inoue, K., & Kohsaka, S. (2013). Purinergic receptors in microglia: Functional modal shifts of microglia mediated by P2 and P1 receptors. *Glia, 61*, 47–54. https://doi.org/10.1002/glia.22358.

Kreutzberg, G. W. (1996). Microglia: A sensor for pathological events in the CNS. *Trends in Neurosciences, 19*, 312–318. https://doi.org/10.1016/0166-2236(96)10049-7.

Kunze, R., Fischer, S., Marti, H. H., & Preissner, K. T. (2023). Brain alarm by self-extracellular nucleic acids: From neuroinflammation to neurodegeneration. *Journal of Biomedical Science, 30*, 64. https://doi.org/10.1186/s12929-023-00954-y.

Lampron, A., Larochelle, A., Laflamme, N., Préfontaine, P., Plante, M.-M., Sánchez, M. G., ... Rivest, S. (2015). Inefficient clearance of myelin debris by microglia impairs remyelinating processes. *The Journal of Experimental Medicine, 212*, 481–495. https://doi.org/10.1084/jem.20141656.

Lassmann, H., Brück, W., & Lucchinetti, C. F. (2007). The immunopathology of multiple sclerosis: An overview. *Brain Pathology (Zurich, Switzerland), 17*, 210–218. https://doi.org/10.1111/j.1750-3639.2007.00064.x.

Lauth, X., von Köckritz-Blickwede, M., McNamara, C. W., Myskowski, S., Zinkernagel, A. S., Beall, B., ... Nizet, V. (2009). M1 Protein allows Group A streptococcal survival in phagocyte extracellular traps through cathelicidin inhibition. *Journal of Innate Immunity, 1*, 202–214. https://doi.org/10.1159/000203645.

Lawson, L. J., Perry, V. H., & Gordon, S. (1992). Turnover of resident microglia in the normal adult mouse brain. *Neuroscience, 48*, 405–415. https://doi.org/10.1016/0306-4522(92)90500-2.

Lawson, L. J., Perry, V. H., Dri, P., & Gordon, S. (1990). Heterogeneity in the distribution and morphology of microglia in the normal adult mouse brain. *Neuroscience, 39*, 151–170. https://doi.org/10.1016/0306-4522(90)90229-w.

Lee, V. M.-Y., & Trojanowski, J. Q. (2006). Mechanisms of Parkinson's disease linked to pathological alpha-synuclein: New targets for drug discovery. *Neuron, 52*, 33–38. https://doi.org/10.1016/j.neuron.2006.09.026.

Lemke, G. (2013). Biology of the TAM receptors. *Cold Spring Harbor Perspectives in Biology, 5*, a009076. https://doi.org/10.1101/cshperspect.a009076.

Leng, F., & Edison, P. (2021). Neuroinflammation and microglial activation in Alzheimer disease: Where do we go from here? *Nature Reviews Neurology, 17*, 157–172. https://doi.org/10.1038/s41582-020-00435-y.

Li, W., Fu, Y., Halliday, G. M., & Sue, C. M. (2021). PARK genes link mitochondrial dysfunction and alpha-synuclein pathology in sporadic Parkinson's disease. *Frontiers in Cell and Developmental Biology, 9*. https://doi.org/10.3389/fcell.2021.612476.

Li, X., Luo, M., Xu, H., Jia, L., Liang, Y., Xu, Q., & Wang, Y. (2024). CAP2 contributes to Parkinson's disease diagnosed by neutrophil extracellular trap-related immune activity. *Frontiers in Immunology, 15*. https://doi.org/10.3389/fimmu.2024.1377409.

Lin, A. M., Rubin, C. J., Khandpur, R., Wang, J. Y., Riblett, M., Yalavarthi, S., ... Bruce, A. T. (2011). Mast cells and neutrophils release IL-17 through extracellular trap formation in psoriasis. *Journal of Immunology (Baltimore, Md. : 1950), 187*, 490–500. https://doi.org/10.4049/JIMMUNOL.1100123.

Ling, E. A., & Wong, W. C. (1993). The origin and nature of ramified and amoeboid microglia: A historical review and current concepts. *Glia, 7*, 9–18. https://doi.org/10.1002/glia.440070105.

Liu, J., Jin, X., Liu, K. J., & Liu, W. (2012). Matrix metalloproteinase-2-mediated occludin degradation and caveolin-1-mediated claudin-5 redistribution contribute to blood–brain barrier damage in early ischemic stroke stage. *The Journal of Neuroscience, 32*, 3044–3057. https://doi.org/10.1523/JNEUROSCI.6409-11.2012.

Liu, S., Ninan, I., Antonova, I., Battaglia, F., Trinchese, F., Narasanna, A., ... Arancio, O. (2004). Alpha-synuclein produces a long-lasting increase in neurotransmitter release. *The EMBO Journal, 23*, 4506–4516. https://doi.org/10.1038/sj.emboj.7600451.

Liu, H., Xu, T., Shi, X., Yin, Y., Yang, X., Wang, J., ... Xu, S. (2025). Neurotoxic domino effect: Dietary silica nanoparticles spark microglial extracellular traps and neuronal pyroptosis. *Journal of Agricultural and Food Chemistry, 73*, 20396–20409. https://doi.org/10.1021/acs.jafc.5c05403.

Liu, J. S.-H., Zhao, M.-L., Brosnan, C. F., & Lee, S. C. (2001). Expression of inducible nitric oxide synthase and nitrotyrosine in multiple sclerosis lesions. *The American Journal of Pathology, 158*, 2057–2066. https://doi.org/10.1016/S0002-9440(10)64677-9.

Lood, C., Blanco, L. P., Purmalek, M. M., Carmona-Rivera, C., De Ravin, S. S., Smith, C. K., ... Kaplan, M. J. (2016). Neutrophil extracellular traps enriched in oxidized mitochondrial DNA are interferogenic and contribute to lupus-like disease. *Nature Medicine, 22*, 146–153. https://doi.org/10.1038/nm.4027.

Lucchinetti, C. F., Popescu, B. F. G., Bunyan, R. F., Moll, N. M., Roemer, S. F., Lassmann, H., ... Ransohoff, R. M. (2011). Inflammatory cortical demyelination in early multiple sclerosis. *The New England Journal of Medicine, 365*, 2188–2197. https://doi.org/10.1056/NEJMoa1100648.

Ma, X., Lin, W. Y., Chen, Y., Stawicki, S., Mukhyala, K., Wu, Y., ... Starovasnik, M. A. (2012). Structural basis for the dual recognition of helical cytokines IL-34 and CSF-1 by CSF-1R. *Structure (London, England: 1993), 20*, 676–687. https://doi.org/10.1016/j.str.2012.02.010.

Manda-Handzlik, A., Bystrzycka, W., Cieloch, A., Glodkowska-Mrowka, E., Jankowska-Steifer, E., Heropolitanska-Pliszka, E., ... Demkow, U. (2020). Nitric oxide and peroxynitrite trigger and enhance release of neutrophil extracellular traps. *Cellular and Molecular Life Sciences (CMLS), 77*, 3059–3075. https://doi.org/10.1007/s00018-019-03331-x.

Martínez-Hernández, M. I., Acosta-Saavedra, L. C., Hernández-Kelly, L. C., Loaeza-Loaeza, J., & Ortega, A. (2023). Microglial activation in metal neurotoxicity: Impact in neurodegenerative diseases. *BioMed Research International, 2023*, 7389508. https://doi.org/10.1155/2023/7389508.

Martinod, K., Demers, M., Fuchs, T. A., Wong, S. L., Brill, A., Gallant, M., ... Wagner, D. D. (2013). Neutrophil histone modification by peptidylarginine deiminase 4 is critical for deep vein thrombosis in mice. *Proceedings of the National Academy of Sciences of the United States of America, 110*, 8674–8679. https://doi.org/10.1073/pnas.1301059110.

Martinod, K., Witsch, T., Erpenbeck, L., Savchenko, A., Hayashi, H., Cherpokova, D., ... Wagner, D. D. (2017). Peptidylarginine deiminase 4 promotes age-related organ fibrosis. *The Journal of Experimental Medicine, 214*, 439–458. https://doi.org/10.1084/jem.20160530.

Mastronardi, F. G., Wood, D. D., Mei, J., Raijmakers, R., Tseveleki, V., Dosch, H.-M., ... Moscarello, M. A. (2006). Increased citrullination of histone H3 in multiple sclerosis brain and animal models of demyelination: A role for tumor necrosis factor-induced peptidylarginine deiminase 4 translocation. *The Journal of Neuroscience, 26*, 11387–11396. https://doi.org/10.1523/JNEUROSCI.3349-06.2006.

Matej, R., Tesar, A., & Rusina, R. (2019). Alzheimer's disease and other neurodegenerative dementias in comorbidity: A clinical and neuropathological overview. *Clinical Biochemistry, 73*, 26–31. https://doi.org/10.1016/j.clinbiochem.2019.08.005.

Maugeri, N., Campana, L., Gavina, M., Covino, C., De Metrio, M., Panciroli, C., ... Manfredi, A. A. (2014). Activated platelets present high mobility group box 1 to neutrophils, inducing autophagy and promoting the extrusion of neutrophil extracellular traps. *Journal of Thrombosis and Haemostasis: JTH, 12*, 2074–2088. https://doi.org/10.1111/jth.12710.

Mazaheri, F., Snaidero, N., Kleinberger, G., Madore, C., Daria, A., Werner, G., ... Haass, C. (2017). TREM2 deficiency impairs chemotaxis and microglial responses to neuronal injury. *EMBO Reports, 18*, 1186–1198. https://doi.org/10.15252/embr.201743922.

Metzler, K. D., Goosmann, C., Lubojemska, A., Zychlinsky, A., & Papayannopoulos, V. (2014). Myeloperoxidase-containing complex regulates neutrophil elastase release and actin dynamics during NETosis. *Cell Reports, 8*, 883–896. https://doi.org/10.1016/J.CELREP.2014.06.044.

Miller, E., & Wachowicz, B., (n.d.) Advances in antioxidative therapy of multiple sclerosis. http://www.eurekaselect.com.

Milligan, K. L., Mann, D., Rump, A., Anderson, V. L., Hsu, A. P., Kuhns, D. B., ... Holland, S. M. (2016). Complete myeloperoxidase deficiency: Beware the "False-Positive" dihydrorhodamine oxidation. *The Journal of Pediatrics, 176*, 204–206. https://doi.org/10.1016/j.jpeds.2016.05.047.

Minohara, M., Matsuoka, T., Li, W., Osoegawa, M., Ishizu, T., Ohyagi, Y., & Kira, J. (2006). Upregulation of myeloperoxidase in patients with opticospinal multiple sclerosis: Positive correlation with disease severity. *Journal of Neuroimmunology, 178*, 156–160. https://doi.org/10.1016/j.jneuroim.2006.05.026.

Mizutani, M., Pino, P. A., Saederup, N., Charo, I. F., Ransohoff, R. M., & Cardona, A. E. (2012). The fractalkine receptor but not CCR2 is present on microglia from embryonic development throughout adulthood. *Journal of Immunology, 188*, 29–36. https://doi.org/10.4049/jimmunol.1100421.

Möllerherm, H., von Köckritz-Blickwede, M., & Branitzki-Heinemann, K. (2016). Antimicrobial activity of mast cells: Role and relevance of extracellular DNA traps. *Frontiers in Immunology, 7*, 207907. https://doi.org/10.3389/FIMMU.2016.00265/BIBTEX.

Morshed, M., Hlushchuk, R., Simon, D., Walls, A. F., Obata-Ninomiya, K., Karasuyama, H., ... Yousefi, S. (2014). NADPH oxidase-independent formation of extracellular DNA traps by basophils. *The Journal of Immunology (Baltimore, Md), 192*, 5314–5323. https://doi.org/10.4049/JIMMUNOL.1303418.

Munir, H., Jones, J. O., Janowitz, T., Hoffmann, M., Euler, M., Martins, C. P., ... Shields, J. D. (2021). Stromal-driven and Amyloid β-dependent induction of neutrophil extracellular traps modulates tumor growth. *Nature Communications, 12*. https://doi.org/10.1038/s41467-021-20982-2.

Naegele, M., Tillack, K., Reinhardt, S., Schippling, S., Martin, R., & Sospedra, M. (2012). Neutrophils in multiple sclerosis are characterized by a primed phenotype. *Journal of Neuroimmunology, 242*, 60–71. https://doi.org/10.1016/j.jneuroim.2011.11.009.

Nahrendorf, M., & Swirski, F. K. (2016). Abandoning M1/M2 for a network model of macrophage function. *Circulation Research, 119*, 414–417. https://doi.org/10.1161/CIRCRESAHA.116.309194.

Nali, L. H., Olival, G. S., Sousa, F. T. G., de Oliveira, A. C. S., Montenegro, H., da Silva, I. T., ... Romano, C. M. (2020). Whole transcriptome analysis of multiple Sclerosis patients reveals active inflammatory profile in relapsing patients and downregulation of neurological repair pathways in secondary progressive cases. *Multiple Sclerosis and Related Disorders, 44*, 102243. https://doi.org/10.1016/j.msard.2020.102243.

Nebeling, F.C., Poll, S., Justus, L.C., Steffen, J., Keppler, K., Mittag, M., & Fuhrmann, M., (n.d.) Microglial motility is modulated by neuronal activity and correlates with dendritic spine plasticity in the hippocampus of awake mice. *eLife, 12*, e83176. https://doi.org/10.7554/eLife.83176.

Neumann, H., Kotter, M. R., & Franklin, R. J. M. (2009). Debris clearance by microglia: An essential link between degeneration and regeneration. *Brain, 132*, 288–295. https://doi.org/10.1093/brain/awn109.

Ng, L. G., Ostuni, R., & Hidalgo, A. (2019). Heterogeneity of neutrophils. *Nature Reviews. Immunology, 19*, 255–265. https://doi.org/10.1038/s41577-019-0141-8.

Nimmerjahn, A., Kirchhoff, F., & Helmchen, F. (2005). Resting microglial cells are highly dynamic surveillants of brain parenchyma in vivo. *Science (New York, N. Y.), 308*, 1314–1318. https://doi.org/10.1126/science.1110647.

Nutma, E., Fancy, N., Weinert, M., Tsartsalis, S., Marzin, M. C., Muirhead, R. C. J., ... Owen, D. R. (2023). Translocator protein is a marker of activated microglia in rodent models but not human neurodegenerative diseases. *Nature Communications, 14*, 5247. https://doi.org/10.1038/s41467-023-40937-z.

Olah, M., Menon, V., Habib, N., Taga, M. F., Ma, Y., Yung, C. J., ... De Jager, P. L. (2020). Single cell RNA sequencing of human microglia uncovers a subset associated with Alzheimer's disease. *Nature Communications, 11*, 6129. https://doi.org/10.1038/s41467-020-19737-2.

Olson, J. K., & Miller, S. D. (2004). Microglia initiate central nervous system innate and adaptive immune responses through multiple TLRs. *The Journal of Immunology (Baltimore, Md) 1950, 173*, 3916–3924. https://doi.org/10.4049/jimmunol.173.6.3916.

Ostendorf, L., Mothes, R., van Koppen, S., Lindquist, R. L., Bellmann-Strobl, J., Asseyer, S., ... Radbruch, H. (2019). Low-density granulocytes are a novel immunopathological feature in both multiple sclerosis and neuromyelitis optica spectrum disorder. *Frontiers in Immunology, 10*, 2725. https://doi.org/10.3389/fimmu.2019.02725.

Paolicelli, R. C., Bolasco, G., Pagani, F., Maggi, L., Scianni, M., Panzanelli, P., ... Gross, C. T. (2011). Synaptic pruning by microglia is necessary for normal brain development. *Science (New York, N. Y.), 333*, 1456–1458. https://doi.org/10.1126/science.1202529.

Papayannopoulos, V. (2018). Neutrophil extracellular traps in immunity and disease. *Nature Reviews. Immunology, 18*, 134–147. https://doi.org/10.1038/nri.2017.105.

Papayannopoulos, V., Metzler, K. D., Hakkim, A., & Zychlinsky, A. (2010). Neutrophil elastase and myeloperoxidase regulate the formation of neutrophil extracellular traps. *The Journal of Cell Biology, 191*, 677–691. https://doi.org/10.1083/JCB.201006052.

Peress, N. S., Fleit, H. B., Perillo, E., Kuljis, R., & Pezzullo, C. (1993). Identification of Fc gamma RI, II and III on normal human brain ramified microglia and on microglia in senile plaques in Alzheimer's disease. *Journal of Neuroimmunology, 48*, 71–79. https://doi.org/10.1016/0165-5728(93)90060-c.

Perry, V. H., Hume, D. A., & Gordon, S. (1985). Immunohistochemical localization of macrophages and microglia in the adult and developing mouse brain. *Neuroscience, 15*, 313–326. https://doi.org/10.1016/0306-4522(85)90215-5.

Petrozziello, T., Mills, A. N., Vaine, C. A., Penney, E. B., Fernandez-Cerado, C., Legarda, G. P. A., ... Sadri-Vakili, G. (2020). Neuroinflammation and histone H3 citrullination are increased in X-linked Dystonia Parkinsonism post-mortem prefrontal cortex. *Neurobiology of Disease, 144*, 105032. https://doi.org/10.1016/j.nbd.2020.105032.

Pieterse, E., Rother, N., Yanginlar, C., Hilbrands, L. B., & van der Vlag, J. (2016). Neutrophils discriminate between lipopolysaccharides of different bacterial sources and selectively release neutrophil extracellular traps. *Frontiers in Immunology, 7*, 484. https://doi.org/10.3389/fimmu.2016.00484.

Pietronigro, E. C., Della Bianca, V., Zenaro, E., & Constantin, G. (2017). NETosis in Alzheimer's disease. *Frontiers in Immunology, 8*. https://doi.org/10.3389/fimmu.2017.00211.

Pilsczek, F. H., Salina, D., Poon, K. K. H., Fahey, C., Yipp, B. G., Sibley, C. D., ... Kubes, P. (2010). A novel mechanism of rapid nuclear neutrophil extracellular trap formation in response to Staphylococcus aureus. *The Journal of Immunology (Baltimore, Md) 1950, 185*, 7413–7425. https://doi.org/10.4049/JIMMUNOL.1000675.

Prineas, J. W., Kwon, E. E., Cho, E. S., Sharer, L. R., Barnett, M. H., Oleszak, E. L., ... Morgan, B. P. (2001). Immunopathology of secondary-progressive multiple sclerosis. *Annals of Neurology, 50*, 646–657. https://doi.org/10.1002/ana.1255.

Prins, M., Eriksson, C., Wierinckx, A., Bol, J. G. J. M., Binnekade, R., Tilders, F. J. H., & Dam, A.-M. V. (2013). Interleukin-1β and interleukin-1 receptor antagonist appear in grey matter additionally to white matter lesions during experimental multiple sclerosis. *PLoS One, 8*, e83835. https://doi.org/10.1371/journal.pone.0083835.

Prinz, M., Jung, S., & Priller, J. (2019). Microglia biology: One century of evolving concepts. *Cell, 179*, 292–311. https://doi.org/10.1016/j.cell.2019.08.053.

Qiao, N., & Shao, H. (2026). Identification of neutrophil extracellular trap-related genes in Alzheimer's disease based on comprehensive bioinformatics analysis. *Computer Methods in Biomechanics and Biomedical Engineering, 29*, 475–488. https://doi.org/10.1080/10255842.2024.2399029.

Ransohoff, R. M. (2016). A polarizing question: Do M1 and M2 microglia exist? *Nature Neuroscience, 19*, 987–991. https://doi.org/10.1038/nn.4338.

Rebeck, G. W., LaDu, M. J., Estus, S., Bu, G., & Weeber, E. J. (2006). The generation and function of soluble apoE receptors in the CNS. *Molecular Neurodegeneration, 1*, 15. https://doi.org/10.1186/1750-1326-1-15.

Rumble, J. M., Huber, A. K., Krishnamoorthy, G., Srinivasan, A., Giles, D. A., Zhang, X., ... Segal, B. M. (2015). Neutrophil-related factors as biomarkers in EAE and MS. *The Journal of Experimental Medicine, 212*, 23–35. https://doi.org/10.1084/jem.20141015.

Saffarzadeh, M., Juenemann, C., Queisser, M. A., Lochnit, G., Barreto, G., Galuska, S. P., ... Preissner, K. T. (2012). Neutrophil extracellular traps directly induce epithelial and endothelial cell death: A predominant role of histones. *PLoS One, 7*. https://doi.org/10.1371/journal.pone.0032366.

Saijo, K., Crotti, A., & Glass, C. K. (2013). Regulation of microglia activation and deactivation by nuclear receptors. *Glia, 61*, 104–111. https://doi.org/10.1002/glia.22423.

Saitoh, T., Komano, J., Saitoh, Y., Misawa, T., Takahama, M., Kozaki, T., ... Akira, S. (2012). Neutrophil extracellular traps mediate a host defense response to human immunodeficiency virus-1. *Cell Host & Microbe, 12*, 109–116. https://doi.org/10.1016/J.CHOM.2012.05.015.

Savchenko, A. S., Borissoff, J. I., Martinod, K., De Meyer, S. F., Gallant, M., Erpenbeck, L., ... Wagner, D. D. (2014). VWF-mediated leukocyte recruitment with chromatin decondensation by PAD4 increases myocardial ischemia/reperfusion injury in mice. *Blood, 123*, 141–148. https://doi.org/10.1182/blood-2013-07-514992.

Scali, C., Prosperi, C., Bracco, L., Piccini, C., Baronti, R., Ginestroni, A., ... Casamenti, F. (2002). Neutrophils CD11b and fibroblasts PGE2 are elevated in Alzheimer's disease. *Neurobiology of Aging, 23*, 523–530. https://doi.org/10.1016/S0197-4580(01)00346-3.

Schauer, C., Janko, C., Munoz, L. E., Zhao, Y., Kienhöfer, D., Frey, B., ... Herrmann, M. (2014). Aggregated neutrophil extracellular traps limit inflammation by degrading cytokines and chemokines. *Nature Medicine, 20*, 511–517. https://doi.org/10.1038/nm.3547.

Schorn, C., Janko, C., Latzko, M., Chaurio, R., Schett, G., & Herrmann, M. (2012). Monosodium urate crystals induce extracellular DNA traps in neutrophils, eosinophils, and basophils but not in mononuclear cells. *Frontiers in Immunology, 3*, 31436. https://doi.org/10.3389/FIMMU.2012.00277/BIBTEX.

Schulz, C., Gomez Perdiguero, E., Chorro, L., Szabo-Rogers, H., Cagnard, N., Kierdorf, K., ... Geissmann, F. (2012). A lineage of myeloid cells independent of Myb and hematopoietic stem cells. *Science (New York, N. Y.), 336*, 86–90. https://doi.org/10.1126/science.1219179.

Shieh, C.-H., Heinrich, A., Serchov, T., van Calker, D., & Biber, K. (2014). P2X7-Dependent, but differentially regulated release of IL-6, CCL2, and TNF-α in cultured mouse microglia. *Glia, 62*, 592–607. https://doi.org/10.1002/glia.22628.

Si, Q., Cosenza, M., Zhao, M.-L., Goldstein, H., & Lee, S. C. (2002). GM-CSF and M-CSF modulate β-chemokine and HIV-1 expression in microglia. *Glia, 39*, 174–183. https://doi.org/10.1002/glia.10095.

Simon, D., Hoesli, S., Roth, N., Staedler, S., Yousefi, S., & Simon, H.-U. (2011). Eosinophil extracellular DNA traps in skin diseases. *The Journal of Allergy and Clinical Immunology, 127*, 194–199. https://doi.org/10.1016/j.jaci.2010.11.002.

Slavik, J. M., Hutchcroft, J. E., & Bierer, B. E. (1999). CD28/CTLA-4 and CD80/CD86 families: Signaling and function. *Immunologic Research, 19*, 1–24. https://doi.org/10.1007/BF02786473.

Smith, J. A., Das, A., Ray, S. K., & Banik, N. L. (2012). Role of pro-inflammatory cytokines released from microglia in neurodegenerative diseases. *Brain Research Bulletin, 87*, 10–20. https://doi.org/10.1016/j.brainresbull.2011.10.004.

Smyth, L. C. D., Murray, H. C., Hill, M., van Leeuwen, E., Highet, B., Magon, N. J., ... Hampton, M. B. (2022). Neutrophil-vascular interactions drive myeloperoxidase accumulation in the brain in Alzheimer's disease. *Acta Neuropathologica Communications, 10*, 38. https://doi.org/10.1186/s40478-022-01347-2.

Song, L., Yang, Y. T., Guo, Q., Zhao, X.-M., & the ZIB Consortium (2022). Cellular transcriptional alterations of peripheral blood in Alzheimer's disease. *BMC Medicine, 20*, 266. https://doi.org/10.1186/s12916-022-02472-4.

Stock, A. J., Kasus-Jacobi, A., & Pereira, H. A. (2018). The role of neutrophil granule proteins in neuroinflammation and Alzheimer's disease. *Journal of Neuroinflammation, 15*, 240. https://doi.org/10.1186/s12974-018-1284-4.

Sun, Z., Zhang, X., So, K.-F., Jiang, W., & Chiu, K. (2024). Targeting microglia in Alzheimer's disease: Pathogenesis and potential therapeutic strategies. *Biomolecules, 14*. https://doi.org/10.3390/biom14070833.

Suzumura, A., Sawada, M., & Marunouchi, T. (1996). Selective induction of interleukin-6 in mouse microglia by granulocyte-macrophage colony-stimulating factor. *Brain Research, 713*, 192–198. https://doi.org/10.1016/0006-8993(95)01535-3.

Tadie, J.-M., Bae, H.-B., Jiang, S., Park, D. W., Bell, C. P., Yang, H., ... Zmijewski, J. W. (2013). HMGB1 promotes neutrophil extracellular trap formation through interactions with Toll-like receptor 4. *The American Journal of Physiology-Lung Cellular and Molecular Physiology, 304*, L342–L349. https://doi.org/10.1152/ajplung.00151.2012.

Takami, S., Nishikawa, H., Minami, M., Nishiyori, A., Sato, M., Akaike, A., & Satoh, M. (1997). Induction of macrophage inflammatory protein MIP-1alpha mRNA on glial cells after focal cerebral ischemia in the rat. *Neuroscience Letters, 227*, 173–176. https://doi.org/10.1016/s0304-3940(97)00338-8.

Tam, W. Y., & Ma, C. H. E. (2014). Bipolar/rod-shaped microglia are proliferating microglia with distinct M1/M2 phenotypes. *Scientific Reports, 4*, 7279. https://doi.org/10.1038/srep07279.

Tang, Y., & Le, W. (2016). Differential roles of M1 and M2 microglia in neurodegenerative diseases. *Molecular Neurobiology, 53*, 1181–1194. https://doi.org/10.1007/s12035-014-9070-5.

Taylor, D. L., Jones, F., Kubota, E. S. F. C. S., & Pocock, J. M. (2005). Stimulation of microglial metabotropic glutamate receptor mGlu2 triggers tumor necrosis factor alpha-induced neurotoxicity in concert with microglial-derived Fas ligand. *The Journal of Neuroscience : the Official Journal of the Society for Neuroscience, 25*, 2952–2964. https://doi.org/10.1523/JNEUROSCI.4456-04.2005.

Tomizawa, H., Arima, M., Miyabe, Y., Furutani, C., Kodama, S., Ito, K., ... Ueki, S. (2025). Characteristics and regulation of human Eosinophil etosis in vitro. *American Journal of Respiratory Cell and Molecular Biology, 72*, 52–61. https://doi.org/10.1165/rcmb.2023-0438OC.

Urban, C. F., Ermert, D., Schmid, M., Abu-Abed, U., Goosmann, C., Nacken, W., ... Zychlinsky, A. (2009). Neutrophil extracellular traps contain calprotectin, a cytosolic protein complex involved in host defense against Candida albicans. *PLoS Pathogens, 5*. https://doi.org/10.1371/JOURNAL.PPAT.1000639.

Urban, C. F., Reichard, U., Brinkmann, V., & Zychlinsky, A. (2006). Neutrophil extracellular traps capture and kill Candida albicans yeast and hyphal forms. *Cellular Microbiology, 8*, 668–676. https://doi.org/10.1111/J.1462-5822.2005.00659.X.

Van Kooten, C., & Banchereau, J. (2000). CD40-CD40 ligand. *Journal of Leukocyte Biology, 67*, 2–17. https://doi.org/10.1002/jlb.67.1.2.

Veroni, C., Gabriele, L., Canini, I., Castiello, L., Coccia, E., Remoli, M. E., ... Agresti, C. (2010). Activation of TNF receptor 2 in microglia promotes induction of anti-inflammatory pathways. *Molecular and Cellular Neurosciences, 45*, 234–244. https://doi.org/10.1016/j.mcn.2010.06.014.

Villanueva, E., Yalavarthi, S., Berthier, C. C., Hodgin, J. B., Khandpur, R., Lin, A. M., ... Kaplan, M. J. (2011). Netting neutrophils induce endothelial damage, infiltrate tissues and expose immunostimulatory molecules in systemic lupus erythematosus. *Journal of immunology (Baltimore, Md.) 1950, 187*, 538–552. https://doi.org/10.4049/jimmunol.1100450.

Von Köckritz-Blickwede, M., Goldmann, O., Thulin, P., Heinemann, K., Norrby-Teglund, A., Rohde, M., & Medina, E. (2008). Phagocytosis-independent antimicrobial activity of mast cells by means of extracellular trap formation. *Blood, 111*, 3070–3080. https://doi.org/10.1182/BLOOD-2007-07-104018.

Wang, Y., Du, C., Zhang, Y., & Zhu, L. (2024). Composition and function of neutrophil extracellular traps. *Biomolecules, 14*, 416. https://doi.org/10.3390/biom14040416.

Wang, C., Wang, Y., Shi, X., Tang, X., Cheng, W., Wang, X., ... Yu, L. (2019). The TRAPs from microglial vesicles protect against listeria infection in the CNS. *Frontiers in Cellular Neuroscience, 13*. https://doi.org/10.3389/fncel.2019.00199.

Warnatsch, A., Ioannou, M., Wang, Q., & Papayannopoulos, V. (2015). Neutrophil extracellular traps license macrophages and Th17 cells for cytokine production in atherosclerosis. *Science (New York, N. Y.), 349*, 316–320. https://doi.org/10.1126/science.aaa8064.

Waubant, E., Lucas, R., Mowry, E., Graves, J., Olsson, T., Alfredsson, L., & Langer-Gould, A. (2019). Environmental and genetic risk factors for MS: An integrated review. *Annals of Clinical and Translational Neurology, 6*, 1905–1922. https://doi.org/10.1002/acn3.50862.

Wculek, S. K., & Malanchi, I. (2015). Neutrophils support lung colonization of metastasis-initiating breast cancer cells. *Nature, 528*, 413–417. https://doi.org/10.1038/nature16140.

Wes, P. D., Holtman, I. R., Boddeke, E. W. G. M., Möller, T., & Eggen, B. J. L. (2016). Next generation transcriptomics and genomics elucidate biological complexity of microglia in health and disease. *Glia, 64*, 197–213. https://doi.org/10.1002/glia.22866.

Yang, Y., Estrada, E. Y., Thompson, J. F., Liu, W., & Rosenberg, G. A. (2007). Matrix metalloproteinase-mediated disruption of tight junction proteins in cerebral vessels is reversed by synthetic matrix metalloproteinase inhibitor in focal ischemia in rat. *Journal of Cerebral Blood Flow and Metabolism, 27*, 697–709. https://doi.org/10.1038/sj.jcbfm.9600375.

Yang, I., Han, S. J., Kaur, G., Crane, C., & Parsa, A. T. (2010). The role of microglia in central nervous system immunity and glioma immunology. *Journal of Clinical Neuroscience : Official Journal of the Neurosurgical Society of Australasia, 17*, 6–10. https://doi.org/10.1016/j.jocn.2009.05.006.

Yang, L., Liu, Q., Zhang, X., Liu, X., Zhou, B., Chen, J., ... Song, E. (2020). DNA of neutrophil extracellular traps promotes cancer metastasis via CCDC25. *Nature*. 2020 5837814 *583*, 133–138. https://doi.org/10.1038/s41586-020-2394-6.

Yipp, B. G., Petri, B., Salina, D., Jenne, C. N., Scott, B. N. V., Zbytnuik, L. D., ... Kubes, P. (2012). Infection-induced NETosis is a dynamic process involving neutrophil multitasking in vivo. *Nature Medicine, 18*, 1386–1393. https://doi.org/10.1038/NM.2847.

Yousefi, S., Gold, J. A., Andina, N., Lee, J. J., Kelly, A. M., Kozlowski, E., ... Simon, H. U. (2008). Catapult-like release of mitochondrial DNA by eosinophils contributes to antibacterial defense. *Nature Medicine, 14*, 949–953. https://doi.org/10.1038/NM.1855.

Yousefi, S., Morshed, M., Amini, P., Stojkov, D., Simon, D., von Gunten, S., ... Simon, H.-U. (2015). Basophils exhibit antibacterial activity through extracellular trap formation. *Allergy, 70*, 1184–1188. https://doi.org/10.1111/all.12662.

Zhang, W. (2023). Role of neuroinflammation in neurodegeneration development. *Signal Transduction and Targeted Therapy*.

Zhang, W., Xiao, D., Mao, Q., & Xia, H. (2023). Role of neuroinflammation in neurodegeneration development. *Signal Transduction and Targeted Therapy, 8*, 267. https://doi.org/10.1038/s41392-023-01486-5.

Ziukelis, E. T., Mak, E., Dounavi, M.-E., Su, L., & T O'Brien, J. (2022). Fractal dimension of the brain in neurodegenerative disease and dementia: A systematic review. *Ageing Research Reviews, 79*, 101651. https://doi.org/10.1016/j.arr.2022.101651.

CHAPTER TWELVE

Microglial polarisation imbalance and receptor-targeted therapeutics in Parkinson's disease

Riddhi Upadhyay and Murugan Sevanan*
Division of Biotechnology, Karunya Institute of Technology and Sciences (Deemed to be University), Coimbatore, Tamil Nadu, India
*Corresponding author. e-mail address: micromurugans@gmail.com

Contents

Abstract

Parkinson's Disease (PD) is a progressive neurodegenerative disease, which is mainly characterised by the selective depletion of dopaminergic neurons in the substantia nigra and deposition of misfolded aggregates of α-synuclein. It is increasingly being observed that neuroinflammation, mitochondrial dysfunction, and lost neurotrophic support are interacting factors that drive disease progression. The aggregated 1-synuclein triggers an anti-inflammatory phenotype and pro-inflammatory phenotypes in activated microglia, which produce cytokines and reactive oxygen species, aggravating stress in neurons. At the same time, mitochondrial dynamic dysfunction increases oxidative injury, which makes neurons sensitive to degeneration. The low concentration of neurotrophic factors,

Advances in Immunology, Volume 171
ISSN 0065-2776, https://doi.org/10.1016/bs.ai.2024.10.003

especially the brain-derived neurotrophic factor (BDNF), impairs the innate ability of the brain to repair itself and maintain its synapses. These pathological processes gradually create a loop of self-feeding, which results in prolonged inflammation, loss of proteostasis, and gradual loss of dopaminergic neurons. This network is interconnected, and understanding it is crucial in the creation of therapies that attempt to restore proteostasis, inhibit inflammation, and increase neurotrophic signalling to delay or prevent PD progression.

Abbervatives

AMPK	AMP-activated protein kinase.
AP-1	Activator protein-1.
Arg1	Arginase-1.
BBB	Blood–brain barrier.
B-CSF	Blood–cerebrospinal fluid barrier.
CaMKKβ	Calcium/calmodulin-dependent protein kinase kinase-β.
CB2	Cannabinoid receptor 2.
CCL2	Chemokine (C-C motif) ligand 2.
CD206	Cluster of differentiation 206.
COX2	Cyclooxygenase-2.
CP	Choroid plexus.
CSF	Cerebrospinal fluid.
DJ-1	Parkinsonism-associated deglycase protein.
ECM	Extracellular matrix.
ERK1/2	Extracellular signal-regulated kinase 1/2.
GM-CSF	Granulocyte-macrophage colony-stimulating factor.
HC	Hippocampus.
IFNγ	Interferon-gamma.
IGF-1	Insulin-like growth factor-1.
IL-1β	Interleukin-1 beta.
IL-2	Interleukin-2.
IL-4	Interleukin-4.
IL-6	Interleukin-6.
IL-8	Interleukin-8.
IL-10	Interleukin-10.
IL-13	Interleukin-13.
IL-17A	Interleukin-17A.
iNOS	Inducible nitric oxide synthase.
JAK/STAT	Janus kinase/Signal transducer and activator of transcription.
JNK	c-Jun N-terminal kinase.
LPS	Lipopolysaccharide.
MAPK	Mitogen-activated protein kinase.
MHC I/II	Major histocompatibility complex class I/II.
MLVs	Meningeal lymphatic vessels.
MMP-3	Matrix metalloproteinase-3.
MPO	Myeloperoxidase.
MyD88	Myeloid differentiation primary response 88.
NF-κB	Nuclear factor kappa-light-chain-enhancer of activated B cells.

NLR	Neutrophil-to-lymphocyte ratio.
PAMPs	Pathogen-associated molecular patterns.
PD	Parkinson's disease.
PET	Positron emission tomography.
PGE2	Prostaglandin E2.
PI3K/Akt	Phosphoinositide 3-kinase/Protein kinase B.
PINK1	PTEN-induced kinase 1.
SN	Substantia nigra.
SNpc	Substantia nigra pars compacta.
STAT1/3/5/6	STAT family transcription factors.
TGF-β	Transforming growth factor-beta.
TLR2/TLR4	Toll-like receptor-2/Toll-like receptor-4.
TNF-α	Tumour necrosis factor-alpha.
TREM2	Triggering receptor expressed on myeloid cells-2.

1. Introduction

Parkinson's Disease (PD) is the second most prevalent neurodegenerative disease in the world and is characterised by motor dysfunction, rigidity, bradykinesia, and postural instability at a spectrum of non-motor symptoms, including cognitive impairment, anosmia, sleep disturbances, and autonomic dysfunction (Mantash, 2019; Aarsland et al., 2021; Callahan, 2024). In the neuropathology of PD, two key characteristics can be identified, namely a gradual degradation of dopaminergic (DA) neurons within the substantia nigra pars compacta (SNpc) and the deposition of intracellular α-synuclein structures called Lewy bodies (Yi et al., 2022). Although these classical observations have been kept at the centre, modern studies have emphasised PD as a multifactorial disorder that occurs due to the integration of neuroinflammation, mitochondrial impairment, oxidative stress, dysregulated proteostasis, and decreased neurotrophic support (Picca et al., 2020). Alpha-synuclein misfolding and aggregation are one of the first and most repeated causes of PD pathology. In physiological conditions, α-synuclein is involved in the dynamics of the synaptic vesicles, release of neurotransmitters, and maintenance of the synaptic unity (Calabresi et al., 2023). Nevertheless, genetic mutations, environmental toxins, and degradation system failures make the α-synuclein take on 2-sheet-based conformations that crystallise and spread in neural networks in a prion-like manner (Vidović & Rikalovic, 2022). These aggregates serve as danger-associated molecular patterns (DAMPs) and stimulate the activation of microglia, the immune cells that are resident in the central nervous system (Colonna & Butovsky, 2017).

Activated microglia undergo a shift towards a pro-inflammatory phenotype, characterised by the upregulation of MHC-II and the release of cytokines such as IL-1β, TNF-α, and IL-6. This chronic neuroinflammatory environment exacerbates neuronal vulnerability by increasing oxidative stress and promoting further α-synuclein misfolding (Gao et al., 2023). The persistent production of reactive oxygen and nitrogen species is a contributing factor to the mitochondrial impairment, destruction of mitochondrial DNA, respiratory complexes, and membrane integrity (Chen et al., 2022). The impaired mitophagy, the choice of autophagic elimination of damaged mitochondria, further increases the formation of ROS and metabolic stress to form a vicious cycle that increases the loss of dopaminergic cells (Ma et al., 2020). Add to these effects the loss of the neurotrophic factor signalling, especially brain-derived neurotrophic factor (BDNF). BDNF plays a vital role in the survival of neurons, axon health, synapse plasticity, and repair (Toader et al., 2025). In PD, the down-regulation of BDNF and the down-regulation of the activation of its receptor TrkB inhibit the ability of the brain to mitigate the permanent damage (Ali et al., 2024). This decrease in neurotrophic support decreases the tissue repair capacity, decreases neuronal resilience, and increases the speed of neurodegeneration. It is especially detrimental that dopaminergic neurons fail to receive enough trophic support, bearing in mind that they are highly metabolically active and vulnerable to the impact of oxidative stress (Chmielarz & Saarma, 2020).

Protein degradation (proteostatic failure) is also a major process that contributes to PD development. There are no checkpoints in the presence of misfolded proteins in case of the overloading of the ubiquitin-proteasome system (UPS) and autophagy-lysosomal pathways by 3-α-synuclein aggregates (Sahoo et al., 2022). The genetic changes in the most important regulators, including Parkin, PINK1, DJ-1, and LRRK2, also impair the proteostasis and the quality of the mitochondria. This leads to the subsequent build-up of dysfunctional mitochondria and aggregated proteins that continue to cause signalling of stress in neurons and microglia (Ge et al., 2020; Ho et al., 2025). These processes are interrelated and create a complex pathophysiology behind PD, including the α-synuclein aggregation, the inflammatory response by microglia, mitochondrial dysfunction, oxidative stress, and reduced BDNF signalling (Chen et al., 2025). Instead of being events that occur in isolation, these mechanisms interact in the form of reinforcing loops that cause the slow yet inexorable process of neurodegeneration to occur. The present studies are currently interested in the therapeutic methods that can improve the changes in disease progression by simultaneously targeting inflammation, restoring proteostasis, and improving neurotrophic pathways (Wareham et al., 2022; Bravo-Jimenez et al., 2025).

2. Microglial dysregulation and immune-barrier crosstalk in Parkinson's disease

Microglia are well known to play neuroprotective functions in the CNS. Nevertheless, the continuous pathological agonists like Lewy body deposition and neuronal death gradually trigger the activation of microglia (Colonna & Butovsky, 2017; Gao et al., 2023). This stimulation leads to the release of the pro-inflammatory cytokines by the microglia, which changes their neurotrophic activities and creates a neurotoxic environment. In the substantia nigra (SN) of PD brains, and in the SN, amygdala, and hippocampus (HC) of PD patients, and in incidental Lewy body dementia, increased numbers of microglia, which adopt an activated amoeboid morphology, have been observed (Woodburn et al., 2021; Ana, 2024). Outstandingly, the morphological and molecular adaptations of microglial cells precede the development of alpha-synuclein accumulation and aggregation, which indicates that the existence of microglial cells in the SN and HC can lead to the activation of microglial cells and neuroinflammation in prodromal PD (Lind-Holm Mogensen et al., 2025). Genetic influences and environmental stressors can impair microglial homeostasis, shifting them from a neuroprotective to a pathogenic state (Zhang et al., 2024). The dysfunctional microglia can be characterised by exhaustion, premature senescence, dysfunctional phagocytosis, and malfunctioning lysosomes, which may sustain cycles of α-synuclein accumulation, mitochondrial dysfunction, sustained neuroinflammation, and synaptic destruction to cause neurodegeneration (Eo et al., 2024). The approach of targeting the homeostasis, metabolism, and early dysfunction of the microglia can delay or prevent the onset of clinical PD. Microglial heterogeneity is the driving force of protective as well as degenerative mechanisms (Noh et al., 2025). Furthermore, dopamine metabolism, as a gene expression of tyrosine hydroxylase, is also greatly downregulated in the SN neurons and glia of patients with PD. The precise analysis of the microglial subpopulations in prodromal and early-stage PD has not been conducted yet, in part due to the invasive nature of the midbrain biopsies and the ethical concerns about them (Harsanyiova et al., 2020).

Ligands that specifically bind markers of microglial activation can be used to assess the activity of microglia in the brain non-invasively using positron emission tomography (PET) and single-photon emission computed tomography (SPECT) (Warden et al., 2023). Those methods facilitate the regional examination of neuroinflammation and especially in fields such as the substantia nigra (SN), which plays a major role in PD pathology (Kouli et al., 2020). One of the most examined markers is the 18 kDa Translocator Protein (TSPO): in the healthy brain, it is barely expressed, but it is highly increased in activated microglia (Yao et al., 2020). Increased TSPO levels were observed in various areas, such as the SN and basal ganglia, and are associated with disease progression and severity. Notably, microglial activation has been detected in the SN, anterior cingulate cortex, and prefrontal cortex of PD patients within the first 7–12 months post-diagnosis, accompanied by increased carbonylated proteins in the cerebrospinal fluid, a sign of oxidative stress and neurodegeneration (Tournier et al., 2020; Muzio et al., 2021). Stokholm et al. (2017) provided key data from a case-control study involving 20 REM sleep behaviour disorder (RBD) patients, who exhibited both microglial activation and diminished nigrostriatal dopamine function. Subsequent follow-up revealed that those with higher baseline microglial activation experienced more pronounced deterioration in the nigrostriatal pathway, suggesting microgliosis may contribute adversely in prodromal PD (Stær et al., 2024). Interpretation of TSPO imaging is complicated by the fact that TSPO is also found on astrocytes and infiltrating immune cells. The most common ligand that is used is 11C-R-PK11195, TSPO, with a weak sensitivity because of low signal-to-noise and not being specific (Salerno et al., 2024). The subsequent improved tracers, such as [18F]DPA-714, have already worked well in the animal models and shown a connection between neuroinflammation and motor symptoms in PD, yet their more extensive clinical validation is pending (Araújo et al., 2022). The brain-peripheral organs communication in PD may occur via a range of interfaces, one of which is the blood-brain barrier (BBB) (Lau et al., 2024). The relationship between BBB dysfunction or an elevated condition of permeability and neurodegenerative diseases like Alzheimer's disease (AD) and PD is being supported by growing evidence. Post-mortem and in vivo PET tracer studies have both shown that PD enhances BBB permeability (Sweeney et al., 2018). The affected regions of the PD brain, such as the substantia nigra and caudate putamen, have more myeloperoxidase (MPO)-positive cells that point to the presence of active neutrophils and macrophages (Gellhaar et al., 2017). MO enzyme is primarily expressed in such cells in response to infection. It is seen in a few cases that the percentage of circulating neutrophils is still higher, and the neutrophil-lymphocyte ratio (NLR) is all the time high in patients of PD, even in prodromal cases, compared to healthy controls (Espejo et al., 2025).

In PD, the choroid plexus (CP) is the blood-cerebrospinal fluid (B-CSF) barrier that plays a central role in brain-immune interactions. The CP has a monolayer of epithelial cells that secretes CSF into the ventricles of the brain, and the large net of fenestrated capillaries allows high vascularisation (Solár et al., 2020). The CP is functionally an integrative centre, which takes in the signals sent by the CNS and peripheral immune cells. This facilitates selective recruitment of inflammation-resolving immune cells, including neutrophils, monocytes and macrophages, especially to inflamed parts of the brain (Dumas et al., 2024). When the brain is inflamed, CP epithelial cells can transiently specialise to support the recruitment, survival, and differentiation of these immune cells, regulating tight junctions to carefully modulate barrier permeability (Xu et al., 2024). Importantly, CP adapts to gut inflammation, such as from bacterial LPS after disruption of gut vascular barriers, by closing itself to block large molecules, as part of an inflammatory cascade. Sustained closure, achieved in a genetic model, led to deficits in short-term memory and anxiety-like behaviours, suggesting a strong association between CP dysfunction and cognitive decline (Li et al., 2023; Zhang et al., 2023). CP dysregulation appears to be a common pathological feature across neurodegenerative diseases, presenting a potential therapeutic target for controlling brain inflammation (Zhang et al., 2023). Although studies show reduced CSF motion in PD patients compared to healthy controls, CP dysfunction or impaired motion in early PD remains unexplored. Moreover, the precise effect of CP impairment on the microglial activity remains unclear, and more studies are needed on these interactions. A recently identified brain-wide drainage system, termed the glymphatic, is important in the clearance of metabolic and protein wastes such as amyloid beta. An impaired glymphatic system, especially in the sort of clearance of alpha-synuclein, could support the accumulation of toxic proteins in PD (Gao et al., 2023). Both neurodegeneration and ageing involve glymphatic dysfunction, which heightens inflammation by hampering cytokine clearance and activating microglia, while neuroinflammation further compromises glymphatic activity, together fueling neurodegenerative progression (Fakorede et al., 2025). MRI studies reveal significantly reduced glymphatic activity in

Table 1 Microglial activation, neuroinflammation in Parkinson's disease.

System	Underlying mechanisms	Implications for PD pathology
Microglial Activation & Dysfunction	Chronic activation leads to cytokine release (IL-1β, TNF-α) Loss of neurotrophic support Impaired α-syn clearance leads to propagation of aggregates Mitochondrial dysfunction & oxidative stress	Sustains cycles of neuroinflammation Promotes α-syn accumulation and synaptic damage Drives early dopaminergic neuron vulnerability Targeting microglial metabolism/homeostasis may delay PD onset
PET/SPECT Biomarkers (TSPO Imaging)	TSPO binding detects activated microglia 11C-PK11195 has low specificity/noise New tracers ([18F]DPA-714, [18F]GE180) show improved sensitivity	Allows early detection of neuroinflammation High baseline TSPO activity predicts faster dopaminergic decline Useful but limited due to non-specific TSPO expression (astrocytes, infiltrating cells)
Blood–Brain Barrier (BBB) Dysfunction	Tight-junction breakdown leads to leakage of proteins/cells MPO enzyme indicates infiltrating immune activation Peripheral immune cells contribute to CNS inflammation	Peripheral inflammation gains access to CNS Promotes oxidative stress and microglial activation Links systemic inflammation with PD progression
Choroid Plexus (CP) / Blood–CSF Barrier Dysfunction	Dynamic modulation of tight junctions Immune training / signalling between periphery & brain Gut–brain axis modifies CP barrier behavior	CP dysfunction may impair immune surveillance Reduced CSF turnover may worsen protein accumulation CP maladaptation may contribute to PD cognitive symptoms

Glymphatic System Impairment	Reduced AQP4 polarisation Impaired CSF–interstitial exchange Sleep disturbances reduce drainage efficiency Ageing reduces glymphatic flow	Accumulation of metabolic waste (α-syn, Aβ) Heightened inflammation due to poor cytokine clearance Glymphatic impairment may be an early prodromal PD marker
Meningeal Lymphatic Vessels (MLVs)	Impaired macromolecule & immune cell trafficking Reduced CSF drainage to deep cervical lymph nodes	Waste retention leads to microglial hyperactivation Contributes to chronic inflammation & neurodegeneration

PD patients, correlating with worsened motor and cognitive symptoms. Although prodromal PD remains unstudied, one report noted no glymphatic activity difference between early and late PD, but the group was small (Ma et al., 2025). Glymphatic function is highest during sleep and declines with age; this leads to less beta-amyloid clearance, dropping 40 % in older mice. The sleep-wake cycle, controlled by the locus coeruleus (LC) and norepinephrine, is crucial for glymphatic activity, and α-synuclein deposits here may explain sleep disorders and glymphatic impairment in PD (Voumvourakis et al., 2023). Research shows that a single night of sleep loss increases amyloid beta and α-synuclein levels. Sleep behaviour disorders, common in prodromal PD, may thus signal glymphatic impairment and higher disease risk (Scott-Massey et al., 2022). Meningeal lymphatic vessels (MLVs) carry waste and immune cells from the brain to lymph nodes. In PD, MLV outflow and lymph node perfusion are reduced, and blocking MLVs in mouse models worsens disease. Ageing further diminishes brain lymphatic drainage, affecting microglial function (Chen et al., 2024) as shown in Table 1.

3. Microglia-activation and phenotypic regulation in Parkinson's disease

Under normal conditions, microglia are in a homeostatic state, constantly monitoring their environment and interacting with nearby cells and blood vessels. Upon detecting pathology, they shift to a reactive state, typically categorised as pro-inflammatory (M1) or anti-inflammatory (M2), though their activation spans a broad spectrum (Wang et al., 2023) as shown in Fig. 1. When triggered, microglia move to areas of injury, and their behaviour may promote or aggravate injury. Homeostatic to reactive transitions involve complicated regulation, and these phenotypes tend to be temporary (Gao et al., 2023). The microglia react, turn amoeboid, grow short processes, an enlarged soma, and express new cell surface receptors, secretions that may stimulate or inhibit disease (Vidal-Itriago et al., 2022). Immunologic processes are delicate in healthy tissue, whereas in disease, the processes are not regulated, causing harmful inflammation. Signals between the blood, brain, endothelium, and the peripheral nervous system continuously modulate the microglial activity, which underscores complicated

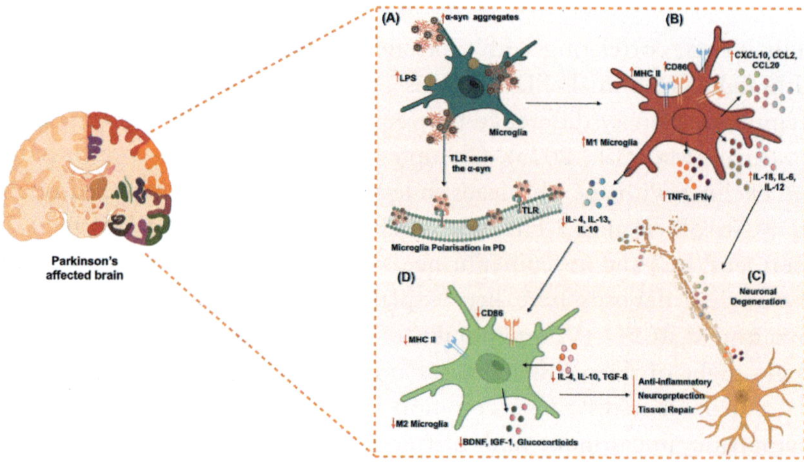

Fig. 1 Microglial activation and impaired polarisation in the Parkinson's disease (PD) brain. (A) Aggregated α-synuclein released from degenerating neurons is sensed by Toll-like receptors (TLRs) on microglia, in combination with inflammatory stimuli such as LPS. This triggers initial microglial activation. (B) Activated microglia shift predominantly toward the pro-inflammatory M1 phenotype, characterised by upregulation of MHC-II and CD86 and the release of cytokines including TNF-α, IL-1β, IL-6, IL-12, IFN-γ, CXCL10, CCL2, and CCL20. These mediators amplify neuroinflammation, increase oxidative stress, and contribute to dopaminergic neuronal degeneration. (C) Sustained M1-driven inflammation promotes progressive neuronal damage and loss of dopaminergic projections typical of PD pathology. (D) Although anti-inflammatory M2 microglia normally secrete neurotrophic and tissue-repair factors such as IL-4, IL-10, TGF-β, BDNF, IGF-1, and glucocorticoids, their activation is suppressed in PD, leading to reduced neurotrophic support and impaired tissue repair. The imbalance between dominant M1 activation and diminished M2 polarisation accelerates neurodegeneration and disease progression.

CNS-immune interactions (Mayer & Fischer, 2024). M1 microglial phenotype is the classical activation state of the microglia, which is characterised by the pro-inflammatory and cytotoxic roles of the immune system as the first line of defence (Zeng et al., 2023; Wang et al., 2023). M1 microglia release pro-inflammatory cytokines (IL-8, IL-6, TNF-α), NO, and chemokines like CCL2. In their expression, they release MHC II, iNOS, CD86, COX2, and generate ROS, PGE2, and RNS (Isik et al., 2023). These activities are useful in destroying pathogens and stimulating adaptive immunity. M1 microglia can develop as a result of M1 to M2 conversion or reaction to stimuli such as alpha-synuclein or amyloid beta (Darwish et al., 2023). They are usually activated through MAPK/AP-1 pathways and inhibition of Kappaß/NF-κB pathways, which promotes the production of pro-inflammatory cytokines (Liu et al., 2017).

Its secretion and accumulation that damages neurons are caused by the aggregation of alpha-synuclein (α-syn) or impaired clearance. Microglia clearance of excess α-syn has been shown, and extracellular α-syn is a DAMP and triggers microglial receptors, such as TLR2, and the NF-κBpathway (Li et al., 2021). This triggers the inflammasome, the release of IL-1β, mitochondrial dysfunction and production of pro-inflammatory cytokines, causing harm to dopaminergic neurons through the NF-κBpathway (Nolan et al., 2020). The result is inflammasome, IL-1B, and mitochondrial dysfunction, accompanied by production of pro-inflammatory cytokines, harming dopaminergic neurons through the NF- between the NF- and the NF pathway (Zhang et al., 2024). Abnormal α-syn also triggers excessive microglial activation, disturbs synaptic and mitochondrial health, and impairs microglial phagocytosis, contributing to neurodegeneration in PD (Eo et al., 2024).

Lipopolysaccharide (LPS) is a key inflammatory stimulus for microglia, causing dopaminergic neuron death by activating the M1 phenotype via TLR4/TLR2 and associated proteins. LPS-activated TLR4 signalling involves MyD88, TRIF, and transcription factors like NF-κB, STAT5, and IRFs, upregulating pro-inflammatory genes (Ye et al., 2020). Interferon gamma (IFNγ) is crucial in immunity, activating microglia and increasing MHC II via the JAK/STAT pathway through IFNγ receptors, which results in gene transcription for inflammatory molecules (Ding et al., 2022). GM-CSF also stimulates microglial activation but can induce both M1 and M2 traits, unlike LPS and IFNγ. TLRs are vital for innate immunity, activated by PAMPs that trigger antigen-presenting cell maturation and inflammatory cytokine release (Chen et al., 2023). TLR4, abundantly found in microglia, responds to diverse PAMPs, such as LPS and viral proteins. Its activation is linked to chronic neuroinflammation in neurodegenerative diseases (Gao et al., 2023). The absence of TLR4 reduces PD-related neuroinflammation via NF-κB, AP-1, and inflammasome pathways, highlighting TLR4 as a therapeutic target. TLR2 detects a wide range of pathogen and damage associated molecules, and misfolded α-synuclein, a key driver of microglia activation and subsequent dopaminergic neuron death in PD (Campolo et al., 2019). TLR2 recognises α-synuclein, increasing ROS, cytokine production, and neuronal loss via NF-κB activation. NF-κB governs inflammatory responses to various stimuli and promotes the pro-inflammatory M1 microglial phenotype (Caplan & Maguire-Zeiss, 2018). Inhibiting its activity can shift microglia to the anti-inflammatory M2 state, providing therapeutic potential. Activation leads NF-κB to induce neuroinflammatory genes like IL-6, TNFα, and COX2. Reducing M1 microglia alleviates inflammation and neuronal loss in PD (Cai et al., 2022; Gao et al., 2023). MAPKs (p38, JNK, ERK1/2) regulate cell survival and inflammation. p38 and JNK drive microglial activation and inflammatory protein production. Their inhibition counters microglial activation and offers anti-inflammatory benefits, positioning the MAPK pathway inactivation as a promising treatment for neuroinflammatory diseases (Canovas & Nebreda, 2021).

The M2 microglia, which includes alternative activation, acquired deactivation, are essential in immunoregulation, inflammation inhibition, and tissue repair. Microglia polarise into the M2 phenotype, and this process removes inflammation and restores homeostasis (Guo et al., 2022). The shift from the classical M1 activation into an anti-inflammatory one is essential to tissue repair and restoration of the ECM. Acute inflammation is suppressed by acquired deactivation, which is caused by the phagocytosis of apoptotic cells or exposure to TGF-β/IL-10 (Pérez & Rius-Pérez, 2022). These M2 states can intersect in disease, which adds to neurodegenerative inflammation. M2 microglia express Arg1 and growth factors (FIZZ1, IGF-1, Ym1) to repair and deposit the matrix, and have receptors such as TREM2 and CD206 (Guo et al., 2022). The M1/M2 paradigm is a simplistic view of the traditional one; the microglial subtypes are more varied, as the omics studies reveal. Three M2 subtypes exist: M2a, M2b, and M2c. Transitioning from M1 to M2, via IL-10, through IL-10 or immunomodulators enhances results (Amici et al., 2017). M1/M2 coexpression can be acquired after injury; pharmacologically induced M2 conversion may become helpful in neurodegenerative therapy. TREM2 facilitates repair and anti-inflammatory expressions through the ERK and DAP12 pathways in microglia (Yu et al., 2025). The JAK/STAT pathway influences microglial phenotype. JAK2/STAT6 enhances M2 genes; STAT1/3 promotes M1. This pathway, when dysregulated, can worsen disease, highlighting the therapeutic importance of targeted interventions (Hu et al., 2021). Histamine/thrombin-induced Ca^{2+} influx activates CaMKKβ/AMPK, essential for the M1-M2 switch and cellular energy balance. AMPK/mitochondrial dysfunction is linked to neurodegeneration (Isik et al., 2023). PI3K/Akt signalling also regulates microglial polarisation; its activation supports the M2 phenotype but can promote inflammation depending on context (He et al., 2022). Rho/ROCK pathway inhibition shifts microglia toward M2, reduces inflammation, restores mitochondria, and may inform therapies. Notch pathway inhibition similarly promotes M2 polarisation and reduces inflammation (Glotfelty et al., 2023).

4. Evidence for neuroinflammation mediated by microglia

M1 phenotype microglia are characterised by an amoeboid morphology and MHC II-positivity. Pro-inflammatory microglia, which express increased MHC I and II, are promoted by DAMPs from dying neurons, inflammatory mediators, misfolded proteins like α-synuclein, and TLR activation (Wendimu & Hooks, 2022). These reactive microglia activate MHC II and are key in antigen presentation and inflammation (Table 2). While these MHC II-positive cells can have various shapes, there is a notable enrichment in reactive amoeboid forms, suggesting a link with pathology (Isik et al., 2023). Aggregated α-synuclein in PD brains correlates with microglial activation. Autopsies reveal that areas with active microglia, like the SNpc and basal ganglia, show higher levels of nitrated α-synuclein (N-α-syn). Enhanced NF-κB expression in the SNpc, especially after N-α-syn stimulation, indicates NF-κB involvement in PD inflammation (Miao & Meng, 2024). Advances like single-cell RNA sequencing (scRNAseq) have revealed increased numbers of reactive, amoeboid microglia in PD midbrains (Smajić et al., 2022).

By using PET imaging to investigate microglial activation in vivo, one can gain an understanding of how neuroinflammation contributes to the pathophysiology of Parkinson's disease. TSPO, which is overbearing in

Table 2 Mechanistic pathways and representative biomarkers in Parkinson's disease.

Mechanism	Biomarkers
Microglial Activation & Neuroinflammation	↑TSPO (PET) ↑MHC-II ↑IL-1β, IL-6, TNF-α ↑CD68 ↑NLRP3 activation
Peripheral Immune Infiltration & Immune–CNS Crosstalk	↑T cell infiltration ($CD4^+$, $CD8^+$) ↑ICAM-1/VCAM-1 ↑CCR2/CCL2 signaling, peripheral cytokines (IL-17, IFN-γ)
Blood–Brain Barrier (BBB) Disruption	Increased BBB permeability ↓Tight junction proteins (claudin-5, occludin, ZO-1) Albumin quotient (CSF/serum) S100B leakage MRI contrast-enhancement
Choroid Plexus & CSF Barrier Dysfunction	Altered AQP1 ↓TTR Changes in epithelial TJ proteins Immune cell trafficking markers CSF cytokine alterations
Glymphatic System Impairment	Altered AQP4 polarization Reduced perivascular CSF–ISF exchange Accumulation of α-synuclein aggregates MRI-DTI glymphatic metrics
Meningeal Lymphatic Dysfunction	Reduced lymphatic vessel integrity ↓VEGFR3 signaling Impaired CSF drainage to deep cervical lymph nodes Accumulation of immune cells at meninges
α-Synuclein Aggregation & Propagation	p-α-syn (Ser129) Oligomeric α-syn CSF α-syn species Seed amplification assay (RT-QuIC) positivity

reactive microglia, became the primary target for PET tracers designed to image neuroinflammation (Ghadery et al., 2019). Recent research using [18 F]-DPA714 examined the function and translation of neuroinflammatory responses in PD patients, evaluating the relationship of imaging biomarkers with clinical status and DAT imaging (Lavisse et al., 2021). Another recent study assessed microglial activation and its link to peripheral immune markers, disease severity, and dopaminergic neuron function using 18F-PBR06 and 18F-FP-DTBZ. 18F-PBR06-PET SUVR was higher in the putamen of early PD patients, particularly ipsilateral to motor onset, and there was a positive correlation between brainstem 18F-PBR06-PET SUVR and 18F-FP-DTBZ-PET SUVR (Liu et al., 2022).

Biomarkers in CSF and blood can clarify PD's neuroinflammatory mechanisms. Elevated CSF oligomeric α-syn and DJ-1 levels are observed in PD patients relative to various neurological controls, and higher DJ-1 in early-stage PD suggests a protective response to early oxidative damage (Peng et al., 2023). Serum cytokine profiles provide prognostic information: a large-cohort study reported TNFα, IL-1ß, IL-2, and IL-10 were upregulated in PD, with a strong pro-inflammatory state linked to worse cognitive and motor outcomes (Fu et al., 2023). Elevated IL-6 correlated with biallelic *PRKN/PINK1* mutations and disease progression (Borsche et al., 2020). Additionally, PD patients exhibited more Th1 cells and higher serum IL-10 and IL-17A, but no important affiliation was observed between microglial activation and peripheral inflammatory markers (Liu et al., 2022).

5. Targeting microglia for Parkinson's disease therapy

TLRs and CB2 receptors are two examples of microglial receptors that can be modified or regulated to provide prospective therapeutic targets for neurodegenerative diseases like Parkinson's disease (Gao et al., 2023) (Fig. 2). In PD patients, the expression of TLR2 varies by disease stage and brain region, correlating with regionally polarisation states of microglia and highlighting TLR2's pivotal role in microglial responses (Gorecki et al., 2021). TLR2 and TLR4 expression can be inhibited by "candesartan cilexetil, an FDA-approved medication for hypertension, cerebrovascular disorders, and chronic heart failure. It may also reverse the pro-inflammatory phenotype of microglia

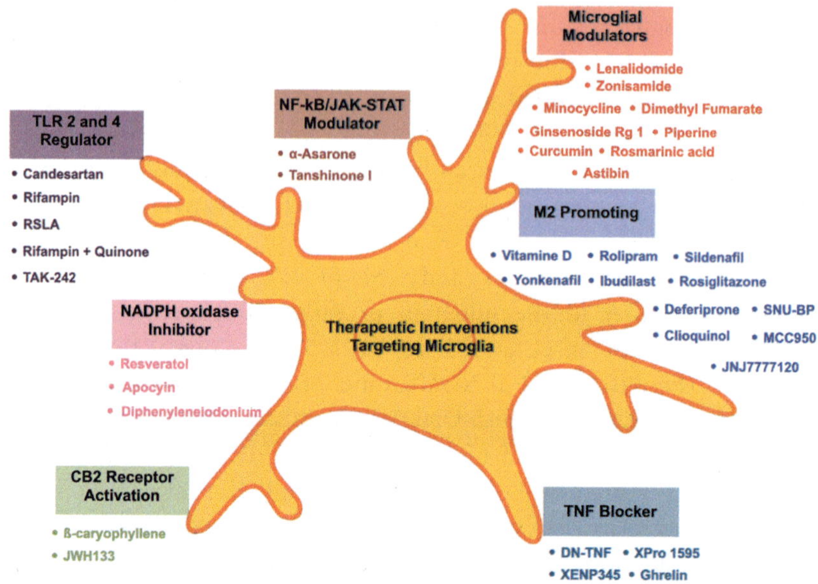

Fig. 2 Therapeutic modulation of microglial receptors and signalling pathways in Parkinson's disease. (A) TLR2 and TLR4 regulators (candesartan, rifampin, rifampicin-quinone, RSLA, TAK-242) modulate pattern-recognition receptor activation and suppress α-synuclein-induced inflammation. (B) CB2 receptor agonists (β-caryophyllene, JWH133) promote anti-inflammatory signalling and protect dopaminergic neurons. (C) NADPH oxidase inhibitors (resveratrol, apocynin, diphenyleneiodonium) reduce ROS-mediated microglial toxicity. (D) NF-κB/JAK-STAT pathways (α-asarone, tanshinone I) inhibit transcriptional drivers of M1 polarisation. (E) microglial modulators (lenalidomide, zonisamide, minocycline, dimethyl fumarate, ginsenoside Rg1, piperine, curcumin, rosmarinic acid, astilbin) suppress inflammatory activation and confer neuroprotection. (F) M2-promoting agents (vitamin D, rolipram, sildenafil, yonkenafil, ibudilast, rosiglitazone, pioglitazone, deferiprone, clioquinol, SNU-BP, MCC950, JNJ7777120) enhance anti-inflammatory phenotype switching, inhibit NLRP3 activation, or provide antioxidant and iron-chelating effects. (G) TNF blockers (DN-TNF, XENP345, XPro1595, ghrelin) reduce pro-inflammatory cytokine signalling, attenuate microglial overactivation, and protect nigrostriatal neurons.

stimulated by oligomeric α-syn (Qie et al., 2020). Also, Rifampin and its autoxidation product, rifampicin quinone, have been demonstrated to inhibit microglial inflammation mediated by TLR2 and P2X7 and induced by α-syn. (Acuña et al., 2019). In MPTP-induced PD" mice, endurance exercise has also been demonstrated to have neuroprotective benefits through the regulation of TLR2 and downstream pathways such as TAK1, MyD88, and TRAF6 (Jang et al., 2017). TLR4 is another promising therapeutic target for modulating microglial activation. Jiang et al. (2020) reported that TAK-242, a small-molecule TLR4 antagonist, notably reduced α-syn-mediated oxidative stress, microglial TNF-α production, and neuronal death in vitro. However, these effects remain to be studied in vivo. An examination by Viveros-Paredes et al. (2017) reported that β-caryophyllene, a natural CB2 receptor agonist, can suppress microglial activation and pro-inflammatory cytokine expression, thereby providing neuroprotection to nigral dopaminergic neurons. Similarly, Chung et al. (2016) reported that JWH133, a selective CB2 receptor agonist, helps protect MPTP-induced PD mice by reducing blood-brain barrier disruption, limiting peripheral immune cell infiltration, and decreasing the production of iNOS and pro-inflammatory cytokines by M1 microglia. JAK/STAT and NF-κB pathways are key to microglial M1 polarisation. Modulating these signals may regulate M1 activation (Li et al., 2021). α-Asarone inhibits NF-κB, reducing M1 polarisation and pro-inflammatory cytokine production, and alleviates Parkinson-like symptoms in MPTP mouse models (Darwish et al., 2023). Tanshinone I also suppresses NF-κB, lowers M1 pro-inflammatory molecules, partially restores M2 markers, and protects against nigrostriatal dopaminergic damage (Zhao et al., 2023). Additionally, some substances, like apocynin, resveratrol, and diphenyleneiodonium, target NADPH oxidase. These substances may prevent microglial activation, reduce the production of different harmful substances, and encourage the microglial phenotype toward an anti-inflammatory state, making them potential candidates for clinical trials in patients with neurodegenerative diseases, including Parkinson's disease. (Liu et al., 2019).

Targeting pro-inflammatory cytokines such as IL-1β and TNF-α may offer new approaches to inhibiting M1 polarisation. In mouse models triggered by MPTP or 6-OHDA, specific inhibition of soluble TNF by intranigral lentiviral delivery of DN-TNF, nigral infusion of DN-TNF compound XENP345, or additional utilisation of DN-TNF inhibitor XPro1595 has been shown to reduce glial activation, protect dopaminergic neurons, and improve behavioural outcomes (Li et al., 2023). Ghrelin, an endogenous ligand for the growth hormone secretagogue receptor 1a, was also evaluated to avoid microglial activation, suppress pro-inflammatory factor production, inhibit iNOS activation, and reduce dopaminergic neuron loss in MPTP-induced" PD mice models (Russo et al., 2022). Its effects appear to be mediated through suppression of MMP-3 expression in stressed dopaminergic neurons. Furthermore, several drugs approved for other disease indications, such as lenalidomide, zonisamide, minocycline, and dimethyl fumarate, as well as various bioactive compounds like ginsenoside Rg1, piperine, curcumin, rosmarinic acid, and astilbin, were found to regulate microglial activation and reduce pro-inflammatory cytokine production in PD mouse models (Liu et al., 2019). These therapies may present alternative treatment options for PD, though their precise mechanisms and signalling pathways need more exploration.

Various potential targets were put out to control microglial activation; CD73-derived adenosine A2A signalling may improve microglia-mediated immune responses(Meng et al., 2019). Inactivation of CD73 substantially reduces adenosine production, inhibits A2A receptor (A2AR)-mediated pro-inflammatory states in microglia, increases dopaminergic neuron activity, and alleviates motor symptoms in animal models of PD (Vincenzi et al., 2023). The activation of microglia is also regulated by the histamine-4 receptor (H4R). The H4R antagonist JNJ7777120 can be infused into the lateral ventricle to enhance Parkinsonian behaviours, inhibit microglial pro-inflammatory activation, stop dopaminergic neuron degeneration, and lessen Lewy body-like neuropathology (Zhou et al., 2019). Another possible target for Parkinson's disease is the NLRP3 inflammasome in microglia, which is activated by fibrillar α-synuclein. In PD mice, oral treatment of the NLRP3 inflammasome inhibitor MCC950 reduced motor impairments and avoided α-synuclein pathology and dopaminergic degeneration (Huang et al., 2023). Other molecules, such as IL-10, cyclic AMP, and vitamin D, that promote an anti-inflammatory phenotype or induce a shift from pro-inflammatory to anti-inflammatory states, potentially have medicinal potential for PD (Saraiva et al., 2020; Fenercioglu, 2024).

PPARs are promising targets in neurodegeneration, as PPAR-γ agonists reduce microglial activation and inflammation, affording neuroprotection (Behl et al., 2021). However, clinical trials of glitazones in PD show mixed results, and more research is needed, including with novel compounds like SNU-BP. Iron chelation therapy (clioquinol, deferiprone) also shows neuroprotective effects in PD models by alleviating iron-related pathology, but mechanisms are uncertain (Negida et al., 2024). Pharmacological microglia modulation carries risk, as microglia serve important roles. The anti-CD22 blocking can revive the function of aged microglia (Aires et al., 2021). In addition to drugs, rTMS and exercise may adjust microglial activity and enhance the results of neurodegeneration, although this has not been investigated completely (Wei et al., 2023).

6. Conclusion

Parkinson's Disease is essentially a system-level disease whereby protein misfolding, immune maladjustment, metabolic stress, and loss of neurotrophic signalling come into play to result in progressive degeneration of dopaminergic neurons. The conceptual framework of the figure reveals the cyclicality of the PD pathology: misfolded α-synuclein triggers microglia and causes chronic inflammation; inflammation and oxidative stress cause damage to mitochondria; mitochondrial breakdown increases oxidative damage; and a failure of the protein degradation process accelerates the α-synuclein deposition. Notably, the deterioration of neurotrophic factors like BDNF makes cells unable to repair themselves and the safety of synapses, which increases neuronal loss. That is, low levels of BDNF greatly limit the inherent ability of the brain to heal the continuous inflammatory and proteotoxic damage, exposing dopaminergic cells to greater susceptibility. This combined knowledge underlines why disease progression cannot be stopped using the monotherapy methods, including only the use of dopamine replacement. More promising therapeutic interventions would be those that reinforce proteostasis, improve mitochondrial quality control, inhibit chronic microglial activation, and repair neurotrophic support. These new approaches, such as α-synuclein immunotherapy, small molecules that act on autophagy signalling, antioxidant-based mitochondrial stabilisers, and BDNF/TrkB agonists, are indicative of this change of focus to multi targeted therapy. In general, PD development is the manifestation of a positive feedback mechanism of inflammation, oxidative stress, mitochondrial dysfunction, and a lack of repair signalling. To stop this cycle, it is necessary to deal with the pathophysiological processes instead of only treating the symptoms. The knowledge of these interrelated pathways can be used in the design of more effective disease-modifying therapies and supports the relevance of integrative mechanistic studies in the case of Parkinson's disease.

Acknowledgements

The authors sincerely acknowledge the Division of Biotechnology, Karunya Institute of Technology and Sciences, for providing the necessary facilities and support that enabled the successful completion of this review.

Author contributions

RU and MS conducted the literature survey and wrote the manuscript. RU designed the study, reviewed the literature, initial draft and edited the paper. MS reviewed the editing and supervised the review work. All authors read and approved the final paper.

Declarations

Competing interest

The authors declare no competing interests.

Ethical approval and consent to participate

Not applicable.

Data availability

All the data have been included in the manuscript.

Consent for publication

Not applicable.

Funding

The authors did not receive any funding for the preparation of this review study.

References

Aarsland, D., Batzu, L., Halliday, G. M., Geurtsen, G. J., Ballard, C., Ray Chaudhuri, K., & Weintraub, D. (2021). Parkinson disease-associated cognitive impairment. *Nature Reviews Disease Primers,* 7(1), 47. https://doi.org/10.1038/s41572-021-00280-3.

Acuña, L., Hamadat, S., Corbalán, N. S., González-Lizárraga, F., Dos-Santos-Pereira, M., Rocca, J., ... Raisman-Vozari, R. (2019). Rifampicin and its derivative rifampicin quinone reduce microglial inflammatory responses and neurodegeneration induced in vitro by α-synuclein fibrillary aggregates. *Cells, 8*(8), 776. https://doi.org/10.3390/cells8080776.

Aires, V., Coulon-Bainier, C., Pavlovic, A., Ebeling, M., Schmucki, R., Schweitzer, C., ... Harde, E. (2021). CD22 blockage restores age-related impairments of microglia surveillance capacity. *Frontiers in Immunology, 12*, 684430. https://doi.org/10.3389/fimmu.2021.684430.

Ali, N. H., Al-Kuraishy, H. M., Al-Gareeb, A. I., Alexiou, A., Papadakis, M., AlAseeri, A. A., ... Batiha, G. E. (2024). BDNF/TrkB activators in Parkinson's disease: A new therapeutic strategy. *Journal of Cellular and Molecular Medicine, 28*(10), e18368. https://doi.org/10.1111/jcmm.18368.

Amici, S. A., Dong, J., & Guerau-de-Arellano, M. (2017). Molecular mechanisms modulating the phenotype of macrophages and microglia. *Frontiers in Immunology, 8*, 1520. https://doi.org/10.3389/fimmu.2017.01520.

Ana, B. (2024). Aged-related changes in microglia and neurodegenerative diseases: Exploring the connection. *Biomedicines, 12*(8), 1737. https://doi.org/10.3390/biomedicines12081737.

Araújo, B., Caridade-Silva, R., Soares-Guedes, C., Martins-Macedo, J., Gomes, E. D., Monteiro, S., & Teixeira, F. G. (2022). Neuroinflammation and Parkinson's disease-from neurodegeneration to therapeutic opportunities. *Cells, 11*(18), 2908. https://doi.org/10.3390/cells11182908.

Behl, T., Madaan, P., Sehgal, A., Singh, S., Sharma, N., Bhatia, S., & Bungau, S. G. (2021). Elucidating the neuroprotective role of PPARs in Parkinson's disease: A neoteric and prospective target. *International Journal of Molecular Sciences, 22*(18), 10161. https://doi.org/10.3390/ijms221810161.

Borsche, M., König, I. R., Delcambre, S., Petrucci, S., Balck, A., Brüggemann, N., ... Klein, C. (2020). Mitochondrial damage-associated inflammation highlights biomarkers in PRKN/PINK1 parkinsonism. *Brain: A Journal of Neurology, 143*(10), 3041–3051. https://doi.org/10.1093/brain/awaa246.

Bravo-Jimenez, M. A., Sharma, S., & Karimi-Abdolrezaee, S. (2025). The integrated stress response in neurodegenerative diseases. *Molecular Neurodegeneration, 20*(1), 20. https://doi.org/10.1186/s13024-025-00811-6.

Cai, Y., Liu, J., Wang, B., Sun, M., & Yang, H. (2022). Microglia in the neuroinflammatory pathogenesis of Alzheimer's disease and related therapeutic targets. *Frontiers in Immunology, 13*, 856376. https://doi.org/10.3389/fimmu.2022.856376.

Calabresi, P., Mechelli, A., Natale, G., Volpicelli-Daley, L., Di Lazzaro, G., & Ghiglieri, V. (2023). Alpha-synuclein in Parkinson's disease and other synucleinopathies: From overt neurodegeneration back to early synaptic dysfunction. *Cell Death & Disease, 14*(3), 176. https://doi.org/10.1038/s41419-023-05672-9.

Callahan, S. M. (2024). The gut-brain symphony: harmony and discord in the microbial orchestra of neural function (Master's thesis, Boston University).

Campolo, M., Paterniti, I., Siracusa, R., Filippone, A., Esposito, E., & Cuzzocrea, S. (2019). TLR4 absence reduces neuroinflammation and inflammasome activation in Parkinson's diseases in vivo model. *Brain, Behavior, and Immunity, 76*, 236–247. https://doi.org/10.1016/j.bbi.2018.12.003.

Canovas, B., & Nebreda, A. R. (2021). Diversity and versatility of p38 kinase signalling in health and disease. *Nature Reviews. Molecular Cell Biology, 22*(5), 346–366. https://doi.org/10.1038/s41580-020-00322-w.

Caplan, I. F., & Maguire-Zeiss, K. A. (2018). Toll-Like receptor 2 signaling and current approaches for therapeutic modulation in synucleinopathies. *Frontiers in Pharmacology, 9*, 417. https://doi.org/10.3389/fphar.2018.00417.

Chen, J., Pan, Y., Liu, Q., Li, G., Chen, G., Li, W., ... Wang, Q. (2024). The interplay between meningeal lymphatic vessels and neuroinflammation in neurodegenerative diseases. *Current Neuropharmacology, 22*(6), 1016–1032. https://doi.org/10.2174/1570159X21666221115150253.

Chen, M. M., Li, Y., Deng, S. L., Zhao, Y., Lian, Z. X., & Yu, K. (2022). Mitochondrial function and reactive oxygen/nitrogen species in skeletal muscle. *Frontiers in Cell and Developmental Biology, 10*, 826981. https://doi.org/10.3389/fcell.2022.826981.

Chen, S., Saeed, A. F., Liu, Q., Jiang, Q., Xu, H., Xiao, G. G., & Duo, Y. (2023). Macrophages in immunoregulation and therapeutics. *Signal Transduction and Targeted Therapy, 8*(1), 207. https://doi.org/10.1038/s41392-023-01452-1.

Chen, X., Zhang, G., Liu, M., He, J., & Zhang, Z. (2025). New perspectives on molecular mechanisms underlying exercise-induced benefits in Parkinson's disease. *NPJ Parkinson's Disease, 11*(1), 256. https://doi.org/10.1038/s41531-025-01113-w.

Chmielarz, P., & Saarma, M. (2020). Neurotrophic factors for disease-modifying treatments of Parkinson's disease: Gaps between basic science and clinical studies. *Pharmacological Reports: PR, 72*(5), 1195–1217. https://doi.org/10.1007/s43440-020-00120-3.

Chung, Y. C., Shin, W. H., Baek, J. Y., Cho, E. J., Baik, H. H., Kim, S. R., ... Jin, B. K. (2016). CB2 receptor activation prevents glial-derived neurotoxic mediator production, BBB leakage and peripheral immune cell infiltration and rescues dopamine neurons in the MPTP model of Parkinson's disease. *Experimental & Molecular Medicine, 48*(1), e205. https://doi.org/10.1038/emm.2015.100.

Colonna, M., & Butovsky, O. (2017). Microglia function in the central nervous system during health and neurodegeneration. *Annual Review of Immunology, 35*, 441–468. https://doi.org/10.1146/annurev-immunol-051116-052358.

Darwish, S. F., Elbadry, A. M. M., Elbokhomy, A. S., Salama, G. A., & Salama, R. M. (2023). The dual face of microglia (M1/M2) as a potential target in the protective effect of nutraceuticals against neurodegenerative diseases. *Frontiers in Aging, 4*, 1231706. https://doi.org/10.3389/fragi.2023.1231706.

Ding, H., Wang, G., Yu, Z., Sun, H., & Wang, L. (2022). Role of interferon-gamma (IFN-γ) and IFN-γ receptor 1/2 (IFNγR1/2) in regulation of immunity, infection, and cancer development: IFN-γ-dependent or independent pathway. *Biomedicine & Pharmacotherapy, 155*, 113683. https://doi.org/10.1016/j.biopha.2022.113683.

Dumas, A. A., Dalmau Gasull, A., & Prinz, M. (2024). Beyond borders: The choroid plexus-immune communication during neuroinflammation. *Signal Transduction and Targeted Therapy, 9*(1), 278. https://doi.org/10.1038/s41392-024-01997-9.

Eo, H., Kim, S., Jung, U. J., & Kim, S. R. (2024). Alpha-synuclein and microglia in Parkinson's disease: From pathogenesis to therapeutic prospects. *Journal of Clinical Medicine, 13*(23), 7243. https://doi.org/10.3390/jcm13237243.

Espejo, E. F., Guerra, M. D., & Castellano, S. (2025). Association between serum myeloperoxidase enzyme activity and Parkinson's disease status. *NPJ Parkinson's Disease, 11*(1), 94. https://doi.org/10.1038/s41531-025-00941-0.

Fakorede, S., Lateef, O. M., Garuba, W. A., Akosile, P. O., Okon, D. A., & Aborode, A. T. (2025). Dual impact of neuroinflammation on cognitive and motor impairments in Alzheimer's disease. *Journal of Alzheimer's Disease Reports, 9*, 25424823251341870. https://doi.org/10.1177/25424823251341870.

Fenercioglu, A. K. (2024). The anti-inflammatory roles of vitamin D for improving human health. *Current Issues in Molecular Biology, 46*(12), 13514–13525. https://doi.org/10.3390/cimb46120807.

Fu, J., Chen, S., Liu, J., Yang, J., Ou, R., Zhang, L., ... Shang, H. (2023). Serum inflammatory cytokines levels and the correlation analyses in Parkinson's disease. *Frontiers in Cell and Developmental Biology, 11*, 1104393. https://doi.org/10.3389/fcell.2023.1104393.

Gao, C., Jiang, J., Tan, Y., & Chen, S. (2023). Microglia in neurodegenerative diseases: Mechanism and potential therapeutic targets. *Signal Transduction and Targeted Therapy, 8*(1), 359. https://doi.org/10.1038/s41392-023-01588-0.

Gao, Y., Liu, K., & Zhu, J. (2023). Glymphatic system: An emerging therapeutic approach for neurological disorders. *Frontiers in Molecular Neuroscience, 16*, 1138769. https://doi.org/10.3389/fnmol.2023.1138769.

Ge, P., Dawson, V. L., & Dawson, T. M. (2020). PINK1 and Parkin mitochondrial quality control: A source of regional vulnerability in Parkinson's disease. *Molecular Neurodegeneration, 15*(1), 20. https://doi.org/10.1186/s13024-020-00367-7.

Gellhaar, S., Sunnemark, D., Eriksson, H., Olson, L., & Galter, D. (2017). Myeloperoxidase-immunoreactive cells are significantly increased in brain areas affected by neurodegeneration in Parkinson's and Alzheimer's disease. *Cell and Tissue Research, 369*(3), 445–454. https://doi.org/10.1007/s00441-017-2626-8.

Ghadery, C., Best, L. A., Pavese, N., Tai, Y. F., & Strafella, A. P. (2019). PET evaluation of microglial activation in non-neurodegenerative brain diseases. *Current Neurology and Neuroscience Reports, 19*(7), 38. https://doi.org/10.1007/s11910-019-0951-x.

Glotfelty, E. J., Tovar-Y-Romo, L. B., Hsueh, S. C., Tweedie, D., Li, Y., Harvey, B. K., ... Greig, N. H. (2023). The RhoA-ROCK1/ROCK2 pathway exacerbates inflammatory signaling in immortalized and primary microglia. *Cells, 12*(10), 1367. https://doi.org/10.3390/cells12101367.

Gorecki, A. M., Anyaegbu, C. C., & Anderton, R. S. (2021). TLR2 and TLR4 in Parkinson's disease pathogenesis: The environment takes a toll on the gut. *Translational Neurodegeneration, 10*(1), 47. https://doi.org/10.1186/s40035-021-00271-0.

Guo, S., Wang, H., & Yin, Y. (2022). Microglia polarization from M1 to M2 in neurodegenerative diseases. *Frontiers in Aging Neuroscience, 14*, 815347. https://doi.org/10.3389/fnagi.2022.815347.

Harsanyiova, J., Buday, T., & Kralova Trancikova, A. (2020). Parkinson's disease and the gut: Future perspectives for early diagnosis. *Frontiers in Neuroscience, 14*, 626. https://doi.org/10.3389/fnins.2020.00626.

He, X., Li, Y., Deng, B., Lin, A., Zhang, G., Ma, M., ... Kang, X. (2022). The PI3K/AKT signalling pathway in inflammation, cell death and glial scar formation after traumatic spinal cord injury: Mechanisms and therapeutic opportunities. *Cell Proliferation, 55*(9), e13275. https://doi.org/10.1111/cpr.13275.

Ho, D. H., Han, S. J., & Son, I. (2025). The multifaceted role of LRRK2 in Parkinson's disease. *Brain Sciences, 15*(4), 407. https://doi.org/10.3390/brainsci15040407.

Hu, X., Li, J., Fu, M., Zhao, X., & Wang, W. (2021). The JAK/STAT signaling pathway: From bench to clinic. *Signal Transduction and Targeted Therapy, 6*(1), 402. https://doi.org/10.1038/s41392-021-00791-1.

Huang, Q., Yang, P., Liu, Y., Ding, J., Lu, M., & Hu, G. (2023). The interplay between α-Synuclein and NLRP3 inflammasome in Parkinson's disease. *Biomedicine & Pharmacotherapy, 168*, 115735. https://doi.org/10.1016/j.biopha.2023.115735.

Isik, S., Yeman Kiyak, B., Akbayir, R., Seyhali, R., & Arpaci, T. (2023). Microglia mediated neuroinflammation in Parkinson's disease. *Cells, 12*(7), 1012. https://doi.org/10.3390/cells12071012.

Jang, Y., Koo, J. H., Kwon, I., Kang, E. B., Um, H. S., Soya, H., & Cho, J. Y. (2017). Neuroprotective effects of endurance exercise against neuroinflammation in MPTP-induced Parkinson's disease mice. *Brain Research, 1655*, 186–193. https://doi.org/10.1016/j.brainres.2016.10.029.

Jiang, L., Xu, Z., Li, H., Wu, M., Wang, F., Liu, S., ... Feng, X. (2020). TAK-242 exerts a neuroprotective effect via suppression of the TLR4/MyD88/TRIF/NF-κB signaling pathway in a neonatal hypoxic-ischemic encephalopathy rat model. *Molecular Medicine Reports, 22*(2), 1440–1448. https://doi.org/10.3892/mmr.2020.11220.

Kouli, A., Camacho, M., Allinson, K., & Williams-Gray, C. H. (2020). Neuroinflammation and protein pathology in Parkinson's disease dementia. *Acta Neuropathologica Communications, 8*(1), 211. https://doi.org/10.1186/s40478-020-01083-5.

Lau, K., Kotzur, R., & Richter, F. (2024). Blood-brain barrier alterations and their impact on Parkinson's disease pathogenesis and therapy. *Translational Neurodegeneration, 13*(1), 37. https://doi.org/10.1186/s40035-024-00430-z.

Lavisse, S., Goutal, S., Wimberley, C., Tonietto, M., Bottlaender, M., Gervais, P., ... Remy, P. (2021). Increased microglial activation in patients with Parkinson disease using [18F]-DPA714 TSPO PET imaging. *Parkinsonism & Related Disorders, 82*, 29–36. https://doi.org/10.1016/j.parkreldis.2020.11.011.

Li, J., Shui, X., Sun, R., Wan, L., Zhang, B., Xiao, B., & Luo, Z. (2021). Microglial phenotypic transition: Signaling pathways and influencing modulators involved in regulation in central nervous system diseases. *Frontiers in Cellular Neuroscience, 15*, 736310. https://doi.org/10.3389/fncel.2021.736310.

Li, J., Ye, F., Xu, X., Xu, P., Wang, P., Zheng, G., ... Shen, H. (2023). Targeting macrophage M1 polarization suppression through PCAF inhibition alleviates autoimmune arthritis via synergistic NF-κB and H3K9Ac blockade. *Journal of Nanobiotechnology, 21*(1), 280. https://doi.org/10.1186/s12951-023-02012-z.

Li, Q., von Ehrlich-Treuenstätt, V., Schardey, J., Wirth, U., Zimmermann, P., Andrassy, J., ... Kühn, F. (2023). Gut barrier dysfunction and bacterial lipopolysaccharides in colorectal cancer. *Journal of Gastrointestinal Surgery: Official Journal of the Society for Surgery of the Alimentary Tract, 27*(7), 1466–1472. https://doi.org/10.1007/s11605-023-05654-4.

Li, Y., Xia, Y., Yin, S., Wan, F., Hu, J., Kou, L., ... Wang, T. (2021). Targeting microglial α-synuclein/TLRs/NF-kappaB/NLRP3 inflammasome axis in Parkinson's disease. *Frontiers in Immunology, 12*, 719807. https://doi.org/10.3389/fimmu.2021.719807.

Lind-Holm Mogensen, F., Seibler, P., Grünewald, A., & Michelucci, A. (2025). Microglial dynamics and neuroinflammation in prodromal and early Parkinson's disease. *Journal of Neuroinflammation, 22*(1), 136. https://doi.org/10.1186/s12974-025-03462-y.

Liu, C. Y., Wang, X., Liu, C., & Zhang, H. L. (2019). Pharmacological targeting of microglial activation: New therapeutic approach. *Frontiers in Cellular Neuroscience, 13*, 514. https://doi.org/10.3389/fncel.2019.00514.

Liu, S. Y., Qiao, H. W., Song, T. B., Liu, X. L., Yao, Y. X., Zhao, C. S., ... Chan, P. (2022). Brain microglia activation and peripheral adaptive immunity in Parkinson's disease: A multimodal PET study. *Journal of Neuroinflammation, 19*(1), 209. https://doi.org/10.1186/s12974-022-02574-z.

Liu, T., Zhang, L., Joo, D., & Sun, S. C. (2017). NF-κB signaling in inflammation. *Signal Transduction and Targeted Therapy, 2*(1), 1–9. https://doi.org/10.1038/sigtrans.2017.23.

Ma, K., Chen, G., Li, W., Kepp, O., Zhu, Y., & Chen, Q. (2020). Mitophagy, mitochondrial homeostasis, and cell fate. *Frontiers in Cell and Developmental Biology, 8*, 467. https://doi.org/10.3389/fcell.2020.00467.

Ma, X., Yan, R., Jian, Y., Zhang, J., Xie, B., Duan, J., ... Ge, W. (2025). Investigating the relationship between glymphatic dysfunction and motor symptoms in Parkinson's disease. *European Journal of Medical Research, 30*(1), 865. https://doi.org/10.1186/s40001-025-03125-x.

Mantash, S. (2019). Cellular and molecular aspects of cell therapy in mouse models of Parkinson's disease and traumatic brain injury (Doctoral dissertation, Université de Poitiers).

Mayer, M. G., & Fischer, T. (2024). Microglia at the blood brain barrier in health and disease. *Frontiers in Cellular Neuroscience, 18*, 1360195. https://doi.org/10.3389/fncel.2024.1360195.

Meng, F., Guo, Z., Hu, Y., Mai, W., Zhang, Z., Zhang, B., ... Gao, Z. (2019). CD73-derived adenosine controls inflammation and neurodegeneration by modulating dopamine signalling. *Brain: a Journal of Neurology, 142*(3), 700–718. https://doi.org/10.1093/brain/awy351.

Miao, Y., & Meng, H. (2024). The involvement of α-synucleinopathy in the disruption of microglial homeostasis contributes to the pathogenesis of Parkinson's disease. *Cell Communication and Signaling: CCS, 22*(1), 31. https://doi.org/10.1186/s12964-023-01402-y.

Muzio, L., Viotti, A., & Martino, G. (2021). Microglia in neuroinflammation and neurodegeneration: From understanding to therapy. *Frontiers in Neuroscience, 15*, 742065.

Negida, A., Hassan, N. M., Aboeldahab, H., Zain, Y. E., Negida, Y., Cadri, S., ... Berman, B. (2024). Efficacy of the iron-chelating agent, deferiprone, in patients with Parkinson's disease: A systematic review and meta-analysis. *CNS Neuroscience & Therapeutics, 30*(2), e14607. https://doi.org/10.1111/cns.14607.

Noh, M. Y., Kwon, H. S., Kwon, M. S., Nahm, M., Jin, H. K., Bae, J. S., & Kim, S. H. (2025). Biomarkers and therapeutic strategies targeting microglia in neurodegenerative diseases: Current status and future directions. *Molecular Neurodegeneration, 20*(1), 82. https://doi.org/10.1186/s13024-025-00867-4.

Nolan, R. A., Reeb, K. L., Rong, Y., Matt, S. M., Johnson, H. S., Runner, K., & Gaskill, P. J. (2020). Dopamine activates NF-κB and primes the NLRP3 inflammasome in primary human macrophages. *Brain, Behavior, & Immunity - Health, 2*, 100030. https://doi.org/10.1016/j.bbih.2019.100030.

Peng, H., Chen, S., Wu, S., Shi, X., Ma, J., Yang, H., & Li, X. (2023). Alpha-synuclein in skin as a high-quality biomarker for Parkinson's disease. *Journal of the Neurological Sciences, 451*, 120730. https://doi.org/10.1016/j.jns.2023.120730.

Picca, A., Calvani, R., Coelho-Junior, H. J., Landi, F., Bernabei, R., & Marzetti, E. (2020). Mitochondrial dysfunction, oxidative stress, and neuroinflammation: Intertwined roads to neurodegeneration. *Antioxidants (Basel, Switzerland), 9*(8), 647. https://doi.org/10.3390/antiox9080647.

Pérez, S., & Rius-Pérez, S. (2022). Macrophage polarization and reprogramming in acute inflammation: A redox perspective. *Antioxidants, 11*(7), 1394. https://doi.org/10.3390/antiox11071394.

Qie, S., Ran, Y., Lu, X., Su, W., Li, W., Xi, J., ... Liu, Z. (2020). Candesartan modulates microglia activation and polarization via NF-κB signaling pathway. *International Journal of Immunopathology and Pharmacology, 34*, 2058738420974900. https://doi.org/10.1177/2058738420974900.

Russo, C., Valle, M. S., Russo, A., & Malaguarnera, L. (2022). The Interplay between Ghrelin and microglia in neuroinflammation: Implications for obesity and neurodegenerative diseases. *International journal of molecular sciences, 23*(21), 13432. https://doi.org/10.3390/ijms232113432.

Sahoo, S., Padhy, A. A., Kumari, V., & Mishra, P. (2022). Role of ubiquitin-proteasome and autophagy-lysosome pathways in α-synuclein aggregate clearance. *Molecular Neurobiology, 59*(9), 5379–5407. https://doi.org/10.1007/s12035-022-02897-1.

Salerno, S., Viviano, M., Baglini, E., Poggetti, V., Giorgini, D., Castagnoli, J., ... Taliani, S. (2024). TSPO radioligands for neuroinflammation: An overview. *Molecules (Basel, Switzerland), 29*(17), 4212. https://doi.org/10.3390/molecules29174212.

Saraiva, M., Vieira, P., & O'Garra, A. (2020). Biology and therapeutic potential of interleukin-10. *The Journal of Experimental Medicine, 217*(1), e20190418. https://doi.org/10.1084/jem.20190418.

Scott-Massey, A., Boag, M. K., Magnier, A., Bispo, D. P. C. F., Khoo, T. K., & Pountney, D. L. (2022). Glymphatic system dysfunction and sleep disturbance may contribute to the pathogenesis and progression of Parkinson's disease. *International Journal of Molecular Sciences, 23*(21), 12928. https://doi.org/10.3390/ijms232112928.

Smajić, S., Prada-Medina, C. A., Landoulsi, Z., Ghelfi, J., Delcambre, S., Dietrich, C., ... Spielmann, M. (2022). Single-cell sequencing of human midbrain reveals glial activation and a Parkinson-specific neuronal state. *Brain: a Journal of Neurology, 145*(3), 964–978. https://doi.org/10.1093/brain/awab446.

Solár, P., Zamani, A., Kubíčková, L., Dubový, P., & Joukal, M. (2020). Choroid plexus and the blood-cerebrospinal fluid barrier in disease. *Fluids and Barriers of the CNS, 17*(1), 35. https://doi.org/10.1186/s12987-020-00196-2.

Stær, K., Iranzo, A., Stokholm, M. G., Hvingelby, V. S., Danielsen, E. H., Østergaard, K., ... Pavese, N. (2024). Microglial activation and progression of nigrostriatal dysfunction in isolated REM sleep behavior disorder. *Movement Disorders: Official Journal of the Movement Disorder Society, 39*(8), 1323–1328. https://doi.org/10.1002/mds.29767.

Stokholm, M. G., Iranzo, A., Østergaard, K., Serradell, M., Otto, M., Svendsen, K. B., ... Pavese, N. (2017). Assessment of neuroinflammation in patients with idiopathic rapid-eye-movement sleep behaviour disorder: A case-control study. *The Lancet Neurology, 16*(10), 789–796. https://doi.org/10.1016/s1474-4422(17)30173-4.

Sweeney, M. D., Sagare, A. P., & Zlokovic, B. V. (2018). Blood-brain barrier breakdown in Alzheimer disease and other neurodegenerative disorders. *Nature Reviews. Neurology, 14*(3), 133–150. https://doi.org/10.1038/nrneurol.2017.188.

Toader, C., Serban, M., Munteanu, O., Covache-Busuioc, R. A., Enyedi, M., Ciurea, A. V., & Tataru, C. P. (2025). From synaptic plasticity to Neurodegeneration: BDNF as a transformative target in medicine. *International Journal of Molecular Sciences, 26*(9), 4271. https://doi.org/10.3390/ijms26094271.

Tournier, B. B., Tsartsalis, S., Ceyzériat, K., Garibotto, V., & Millet, P. (2020). Vivo TSPO signal and neuroinflammation in Alzheimer's disease. *Cells, 9*(9), 1941. https://doi.org/10.3390/cells9091941.

Vidal-Itriago, A., Radford, R. A. W., Aramideh, J. A., Maurel, C., Scherer, N. M., Don, E. K., ... Morsch, M. (2022). Microglia morphophysiological diversity and its implications for the CNS. *Frontiers in Immunology, 13*, 997786. https://doi.org/10.3389/fimmu.2022.997786.

Vidović, M., & Rikalovic, M. G. (2022). Alpha-synuclein aggregation pathway in Parkinson's disease: Current status and novel therapeutic approaches. *Cells, 11*(11), 1732. https://doi.org/10.3390/cells11111732.

Vincenzi, F., Pasquini, S., Contri, C., Cappello, M., Nigro, M., Travagli, A., & Varani, K. (2023). Pharmacology of adenosine receptors: Recent advancements. *Biomolecules, 13*(9), 1387. https://doi.org/10.3390/biom13091387.

Viveros-Paredes, J. M., González-Castañeda, R. E., Gertsch, J., Chaparro-Huerta, V., López-Roa, R. I., Vázquez-Valls, E., ... Flores-Soto, M. E. (2017). Neuroprotective effects of β-caryophyllene against dopaminergic neuron injury in a murine model of Parkinson's disease induced by MPTP. *Pharmaceuticals (Basel, Switzerland), 10*(3), 60. https://doi.org/10.3390/ph10030060.

Voumvourakis, K. I., Sideri, E., Papadimitropoulos, G. N., Tsantzali, I., Hewlett, P., Kitsos, D., ... Paraskevas, G. P. (2023). The dynamic relationship between the glymphatic system, aging, memory, and sleep. *Biomedicines, 11*(8), 2092. https://doi.org/10.3390/biomedicines11082092.

Wang, J., He, W., & Zhang, J. (2023). A richer and more diverse future for microglia phenotypes. *Heliyon, 9*(4), https://doi.org/10.1016/j.heliyon.2023.e14713.

Warden, A. S., Han, C., Hansen, E., Trescott, S., Nguyen, C., Kim, R., & Coufal, N. G. (2023). Tools for studying human microglia: In vitro and in vivo strategies. *Brain, Behavior, and Immunity, 107*, 369–382. https://doi.org/10.1016/j.bbi.2022.10.008.

Wareham, L. K., Liddelow, S. A., Temple, S., Benowitz, L. I., Di Polo, A., Wellington, C., ... Calkins, D. J. (2022). Solving neurodegeneration: Common mechanisms and strategies for new treatments. *Molecular Neurodegeneration, 17*(1), 23. https://doi.org/10.1186/s13024-022-00524-0.

Wei, J. A., Liu, L., Song, X., Lin, B., Cui, J., Luo, L., & Zhang, L. (2023). Physical exercise modulates the microglial complement pathway in mice to relieve cortical circuitry deficits induced by mutant human TDP-43. *Cell Reports, 42*(3), https://doi.org/10.1016/j.celrep.2023.112240.

Wendimu, M. Y., & Hooks, S. B. (2022). Microglia phenotypes in aging and neurodegenerative diseases. *Cells, 11*(13), 2091. https://doi.org/10.3390/cells11132091.

Woodburn, S. C., Bollinger, J. L., & Wohleb, E. S. (2021). The semantics of microglia activation: Neuroinflammation, homeostasis, and stress. *Journal of Neuroinflammation, 18*(1), 258. https://doi.org/10.1186/s12974-021-02309-6.

Xu, H., Lotfy, P., Gelb, S., Pragana, A., Hehnly, C., Byer, L. I. J., ... Lehtinen, M. K. (2024). The choroid plexus synergizes with immune cells during neuroinflammation. *Cell, 187*(18), 4946–4963.e17. https://doi.org/10.1016/j.cell.2024.07.002.

Yao, R., Pan, R., Shang, C., Li, X., Cheng, J., Xu, J., & Li, Y. (2020). Translocator protein 18 kDa (TSPO) deficiency inhibits microglial activation and impairs mitochondrial function. *Frontiers in Pharmacology, 11*, 986. https://doi.org/10.3389/fphar.2020.00986.

Ye, X., Zhu, M., Che, X., Wang, H., Liang, X. J., Wu, C., & Yang, J. (2020). Lipopolysaccharide induces neuroinflammation in microglia by activating the MTOR pathway and downregulating Vps34 to inhibit autophagosome formation. *Journal of Neuroinflammation, 17*(1), 18. https://doi.org/10.1186/s12974-019-1644-8.

Yi, S., Wang, L., Wang, H., Ho, M. S., & Zhang, S. (2022). Pathogenesis of α-synuclein in Parkinson's disease: From a neuron-glia crosstalk perspective. *International Journal of Molecular Sciences, 23*(23), 14753. https://doi.org/10.3390/ijms232314753.

Yu, H., Zhang, L., Song, B., Ren, K., Chen, X., Dai, Y., ... Wei, Z. (2025). TREM2-mediated regulation of microglial activity: A promising target for the treatment of ischemic stroke. *Journal of Translational Medicine, 23*(1), 782. https://doi.org/10.1186/s12967-025-06799-3.

Zeng, J., Bao, T., Yang, K., Zhu, X., Wang, S., Xiang, W., ... Ge, J. (2023). The mechanism of microglia-mediated immune inflammation in ischemic stroke and the role of natural botanical components in regulating microglia: A review. *Frontiers in Immunology, 13*, 1047550. https://doi.org/10.3389/fimmu.2022.1047550.

Zhang, J., Xie, D., Jiao, D., Zhou, S., Liu, S., Ju, Z., & Zhao, C. (2024). From inflammatory signaling to neuronal damage: Exploring NLR inflammasomes in ageing neurological disorders. *Heliyon, 10*(12), https://doi.org/10.1016/j.heliyon.2024.e32688.

Zhang, M., Liang, C., Chen, X., Cai, Y., & Cui, L. (2024). Interplay between microglia and environmental risk factors in Alzheimer's disease. *Neural Regeneration Research, 19*(8), 1718–1727. https://doi.org/10.4103/1673-5374.389745.

Zhang, W., Xiao, D., Mao, Q., & Xia, H. (2023). Role of neuroinflammation in neurodegeneration development. *Signal Transduction and Targeted Therapy, 8*(1), 267. https://doi.org/10.1038/s41392-023-01486-5.

Zhao, J., Liu, H., Hong, Z., Luo, W., Mu, W., Hou, X., ... Zhan, X. (2023). Tanshinone I specifically suppresses NLRP3 inflammasome activation by disrupting the association of NLRP3 and ASC. *Molecular Medicine (Cambridge, Mass.), 29*(1), 84. https://doi.org/10.1186/s10020-023-00671-0.

Zhou, P., Homberg, J. R., Fang, Q., Wang, J., Li, W., Meng, X., ... Liu, C. (2019). Histamine-4 receptor antagonist JNJ7777120 inhibits pro-inflammatory microglia and prevents the progression of Parkinson-like pathology and behaviour in a rat model. *Brain, Behavior, and Immunity, 76*, 61–73. https://doi.org/10.1016/j.bbi.2018.11.006.

CHAPTER THIRTEEN

Microglial advances in psychiatric disorders

Jemmyson R. de Jesus[a,b,*], Iare S. Ribeiro[a,b], Marcos V.S. Pereira[a,b], Wesley C.P. Aquino[a,b], and Lucas H.M. Alfredo[a,b]

[a]Research Laboratory in bionanomaterials, LPbio, Department of Chemistry, Federal University of Viçosa, Viçosa, MG, Brazil

[b]National Institute of Science and Technology of Bioanalytics-Lauro Kubota (INCTBio-LK), Campinas, SP, Brazil

*Corresponding author. e-mail address: jemmyson.jesus@ufv.br

Contents

Abstract

Psychiatric disorders constitute a major global challenge to public health, characterized by complex and multifactorial etiologies involving genetic, environmental, and neurobiological factors. In recent years, growing evidence has highlighted the central role of microglia, the resident immune cells of the central nervous system, in regulating brain homeostasis and in the pathophysiology of neuropsychiatric conditions. Beyond their classic immune functions, microglia actively participate in synaptic pruning, neurogenesis, and the modulation of neural circuits. Dysregulation of microglial activity, particularly chronic pro-inflammatory activation, has been strongly associated with disorders such as major depression, schizophrenia, bipolar disorder, and neurodegenerative diseases, contributing to impaired synaptic plasticity, neuroinflammation, and behavioral dysfunction. This chapter discusses recent advances in microglial biology, emphasizing its functional heterogeneity and dynamic phenotypic states. This chapter

Advances in Immunology, Volume 171
ISSN 0065-2776, https://doi.org/10.1016/bs.ai.2026.04.007

explores the main molecular pathways involved in microglia-mediated synaptic remodeling and their implications for the progression of neuropsychiatric disorders. Furthermore, emerging therapeutic strategies targeting microglia were discussed, including anti-inflammatory approaches, functional reprogramming, neuromodulation techniques, and microglial replacement or niche engineering. These advances support a paradigm shift from indiscriminate microglia inhibition to the precise modulation of specific functional states. Understanding and targeting microglia dynamics may provide innovative and more effective therapeutic pathways for the treatment of psychiatric disorders.

Abbreviation

Aβ	Amyloid-beta.
AI	Artificial intelligence.
APP	Amyloid precursor protein.
Arg1	Arginase−1.
ASC	Apoptosis-associated speck-like protein containing a CARD.
ASD	Autism Spectrum Disorder.
ATP−5A	ATP synthase alpha subunit.
BBB	Blood-brain barrier.
BDNF	Brain-derived neurotrophic factor.
BLZ945	CSF1R inhibitor.
C1q	Complement component 1q.
C3	Complement component 3.
CAR-M	Chimeric antigen receptor-macrophage.
Ccp1	Cytosolic carboxypeptidase 1.
CD11b	Cluster of differentiation 11b.
CD18	Cluster of differentiation 18.
CD86	Cluster of differentiation 86.
CGI-S	Clinical Global Impression Scale.Severity.
circDYM	Circular RNA DYM.
circRNA	Circular RNA.
CMKLR1	Chemokine-like receptor 1.
CNS	Central nervous system.
COX1	Cyclooxygenase−1.
CR3	Complement receptor 3.
CREB	cAMP response element-binding protein.
CRISPR	Clustered regularly interspaced short palindromic repeats.
CRP	C-reactive protein.
CSDS	Chronic social defeat stress.
CSF1	Colony stimulating factor 1.
CSF1R	Colony stimulating factor receptor.
CTLA−4	Cytotoxic T-lymphocyte-associated protein 4.
CUMS / CUS	Chronic unpredictable (mild) stress.
CX3CL1	C-X3-C motif chemokine ligand 1.
CX3CR1	C-X3-C motif chemokine receptor 1.
DAM	Disease-associated microglia.

DBS	Deep brain stimulation.
DCX	Doublecortin.
Drp−1	Dynamin-related protein 1.
ECS	Electroconvulsive stimulation.
ECT	Electroconvulsive therapy.
EP2	Prostaglandin E2 receptor 2.
ERK	Extracellular signal-regulated kinase.
EVs	Extracellular vesicles.
GENUS	Gamma entrainment using sensory stimuli.
HAM-D / HAM-D 17	Hamilton Depression Rating Scale.
HDAC3	Histone deacetylase 3.
HIPP	Hippocampus.
HMGB1	High mobility group box 1.
Hv1	Voltage-gated hydrogen channel 1.
IF	Immunofluorescence.
IFNγ	Interferon gamma.
IL−1β	Interleukin−1 beta.
IL−4	Interleukin−4.
IL−6	Interleukin 6.
IL−10	Interleukin−10.
IL−18	Interleukin−18.
IL−34	Interleukin−34.
IL4Rα	Interleukin−4 receptor alpha.
iPSCs	Induced pluripotent stem cells.
LAG3	Lymphocyte-activation gene 3.
LFP	Local Field Potential.
LPS	Lipopolysaccharide.
LRP1	Low-density lipoprotein receptor-related protein 1.
LRRK2	Leucine-rich repeat kinase 2.
M1	Pro-inflammatory state.
M2	Anti-inflammatory or resolving state.
MADRS	Montgomery-Åsberg Depression Rating Scale.
MCLs	Mannosylated clodronate liposomes.
MDD	Major depressive disorder.
MeCP2	Methyl-CpG-binding protein 2.
mPFC	Medial prefrontal cortex.
MT	Melatonin.
NF-κB	Nuclear factor kappa B.
NIR	Near-Infrared.
NLRP3	NLR family pyrin domain containing 3.
NRBP1	Nuclear receptor binding protein 1.
OGD/R	Oxygen-glucose deprivation/reoxygenation.
PANSS	Positive and Negative Syndrome Scale.
PDE4	Phosphodiesterase 4.
PGE2	Prostaglandin E2.
PLX3397	Pexidartinib (CSF1R inhibitor).
PLX5622	CSF1R inhibitor.

Prrc2a	Proline-rich coiled-coil 2 A.
PSD−95	Postsynaptic density protein 95.
RCG	Rabies virus glycoprotein control peptide.
RCT	Randomized clinical trial.
RNA	Ribonucleic acid.
ROS	Reactive oxygen species.
RPE	Retinal pigment epithelium.
rTMS	Repetitive transcranial magnetic stimulation.
RVG	Rabies virus glycoprotein.
SERCA	Sarco/endoplasmic reticulum Ca^{2+}-ATPase.
SIRT1	Sirtuin 1.
Smo	Smoothened.
STAT6	Signal transducer and activator of transcription 6.
TAF1	TATA-box binding protein associated factor 1.
tDCS	Transcranial direct current stimulation.
TNF-α	Tumor necrosis factor-alpha.
TRD	Treatment-resistant depression.
TrkB	Tropomyosin receptor kinase B.

1. Introduction

Psychiatric disorders represent a major global health challenge, affecting hundreds of millions of people worldwide and contributing substantially to disability, reduced quality of life, and increased socioeconomic impact (Fan et al., 2025). Conditions such as major depressive disorder, schizophrenia, bipolar disorder, and anxiety disorders are characterized by complex and multifactorial etiologies involving genetic, environmental, and neurobiological factors (Astorino et al., 2025). Despite decades of research, the precise mechanisms underlying these disorders remain incompletely understood, limiting the development of effective and targeted therapeutic strategies.

In recent years, increasing attention has been given to the role of neuroinflammation in the pathophysiology of psychiatric disorders (Gorji, 2022; Hassamal, 2023; Kip & Parr-Brownlie, 2023). Among the cellular mediators involved in neuroimmune responses, microglia (the resident immune cells of the central nervous system) have emerged as a key regulator of brain homeostasis and neural function (Colonna & Butovsky, 2017). Under physiological conditions, microglia continuously monitor the neural environment, participate in synaptic remodeling, and contribute to the maintenance of neuronal networks (Müller et al., 2025). However, when dysregulated or chronically activated, these cells can produce pro-inflammatory cytokines, reactive oxygen species, and other mediators capable of altering neuronal signaling and synaptic plasticity (Gao et al., 2023a).

Recent evidence suggests that abnormal microglia activation is closely associated with the development and progression of several psychiatric disorders (Rawani et al., 2024; Xia et al., 2025a). In major depressive disorder, microglia-mediated neuroinflammation has been linked to alterations in neurotransmitter systems, synaptic connectivity, and stress-related neuroendocrine pathways (Xia et al., 2025a). These alterations may contribute to behavioral symptoms such as mood dysregulation and cognitive impairment. In fact, some studies propose that depression may, at least in part, be considered a microglia-associated disorder, highlighting the central role of these cells in regulating inflammatory signaling and neural circuit function (Chen et al., 2026a; Wang et al., 2022a).

Similarly, microglial dysfunction has been implicated in the pathophysiology of other psychiatric conditions, including schizophrenia (Chen et al., 2026a; Wang et al., 2022a) and bipolar disorder (Sneeboer et al., 2019). In schizophrenia, evidence indicates that activated microglia can release inflammatory mediators and free radicals that contribute to synaptic alterations and cognitive deficits, suggesting that neuroimmune dysregulation may play a critical role in disease progression (Chen et al., 2026a; Wang et al., 2022a). Furthermore, environmental stressors (recognized as risk factors for psychiatric disorders) have been shown to induce microglial activation in important brain regions such as the hippocampus and prefrontal cortex, further reinforcing the link between stress, neuroinflammation, and mental health disorders (Calcia et al., 2016). These findings have contributed to a paradigm shift in psychiatric research, moving beyond traditional neurotransmitter-based models toward a more integrated neuroimmune framework. From this perspective, microglia are increasingly recognized not only as mediators of neuroinflammation but also as active modulators of synaptic plasticity, neural connectivity, and behavioral regulation (Maziz et al., 2025). Consequently, targeting microglial signaling pathways has emerged as a promising therapeutic strategy for the treatment of psychiatric disorders.

This chapter discusses recent advances in understanding microglial biology in psychiatric disorders, highlighting emerging mechanisms that link microglial dysfunction to neuropsychiatric pathology and exploring the potential of microglia-targeted approaches for the development of new therapeutic interventions.

2. Biological functions of microglia

Microglia are neuroglial cells that use receptors to dynamically monitor the brain microenvironment, forming the main line of immune defense in the central nervous system (CNS) (Fig. 1) (Augusto-Oliveira et al., 2022). They are macrophages that maintain cellular homeostasis by phagocytosing misfolded proteins, as well as debris and dying cells (Gao et al., 2023a). Their role in the non-inflammatory elimination of apoptotic neurons greatly contributes to the formation and maintenance of synapses (Provenzano et al., 2021).

Although microglia were long regarded as a relatively homogeneous population predominantly detrimental activation, recent demonstrated that these cells adopt multiple dynamic functional states (Fig. 1) (Gao et al., 2023a; Provenzano et al., 2021). This phenotypic diversity is closely associated with neurodevelopment, aging, and disease processes, and play a fundamental in mediating neuroprotective responses (Merighi et al., 2022). The dynamic remodeling of microglial processes, together with the release

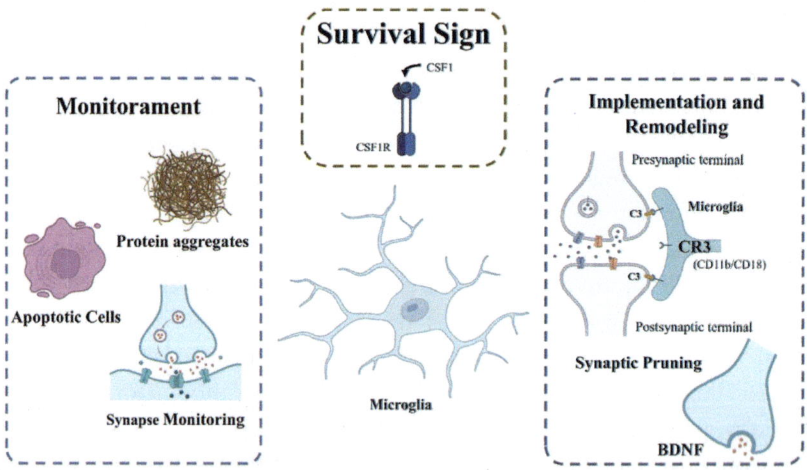

Fig. 1 Schematic representation of the microglial unit and its biological functions. In the center, the branched morphology is maintained by CSF1R receptor signaling, via CSF1, ensuring self-renewal and cellular homeostasis. Microglial monitoring, exemplified by the complement receptor CR3 (CD11b/CD18), observes the microenvironment for the detection of C3 signals, apoptotic neurons, and protein residues. Implementation and remodeling ensure circuit refinement through CR3-mediated synaptic pruning and BDNF-dependent neuromodulation, promoting interneuron maturation and memory, and supporting development. *Figure created with BioRender.com.*

of soluble factors, enables these cells to participate in neurogenesis, glycogenesis, and vasculogenesis, as well as synaptic modulation and myelination (Paolicelli et al., 2022).

The development and maintenance of microglia fundamentally depend on signaling through the colony-stimulating factor receptor (CSF1R) and its ligand (Fig. 1) (Ni et al., 2025). Pharmacological or genetic inhibitory interventions of CSF1R leads to a marked depletion of microglia, demonstrating their strong dependence on this pathway (Chadarevian et al., 2026b; Chung et al., 2023). This signaling axis ensures the microglia's continuous self-renewal capacity, allowing rapid repopulation even after massive depletion by CSF1R antagonists (Paolicelli et al., 2022).

Established within the brain parenchyma, microglia constantly survey their local environment, detecting and responding to subtle alterations in cerebral homeostasis. Although microglial activation was historically categorized into pro-inflammatory (M1) and anti-inflammatory or resolving (M2) states, advances in single-cell technologies have demonstrate that this classification is overly simplistic and does not capture the full functional complexity of these cells (Gao et al., 2023a). Instead, microglia exhibit a broad spectrum of dynamic states, which underpin their diverse roles in brain physiology. Among these functions, microglia are essential for synaptic remodeling, including the elimination of excess synapses and the refinement of neural circuits through synaptic pruning (Chung et al., 2023).

Synaptic pruning a critical developmental process in which microglia selectively eliminate unnecessary excitatory and inhibitory synaptic connections by microglia, thereby promoting the maturation and efficiency of neuronal networks (Liu et al., 2021; Mordelt & de Witte, 2023). This process is primarily mediated by the complements system. Specifically, complement component C3 is deposited at synapses destined for elimination, serving as an "eat-me" signal. Microglial phagocytosis is then triggered through recognition of C3 by the complement receptor 3 (CR3). This interaction occurs via the CD11b and CD18 subunits expressed on microglial cells, enabling targeted synaptic engulfment (de Deus et al., 2024, Mordelt & de Witte, 2023). Complementing their role in synaptic pruning, microglia play a vital role in modulating synaptic plasticity, ensuring the functioning of neural circuits. In particular, microglia-derived brain-derived neurotrophic factor (BDNF) plays a critical role in the functional maturation of inhibitory interneurons and in the closure of critical periods during neurodevelopment (Komori et al., 2024). BDNF-mediated signaling mediated is essential for activity-dependent synaptic plasticity and for maintaining the homeostasis of inhibitory neurotransmission throughout the brain–spinal axis.

With its multiple biological functions, microglia establish itself as an immunological sentinel and an essential architectural basis for healthy brain function. Understanding its biological structure is crucial for a deeper comprehension of how dysregulation in it signaling pathways contributes to vulnerability and the progression of psychiatric disorders (Akhmetzyanova et al., 2026; Hendricus Maes & Briedé, 2026).

3. Microglia in behavioral regulation and neuropsychiatric disorders

The traditional view of microglia as mere resident immune cells of then CNS has evolved to recognize their vital role as active regulators of neural circuitry (Di Pietro et al., 2026). Under physiological conditions, microglia exhibit a highly ramified morphology, characteristic of their homeostatic state, which enables continuous surveillance of the brain parenchyma. This functional versatility is reflected in distinct morphological changes, allowing microglia to transition between maintaining neuronal health and responding to injury or pathological stimuli, as illustrated in Fig. 2 (Flury et al., 2026; Rao et al., 2025).

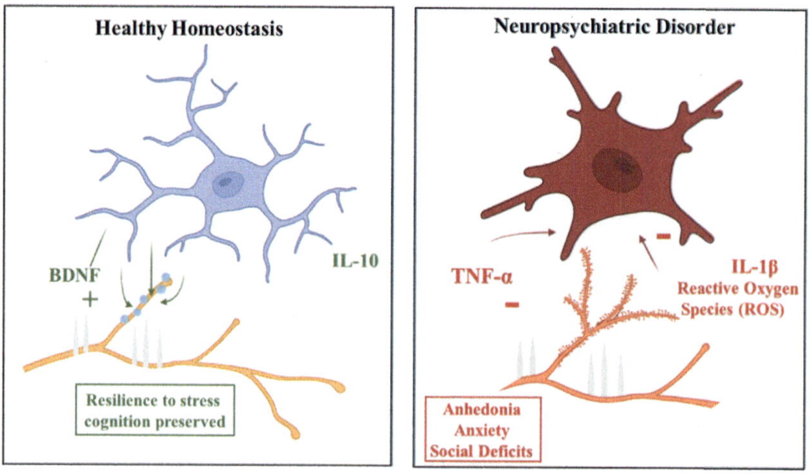

Fig. 2 Comparison between microglial homeostatic functions and its pro-inflammatory activation in neuropsychiatric disorders. *Figure created with BioRender.com.*

As illustrated, microglia play a dual and dynamic role in the CNS, transitioning between supportive and neurotoxic states in response to changes in the microenvironment (Ghimire et al., 2025). Under physiological conditions (healthy homeostasis, Fig. 2), microglia exhibit a ramified morphology, characterized by thin processes that continuously monitor synaptic integrity. In this homeostatic state, the microglia secrete neurotrophic factors such as brain-derived neurotrophic factor (BDNF) and anti-inflammatory cytokines (e.g., IL-10), thereby promoting synaptic plasticity and resilience to stress. Conversely, in neuropsychiatric disorder, microglia adopt an activated or *primed* state, characterized by an amoeboid morphology with retracted processes (Sprenger et al., 2025). This phenotypic transition is associated with the release of pro-inflammatory mediators, including tumor necrosis factor-alpha (TNF-α), interleukin-1 beta (IL-1β) (represented as IL-18, a member of the same cytokine family), and reactive oxygen species (ROS). The resulting neuroinflammatory environment disrupts neuronal communication and leads to aberrant synaptic pruning, which is clinically correlating with symptoms such as anhedonia, anxiety, and social deficits (Jäntti et al., 2026; Kang et al., 2025).

Table 1 summarizes some molecular pathways and functional states of microglia in the brain associated with neuropsychiatric disorders.

In general, the various pathways summarized in Table 1 highlight that microglial activity is not a binary 'on-off' state, but rather a finely tuned regulated spectrum of molecular responses. Mechanisms ranging from stabilization of transcripts by *Prrc2a* to the metabolic regulation via the Chemerin/CMKLR1 axis enable microglia to dynamically transition between functions such as synaptic pruning and tissue repair. The disruption of this delicate homeostatic balance, whether through genetic mutations or chronic environmental stressors, marks the transition from a protective to a maladaptive phenotype, setting the stage for the circuit-level impairments observed in neuropsychiatric disorders (Leavy et al., 2024a).

3.1 Homeostatic functions and synaptic refinement

Throughout development and adult life, microglia play a crucial role in synaptic pruning, a process mediated by the complement system, specifically C1q and C3. This refinement is essential for proper synaptic plasticity, allowing neuronal connections to be strengthened or eliminated based on experience and learning. Any imbalance in this function can result in aberrant connectivity, frequently observed in disorders such as Autism Spectrum Disorder (ASD) and schizophrenia (Choi et al., 2026; Santos et al., 2022).

Table 1 Overview of molecular pathways and microglial functional states in the central nervous system.

Mechanism/path	Pathway stimulus	Microglia response	Functional consequence	References
IL−34 axis	RPE	Recruitment of microglia/ macrophages to the site of injury via IL−34	Impaired microglial maintenance	Naggan et al. (2023)
Hv1–SERCA–Ca^{2+}	Hv1 activation	Intracellular alkalization	Pro-inflammatory phenotype	Sharma et al. (2026)
Ccp1 / Cytoskeleton	*Ccp1* Mutation	Impaired motility and phagocytic deficits	Maladaptive response and motor impairments	Pérez-Boyero et al. (2026)
Smo	Non-canonical Smo Activation	Regulation of innate immune response and phagocytosis	Effective pathogen defense and anti-inflammatory activity	El Mesaoudi et al. (2026)
SIRT1-HMGB1 Axis	Chronic Heroin	SIRT1/HMGB1 induction	Cognitive impairment; Hippocampal apoptosis	Li et al. (2026)
LRRK2-G2019S / NLRP3	LRRK2 Mutation	Increased nuclear ASC speck formation	Neuroinflammation; dopaminergic loss	Ballotto et al. (2026)
Chemerin / CMKLR1 Axis	OGD/R (Ischemia)	Chemerin expression shift; CMKLR1 downregulation	Altered mitochondrial dynamics and impaired autophagy	Long et al. (2025)
Prrc2a / RNA Reg.	*Prrc2a* Gene Deletion	Abnormal transcriptomic *activation; Altered morphology*	Purkinje cell dysfunction and *motor coordination defects*	Li et al. (2025)

Abbreviations: DAM: Disease-Associated Microglia; RPE: Retinal Pigment Epithelium; Smo: Smoothened; LRRK2 Mutation: Parkinson's Model; OGD/R: Ischemia Model.

In parallel with the complement system, the maintenance of synaptic homeostasis critically depends on the CX3CL1-CX3CR1 (Fractalkine) signaling axis. CX3CL1 is a chemokine constitutively expressed by neurons that acts as a maintenance signal by binding to its exclusive receptor, CX3CR1, on microglia (Fu et al., 2024; Perrone et al., 2023). Recent studies have demonstrated that disrupting this neuron–microglia communication, whether through genetic knockout or chronic stress, results in a failure of experience-dependent plasticity. Without this neuronal feedback, microglia exhibit dysfunctional monitoring activity, leading to deficits in synaptic maturation and altered connectivity, particularly within the hippocampus, which phenotypically manifests as cognitive impairment and reduced stress resilience (Li et al., 2025a; Trettel et al., 2020). Importantly, these alterations have been directly associated with neuropsychiatric disorders, such as major depressive disorder and schizophrenia, in which disrupted hippocampal connectivity and synaptic dysfunction underlie cognitive deficits, anhedonia, and reduced stress resilience (Han et al., 2024).

According to Han et al., the C1q/C3-CR3 complement signaling pathway plays a decisive role in mediating anomalous microglial synaptic phagocytosis in depressive contexts. Using LPS-induced experimental models, the authors discussed how microglial activation does not merely accompany the inflammatory state but actively drives the loss of neuronal synapses in the hippocampal dentate gyrus. The core of this discussion lies in the fact that this dysfunctional engulfment of dendritic spines is the underlying mechanism for behavioral impairments such as anxiety and anhedonia. Furthermore, the study demonstrates that neutralizing the C1q protein can interrupt this cycle of synaptic degradation, suggesting that specific modulation of complement proteins may reverse cognitive and emotional deficits by preserving the integrity of neural networks (Han et al., 2024).

Expanding therapeutic perspectives, Zhao et al. demonstrated that intervention in the phosphodiesterase 4 (PDE4) pathway offers a promising strategy to mitigate excessive synaptic pruning (Zhao et al., 2025). The authors discuss how inflammatory stimuli mediated by the HMGB1 (High-Mobility Group Box−1) protein act as a trigger for elevated C1q and C3 levels, promoting microglial activation and subsequent synaptic degradation. In this context, the development of the PDE4 inhibitor, A06, revealed significant antidepressant effects by reducing HMGB1 levels and suppressing neuroinflammation. The relevance of this mechanism was confirmed by the observation that C1q overexpression reverses the protective effects of A06, reinforcing that the preservation of synaptic integrity (evidenced by increased PSD−95 protein levels) is dependent on the regulation of this pathway (Zhao et al., 2025). Therefore, the transition to a pro-inflammatory state, as represented in Fig. 1, can be pharmacologically modulated. These studies suggest that PDE4 inhibition not only reduces systemic inflammation but specifically protects the synaptic architecture necessary for the regulation of behavior and emotions.

3.2 Transition to the pro-inflammatory state

Under chronic stress or pathological stimuli, microglia transition from a state of vigilance to an activated or amoeboid state. This morphological change is accompanied by a profound functional alteration, characterized mainly by the release of cytokines. The secretion of factors such as TNF-α, IL-1β, and IL-6 promotes a neuroinflammatory environment that interferes with signaling of essential neurotransmitter, such as serotonin and glutamate (Depp et al., 2025a; Hu & Gao, 2025).

The severity of this metabolic dysregulation is illustrated by the critical role of the microglial enzyme indoleamine-2,3-dioxygenase 1 (IDO1). Sugisawa et al. demonstrated that the uncontrolled activation of IDO1 in microglia leads to the excessive production of quinolinic acid, a neurotoxic metabolite of the kynurenine pathway. This compound not only promotes excitotoxicity but also disrupts cerebral energy metabolism by inhibiting hexokinase 1 (HK1), thereby reducing the production of adenosine triphosphate (ATP), the primary cellular energy currency. The importance of rigorous regulation of this pathway is reinforced by the presence of endogenous protective mechanisms, such as the nociceptor-derived hormone Reg3γ, which acts specifically on microglia to suppress IDO1. Failure in these control mechanisms exacerbates neurotoxicity and promotes central neuroinflammation (Sugisawa et al., 2022). In this context, He et al. demonstrated that novel pharmacological interventions targeting the NLRP3 inflammasome, a important molecular precursor to TNF-α and IL-1β, represent a promising strategy to mitigate microglial-induced synaptic loss. Specifically, inhibition of this pathway prevents the transition of microglia to a hyperactive amoeboid state, even under chronic stress conditions. By limiting the excessive production of these pro-inflammatory cytokines, such interventions effectively preserve hippocampal synaptic integrity and prevent the behavioral deficits typically associated with sustained microglial activation (He et al., 2023). This microglial activation has been directly correlated with the pathophysiology of major depressive disorder and anxiety, resulting in behavioral dysfunction. Chronic neuroinflammation can induce "sickness behavior," which shares symptoms with clinical depression, including anhedonia and social withdrawal (Shen et al., 2026; Wang et al., 2025).

The search for strategies that limit secretion of pro-inflammatory cytokine by microglia has driven the investigation of new chemical entities with high specificity. Given the urgency in developing effective drugs for neurodegenerative and neuropsychiatric disease, molecular hybridization emerges as a strategic tool. Recently, Wang et al. (2022a) developed isatin-chalcone hybrid derivatives, standing out for its high potency in microglia (IC50 = 1.6 μM) and high safety profile (Therapeutic Index = 21.6). This derivative significantly reduced TNF-α and IL-6 levels, an effect attributed *in silico* to its interaction with key inflammatory targets such as TLR4/MD2 and p38. Additionally, pharmacokinetic predictions indicate favorable physicochemical properties for blood-brain barrier permeability, validating its potential as a therapeutic candidate for the CNS (Wang et al., 2025).

In general, the development of multi-target hybrid molecules represents a robust strategy for selectively modulating microglial reactivity (Zhou et al., 2026). Integrating high inhibitory potency with validated safety profiles and blood-brain barrier permeability is essential to bridge the gap between chemical synthesis and therapeutic application. Thus, the design of new chemical entities capable of silencing pro-inflammatory signaling without compromising cellular viability establishes a promising path for the treatment of neuropsychiatric and neurodegenerative disorders (Akhmetzyanova et al., 2026; Hendricus Maes & Briedé, 2026).

Ultimately, the integration of these therapeutic advances ranging from the inhibition of the complement-mediated synaptic pruning to the modulation of the NLRP3 inflammasome and the kynurenine pathway is synthesized in (Fig. 3).

Fig. 3 illustrates the transition from a maladaptive, pro-inflammatory microglial state, associated with psychiatric symptomatology, back to a homeostatic phenotype. By targeting these specific molecular hubs, often through compounds designed for optimal blood-brain barrier permeability, it is possible to mitigate neuroinflammation, restore neurotrophic support via BDNF, and re-establish the CX3CL1-CX3CR1 signaling axis essential for experience-dependent plasticity. Collectively, these interventions promote the recovery of neuronal circuit function and alleviate clinical symptoms such as anhedonia and social deficits, highlighting the potential of microglia-centered therapies as a cornerstone for future neuropsychiatric treatments.

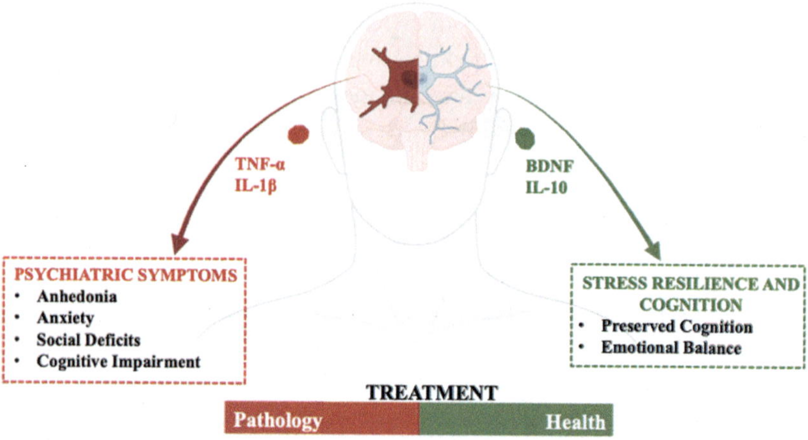

Fig. 3 Schematic representation of pharmacological modulation of microglial phenotypes. *Figure created with BioRender.com.*

4. Advances in therapeutic strategies targeting microglia

Recent advances in neuroimmunology have reframed the perception of microglia not as cells to be largely suppressed, but as dynamic and adaptive regulators of brain function that can be therapeutically modulated in neuropsychiatric disorders (Feiger et al., 2022). This emerging paradigm encompasses four major and complementary strategies: (i) anti-inflammatory approaches aimed at containing excessive microglial activation; (ii) functional reprogramming of microglia through precision-targeted therapies; (iii) microglia-mediated neuromodulation, including brain stimulation techniques; and (iv) cellular replacement and microglial niche engineering (Borst et al., 2021).

This conceptual shift is grounded in growing evidence that microglia play multifaceted roles beyond neuroinflammation, including the regulation of synaptic plasticity, the formation and remodeling of neural circuits, and the control of neurogenesis in brain regions associated with mood and behavior (Zhu et al., 2023).

Accordingly, the most promising therapeutic approaches no longer rely on indiscriminate microglial inhibition, but rather on the selective modulation of distinct microglial states. Depending on the context, the same microglial population may contribute either to inflammatory damage or to neuroprotective and antidepressant effects (Singhal & Baune, 2017; Zhang et al., 2021).

4.1 Anti-inflammatory strategies and the containment of microglial activation

Initial strategies targeting microglia focused primarily on anti-inflammatory approaches, based on the premise that sustained microglial activation contributes to emotional and cognitive dysfunction (Marwaha et al., 2023; Wang et al., 2020). In this context, minocycline has emerged as a prominent example of pharmacological repositioning. In a chronic unpredictable stress model, Wang et al. observed that minocycline improved depressive-like behaviors and reduced the translocation/release of high mobility group box 1 (HMGB1) by microglia and neurons in the hippocampus. These findings support the hypothesis that microglial activation contributes to the inflammatory signaling associated with the depressive phenotype (Wang et al., 2020).

Similarly, strategies involving microglial depletion or functional inhibition, particularly through targeting the colony-stimulating factor 1 receptor (CSF1R), have shown significant effect on behavioral, inflammatory, synaptic, and neurodegenerative benefit across various multiple preclinical models (Deng et al., 2023). However, despite these promising findings, translational evidence in humans remains limited, highlighting the need for further clinical investigation (Green et al., 2020).

Beyond classic anti-inflammatory drugs and CSF1R inhibitors, more recent strategies have also sought to contain microglial inflammatory activation through targeted molecular delivery systems. In this scenario, various compounds and microglia-targeted platforms have been evaluated in both preclinical and clinical studies, as summarized in Table 2.

4.2 Functional reprogramming of microglia and targeted precision therapies

Beyond approaches aimed at the non-specific suppression of inflammation, the concept that microglia can be functionally reprogrammed into states more conducive to plasticity, neurogenesis, and tissue repair has gained significant traction. From this perspective, a wide range of stimuli ranging from immunoregulatory signals to antidepressant drugs, may converge to induce microglial phenotypes with neuroprotective properties.

Among these strategies, interleukin-4 (IL-4) stands out for its ability to induce polarization of hippocampal microglia towards an Arg1 + phenotype, associated with pro-neurogenic properties (Zhang et al., 2021). Increased IL-4 signaling promotes activation of the IL4Rα/STAT6 pathway in microglia, reducing pro-inflammatory mediators and favoring the restoration

Table 2 Therapeutic strategies for the regulation of microglial activation and neuroinflammatory responses.

Strategy/compound	Approach	Findings	Assay	References
Minocycline	*In vivo* and in vitro model	Minocycline attenuated stress-induced depressive behaviors	Behavioral assays, Immunohistochemistry, Western blotting, and Phagocytosis assay	Bassett et al. (2021)
Minocycline (200 mg/d) + standard antidepressant	Multicenter, double-blind RCT	Minocycline was well-tolerated but not superior to placebo in reducing depressive symptoms after 6 weeks	Clinical rating scales (Primary: MADRS; Screening: HAMD-17, CGI-S).	Hellmann-Regen et al. (2022)
Minocycline	RCT (207 early-schizophrenia patients)	No improvement in depressive or negative symptoms with minocycline	Clinical scales (PANSS, Calgary) & blood biomarkers (IL-6, CRP, TNF-α)	Krynicki et al. (2021)
Minocycline (50 mg/kg)	*In vivo* (CUMS mouse model)	Prevented anxiety and circuit impairments via microglial inhibition	Behavior, Western blot, IF, LFP	Tabassum et al. (2022)
Minocycline (200 mg/day) + antidepressants	4-Week RCT (39 TRD patients)	Efficacy only in patients with CRP ≥ 3 mg/L	HAM-D-17, CRP, IL-6, IFNγ	Nettis et al. (2021)
CAR-M-UZPM (melatonin delivery system)	*In vitro* and in vivo	Crosses BBB, inhibits M1 microglia, prevents depression	CD86 binding & inflammatory markers	Liu et al. (2022)
RVG-circDYM-EVs and RCG-circDYM-EVs	*In vivo* (CUS mouse model) & in vitro (HEK 293 T cells)	Crosses BBB, reduces neuroinflammation & depressive behaviors via TAF1	EV characterization, behavior and inflammatory markers	Yu et al. (2022)

Abbreviation: BBB: Blood-Brain Barrier; CAR: Chimeric Antigen Receptor; CD86: Cluster of Differentiation 86; CGI-S: Clinical Global Impression Scale – Severity; circRNA: Circular RNA; CRP: C-reactive protein; CUMS / CUS: Chronic Unpredictable Mild Stress / Chronic Unpredictable Stress; EVs: Extracellular Vesicles; HAMD−17 / HAM-D−17: Hamilton Depression Rating Scale; IF: Immunofluorescence; IFNγ: Interferon gamma; IL−6: Interleukin 6; LFP: Local Field Potential; MADRS: Montgomery-Åsberg Depression Rating Scale; MT: Melatonin; NIR: Near-Infrared; PANSS: Positive and Negative Syndrome Scale; RCT: Randomized Clinical Trial; TAF1: TATA-box binding protein associated factor 1; TNF-α: Tumor necrosis factor alpha; TRD: Treatment-Resistant Depression.

of neurogenesis. Crucially, these effects depend on BDNF/TrkB signaling, highlighting that microglia are not merely "silenced" but actively producing trophic factors (Olaolu et al., 2025).

In parallel, drugs such as (R)-ketamine have demonstrated profound effects on microglial reprogramming. (Yao et al., 2022) revealed that the sustained antidepressant action of (R)-ketamine involves a specific microglial response in the medial prefrontal cortex (mPFC). (R)-ketamine activates the ERK–NRBP1–CREB signaling pathway in microglia and reduces levels of the transcriptional repressor MeCP2, culminating in increased BDNF expression. Thus, (R)-ketamine reprograms microglia to a functional state more permissive to neuroplasticity. The relevance of this pathway has been demonstrated in vivo: microglial depletion (with PLX3397) or BDNF transcription blockade completely abolished the antidepressant effects and restored dendritic spine density (Yao et al., 2022).

Although they act through distinct initial pathways, IL-4 and (R)-ketamine converge on a fundamental principle: the modulation of microglia functions as a mechanism for inducing cellular states capable of sustaining behavioral adaptation. However, the re-education of this cellular network does not have to depend exclusively on chemical interventions and can be achieved through the direct alteration of the electrical and oscillatory activity of the brain.

4.3 Microglial-mediated neuromodulation (brain stimulation)

Brain stimulation strategies have assumed an increasing role among biological approaches for depression, especially in cases with an insufficient response to conventional pharmacological therapies (Gao et al., 2026; Peng et al., 2026). This category includes non-invasive modalities, such as repetitive transcranial magnetic stimulation (rTMS) and transcranial direct current stimulation (tDCS), as well as more complex interventions, such as electroconvulsive therapy (ECT) and deep brain stimulation (DBS) (Marwaha et al., 2023). Although these techniques differ in their degree of invasiveness, intensity, and clinical applicability, they all share the principle that the targeted modulation of neural circuit activity can produce relevant antidepressant effects through the reorganization of the neuroinflammatory environment (Kim et al., 2026).

In the experimental context, electroconvulsive stimulation (ECS) considered the preclinical analog of ECT, appears to require microglia not for the onset of the depressive phenotype induced by chronic unpredictable stress (CUS), but rather for the therapeutic response to the procedure itself

(Acero González et al., 2023; Wennström et al., 2003). Mechanistically, Rimmerman et al. (Rimmerman et al., 2022) demonstrated that ECS reversed the decline and morphological alterations of microglia in the dentate gyrus a hippocampal subregion strongly involved in adult neurogenesis increased the expression of genes linked to neurogenesis, and reduced genes associated with immune checkpoints, most notably LAG3, the only microglial transcript significantly modulated by ECS. Since LAG3 acts as an immune brake, its reduction suggests that ECS restores a more functional microglial state, capable of sustaining hippocampal neurogenesis. In this model, ECS appears to exert part of its antidepressant action by alleviating microglial suppression/checkpoints and restoring a microglial activity compatible with supporting newly generated DCX + neurons in the hippocampus (Rimmerman et al., 2022).

Gamma entrainment has also emerged as a promising strategy to restore disrupted oscillatory patterns while simultaneously modulating broader processes within the cerebral microenvironment (Wang et al., 2026). Experimental studies suggest that this induction can increase coherence between brain areas, influence gene expression in glia, promote synaptic plasticity, and recruit microglial responses with potential neuroprotective effects. Nevertheless, its mechanisms remain only partially elucidated and appear to depend on the frequency employed, the recruited circuit, and the pathological context (Adaikkan et al., 2019; Adaikkan & Tsai, 2020; Guan et al., 2022).

In Alzheimer's disease models, gamma entrainment increases microglial phagocytic activity by inducing a shift toward a profile compatible with the clearance of amyloid-beta (Aβ) (Stramucci et al., 2025) described that the induction of gamma rhythms via GENUS (gamma entrainment using sensory stimuli) through sensory or optogenetic stimulation was associated with the transformation of microglia into a phagocytic state, characterized by increased cell body size and shortening of processes (Park et al., 2019). This effect occurred in parallel with moderate vasodilation and increased colocalization between Aβ and its clearance receptor LRP1 (low-density lipoprotein receptor-related protein 1). Thus, the benefit of gamma entrainment arises from the combination of decreased neuronal amyloid generation and enhanced Aβ removal by both microglia and the endothelium (Guan et al., 2022).

Furthermore, in post-stroke models, the beneficial effect of gamma entrainment on anxiety susceptibility stems from the attenuation of a microglial pro-inflammatory cascade (Pellegrino et al., 2019). According to Zhu et al. (Zhu et al., 2022) the combination of photothrombosis and environmental stress was accompanied by microglial hyperactivation and increased HDAC3 levels. This alteration favored the activation of the NF-κB pathway through p65 deacetylation, thereby increasing microglial PGE2 production. Local excess of PGE2, in turn, was associated with increased anxiety via the EP2 receptor in the amygdala. In this context, intermittent visual gamma stimulation attenuated anxious behavior by modulating the HDAC3/COX1/PGE2/EP2 axis (Zhu et al., 2022).

These findings highlight a shift in the therapeutic paradigm: from the global suppression of microglial activity toward a precise functional orchestration. Whether through pharmacological reprogramming or the modulation of neural oscillations, the goal is to restore a microglial homeostatic state capable of supporting structural plasticity and emotional resilience.

4.4 Cellular replacement and microglial niche engineering

With the recognition of microglial repopulation capacity, strategies focused on niche reconstruction including pharmacologically induced renewal and transplant-based approaches have emerged as promising therapeutic alternatives (Chadarevian et al., 2026b; Zhang et al., 2025a). Among these, the most established method is endogenous repopulation via CSF1R inhibition. Since adult microglia critically depend on CSF1R signaling for survival, the administration of inhibitors such as PLX3397 or PLX5622 promotes a robust depletion of the resident population (Zhang et al., 2025a). Crucially, as demonstrated by Green et al., once treatment is discontinued, the microglial compartment is rapidly reconstituted through the proliferation of surviving cells, without peripheral contribution. These repopulated microglia gradually acquire characteristics indistinguishable from the original population including density, morphology, and transcriptional profiles effectively "resetting" the niche. This renewal has been associated with the reversal of age-related cognitive deficits and improved recovery following traumatic brain injury, suggesting that replacing a dysfunctional population with a homeostatic one is biologically beneficial (Green et al., 2020).

Despite its efficacy, this approach faces challenges regarding specificity. Recently, it has been emphasized that, since CSF1R is also expressed in other myeloid cells, the systemic effects of these inhibitors must be interpreted with caution. Moving beyond endogenous renewal, a more recent frontier involves the xenotransplantation of human microglia derived from induced pluripotent stem cells (iPSCs). Through protocols like MIGRATE, microglial progenitors are transplanted into the brains of hosts previously subjected to partial depletion (e.g., via the inhibitor BLZ945). The survival and integration of these cells depend on a humanized environment, such as the expression of human CSF1. Once engafted, these cells colonize extensive areas and acquire a transcriptional signature close to in vivo human microglia. This system is particularly valuable for investigating how human genetic variants modulate microglial biology in neurological diseases (Fattorelli et al., 2021).

These advances indicate that microglial-targeted therapies have evolved from non-specific anti-inflammatory suppression toward a refined orchestration of the cellular environment. Whether through functional reprogramming, targeted molecular delivery, or niche remodeling, the goal is to restore microglial homeostasis to support neuroplasticity. The primary challenge remains translational. In other words, the field now requires precise biomarkers to identify specific microglial states and define the ideal therapeutic window for each patient (Casali & Reed-Geaghan, 2021; Eme-Scolan & Dando, 2020).

5. Outlook

While microglia have emerged as a cornerstone for therapeutic innovation in neuropsychiatric disorders, significant challenges remain. The spatiotemporal complexity of microglial phenotypes (Javanmehr et al., 2022) and their functional variability across sex and age (Stojiljkovic et al., 2024) demand a move away from generalized inhibition (Fumagalli et al., 2025; Ishikawa et al., 2025; Malvaso et al., 2023). Translational hurdles, such as the limited specificity of current clinical tools (Cavalcanti et al., 2025) and the restrictive permeability of the blood-brain barrier (Silva et al., 2025), still hinder the clinical application of preclinical findings Volonté et al., 2026).

In order to mitigate these limitations, recent studies have proposed promising microglia-targeted therapeutic strategies, including microglial phenotypic reprogramming (Bai et al., 2025), inhibition of inflammatory signaling pathways (Noh et al., 2025), controlled microglial depletion (Boland & Kokiko-Cochran, 2024), neutralization of components of the complement system (Xu et al., 2023) and nanocarrier-based delivery systems capable of crossing the blood-brain barrier (Yong et al., 2025).

Furthermore, CRISPR-based functional characterization allows for the systematic identification of molecular regulators of microglial states (Dräger et al., 2022).

Ultimately, the future of neuroimmunology lies in precision medicine. By integrating AI-based multi-omics with specific cellular biomarkers, it will be possible to stratify patients and deliver personalized interventions that selectively modulate microglial states (Hampel et al., 2020; Hou et al., 2026), enabling the identification of subgroups based on specific molecular and cellular biomarkers and allowing more selective, personalized therapeutic interventions. This shift in approach, toward the targeted orchestration of the neuroinflammatory environment, will be crucial in translating experimental advances into effective clinical therapies.

6. Conclusion

In general, microglia have emerged as central regulators of brain function, connecting neuroimmune signaling, synaptic plasticity, and behavioral outcomes. Rather than acting solely as mediators of neuroinflammation, these cells exhibit significant functional plasticity, dynamically transitioning between homeostatic and reactive states in response to environmental and pathological stimuli. Disruption of this finely tuned balance directly contributes to the pathophysiology of psychiatric disorders, including depression, schizophrenia, and anxiety-related conditions, through mechanisms involving aberrant synaptic pruning, impaired neurogenesis, and chronic neuroinflammation. Recent advances have redefined therapeutic strategies targeting microglia, shifting from broad anti-inflammatory approaches to more refined interventions aimed at modulating specific molecular pathways and cellular states. Strategies such as microglial reprogramming, inflammasome inhibition, complement pathway modulation, and targeted drug delivery across the blood-brain barrier demonstrate significant potential in restoring the integrity of neural circuits and improving behavioral outcomes. However, important challenges persist, particularly regarding the translation of preclinical findings into clinical applications, the identification of reliable biomarkers, and the development of highly specific therapeutic tools. Progress in this area will depend on a deeper understanding of microglial heterogeneity, including spatial, temporal, and individual variability, as well as the integration of emerging technologies such as multiomics, organoid models, and precision medicine approaches. Ultimately, targeting microglia with greater specificity and context-dependent precision holds great promise for advancing the treatment of neuropsychiatric disorders and bridging the gap between experimental research and clinical practice.

Acknowledgements

JRJ is grateful to the Conselho Nacional de Desenvolvimento Científico e Tecnológico (CNPq, grant 405828/2022–5 and 408338/2024–5), and to the Fundaç ão de Amparo à Pesquisa do Estado de Minas (FAPEMIG, grants APQ−01786–22, APQ−05429–23, RED−00144–22, APQ−03853–25, BDT−00004–25) for their financial support.

References

Acero González, Á. R., Guzmán Sabogal, Y. R., Salamanca Dimas, H., Páez Avendaño, V., Pineda Carrascal, E., Izquierdo Polanco, J., & Ayala Escudero, A. (2023). Clinical experience of electroconvulsive therapy with anaesthetic and muscle relaxant at the Clínica Universidad de La Sabana: 2009–2017. *Revista Colombiana de Psiquiatría (English Ed.), 52*(2), 101–106. https://doi.org/10.1016/j.rcpeng.2021.01.004.

Adaikkan, C., Middleton, S. J., Marco, A., Pao, P.-C., Mathys, H., Kim, D. N.-W., ... Tsai, L.-H. (2019). Gamma entrainment binds higher-order brain regions and offers neuroprotection. *Neuron, 102*(5), 929–943.e8. https://doi.org/10.1016/j.neuron.2019.04.011.

Adaikkan, C., & Tsai, L.-H. (2020). Gamma entrainment: Impact on neurocircuits, glia, and therapeutic opportunities. *Trends in Neurosciences, 43*(1), 24–41. https://doi.org/10.1016/j.tins.2019.11.001.

Akhmetzyanova, E. R., Rizvanov, A. A., & Mukhamedshina, Y. O. (2026). The main signaling pathways determining the microglia responses in spinal cord injury: Potential effectors among known pharmaceuticals. *Experimental Neurology, 396*, 115523. https://doi.org/10.1016/j.expneurol.2025.115523.

Astorino, M. F., Calabrò, M., Infortuna, C., Muscatello, M. R. A., Briuglia, S., Cicero, N., ... Crisafulli, C. (2025). The multifaceted etiology of mental disorders with a focus on trace elements, a review of recent literature. *American Journal of Medical Genetics Part B: Neuropsychiatric Genetics, 198*(8), 168–189. https://doi.org/10.1002/ajmg.b.33045.

Augusto-Oliveira, M., Arrifano, G. P., Delage, C. I., Tremblay, M., Crespo-Lopez, M. E., & Verkhratsky, A. (2022). Plasticity of microglia. *Biological Reviews, 97*(1), 217–250. https://doi.org/10.1111/brv.12797.

Bai, Y., Wang, X., Qi, F., Zuo, X., & Zou, G. (2025). Mechanisms of action of retinal microglia in diabetic retinopathy (Review). *International Journal of Molecular Medicine, 56*(6), 1–12. https://doi.org/10.3892/ijmm.2025.5643.

Ballotto, L., Baratta, T., Winterberg, H., Dusanter, C., Sambin, S., Corvol, J. C., ... Novello, S. (2026). Nuclear ASC speck formation in microglia is associated with inflammasome priming and is exacerbated in LRRK2-G2019S Parkinson's disease. *Neurobiology of Disease, 218*, 107237. https://doi.org/10.1016/j.nbd.2025.107237.

Bassett, B., Subramaniyam, S., Fan, Y., Varney, S., Pan, H., Carneiro, A. M. D., & Chung, C. Y. (2021). Minocycline alleviates depression-like symptoms by rescuing decrease in neurogenesis in dorsal hippocampus via blocking microglia activation/phagocytosis. *Brain, Behavior, and Immunity, 91*, 519–530. https://doi.org/10.1016/j.bbi.2020.11.009.

Boland, R., & Kokiko-Cochran, O. N. (2024). Deplete and repeat: Microglial CSF1R inhibition and traumatic brain injury. *Frontiers in Cellular Neuroscience, 18*. https://doi.org/10.3389/fncel.2024.1352790.

Borst, K., Dumas, A. A., & Prinz, M. (2021). Microglia: Immune and non-immune functions. *Immunity, 54*(10), 2194–2208. https://doi.org/10.1016/j.immuni.2021.09.014.

Calcia, M. A., Bonsall, D. R., Bloomfield, P. S., Selvaraj, S., Barichello, T., & Howes, O. D. (2016). Stress and neuroinflammation: A systematic review of the effects of stress on microglia and the implications for mental illness. *Psychopharmacology, 233*(9), 1637–1650. https://doi.org/10.1007/s00213-016-4218-9.

Casali, B. T., & Reed-Geaghan, E. G. (2021). Microglial function and regulation during development, homeostasis and Alzheimer's disease. *Cells, 10*(4), 957. https://doi.org/10.3390/cells10040957.

Cavalcanti, R. R., Almeida, F. M., Martinez, A. M. B., & Freria, C. M. (2025). Neuroinflammation: Targeting microglia for neuroprotection and repair after spinal cord injury. *Frontiers in Immunology, 16*. https://doi.org/10.3389/fimmu.2025.1670650.

Chadarevian, J. P., Nguyen, J., Le, L., Ayala, L. A., Chadarevian, A. L., Zhou, C., ... Blurton-Jones, M. (2026b). CSF1R inhibitor-resistant model for CNS-wide microglia replacement strategies. *Molecular Therapy, 34*(2), 832–849. https://doi.org/10.1016/j.ymthe.2025.10.051.

Chen, Y.-J., Zhu, Q.-Q., Xie, M.-R., Zhang, D., Shuai, Y.-F., Li, Y., ... Li, B. (2026a). Microglia associated research in depression: An exploratory trends analysis. *Frontiers in Aging Neuroscience, 18*. https://doi.org/10.3389/fnagi.2026.1757943.

Choi, T.-Y., Gunawan, A., Seo, D., Park, J., Ahn, E. H., Suh, S. W., ... Choi, K. (2026). Applying biologically anchored subtypes to advance precision medicine in autism spectrum disorder. *Neurobiology of Disease, 218*, 107219. https://doi.org/10.1016/j.nbd.2025.107219.

Chung, H.-Y., Wickel, J., Hahn, N., Mein, N., Schwarzbrunn, M., Koch, P., ... Geis, C. (2023). Microglia mediate neurocognitive deficits by eliminating C1q-tagged synapses in sepsis-associated encephalopathy. *Science Advances, 9*(21), https://doi.org/10.1126/sciadv.abq7806.

Colonna, M., & Butovsky, O. (2017). Microglia function in the central nervous system during health and neurodegeneration. *Annual Review of Immunology, 35*(1), 441–468. https://doi.org/10.1146/annurev-immunol-051116-052358.

de Deus, J. L., Faborode, O. S., & Nandi, S. (2024). Synaptic pruning by microglia: Lessons from genetic studies in mice. *Developmental Neuroscience, 47*(5), 362–382. https://doi.org/10.1159/000541379.

Deng, Q., Gupta, A., Jeon, H., Nam, J. H., Yilmaz, A. S., Chang, W., ... Chung, D. (2023). graph-GPA 2.0: Improving multi-disease genetic analysis with integration of functional annotation data. *Frontiers in Genetics, 14*. https://doi.org/10.3389/fgene.2023.1079198.

Depp, C., Doman, J. L., Hingerl, M., Xia, J., & Stevens, B. (2025a). Microglia transcriptional states and their functional significance: Context drives diversity. *Immunity, 58*(5), 1052–1067. https://doi.org/10.1016/j.immuni.2025.04.009.

Di Pietro, A. A., Powley, S., Perciballi, E., Stewart, M., Therrien, M., & Scott-Hewitt, N. (2026). Microglia in systemic neuroimmune communication: functions beyond phagocytosis. *Trends in Immunology*. https://doi.org/10.1016/j.it.2025.12.002.

Dräger, N. M., Sattler, S. M., Huang, C. T.-L., Teter, O. M., Leng, K., Hashemi, S. H., ... Kampmann, M. (2022). A CRISPRi/a platform in human iPSC-derived microglia uncovers regulators of disease states. *Nature Neuroscience, 25*(9), 1149–1162. https://doi.org/10.1038/s41593-022-01131-4.

El Mesaoudi, A., Kassoussi, A., Zahaf, A., Ayadi, M., Naglieri, S., Marie, C., ... Traiffort, E. (2026). Smoothened-mediated signaling contributes to immune and non-immune functions of microglia. *Brain, Behavior, and Immunity, 132*, 106226. https://doi.org/10.1016/j.bbi.2025.106226.

Eme-Scolan, E., & Dando, S. J. (2020). Tools and approaches for studying microglia in vivo. *Frontiers in Immunology, 11*. https://doi.org/10.3389/fimmu.2020.583647.

Fan, Y., Fan, A., Yang, Z., & Fan, D. (2025). Global burden of mental disorders in 204 countries and territories, 1990–2021: results from the global burden of disease study 2021. *BMC Psychiatry, 25*(1), 486. https://doi.org/10.1186/s12888-025-06932-y.

Fattorelli, N., Martinez-Muriana, A., Wolfs, L., Geric, I., De Strooper, B., & Mancuso, R. (2021). Stem-cell-derived human microglia transplanted into mouse brain to study human disease. *Nature Protocols, 16*(2), 1013–1033. https://doi.org/10.1038/s41596-020-00447-4.

Feiger, J. A., Snyder, R. L., Walsh, M. J., Cissne, M., Cwiek, A., Al-Momani, S. I., & Chiou, K. S. (2022). The role of neuroinflammation in neuropsychiatric disorders following traumatic brain injury: A systematic review. *Journal of Head Trauma Rehabilitation, 37*(5), E370–E382. https://doi.org/10.1097/HTR.0000000000000754.

Flury, A., St-Pierre, M.-K., Ayata, P., & Tremblay, M.-È. (2026). Evolving insights into the identity and function of dark microglia. *Trends in Neurosciences, 49*(1), 20–34. https://doi.org/10.1016/j.tins.2025.11.002.

Fu, G.-Q., Wang, Y.-Y., Xu, Y.-M., Bian, M.-M., Zhang, L., Yan, H.-Z., ... Lü, H.-Z. (2024). Exosomes derived from vMIP-II-Lamp2b gene-modified M2 cells provide neuroprotection by targeting the injured spinal cord, inhibiting chemokine signals and modulating microglia/macrophage polarization in mice. *Experimental Neurology, 377*, 114784. https://doi.org/10.1016/j.expneurol.2024.114784.

Fumagalli, L., Nazlie Mohebiany, A., Premereur, J., Polanco Miquel, P., Bijnens, B., Van de Walle, P., ... Mancuso, R. (2025). Microglia heterogeneity, modeling and cell-state annotation in development and neurodegeneration. *Nature Neuroscience, 28*(7), 1381–1392. https://doi.org/10.1038/s41593-025-01931-4.

Gao, C., Jiang, J., Tan, Y., & Chen, S. (2023a). Microglia in neurodegenerative diseases: Mechanism and potential therapeutic targets. *Signal Transduction and Targeted Therapy, 8*(1), 359. https://doi.org/10.1038/s41392-023-01588-0.

Gao, J., Liang, Y., Rong, P., Wang, Y., & Chen, H. (2026). Auricular stimulation therapy: An evidence-based practice strategy for depression. *Current Opinion in Pharmacology, 87*, 102607. https://doi.org/10.1016/j.coph.2026.102607.

Ghimire, A., Rehman, S. A., Subhani, A., Khan, M. A., Rahman, Z., Iqubal, M. K., & Iqubal, A. (2025). Mechanism of microglia-mediated neuroinflammation, associated cognitive dysfunction, and therapeutic updates in Alzheimer's disease. *HLife, 3*(2), 64–81. https://doi.org/10.1016/j.hlife.2024.11.006.

Gorji, A. (2022). Neuroinflammation: The pathogenic mechanism of neurological disorders. *International Journal of Molecular Sciences, 23*(10), 5744. https://doi.org/10.3390/ijms23105744.

Green, K. N., Crapser, J. D., & Hohsfield, L. A. (2020). To kill a microglia: A case for CSF1R inhibitors. *Trends in Immunology, 41*(9), 771–784. https://doi.org/10.1016/j.it.2020.07.001.

Guan, A., Wang, S., Huang, A., Qiu, C., Li, Y., Li, X., ... Deng, B. (2022). The role of gamma oscillations in central nervous system diseases: Mechanism and treatment. *Frontiers in Cellular Neuroscience, 16*. https://doi.org/10.3389/fncel.2022.962957.

Hampel, H., Caraci, F., Cuello, A. C., Caruso, G., Nisticò, R., Corbo, M., ... Lista, S. (2020). A path toward precision medicine for neuroinflammatory mechanisms in Alzheimer's disease. *Frontiers in Immunology, 11*. https://doi.org/10.3389/fimmu.2020.00456.

Han, Q.-Q., Shen, S.-Y., Liang, L.-F., Chen, X.-R., & Yu, J. (2024). Complement C1q/C3-CR3 signaling pathway mediates abnormal microglial phagocytosis of synapses in a mouse model of depression. *Brain, Behavior, and Immunity, 119*, 454–464. https://doi.org/10.1016/j.bbi.2024.04.018.

Hassamal, S. (2023). Chronic stress, neuroinflammation, and depression: An overview of pathophysiological mechanisms and emerging anti-inflammatories. *Frontiers in Psychiatry, 14*. https://doi.org/10.3389/fpsyt.2023.1130989.

He, H., Xie, X., Zhang, J., Mo, L., Kang, X., Zhang, Y., ... You, Z. (2023). Patchouli alcohol ameliorates depression-like behaviors through inhibiting NLRP3-mediated neuroinflammation in male stress-exposed mice. *Journal of Affective Disorders, 326*, 120–131. https://doi.org/10.1016/j.jad.2023.01.065.

Hellmann-Regen, J., Clemens, V., Grözinger, M., Kornhuber, J., Reif, A., Prvulovic, D., ... Heuser, I. (2022). Effect of minocycline on depressive symptoms in patients with treatment-resistant depression: A randomized clinical trial. *JAMA Network Open, 5*(9), e2230367. https://doi.org/10.1001/jamanetworkopen.2022.30367.

Hendricus Maes, K. J., & Briedé, J. J. (2026). Repurposing immunomodulatory drugs targeting microglia for amyotrophic lateral sclerosis. *Brain Research, 1870*, 150032. https://doi.org/10.1016/j.brainres.2025.150032.

Hou, K., An, Z., Xu, Y., Wang, J., Zhou, M., Liu, Y., ... Wei, J. (2026). Parkinson's disease: Spatiotemporal regulation and therapeutic prospects of TREM2-mediated microglial responses. *Npj Parkinson's Disease, 12*(1), 37. https://doi.org/10.1038/s41531-025-01247-x.

Hu, Y., & Gao, J. (2025). The role of polarization dynamics in macrophages and microglia on the inflammatory microenvironment of spinal cord injury. *Molecular and Cellular Neuroscience, 135*, 104054. https://doi.org/10.1016/j.mcn.2025.104054.

Ishikawa, K., Fujikawa, R., Okita, K., Kimura, F., Watanabe, T., Katsurabayashi, S., & Iwasaki, K. (2025). Microglia in brain aging and age-related diseases: Friends or foes? *International Journal of Molecular Sciences, 26*(23), 11494. https://doi.org/10.3390/ijms262311494.

Jäntti, H., Michels, S., Cherubini, E., Giniatullin, R., & Malm, T. (2026). Non-neuronal mechanisms in autism spectrum disorder (ASD): Microglia and astrocytes at the crossroads with neurons. *Brain, Behavior, and Immunity, 133*, 106275. https://doi.org/10.1016/j.bbi.2026.106275.

Javanmehr, N., Saleki, K., Alijanizadeh, P., & Rezaei, N. (2022). Microglia dynamics in aging-related neurobehavioral and neuroinflammatory diseases. *Journal of Neuroinflammation, 19*(1), 273. https://doi.org/10.1186/s12974-022-02637-1.

Kang, X., Tian, J., Shu, Q., Cheng, T., Wang, S., & Hu, Y. (2025). Microglia-neuron crosstalk in Alzheimer's disease: An exploration of molecular mechanisms and pathological implications. *Neuroscience, 583*, 1–9. https://doi.org/10.1016/j.neuroscience.2025.07.019.

Kim, K., Krishnan, G. P., Kim, J., Arroyo, S., Bazhenov, M., & Ganguly, K. (2026). Effects of low-frequency burst stimulation of the motor thalamus on cortical neural co-firing. *Brain Stimulation, 19*(1), 103018. https://doi.org/10.1016/j.brs.2025.103018.

Kip, E., & Parr-Brownlie, L. C. (2023). Healthy lifestyles and wellbeing reduce neuroinflammation and prevent neurodegenerative and psychiatric disorders. *Frontiers in Neuroscience, 17*. https://doi.org/10.3389/fnins.2023.1092537.

Komori, T., Okamura, K., Ikehara, M., Yamamuro, K., Endo, N., Okumura, K., ... Makinodan, M. (2024). Brain-derived neurotrophic factor from microglia regulates neuronal development in the medial prefrontal cortex and its associated social behavior. *Molecular Psychiatry, 29*(5), 1338–1349. https://doi.org/10.1038/s41380-024-02413-y.

Krynicki, C. R., Dazzan, P., Pariante, C. M., Barnes, N. M., Vincent, R. C., Roberts, A., ... BeneMin Study team (2021). Deconstructing depression and negative symptoms of schizophrenia; differential and longitudinal immune correlates, and response to minocycline treatment. *Brain, Behavior, and Immunity, 91*, 498–504. https://doi.org/10.1016/j.bbi.2020.10.026.

Leavy, A., Phelan, J., & Jimenez-Mateos, E. M. (2024a). Contribution of microglia to the epileptiform activity that results from neonatal hypoxia. *Neuropharmacology, 253*, 109968. https://doi.org/10.1016/j.neuropharm.2024.109968.

Li, C., Wei, Y., Yin, D., Zhao, C., Chen, G., Wang, Q., ... Xia, B. (2026). The SIRT1-HMGB1 pathway in hippocampal microglia is involved in chronic heroin-induced cognitive impairment. *Pharmacology, Biochemistry, and Behavior, 260*, 174155. https://doi.org/10.1016/j.pbb.2026.174155.

Li, W., Yong-Yan, X., Jia-Xin, M., Shu-Chao, G., & Li-Ping, H. (2025a). Senescent microglia: The hidden culprits accelerating Alzheimer's disease. *Brain Research, 1851*, 149480. https://doi.org/10.1016/j.brainres.2025.149480.

Li, X., Yang, P., Dong, B., Jiang, L., Xiu, R., Guo, J., ... Yuan, Z. (2025). Microglial Prrc2a regulates microglia-neuron interaction in cerebellum and motor functions in mice. *IScience, 28*(12), 113949. https://doi.org/10.1016/j.isci.2025.113949.

Liu, Y., Hu, P., Zheng, Z., Zhong, D., Xie, W., Tang, Z., ... Wang, X. (2022). Photoresponsive vaccine-like CAR-M system with high-efficiency central immune regulation for inflammation-related depression. *Advanced Materials, 34*(11), https://doi.org/10.1002/adma.202108525.

Liu, Y.-J., Spangenberg, E. E., Tang, B., Holmes, T. C., Green, K. N., & Xu, X. (2021). Microglia elimination increases neural circuit connectivity and activity in adult mouse cortex. *The Journal of Neuroscience, 41*(6), 1274–1287. https://doi.org/10.1523/JNEUROSCI.2140-20.2020.

Long, P.-Y., Tang, Z., Cai, N., Yan, Z.-Q., Gao, X., Wang, Z.-W., ... Xiao, Y. (2025). Chemerin-CMKLR1 differentially mediated OGD/R-induced mitochondrial dysfunction, oxidative stress, and autophagy in microglia and neurons. *Biomedicine & Pharmacotherapy, 192*, 118702. https://doi.org/10.1016/j.biopha.2025.118702.

Malvaso, A., Gatti, A., Negro, G., Calatozzolo, C., Medici, V., & Poloni, T. E. (2023). Microglial senescence and activation in healthy aging and Alzheimer's disease: Systematic review and neuropathological scoring. *Cells, 12*(24), 2824. https://doi.org/10.3390/cells12242824.

Marwaha, S., Palmer, E., Suppes, T., Cons, E., Young, A. H., & Upthegrove, R. (2023). Novel and emerging treatments for major depression. *The Lancet, 401*(10371), 141–153. https://doi.org/10.1016/S0140-6736(22)02080-3.

Maziz, M. N. H., Chakravarthi, S., Aung, T., Htoo, P. M., Shwe, W. H., Gupalo, S., ... Kodali, M. (2025). Microglia-mediated neuroinflammation through phosphatidylinositol 3-kinase signaling causes cognitive dysfunction. *International Journal of Molecular Sciences, 26*(15), 7212. https://doi.org/10.3390/ijms26157212.

Merighi, S., Nigro, M., Travagli, A., & Gessi, S. (2022). Microglia and Alzheimer's disease. *International Journal of Molecular Sciences, 23*(21), 12990. https://doi.org/10.3390/ijms232112990.

Mordelt, A., & de Witte, L. D. (2023). Microglia-mediated synaptic pruning as a key deficit in neurodevelopmental disorders: Hype or hope? *Current Opinion in Neurobiology, 79*, 102674. https://doi.org/10.1016/j.conb.2022.102674.

Müller, L., Di Benedetto, S., & Müller, V. (2025). The dual nature of neuroinflammation in networked brain. *Frontiers in Immunology, 16*. https://doi.org/10.3389/fimmu.2025.1659947.

Naggan, L., Robinson, E., Dinur, E., Goldenberg, H., Kozela, E., & Yirmiya, R. (2023). Suicide in bipolar disorder patients is associated with hippocampal microglia activation and reduction of lymphocytes-activation gene 3 (LAG3) microglial checkpoint expression. *Brain, Behavior, and Immunity, 110*, 185–194. https://doi.org/10.1016/j.bbi.2023.02.021.

Nettis, M. A., Lombardo, G., Hastings, C., Zajkowska, Z., Mariani, N., Nikkheslat, N., ... Mondelli, V. (2021). Augmentation therapy with minocycline in treatment-resistant depression patients with low-grade peripheral inflammation: Results from a double-blind randomised clinical trial. *Neuropsychopharmacology: Official Publication of the American College of Neuropsychopharmacology, 46*(5), 939–948. https://doi.org/10.1038/s41386-020-00948-6.

Ni, R.-J., Yuan, W.-J., Wang, Y.-Y., Yang, X., Wei, J.-X., Zhao, L.-S., ... Ma, X.-H. (2025). Microglia-mediated inflammation and synaptic pruning contribute to sleep deprivation-induced mania in a sex-specific manner. *Translational Psychiatry, 15*(1), 285. https://doi.org/10.1038/s41398-025-03525-x.

Noh, M.-Y., Kwon, H. S., Kwon, M.-S., Nahm, M., Jin, H. K., Bae, J., & Kim, S. H. (2025). Biomarkers and therapeutic strategies targeting microglia in neurodegenerative diseases: current status and future directions. *Molecular Neurodegeneration, 20*(1), 82. https://doi.org/10.1186/s13024-025-00867-4.

Olaolu, D. O., Davids, P. H., Dealtry, P. Gill B., Morenikeji, M. O., Obishakin, D. E. T., Iliayasu, M. B., ... Ajonijebu, D. C. D. (2025). Iloprost treatment enhanced IL-4 signalling to reverse trypanosome-induced cognitive deficits and suppressed neuroinflammation in mice. *International Journal of Infectious Diseases, 152*, 107622. https://doi.org/10.1016/j.ijid.2024.107622.

Paolicelli, R. C., Sierra, A., Stevens, B., Tremblay, M.-E., Aguzzi, A., Ajami, B., ... Wyss-Coray, T. (2022). Microglia states and nomenclature: A field at its crossroads. *Neuron, 110*(21), 3458–3483. https://doi.org/10.1016/j.neuron.2022.10.020.

Park, M., Ryu, S., Lee, J., Jung, J., & Kim, T. (2019). Improved sleep-wake behavior after gamma entrainment with acoustic stimulation in a mouse model of Alzheimer's disease. *IBRO Reports, 6*, S437. https://doi.org/10.1016/j.ibror.2019.07.1385.

Pellegrino, G., Arcara, G., Cortese, A. M., Weis, L., Di Tomasso, S., Marioni, G., ... Piccione, F. (2019). Cortical gamma-synchrony measured with magnetoencephalography is a marker of clinical status and predicts clinical outcome in stroke survivors. *NeuroImage: Clinical, 24*, 102092. https://doi.org/10.1016/j.nicl.2019.102092.

Peng, Y., Webster, L., Lankappa, S., Morriss, R., & Briley, P. M. (2026). Augmentation strategies for transcranial magnetic stimulation (TMS) in the treatment of unipolar depression: A scoping review. *Journal of Affective Disorders Reports*, 101058. https://doi.org/10.1016/j.jadr.2026.101058.

Pérez-Boyero, D., de la Mata, A., Castillo-Sanchez, J., Reverte, I., Yanguas-Casás, N., Ávila-Zarza, C., ... Díaz, D. (2026). Model of selective neurodegeneration driven by a Ccp1 mutation leads to atypical microglia with an increased response to pathological stimuli. *Brain, Behavior, and Immunity, 133*, 106248. https://doi.org/10.1016/j.bbi.2025.106248.

Perrone, M., Pagano, M., Belardo, C., Ricciardi, F., Ricciardi, F., Fusco, A., ... Guida, F. (2023). Potential role of the hydroxyl carboxylic acid receptor type 2 (HCAR2) in microglia pathophysiology: A possible cross-talk with C-X-C chemokine receptor 1 (CXCR1). *Neuropharmacology, 228*, 109456. https://doi.org/10.1016/j.neuropharm.2023.109456.

Provenzano, F., Pérez, M. J., & Deleidi, M. (2021). Redefining microglial identity in health and disease at single-cell resolution. *Trends in Molecular Medicine, 27*(1), 47–59. https://doi.org/10.1016/j.molmed.2020.09.001.

Rao, Y., Bai, Y., Li, X., Du, B., & Peng, B. (2025). The evolution of microglia replacement: A new paradigm for CNS disease therapy. *Cell Stem Cell, 32*(12), 1807–1832. https://doi.org/10.1016/j.stem.2025.10.014.

Rawani, N. S., Chan, A. W., Todd, K. G., Baker, G. B., & Dursun, S. M. (2024). The role of neuroglia in the development and progression of schizophrenia. *Biomolecules, 15*(1), 10. https://doi.org/10.3390/biom15010010.

Rimmerman, N., Verdiger, H., Goldenberg, H., Naggan, L., Robinson, E., Kozela, E., ... Yirmiya, R. (2022). Microglia and their LAG3 checkpoint underlie the antidepressant and neurogenesis-enhancing effects of electroconvulsive stimulation. *Molecular Psychiatry, 27*(2), 1120–1135. https://doi.org/10.1038/s41380-021-01338-0.

Santos, S., Ferreira, H., Martins, J., Gonçalves, J., & Castelo-Branco, M. (2022). Male sex bias in early and late onset neurodevelopmental disorders: Shared aspects and differences in autism spectrum disorder, attention deficit/hyperactivity disorder, and schizophrenia. *Neuroscience & Biobehavioral Reviews, 135*, 104577. https://doi.org/10.1016/j.neubiorev.2022.104577.

Sharma, A., Yadav, P., Yadav, S., Kumar, V., Ravendra singh, K., Ranawat, M., & Kshatri, A. S. (2026). A NOX2-independent mechanism of Hv1 channel activation promotes inflammatory cytokine release from BV-2 microglia via intracellular Ca2+ mobilisation. *Cell Calcium, 134*, 103122. https://doi.org/10.1016/j.ceca.2026.103122.

Shen, X., Ji, W., Zheng, H., Yu, B., Wan, Y., Cai, H., ... Zhong, H. (2026). Peripheral cytokine dysregulation, microglial dysfunction in adolescent major depressive disorder: Neuroimmune crosstalk implications. *Psychoneuroendocrinology, 183*, 107656. https://doi.org/10.1016/j.psyneuen.2025.107656.

Silva, P. R., da, Barbosa, N. M. M. V., Leite, J. M., da, S., Alves, L. P., Andrade, J. C., ... Scotti, L. (2025). Microglia-targeted nanotherapeutics in major depressive disorder: An integrative perspective on neuroinflammation and drug delivery. *Pharmaceutics, 18*(1), 27. https://doi.org/10.3390/pharmaceutics18010027.

Singhal, G., & Baune, B. T. (2017). Microglia: An interface between the loss of neuroplasticity and depression. *Frontiers in Cellular Neuroscience, 11*, 270. https://doi.org/10.3389/fncel.2017.00270.

Sneeboer, M. A. M., Snijders, G. J. L. J., Berdowski, W. M., Fernández-Andreu, A., van Mierlo, H. C., Berdenis van Berlekom, A., ... de Witte, L. D. (2019). Microglia in postmortem brain tissue of patients with bipolar disorder are not immune activated. *Translational Psychiatry, 9*(1), 153. https://doi.org/10.1038/s41398-019-0490-x.

Sprenger, K. G., Lietzke, E. E., Melchior, J. T., & Bruce, K. D. (2025). Lipid and lipoprotein metabolism in microglia: Alzheimer's disease mechanisms and interventions. *Journal of Lipid Research, 66*(10), 100872. https://doi.org/10.1016/j.jlr.2025.100872.

Stojiljkovic, M. R., Schmeer, C., & Witte, O. W. (2024). Senescence and aging differentially alter key metabolic pathways in murine brain microglia. *Neuroscience Letters, 828*, 137751. https://doi.org/10.1016/j.neulet.2024.137751.

Stramucci, G., Smeralda, C. L., Giannotta, A., Neri, F., Cinti, A., Benelli, A., ... Santarnecchi, E. (2025). Gamma frequency-transcranial alternating current stimulation improves memory and entrains gamma oscillations in moderate but not mild Alzheimer's disease patients. *Brain Stimulation, 18*(1), 552. https://doi.org/10.1016/j.brs.2024.12.980.

Sugisawa, E., Kondo, T., Kumagai, Y., Kato, H., Takayama, Y., Isohashi, K., ... Maruyama, K. (2022). Nociceptor-derived Reg3γ prevents endotoxic death by targeting kynurenine pathway in microglia. *Cell Reports, 38*(10), 110462. https://doi.org/10.1016/j.celrep.2022.110462.

Tabassum, S., Misrani, A., Huo, Q., Ahmed, A., Long, C., & Yang, L. (2022). Minocycline ameliorates chronic unpredictable mild stress-induced neuroinflammation and abnormal mPFC-HIPP oscillations in mice. *Molecular Neurobiology, 59*(11), 6874–6895. https://doi.org/10.1007/s12035-022-03018-8.

Trettel, F., Di Castro, M. A., & Limatola, C. (2020). Chemokines: Key molecules that orchestrate communication among neurons, microglia and astrocytes to preserve brain function. *Neuroscience, 439*, 230–240. https://doi.org/10.1016/j.neuroscience.2019.07.035.

Volonté, C., Hu, G., Shaw, C. A., Viegas, C., dos Santos, J. A., Vaz, S. H., ... Franco, R. (2026). Neuroprotection beyond neurons: Integrated biomarker-based and astroglia- or microglia-targeted approaches to combat neurodegenerative diseases. *Exploration of Neuroprotective Therapy, 6*. https://doi.org/10.37349/ent.2026.1004136.

Wang, B., Huang, X., Pan, X., Zhang, T., Hou, C., Su, W.-J., ... Wang, Y.-X. (2020). Minocycline prevents the depressive-like behavior through inhibiting the release of HMGB1 from microglia and neurons. *Brain, Behavior, and Immunity, 88*, 132–143. https://doi.org/10.1016/j.bbi.2020.06.019.

Wang, H., He, Y., Sun, Z., Ren, S., Liu, M., Wang, G., & Yang, J. (2022a). Microglia in depression: An overview of microglia in the pathogenesis and treatment of depression. *Journal of Neuroinflammation, 19*(1), 132. https://doi.org/10.1186/s12974-022-02492-0.

Wang, H., Shi, X., Qi, Y., Gao, M., & Zhao, Y. (2026). Gamma entrainment modulates cognitive impaired subgroup of depression: Evidence from EEG microstate dynamics. *Journal of Affective Disorders, 397*, 120971. https://doi.org/10.1016/j.jad.2025.120971.

Wang, R., Zhang, Z., Jiang, W., Liu, J., Tian, C., & Wang, M. (2025). Novel Isatin–chalcone hybrid molecules: Design, synthesis and anti-neuroinflammatory activity evaluation. *Molecules (Basel, Switzerland), 30*(7), 1421. https://doi.org/10.3390/molecules30071421.

Wang, Y.-F., Chen, C.-Y., Lei, L., & Zhang, Y. (2025). Regulation of the microglial polarization for alleviating neuroinflammation in the pathogenesis and therapeutics of major depressive disorder. *Life Sciences, 362*, 123373. https://doi.org/10.1016/j.lfs.2025.123373.

Wennström, M., Hellsten, J., Ekdahl, C. T., & Tingström, A. (2003). Electroconvulsive seizures induce proliferation of NG2-expressing glial cells in adult rat hippocampus. *Biological Psychiatry, 54*(10), 1015–1024. https://doi.org/10.1016/S0006-3223(03)00693-0.

Xia, X., Li, K., Zou, W., & Wang, L. (2025a). The central role of microglia in major depressive disorder and its potential as a therapeutic target. *Frontiers in Behavioral Neuroscience, 19*. https://doi.org/10.3389/fnbeh.2025.1598178.

Xu, F., Han, L., Wang, Y., Deng, D., Ding, Y., Zhao, S., ... Chen, X. (2023). Prolonged anesthesia induces neuroinflammation and complement-mediated microglial synaptic elimination involved in neurocognitive dysfunction and anxiety-like behaviors. *BMC Medicine, 21*(1), 7. https://doi.org/10.1186/s12916-022-02705-6.

Yao, W., Cao, Q., Luo, S., He, L., Yang, C., Chen, J., ... Zhang, J. (2022). Microglial ERK-NRBP1-CREB-BDNF signaling in sustained antidepressant actions of (R)-ketamine. *Molecular Psychiatry, 27*(3), 1618–1629. https://doi.org/10.1038/s41380-021-01377-7.

Yong, J., Hakobyan, K., Mahmud, S. A. Z., Johnson, D. J., Lee, J., Diwan, A. D., ... Mao, G. (2025). Challenges and opportunities in nanotherapeutics targeted for central nervous system disorders. *Nanoscale, 17*(43), 24860–24896. https://doi.org/10.1039/D5NR02463C.

Yu, X., Bai, Y., Han, B., Ju, M., Tang, T., Shen, L., ... Yao, H. (2022). Extracellular vesicle-mediated delivery of circDYM alleviates CUS-induced depressive-like behaviours. *Journal of Extracellular Vesicles, 11*(1), https://doi.org/10.1002/jev2.12185.

Zhang, J., Huang, X., Li, M., Zhang, W., & Yang, H. (2025a). CSF1R inhibition agents protect against cisplatin ototoxicity and synergize with immunotherapy for head and neck squamous cell carcinoma. *International Immunopharmacology, 152*, 114428. https://doi.org/10.1016/j.intimp.2025.114428.

Zhang, J., Rong, P., Zhang, L., He, H., Zhou, T., Fan, Y., ... You, Z. (2021). IL4-Driven microglia modulate stress resilience through BDNF-dependent neurogenesis. *Science Advances*, 7(12), https://doi.org/10.1126/sciadv.abb9888.

Zhao, Q., Zeng, C., Luo, F., Xian, Z., Wen, H., Tu, X., ... Wang, H. (2025). PDE4 inhibition alleviates HMGB1/C1q/C3-mediated excessive phagocytic pruning of synapses by microglia and depressive-like behaviors in mice. *Brain, Behavior, and Immunity, 126*, 126–143. https://doi.org/10.1016/j.bbi.2025.02.007.

Zhou, J., Zheng, L., Zheng, Z., Ding, K., Fu, Z., & Ni, Y. (2026). The characteristic of microglia and gut-microglia-brain axis: Implications for cognitive impairment and therapeutic strategies. *The Journal of Nutritional Biochemistry*, 110351. https://doi.org/10.1016/j.jnutbio.2026.110351.

Zhu, H., Guan, A., Liu, J., Peng, L., Zhang, Z., & Wang, S. (2023). Noteworthy perspectives on microglia in neuropsychiatric disorders. *Journal of Neuroinflammation, 20*(1), 223. https://doi.org/10.1186/s12974-023-02901-y.

Zhu, H., Guo, Y., Huang, A., Shen, H., Chen, Y., Song, J., ... Deng, B. (2022). HDAC3-regulated PGE2 production by microglia induces phobic anxiety susceptibility after stroke and pointedly exploiting a signal-targeted gamma visual stimulation new therapy. *Frontiers in Immunology, 13*. https://doi.org/10.3389/fimmu.2022.845678.

CHAPTER FOURTEEN

Neuroinflammation and vaccination strategy in Parkinson's disease

Yukti, Sanyukta Sharma, Ateendra Kumar Dubey, Anushka Sharma, and Vijay Kumar Prajapati*
Department of Biochemistry, University of Delhi South Campus, Dhaula Kuan, New Delhi, India
*Corresponding author. e-mail address: vkp@south.du.ac.in

Contents

Abstract

Parkinson's disease (PD) is a neurodegenerative disorder characterized by loss of dopaminergic neurons in the substantia nigra. Other neuropathological hallmarks include α-synuclein aggregation, Lewy bodies, Lewy neurites, and neuroinflammation in the brain. It has been proposed that the α-synuclein pathology starts in the gut with the non-motor symptoms, and then it propagates to the brain via the

Advances in Immunology, Volume 171
ISSN 0065-2776, https://doi.org/10.1016/bs.ai.2026.04.006

vagus nerve causing motor symptoms. The immune cells in the brain, namely microglia and astrocytes trigger innate immune responses and the infiltrating T cells are a part of adaptive immune response. The production of cytokines and chemokines enhances neuroinflammation. In the periphery, the monocytes and CD4+ and CD8+ T cells activation increases, causing inflammation. As inflammation is the key pathological hallmark of PD, it has emerged as an attractive target for immunotherapies. The active and passive immunotherapeutic drugs target the α-syn aggregates to overcome neuroinflammation and other motor and non-motor symptoms.

1. Introduction

Parkinson's disease (PD) is among the most prevalent neurodegenerative disorders that affects 6.1 million people worldwide (Ray Dorsey et al., 2018). It is characterized by sustained neuroinflammation and loss of dopamine-producing neurons in the substantia nigra pars compacta (SNpc) due to the accumulation of misfolded alpha-synuclein (α-syn) protein and the development of proteinaceous inclusions in Lewy bodies and Lewy neurites in the brain and periphery (Maroteaux et al., 1988). Before the onset of the disease, there is an asymptomatic phase that is different from the standard motor and non-motor PD symptoms (Mahlknecht et al., 2015). As the disease progresses, the patients face certain discomforting symptoms such as speech deficits, gait disturbance, bradykinesia, tremor, followed by hyposmia, constipation, cognitive impairment, sleep disorders, and depression(Schapira et al., 2017; Moustafa et al., 2016). A meta-analysis study showed that with increasing age, the probability of a person having PD rises, with a peak between the ages of 70–79. The entire population worldwide has an overall prevalence of 0.3 %, but for the aged population of around 80 years of age, it is > 3 % (Poewe et al., 2017). Some studies report that the disease is more common in males as compared to females, while others record no difference or more cases in females. Other factors playing a role are environmental changes, lifestyle, diet, ethnicity, and genotype (Pringsheim et al., 2014). The Braak's group presented the PD model in which the disease progresses in two stages. Stage 1 is characterised by the presence of aggregated α-syn in the olfactory bulb, while in stage 2, the pathological features affect the medulla oblongata. The later stage is usually a pre-symptomatic phase with REM sleep as a main symptom. At stage 4, the PD-related lesions spread in the anteromedial temporal mesocortex. In stage 5, the disease spreads from the temporal mesocortex to the areas that help the brain to process sensory information. Stage 6 damages involve the impairment of primary motor and sensory regions of the brain and affect the entire cerebral cortex (Braak et al., 2003).

The pathophysiology involves many key players that together contribute towards the progression of the disease. Along with the aggregation of α-synuclein and neuroinflammation, there is a defect in the lysosomal transport, mitochondria, and synaptic transport. The degeneration of the dopaminergic neurons in the substantia nigra pars compacta (SNpc) relates to the excessive beta oscillatory activity, resulting in the motor symptoms of PD (Surmeier, 2018). α-Syn is a 140-amino acid protein that forms intraneuronal aggregates in the case of synucleinopathies. The autosomal dominant early-onset of PD is due to certain missense mutations such as Ala53Thr, Ala30Pro and Glu46Lys in the α-syn protein (Polymeropoulos et al., 1997; Krüger et al., 1998; Zarranz et al., 2004). There is a key role of adaptive and innate immune pathways in the pathology of PD. In the brain, the expression of specialized immune cells- microglia and astrocytes increases with neuroinflammation. Histological studies of the substantia nigra in diseased patients revealed an increase in the density of infiltrating T lymphocytes, astrocytes and activated microglia. This is accompanied by elevated levels of tumor necrosis factor (TNF), interleukin (IL)-1 and IL-6 (Lema Tomé et al., 2013). This can, in turn, promote α-synuclein misfolding and aggregation and vice versa. The immunotherapies directed against aggregated α-synuclein can be classified as active or passive immunization. Active immunization enables the humoral immune system to produce a specific response upon injecting the antigen. On the other hand, passive immunization involves the direct and repeated administration of engineered antibodies (Baxter, 2007). The Thy1-aSyn (line 61) mouse line and model has been extensively studied as it develops an inflammatory phenotype characterised by the activation of key immune cells- microglia, elevated TNF-α, toll-like receptors (TLRs), MHCII, and T-cells in blood throughout aging (Watson et al., 2012). Several other transgenic mouse and rat model studies have reported the generation of an immune response with increased cytokines in the CSF and activated monocytes in the periphery (Gomez-Isla et al., 2003; Krashia et al., 2019). The model animals have been insightful in the identification of various inflammation-related targets and in the development of inhibitors that show anti-inflammatory action.

2. Mechanistic basis of neuroinflammation in PD

2.1 CNS immune activation

In PD, structural alterations due to phosphorylation, nitration, truncation, etc., cause fibrillation of the endogenous protein α-syn, which acts as a damage-associated molecular pattern (DAMP). Under normal conditions, these misfolded proteins are taken up by microglia and/or infiltrating macrophages (CD163+ /CCR2+) and astrocytes. Microglia are responsible for maintaining a protective environment in the brain by antibody-mediated clearance of α-synuclein in PD. The regional density and function of microglial cells differ, with a higher density in gray matter than in white matter. Also, gray matter microglia show higher expression of type-I interferon genes, while white matter microglia show higher expression of genes belonging to the nuclear factor kappa B (NF-κB) pathway (Zhu et al., 2022). The presence of misfolded proteins triggers the secretion of pro-inflammatory cytokines (IL-1β, TNF-α, IL-12, IL-23) by M1 microglia (Orihuela et al., 2016). This increases ROS production and enhances phagocytic activity. The monomeric form of α-synuclein is taken up via the monosialotetrahexosylganglioside (GM-1) receptor, while aggregated α-synuclein is taken up by clathrin for phagocytosis. On the other hand, the presence of anti-inflammatory cytokines (IL-10, IL-4, IL-13, TGF-β) triggers the neuroprotective M2 microglia phenotype (Park et al., 2009; Scheiblich et al., 2021).

α-synuclein fibrils or oligomers activate microglial cells via the interaction with Toll-like receptor 4 (TLR4) or TLR. This causes NF-κB translocation and NLRP3 inflammasome activation. Reactive microglia are concentrated in the substantia nigra of PD patients along with higher levels of pro-inflammatory cytokines, such as tumor necrosis factor-α (TNF-α), interleukin-1β (IL-1β), interleukin-6 (IL-6), and interferon-gamma (IFN-γ). Studies also show that α-synuclein activates the enzyme phosphate oxidase (PHOX), which generates ROS, and that Galectin-3, which regulates inflammation in microglia, is upregulated. Microglia act as the major APCs in the brain and show elevated MHC class II expression and high CD4 T cell proliferation (Zhang et al., 2007; Boza-Serrano et al., 2014; Zhu et al., 2022). The microglial phagocytosis is mediated by the interaction of the aggregated α-syn with the complement receptors- CR3 and CR4. Mouse models show increased production of oxygen radicals and NOX activation, driven by CD11b. The CR4 specifically recognises fibrillar microglia. The NLRP3 inflammasome activation is triggered by α-syn interaction with CD36 and Fyn kinase. Other pathways activated by α-syn that produce pro-inflammatory signals include p38 MAPK, NFκB, and ERK. Thus, the increased accumulation of misfolded antigenic α-syn in synapses activates immune responses. Microglial activation, in turn, contributes to α-syn pathology, thereby worsening the disease. The inflammasome-induced phagocytosis enhances α-syn truncation via the induction of caspase-1 expression. It also promotes further oxidation or nitration of α-syn, causing aggregation. So, elevated microglial activation can be toxic, leading to synaptic loss (Stefanova, 2022; Harms et al., 2021).

2.2 Peripheral immunity

Apart from microglia, there is an increase in the expression of myeloid cells, such as CD163 and CCR2 in PD. The postmortem brains and rodent PD models showed an elevation in the number of cells expressing scavenger receptor CD163. This suggests CCR2+ monocyte/macrophage infiltration into the inflamed PD brain. Also, the patients' blood showed enrichment for CCL2, and monocytes exhibited upregulation of CCR2. The transcriptomic analysis of diseased patients revealed differential expression of certain genes, namely HLA-DQB1 (MHC II system), MYD88 (associated with TLR2 and 4), REL (member of the NFκB transcription factors), and TNF (Zhu et al., 2022; Su et al., 2022). Postmortem PD brain tissue has revealed the prominent expression of HLA-DR, which is a component of MHC II. MHC II proteins are expressed on the infiltrating monocytes and monocyte-derived macrophages in the periphery and microglia in the CNS. HLA-DR expression is seen near the neurons with α-syn aggregation, along with CD4+ and CD8+ T cells in SN. The elevation of T cell-derived IFN-γ and TNF in blood, brain, and CSF is due to the $MHCII^{+}$-APC interaction. Studies show an overall imbalance in the number of Th cells. Also, studies show that the ability of Treg cells to inhibit Teff cells decreases, modulating inflammatory responses (McGeer et al., 1988; Zhu et al., 2022).

A study by Yun Su et al. revealed dysregulation of distinct PBMC subpopulations in patients with PD, highlighting the importance of the innate immune system. Classical monocytes (CD14+) were more numerous than intermediate and nonclassical monocytes. This can be due to CCR2-mediated migration from the bone marrow into the bloodstream, and C–C chemokine receptor type 2 (CCR2) was found to be upregulated on CD14+ monocytes along with its ligand, C–C motif ligand 2 (CCL2). Also, α-synuclein stimulation led to elevated expression of TNF-α, IL-1β, and IL-6, suggesting an inflammatory response upon monocyte activation. Similarly, Julia C. Greenland et al. found a higher proportion of classical monocytes that secrete inflammatory cytokines in response to TLR binding and activate the NOD-like receptor protein 3 (NLRP3) inflammasome, which in turn activates caspase-1, leading to activation of pro-inflammatory cytokines.(Greenland et al., 2025).

T cell migration to the CNS via the BBB is facilitated by C-X-C motif chemokine receptor 3 (CXCR3) binding to the ligands- CXCL10, CXCL9, and CXCL11 in experimental autoimmune encephalomyelitis (EAE) (Sporici & Issekutz, 2010). Also, cell adhesion to the VCAM-1 is mediated by α4β1-integrin on Th1 and Th17 cells. Several studies have related T cell infiltration to dopaminergic neuron loss (Sonar & Lal, 2017; Brochard et al., 2009). The cerebrospinal fluid (CSF) plays an important role in immune surveillance due to the abundance of T cells, as well as the presence of B cells and myeloid cells. PD mouse models and postmortem brain samples from patients showed elevated levels of T cells and pro-inflammatory cytokines, including interleukin-2 (IL-2), IL-6, and TNF-α. The T cells recognize epitopes in the Y39 and S129 regions of α-synuclein and generate an adaptive immune response in which CD4 and CD8 cytotoxic T cells secrete IFNγ (Zhu et al., 2022). High T cell responses and cytokines (IFN-γ, IL-5, and IL-10) are found in patients after PD diagnosis. HLA alleles, DRB5*01 and DRB1*15:01, are HLA class II variants that have high affinity for α-synuclein Y39 region. HLA class I allele A*11:01 interacts with a shorter α-synuclein peptide in the Y39 region with high affinity (Yu et al., 2021). The MHCII antigen presentation and activation of the CD4 T-cells is found in the areas of neurodegeneration. The Fas/FasL-dependent dopaminergic neurotoxicity is caused due to CD4 T-cell infiltration into the SNpc in MPTP neurotoxin mouse model (Brochard et al., 2009). Upon MHCII KO, the number of CD8 T-cells increase and it also reverses CD11b microgliosis and IgG deposition (Madsen et al., 1999).

2.3 Interactions between α-synuclein pathology and immune activation

AAV2-SYN model of PD showed that the overexpression of human full-length α-syn can induce inflammation via NF-κB activation, microglial activation, IgG deposition, lymphocyte infiltration, and gradual degeneration of dopaminergic neurons (Cao et al., 2010). The 6-OHDA and 1-methyl-4-phenyl-1,2,3,6-tetrahydropyridine (MPTP) neurotoxic models have explored the importance of pro-inflammatory cytokine neutralization in preventing reactive microgliosis (Harms et al., 2011). Inflammation in the olfactory bulb and gastrointestinal tract contributes PD pathology by promoting the early misfolding of α-synuclein. This involves various cytokines, reactive oxygen species (ROS), chemokines, and complement proteins regulating the innate and adaptive immune system. Although it is usually not known if the aggregation of the misfolded protein triggers neuroinflammation or vice versa. In PD, the aggregated α-syn is taken up by microglial cells that further creates a positive loop of degeneration of dopaminergic cells. Also, post translational modifications such as phosphorylation of α-syn at serine 87 (S87-P) and serine 129 (S129-P) leads to uncontrolled activation of microglia (Anderson et al., 2006). There are prion-like mechanisms, involving Aβ plaques, proposed for the spreading of α-syn. Aβ plaques and α-syn pathology have together contributed towards the activation of microglia, causing neuroinflammation and oxidative stress. The orphan receptor Nurr1, is responsible for maintaining the dopaminergic neurons and the loss of this receptor leads to the activation of the NF-kB signaling cascade in astrocytes and microglia, which further have neurotoxic effects (Lema Tomé et al., 2013).

There are two mechanisms proposed which are responsible for the spread of synucleinopathy. First is from the olfactory bulb to the midbrain and second is from the enteric nervous system (ENS) to the central nervous system (CNS), that is from the gastrointestinal tract to the brain via the spinal cord. The histological studies of PD patients show the spread of α-syn abnormality to the olfactory regions like the periamygdaloid, piriform, and entorhinal cortices. The olfactory epithelium makes contact with the exogenous particles in the air, and the olfactory epithelium neurons project their axons into the glomerular layer of the OB (Loseva et al., 2009). The microglia present in the olfactory bulb can sense the external pathogens, toxins, viruses, nanoparticles and microparticle, and can promote possible neuroinflammation. So, the entry of neurotropic particles causing diseases such as influenza, allergic rhinitis and asthma, that occurs via the olfactory route may contribute to PD-related inflammation in distant brain regions. This is because the activated microglia produce ROS and cytokines that disrupt the blood-brain barrier (BBB) (Bower et al., 2006; Rohn & Catlin, 2011). H5N1 viral infection in C57Bl/6 mice by intranasal inoculation leads to the immune response that persisted at least 2 months and phosphorylated α-syn (pSer129) was observed in the OB, locus coeruleus, hippocampus, and brainstem (Jang et al., 2009). PD patients experience constipation, dysphagia, and gastroesophageal reflux, and also histological studies revealed the accumulation of α-syn in the ENS. α-synuclein pathology spreads through the

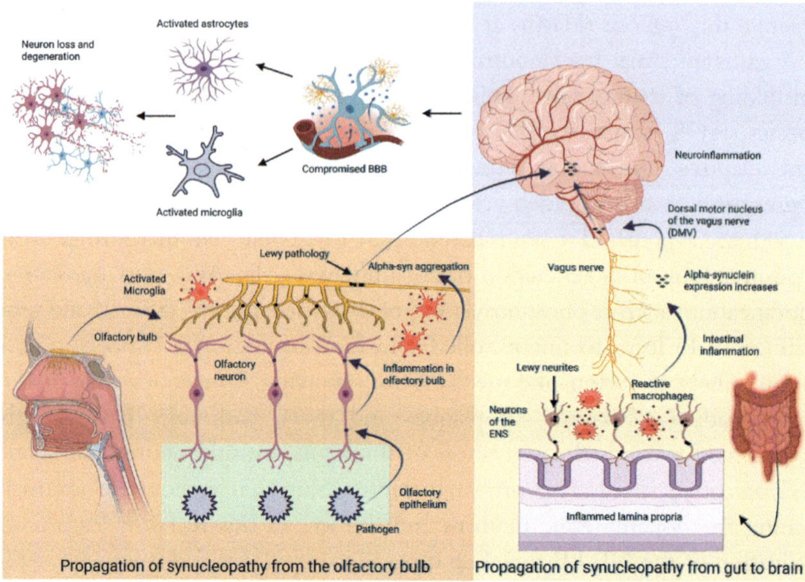

Fig. 1 Spread of parkinson's disease via the olfactory bulb and the gastrointestinal tract to the brain.

vagus nerve to the dorsal motor nucleus (DMV) and finally the substantia nigra. Infection in the intestine causes inflammation and if left untreated, it causes dysbiosis of the gut microbiome and permeability of intestine increases. This causes the inflammatory factors to leak from the gut to the systemic circulation and activation of APCs (Cersosimo & Benarroch, 2012) (Fig. 1).

3. Immune system and PD

3.1 Blood–brain barrier (BBB) dysfunction

Brain is the control center of the body and a main part of the central nervous system. The CNS plays a key role in the control and coordination of all the processes inside the body. The Spinal cord and brain are the two main principal organs that play a crucial role in CNS. The brain is located in the cranial cavity and the average adult human brain weighs about 1.3–1.4 kg. It has about 644 kilometers of blood vessels, which provide oxygen, energy, metabolites, and nutrients to brain cells and simultaneously remove carbon dioxide as well as other metabolite waste from the circulating system (Sweeney et al., 2018). The separation of circulating blood from the extracellular fluid of the central nervous system is regulated by the blood-brain barrier (BBB). The BBB is a highly selective, semipermeable barrier that primarily maintains brain homeostasis. Approximately 20 % of the body's total glucose and oxygen consumption is required by the brain (Alahmari, 2021). Neurovascular Coupling is a process where cerebral blood flow is precisely matched to neuronal activity, which ensures adequate delivery of oxygen and metabolites to meet the high metabolic demands. It is regulated by a specialized barrier layer, known as the BBB, which is located at the primary interface between blood and neural tissues. The BBB includes Brain microvascular endothelial cells, Pericytes, Astrocytic end-feet and Basement membrane (Daneman & Prat, 2015). Blood–brain barrier dysfunction can cause loss of structural integrity or regulatory function, which will lead to abnormal permeability between the bloodstream and the central nervous system (CNS) (Sweeney et al., 2018). This leads to neuroinflammation, ischemia, hypoxia, oxidative stress, mitochondrial dysfunction, aging, infections, and neurodegenerative diseases (Zierfuss et al., 2024). In Multiple sclerosis, the CNS is severely affected and causes chronic inflammatory diseases. Relapsing remitting multiple sclerosis is characterized by bouts of neurological deterioration (ie, relapses) followed by a variable degree of recovery (ie, remission). In Multiple Sclerosis, BBB dysfunction plays central role in disease development. This leads to increased permeability of the tight junction, loss of endothelial integrity and enhanced transcellular and paracellular transport (Daneman & Prat, 2015; Zierfuss et al., 2024). This breakdown allows peripheral immune cells, such as autoreactive $CD4^+$ and $CD8^+$ T cells, B cells, macrophages, and monocytes to enter the CNS, and recognize myelin antigens to initiate inflammation (Balasa et al., 2021; Bennett et al., 2010).

3.2 Role of T cells (Th17/Treg balance) and B-cell–mediated responses

Immunity is the efficiency or ability of an organism to fight against disease-causing organisms such as bacteria, virus, fungi, parasites and abnormal cells. The immune system works together with the help of immune cells, molecules and tissues to prevent infection and promote physiological homeostasis. Immunity is further classified into two different types, on the basis of specificity and origin i.e, innate and adaptive immunity. Innate immunity is present from birth and non-specific, while the adaptive immunity is adapted after exposure to the antigens and is highly specific (Pulendran & Davis, 2020). The cells that play an important role in mediating the immune responses are monocytes, neutrophils, macrophages, natural killer cells, mast cells, basophils and eosinophils. Parkinson's disease (PD) is a neurodegenerative disorder characterized by motor impairments such as muscular rigidity, tremor, bradykinesia, and postural instability, along with non-motor symptoms including cognitive impairment, depression, sleep disorders, and autonomic dysfunction (Poewe et al., 2017). Loss of dopaminergic neurons, a neurotransmitter that is essential for motor control, leads to decreased dopamine levels, resulting in impaired communication within the basal ganglia circuitry that regulates movement (Kalia & Lang, 2015; Poewe et al., 2017). In Parkinson's disease, strong neuroinflammatory processes occur involving microglial activation, infiltration of peripheral T cells, and dysregulation of cytokine production (Hirsch & Hunot, 2009). A key pathological feature of PD is the misfolding and aggregation of α-synuclein protein, which forms intracellular inclusions known as Lewy bodies. Misfolded α-synuclein can trigger immune activation and stimulate both $CD4^+$ T helper cells and $CD8^+$ cytotoxic T cells (Sulzer et al., 2017).

$CD4^+$ T helper cells differentiate into several subsets, including Th1, Th17, and regulatory T cells (Tregs). $CD8^+$ cytotoxic T cells recognize neuronal antigens presented on MHC-I molecules and release cytotoxic molecules such as perforin and granzymes that contribute to neuronal injury (Sulzer et al., 2017; Brochard et al., 2009). Regulatory T cells are characterized by the expression of $CD4^+$, $CD25^+$, and the transcription factor FOXP3, which acts as the master regulator of Treg function. The main role of T regulatory cells is to suppress excessive immune responses and maintain immune tolerance, thereby providing protective effects against neuroinflammation (Gendelman et al., 2017). Th17 cells are a subset of $CD4^+$ T helper cells that play a pro-inflammatory role. These cells produce cytokines such as interleukin-17 (IL-17), interleukin-21 (IL-21), and interleukin-22 (IL-22). Differentiation of Th17 cells is typically driven by cytokines including interleukin-6 (IL-6), transforming growth factor-β (TGF-β), and interleukin-23 (IL-23) (Korn et al., 2009). Th17 cells contribute significantly to neuroinflammation in Parkinson's disease and are involved in neuronal damage. IL-17 produced by Th17 cells can activate microglial cells, which in turn release pro-inflammatory cytokines such as TNF-α, IL-1β, and IL-6, amplifying neuroinflammatory responses (Storelli et al., 2019). Activated microglia release inflammatory mediators, such as nitric oxide and reactive oxygen species, which are toxic molecules that contribute to the degeneration of dopaminergic neurons (Hirsch & Hunot, 2009). Th17-mediated inflammation can also increase blood–brain barrier permeability, allowing peripheral immune cells to infiltrate the brain and further aggravate neuroinflammation (Storelli et al., 2019). The balance between pro-inflammatory Th17 cells and anti-inflammatory regulatory T cells plays an important role in controlling immune responses. In Parkinson's disease, this balance is disrupted. Th17 cells are increased in the peripheral blood of PD patients, and elevated levels of IL-17 have been observed (Sommer et al., 2018). IL-17 promotes microglial activation and increases production of TNF-α and IL-1β, leading to oxidative stress, blood–brain barrier disruption, and dopaminergic neuronal death (Storelli et al., 2019).

Conversely, regulatory T cells are reduced or functionally impaired in Parkinson's disease, resulting in diminished immunosuppressive activity. T regulatory cells normally suppress Th17 expansion, inhibit microglial activation, reduce pro-inflammatory cytokine production, and promote neuroprotective anti-inflammatory responses such as M2 microglial polarization (Gendelman et al., 2017). However, in PD the imbalance between Th17 and Treg cells leads to chronic inflammation, persistent microglial activation, and progressive neuronal degeneration. Misfolded α-synuclein aggregates can also activate the peripheral immune system and stimulate B-cell responses. B cells differentiate into plasma cells and memory cells. Plasma cells produce antibodies against α-synuclein, which form antigen–antibody complexes and contribute to inflammatory responses (Wahner et al., 2007). B cells can also function as antigen-presenting cells by presenting α-synuclein peptides to $CD4^+$ T cells via MHC-II molecules, thereby promoting further T-cell activation (Lindestam Arlehamn et al., 2020). Additionally, B cells secrete pro-inflammatory cytokines such as IL-6 and TNF-α that further contribute to neuroinflammation in Parkinson's disease (Lindestam Arlehamn et al., 2020).

3.3 Systemic inflammation as a driver of central neuroinflammation

Systemic inflammation occurs due to continuous activation of the peripheral immune system and is characterized by increased circulating pro-inflammatory cytokines such as tumor necrosis factor-alpha (TNF-α), interleukin-1 beta (IL-1β), interleukin-6 (IL-6), and the activation of circulating immune cells. Systemic inflammation plays an important role in amplifying central neuroinflammation in Parkinson's disease through complex interactions between the peripheral immune system, the blood–brain barrier (BBB), and resident immune cells of the central nervous system (Perry et al., 2010; Hirsch & Hunot, 2009). In Parkinson's disease, α-synuclein exists in a misfolded and aggregated form, which accumulates in neuronal cells and acts as a damage-associated molecular pattern (DAMP). These aggregated proteins can activate the peripheral immune system and trigger inflammatory responses (Sulzer et al., 2017). Activation of the peripheral immune system results in stimulation of immune cells including monocytes, macrophages, dendritic cells, $CD4^+$ T lymphocytes, $CD8^+$ T lymphocytes, Th1 cells, Th17 cells, and B lymphocytes (Lindestam Arlehamn et al., 2020). These activated immune cells produce pro-inflammatory cytokines such as TNF-α, IL-1β, IL-6, and interferon-gamma (IFN-γ), which contribute to systemic inflammation and promote neuroinflammatory processes (Hirsch & Hunot, 2009; Tansey & Romero-Ramos, 2019).

The blood–brain barrier is a highly selective barrier formed by brain microvascular endothelial cells connected by tight junction proteins such as claudin-5 and occludin, along with astrocytic end-feet and pericytes (Daneman & Prat, 2015). During systemic inflammation, circulating pro-inflammatory cytokines can disrupt the integrity of the blood–brain barrier by altering tight junction proteins and increasing BBB permeability (Varatharaj & Galea, 2017). Oxidative stress generated during inflammation can also damage endothelial cells, leading to the activation of matrix metalloproteinases such as MMP-2 and MMP-9, which degrade BBB structural components and further compromise barrier integrity (Varatharaj & Galea, 2017). Increased permeability of the BBB allows peripheral immune cells such as monocytes, $CD4^+$ T cells, $CD8^+$ T cells, and B cells to infiltrate the central nervous system (Brochard et al., 2009). Th1 cells contribute to neuroinflammation by releasing interferon-gamma, which activates microglia in the brain (Storelli et al., 2019). Th17 cells release interleukin-17 (IL-17), a pro-inflammatory cytokine that promotes inflammatory responses and contributes to neuronal damage (Sommer et al., 2018). $CD8^+$ cytotoxic T cells can directly induce dopaminergic neuronal death through the release of cytotoxic molecules such as perforin and granzymes (Sulzer et al., 2017). B cells produce antibodies against α-synuclein, which form antigen–antibody complexes and activate complement pathways, further promoting inflammation (Lindestam Arlehamn et al., 2020). Microglia are the resident immune cells of the central nervous system. Once activated, microglial cells release pro-inflammatory mediators including TNF-α, IL-1β, IL-6, reactive oxygen species (ROS), and nitric oxide (NO), which amplify inflammatory signaling pathways and contribute to neuronal injury (Hirsch & Hunot, 2009). This inflammatory cascade leads to degeneration of dopaminergic neurons in the substantia nigra, which occurs due to oxidative stress, mitochondrial dysfunction, excitotoxicity, and immune-mediated cytotoxicity (Kalia & Lang, 2015). Systemic inflammation further contributes to neuroinflammation by promoting BBB disruption, immune cell infiltration, microglial activation, and neuronal damage. This inflammatory environment can promote further release of misfolded α-synuclein, which in turn activates the peripheral immune system, creating a self-propagating inflammatory cycle (Tansey & Romero-Ramos, 2019). Under normal physiological conditions, regulatory T cells (Tregs) suppress excessive immune responses by releasing anti-inflammatory cytokines such as interleukin-10 (IL-10) and transforming growth factor-beta (TGF-β). However, in Parkinson's disease the number or functional activity of regulatory T cells is reduced, leading to impaired immunosuppression and dominance of pro-inflammatory immune responses (Gendelman et al., 2017). This imbalance between pro-inflammatory and anti-inflammatory immune responses contributes to chronic neuroinflammation and progressive neuronal degeneration in Parkinson's disease (Fig. 2).

3.4 Biomarkers linking peripheral immune activation to PD progression

There are the various biomarkers which are responsible for the progressions of Parkinson's disease from systemic to the central nervous system. These can be detected in the blood, serum, plasma and cerebrospinal fluids. There include the proinflammatory and anti-inflammatory cytokines, alpha-synuclein, immune cells biomarkers, C-reactive proteins, chemokines, blood-brain barrier dysfunctions, oxidative stress, monocytes activations and neurodegeneration associated peripheral biomarkers (Poewe et al., 2017; Tansey & Romero-Ramos, 2019). As we all know, the misfolded alpha-synuclein get accumulated and will act as a damage-associated molecular pattern for the activations of various immune cells (Sulzer et al., 2017). These immune cells are responsible for the productions of cytokines and increases the amount of circulating cytokines that are the strongest

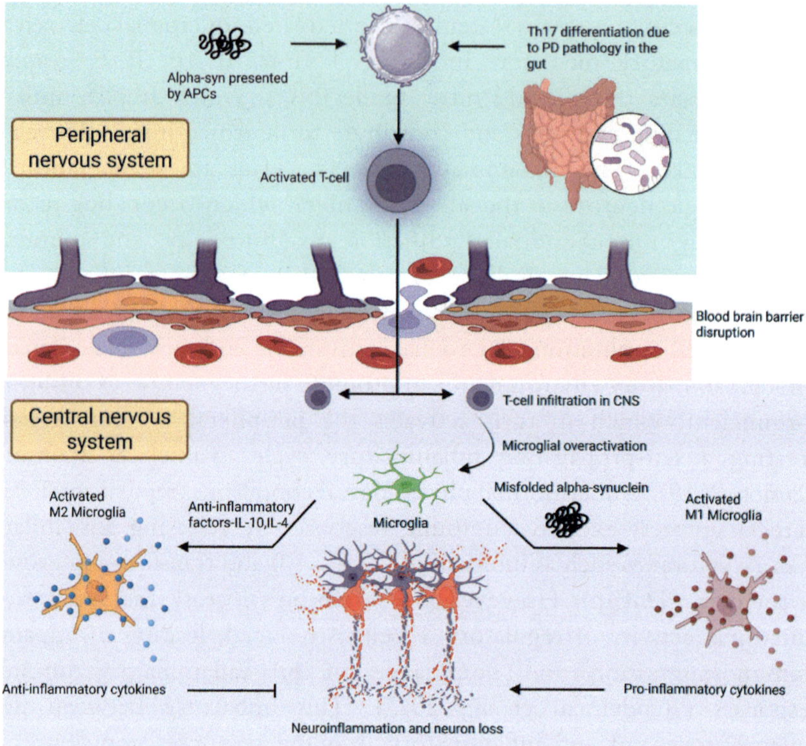

Fig. 2 The role of peripheral and central nervous system in neuroinflammation and neuron degeneration.

indicators of systemic immune activations in Parkinson's disease (Hirsch & Hunot, 2009). Some of the important cytokine biomarkers are the tumor necrosis factor alpha, interleukin-1 beta, interleukin-6, interferon gamma, and interleukin-17 (Tansey & Romero-Ramos, 2019). The tumor necrosis factors are present in the serum and cerebrospinal fluids in the Parkinson's disease patients and it is responsible for the disease severity, progression of disease, blood-brain barrier dysfunctions and microglial activations (Hirsch & Hunot, 2009). Interleukin-1 beta acts as an active inflammatory cytokine and is responsible for inflammation and dopaminergic neuron degradation (Tansey & Romero-Ramos, 2019). Interleukin-6, which is a major biomarker of systemic inflammations, is responsible for the fast disease progression (Qin et al., 2016). Interferon gamma, which is released by the TH1 cells activates the microglial cells and promotes neurotoxicity

(Brochard et al., 2009). Interleukin-17, which is produced by the TH17 cells is responsible for the autoimmune mediated neurodegeneration (Sommer et al., 2018). There are some anti-inflammatory cytokines also such as the interleukin-10 and the TGF-beta, produced by the T regulatory cells and their lower number indicates that there is a reduced T-regulatory cell function (Gendelman et al., 2017). These are responsible for maintaining the immune tolerance and reduction in their levels is related to increased neuroinflammation (Gendelman et al., 2017).

The alpha-synuclein biomarkers, which is a central and the most important Parkinson's disease biomarker, is produced in the misfolded form and then get accumulated. It is present in the blood and the cerebrospinal fluid. Its misfolded accumulated form acts as a damage-associated molecular pattern, activating the peripheral immune cells, and its higher oligomeric form will increase the disease severity (Sulzer et al., 2017; Poewe et al., 2017). The C-reactive protein biomarker is a related to systemic inflammation, and its elevated levels in Parkinson's correlates with the motor symptoms severity (Qin et al., 2016). The chemokine biomarkers recruit the immune cells in the central nervous system like CCL2 (which recruits the monocytes), CXCL10 (which recruits the T cells) and CCL5 (which promotes the immune infiltration). Their elevated levels indicate the peripheral to central immune signaling (Tansey & Romero-Ramos, 2019). The blood-brain barrier dysfunction biomarkers allow the immune cells infiltration such as the matrix metalloproteinases 9, matrix metalloproteinases 2, S100B proteins, ICAM-1, and VCAM-1. Their elevated levels generally indicate that there is an increase in blood-brain barrier permeability (Varatharaj & Galea, 2017). The systemic inflammation generally increases the oxidative stress due to the production of nitric oxide, reactive oxygen species, and malondialdehyde which indicates the oxidative neuronal damage (Dias et al., 2013). Monocyte activation biomarkers include CD14, CD16, HLA-DR, and soluble CD16. The soluble CD16 is a strong biomarker in the monocyte activations in Parkinson's disease (Grozdanov et al., 2014). The neurodegeneration-associated peripheral markers are the neurofilament light chain and glial fibrillary acidic proteins. Their higher levels correlate with the disease progressions and these reflect the neuronal damage, but can be measured peripherally, mostly (Hansson et al., 2017).

4. Modulation of neuroinflammation as a therapeutic target

4.1 Anti-inflammatory drugs (NSAIDs, corticosteroids, microglial inhibitors)

In neurodegenerative diseases, neuroinflammation is one of the major causes of neuronal damage. Therefore, reducing neuroinflammation in the nervous system can be an effective therapeutic approach to limit neural inflammation. Several strategies can be used such as anti-inflammatory drugs, microglial inhibitors, cytokine-targeted therapies, nutraceuticals, and metabolic modulators to reduce the impact of neurodegenerative diseases (Glass et al., 2010; Tansey & Romero-Ramos, 2019). However, there are some limitations associated with these therapies, including systemic immunosuppression, which may weaken the normal immune system and increase the risk of several infections (Glass et al., 2010). Therefore, these therapies should ideally target brain inflammation specifically while minimizing systemic immune suppression. Hence, therapies must aim to reduce brain inflammation without significantly affecting overall immune functions. There are several anti-inflammatory drugs (NSAIDs -non-steroidal anti-inflammatory drugs), which reduce inflammation by inhibiting the cyclooxygenase enzymes COX-1 and COX-2. These enzymes are responsible for the production of prostaglandins, which are key mediators of inflammation (Cote et al., 2015). In neuroinflammation, NSAIDs may reduce microglial activation and consequently decrease the release of pro-inflammatory cytokines while also lowering oxidative stress (Cote et al., 2015). Some examples of NSAIDs are aspirin, Ibuprofen, Diclofenac, Celecoxib and Naproxen. NSAIDs generally inhibit the enzyme, Cyclooxygenase (COX-1 and COX-2) affecting the arachidonic acid pathway as COXs are responsible for converting arachidonic acid into prostaglandins. It also leads to reduced prostaglandin synthesis and thereby decreasing inflammation, pain, and fever. Corticosteroids can also be used as strong anti-inflammatory agents that suppress immune responses at the gene-expression level. They inhibit the production of inflammatory cytokines such as interleukin-1, interleukin-6, and TNF-alpha, and they also reduce leukocyte migration (Barnes, 2016). Some examples of corticosteroids are Prednisone, Dexamethasone, Hydrocortisone, Methylprednisolone and Betamethasone. It generally binds to the Glucocorticoid Receptor inside the cell and regulate the gene transcription to suppress inflammatory pathways. Prednisone acts through the glucocorticoid receptor signalling pathway to inhibit the Phospholipase A2 which in turn decreases the production of arachidonic acid–derived mediators, reducing inflammation and immune responses. Dexamethasone binds to intracellular glucocorticoid receptors and suppresses the NF-κB Signalling Pathway, reducing the expression of pro-inflammatory cytokines and inflammatory mediators. Microglial inhibitors can also be used as therapeutic agents because microglial cells are the resident immune cells of the brain and the central nervous system. When excessively activated, microglia release pro-inflammatory cytokines, reactive oxygen species, and nitric oxide (Block et al., 2007). Therefore, the use of microglial inhibitors can reduce the effects of excessive microglial activation. These inhibitors may prevent excessive activation and promote a shift of microglia from a pro-inflammatory phenotype toward a protective or anti-inflammatory phenotype, thereby reducing chronic neuroinflammation (Tang & Le, 2016). Some examples of microglial inhibitors are Minocycline, Ibudilast and Propentofylline. Microglial inhibitors suppress the activation of microglia by blocking inflammatory signaling pathways such as the NF-κB Signaling Pathway and the MAPK Signaling Pathway. Minocycline inhibits microglial activation by suppressing the NF-κB Signaling Pathway which in result decreases the production of pro-inflammatory cytokines and reduces neuroinflammation. Ibudilast inhibits Phosphodiesterase-4 (PDE-4) and modulates glial cell activation pathways, reducing the release of inflammatory mediators such as TNF-α and IL-1β from microglia. However, long-term use of these drugs can increase the risk of systemic immunosuppression, which may elevate susceptibility to infections and metabolic side effects (Glass et al., 2010). Additionally, the ability of many anti-inflammatory drugs to cross the blood–brain barrier is limited, and prolonged use may also cause gastrointestinal and cardiovascular side effects (Cote et al., 2015).

4.2 Cytokine-targeted therapies (IL-1, IL-6, TNF blockers)

wIn Parkinson's disease, when the microglial cells in the brain area get activated, they release cytokines such as interleukin-1, interleukin-6, and tumor necrosis factor-alpha. These cytokines are responsible for neuroinflammation and they also promote neuronal damage, increase oxidative stress, and contribute to blood–brain barrier destruction (Hirsch & Hunot, 2009; Block et al., 2007). If we target these cytokines, the inflammatory responses can be reduced. In cytokine-targeted therapy, modulation of neuroinflammation specifically blocks the pro-inflammatory cytokines that drive chronic neuroinflammation and neurodegenerative diseases such as Parkinson's disease and Alzheimer's disease (Tansey & Romero-Ramos, 2019). In this approach, interleukin-1 blockers such as Canakinumab and

Rilonacept can be used because IL-1 is a key mediator of inflammatory cascades in the brain. By blocking interleukin-1, microglial activation can be reduced, neuronal apoptosis can be decreased, and inflammatory signalling can be lowered (Dinarello, 2011). Another strategy is the use of interleukin-6 inhibitors such as Tocilizumab and Sarilumab. IL-6 contributes to chronic inflammation and immune cell activation. By inhibiting interleukin-6, inflammatory cytokine production can be reduced and peripheral immune cell infiltration into the central nervous system through the blood–brain barrier can also be limited (Tanaka et al., 2014). Tumor necrosis factor-alpha (TNF-α) is a central pro-inflammatory cytokine involved in neuronal injury. By blocking TNF-α with the inhibitors such as Infliximab, Adalimumab, Etanercept and Golimumab, neurotoxicity can be decreased, oxidative stress can be reduced, and synaptic functions can be protected (McCoy & Tansey, 2008). TNF-α inhibitors are widely used in autoimmune diseases and are being explored as potential therapeutic agents in neurodegenerative disorders (McCoy & Tansey, 2008). Cytokine-targeted therapy is more specific than general anti-inflammatory drugs because it blocks particular inflammatory mediators rather than suppressing the entire immune system. However, it also has certain limitations such as systemic immunosuppression, which may increase susceptibility to various infections and may interfere with normal immune responses (Glass et al., 2010).

4.3 Nutraceutical and metabolic modulators with neuroimmune benefits

Nutraceuticals and metabolic modulators are natural or metabolism-regulating compounds that help in reducing neuroinflammation and protecting the neurons of the central nervous system. They are considered promising therapeutic approaches to reduce neuroinflammation and provide neuroimmune benefits with fewer side effects compared to conventional anti-inflammatory drugs (Vauzour et al., 2010). As we know, in neurodegenerative diseases such as Parkinson's disease, there is chronic activation of microglial cells that are resident in the brain, which leads to the release of pro-inflammatory cytokines, oxidative stress, and mitochondrial dysfunction that are responsible for chronic neuroinflammation (Hirsch & Hunot, 2009). Nutraceuticals and metabolic modulators help in reducing these processes through multiple mechanisms. In this approach, antioxidants can be used, which are responsible for reducing oxidative stress by neutralizing reactive oxygen species, which are major contributors to neuronal damage. Examples include vitamin C, vitamin E, polyphenols, and coenzyme Q10 (Dias et al., 2013). These compounds are associated with benefits such as reducing oxidative stress, protecting dopaminergic neurons, and decreasing inflammatory signaling (Beal, 2003). Omega-3 fatty acids can also be used because they possess strong anti-inflammatory properties. Omega-3 fatty acids reduce the production of pro-inflammatory cytokines such as interleukin-1, interleukin-6, and TNF-alpha, while promoting anti-inflammatory cytokines and improving neuronal membrane stability (Calder, 2015). They also help regulate microglial activation and support neuronal survival (Calder, 2015). Mitochondrial metabolic modulators can also be used in cases of mitochondrial dysfunction, which is a key feature of neurodegeneration (Exner et al., 2012). These metabolic modulators improve mitochondrial function and energy production. Examples include coenzyme Q10, NAD^+ precursors, and creatine. These compounds help improve ATP production, reduce oxidative stress, and protect neurons from degeneration (Beal, 2003; Exner et al., 2012).

Plant-derived anti-inflammatory compounds may also be beneficial, such as curcumin and flavonoids. These compounds help reduce neuroinflammation by inhibiting inflammatory pathways such as NF-κB, reducing excessive microglial activation, and lowering cytokine production (Aggarwal & Harikumar, 2009; Vauzour et al., 2010). Their significance lies in reducing neuroinflammation, protecting neurons from damage, improving mitochondrial function, and supporting neuroimmune balance, which may help reduce the symptoms of Parkinson's disease and other neurodegenerative disorders. Their advantages include relatively fewer side effects, safety for long-term use, and support for overall brain health. However, their limitations include lower potency compared to pharmaceutical drugs, limited bioavailability, and the inability to completely stop disease progression when used alone (Vauzour et al., 2010) (Table 1).

4.4 Limitations of systemic immunosuppression

Targeting neuroinflammation is an important strategy in neurodegenerative diseases such as Parkinson's disease and Alzheimer's disease. However, many anti-inflammatory and cytokine-targeted therapies suppress the immune system not only in the brain but also in the body (Glass et al., 2010; Tansey & Romero-Ramos, 2019). This systemic immunosuppression has several limitations. It is responsible for increased risk of infections, impaired immune surveillance, poor specificity, blood–brain barrier challenges, long-term side effects, and interference with beneficial inflammatory responses (Ransohoff, 2016). It increases the risk of infections by

Table 1 Drugs targeting neuroinflammation in Parkinson's disease.

S.No.	Category of drugs	Group	Example	Mechanism of action
1	Anti-inflammatory drugs	NSAIDs,	Aspirin, Ibuprofen, Diclofenac, Celecoxib and Naproxen	Inhibit Cyclooxygenase (COX-1 and COX-2).
		Corticosteroids	Prednisone, Dexamethasone, Hydrocortisone, Methylprednisolone and Betamethasone	Bind to the Glucocorticoid Receptor inside cells and regulate gene transcription to suppress inflammatory pathways
		Microglial inhibitors	Minocycline, Ibudilast and Propentofylline	Inhibit microglial activation by blocking inflammatory signalling pathways such as the NF-κB and the MAPK.
2	Cytokine-targeted therapies	IL-1 blockers	Canakinumab and Rilonacept	Reduce microglial activation.
		IL-6 blockers	Tocilizumab and Sarilumab	Reduce peripheral immune cell infiltration.
		TNF blockers	Infliximab, Adalimumab, Etanercept and Golimumab	Reduce oxidative stress and neurotoxicity.
3	Nutraceuticals and metabolic modulators	Antioxidants	Vitamin C, vitamin E, polyphenols	Reduce oxidative stress by neutralising reactive oxygen species.
			Omega-3 fatty acids	Reduce the production of pro-inflammatory cytokines such as interleukin-1, interleukin-6, and TNF-alpha, while promoting anti-inflammatory cytokines.
		Mitochondrial metabolic modulators	Coenzyme Q10, NAD^+ precursors, and creatine	Improve ATP production, and reduce oxidative stress
		Plant-derived anti-inflammatory compounds	Curcumin and flavonoids	Inhibit NF-κB, reduce excessive microglial activation, and cytokine production

suppressing immune responses and reducing the body's ability to fight against bacterial, viral, and fungal infections. Patients become more susceptible to opportunistic infections because of the weakened immune system (Ransohoff, 2016). Impaired immune surveillance is another limitation. The immune system normally plays a role in clearing abnormal proteins such as α-synuclein aggregates and detecting and eliminating malignant cells. Excessive immunosuppression may reduce the body's natural protective mechanisms (Tansey & Romero-Ramos, 2019). Poor specificity is also a major issue. Systemic drugs do not selectively target only the brain but also affect peripheral immune cells. Lack of specificity can lead to disturbances in normal immune homeostasis outside the central nervous system (Glass et al., 2010). Long-term side effects are another concern. Chronic immunosuppression may lead to metabolic disturbances, gastrointestinal problems, cardiovascular complications, and hormonal imbalances (Ransohoff, 2016). Therefore, modern therapeutic strategies aim to develop brain-specific targeted immunomodulation that reduces harmful neuroinflammation without compromising overall immune functions (Tansey & Romero-Ramos, 2019).

5. Immunotherapeutic and vaccination strategies in PD

5.1 Vaccination and Parkinson's disease

Immune activation refers to the immunophysiological process by which the host immune system is stimulated in response to potential threats such as an antigen from pathogen or from donor, tumour cells or vaccine antigens. Immune modulation refers to fine tuning or modification of immune response by changing or regulating it either by supressing it through immunosuppressant or by elevating it through immune response simulants in order to balance the immune response and manage or reverse the pathophysiological change presented in disease or disorder. Parkinson's Disease (PD) involves aggregation of alpha synuclein pathological forms in Lewy bodies and Lewy neurites and can potentially induce autoimmune response that accelerates PD progression involving binding with TLRs that subsequently leads to induction of release of pro-inflammatory cytokines from microglia causing neuroinflammation (Su & Zhou, 2021). Therefore, a number of active and passive immunotherapeutic approaches are being explored that aim at modulating this imbalance created by protein aggregation by using immunotherapeutic vaccines and passive mAb based approach for eliminating pathological alpha synuclein. PD, the 2nd most common neurodegenerative disorder is characterised by loss of dopaminergic neurons of substantia nigra pars compacts due to misfolding, accumulation and spread of SNCA gene encoded 140 aa long alpha synuclein protein aggregates that gradually form fibrils and then Lewy bodies in the soma or cell body of dopaminergic neurons and Lewy neurites in the neuronal processes including axons and dendrites (Mor et al., 2016). Under normal physiological state this protein is associated with a number of functions including intracellular trafficking, functioning of mitochondrion, dynamics of synaptic vesicle among others. Exact pathophysiological mechanism involved in onset and progression of PD is not completely elucidated yet it is evident that alpha synuclein and the gene encoding it are directly involved in its pathophysiology like prions considering that mutation in SNCA gene is associated with familial autosomal dominant PD. Therefore, alpha synuclein holds potential as a therapeutic target and by targeting alpha synuclein, by immunisation, the production and gradual spread of misfolded alpha synuclein and thus progression of PD can be retarded (Alfaidi et al., 2025).

Prophylaxis of a disease before its onset or exposure to causative pathogen is a common strategy that serves as basis for immunisation with most vaccines developed against infectious pathogenic diseases with exception of some post exposure pathogenic disease vaccines. However, unlike prophylactic vaccines that aim at preventing the disease by providing exposure to antigen and impart memory to immune system before one is exposed to actual infection, the strategy is not relevant in case of Parkinson's disease at least based on current understanding of PD and on basis of fact that most current PD vaccines under investigation focus of immunisation against PD through therapeutic vaccination instead of PD considering that alpha synuclein prophylactic vaccine could trigger auto-immunity in healthy individuals and that PD is largely sporadic with only 15 % of cases being familial (Pankratz & Foroud, 2007). Even in case of familial PD, the prophylactic vaccination for PD is not a relevant strategy considering that familial PD can occur due to mutation in various genes and not necessarily SNCA gene making prophylactic targeting challenging (Nuytemans et al., 2010). Moreover, typical onset of the disease in familial cases is around middle ages making prophylactic vaccines unsafe (due to potential auto-immunity development against normal self-antigen) before the onset of PD in genetically predisposed individuals as alpha synuclein has normal physiological roles in normal individuals even with genetic predisposition of PD. Apart for these factors, there can be many other possible reasons due to which most PD vaccines currently under development or in clinical trials are therapeutic and not prophylactic in nature unlike vaccines against pathogenic diseases. Some of the therapeutic vaccines developed against alpha synuclein currently in different phases of clinical trials include UB-312, AFFITOPE PD01A, PD03A, and ACI-7104.056 (Romero-Ramos et al., 2014; Alfaidi et al., 2025).

5.2 Active and passive immunization approaches

5.2.1 Active immunization

A number of different active immunisation-based vaccination strategies are currently being explored as therapeutics to slow down the progression of PD. Some of the vaccines have reached different phases of clinical trials and are developed by different biopharmaceutical enterprises involving different strategies. A number of peptide-based vaccines targeting alpha synuclein aggregation are under research and development and some of the vaccines have even reached the clinical trials. In a study by Ghochikyan et al., short sequences of engineered peptide vaccines were developed from B-cell epitopes connected to a non-self-carrier in order to increase immunogenicity and prevent T-cell tolerance and autoimmunity. Mice were immunised with engineered peptide vaccine, and they developed high titres of alpha synuclein specific antibodies in plasma that were able to recognise alpha synuclein aggregates in vitro and in vivo. These antibodies were found to enter CNS and bind aggregates of alpha synuclein. Additionally, the antibody response was epitope specific and did not cross react with human alpha synuclein (hα-Syn) indicating that peptide based engineered vaccines can effectively target alpha synuclein aggregates in Lewy bodies and Lewy neurites and hence reduce progression of PD (Ghochikyan et al., 2014). One of the synthetic peptide-based vaccine is UB-312, developed by Vaxxinity is alpha syn peptide conjugated to 'T' helper peptide, designed against alpha synuclein C-terminal epitope 97–135. It resulted in serum antibody production against antigen oligomeric and fibrillar forms with peak titres at week 29 that stayed above baseline up to week 45 (Alfaidi et al., 2025; Nimmo et al., 2022). Under Phase I trial, of the 50 healthy participants aged between 40–80 years of both sex that were enrolled in 44 week randomised, placebo-controlled double blind trial, 23 participants received all 3 doses of UB-312 intramuscularly at weeks 1, 5 and 12 with variable doses in 7 cohorts starting from 40 μg till 2000 μg in 7th cohort for 12 weeks followed by 32 weeks of follow up period (ClinicalTrials.gov: NCT04075318). General treatment-emergent adverse effects (TEAE) of mild, transient and self-resolving nature including headache, local puncture site pain, nasopharyngitis and fatigue were observed. Participants receiving dosage regimen of 300/300/300 μg of vaccine had detectable levels of antibodies in serum and CSF (Yu et al., 2022).

Further, under the phase 1 clinical trials of UB-312 that was conducted to assess safety, tolerability and immunogenicity of UB-312, 6 healthy individuals received placebo and 14 participants with PD received 2 different dosage regimens of UB-312 in two groups of 6 individuals each. Group 1 received dosage regimens of 300 μg /100 μg /100 μg while second group of participants with PD received dosage regimens of 7300 μg /300 μg /300 μg. Most TEAE were of mild to moderate severity comprising of headache, local pain post lumbar puncture and fatigue in similar frequency in all 14 participants with PD and 5 of 6 participants in placebo group (Eijsvogel et al., 2024). Analyis of blood, urine and other vital signs including electrocardiogram had no concerning deviations. Furthermore, in participants with PD with detectable UB-312 induced antibodies in Cerebrospinal fluid (CSF), reduction in amount of alpha synuclein aggregation and phosphorylated alpha synuclein was reported indicating potential therapeutic activity of vaccine in these participants (Alfaidi et al., 2025).

Like UB312, other peptide-based vaccines that targets alpha-syn oligomers and have reached clinical trials include AFFITOPE PD01A (AFF008) and PD03A (AFF011), developed by AFFiRiS. Both vaccines are engineered to elicit a selective humoral response against pathological alpha-synuclein species while preventing autoreactive T cell activation and deleterious neuroinflammation. PD01A is an engineered octamer peptide vaccine based on the C-terminal region of alpha synuclein, an exposed region in aggregated conformations allowing for selective targeting of oligomeric alpha syn and restricting interaction with physiological monomeric alpha syn. It is conjugated with carrier protein namely keyhole limpet haemocyanin (KLH) and absorbed onto aluminium hydroxide. KLH provides T-helper epitope while the PD01 antigen is involved in providing specificity to humoral response by acting as B-cell epitope (Volc et al., 2020). A series of trials were conducted under phase I evaluating safety, tolerability and immunogenicity of PD01A in patients with PD, validated by dopamine transporter single-photon emission computed tomography (DaT-SPECT). Under these trials, 32 participants with PD were enrolled of which 21 patients were suitable for immunisation and stayed throughout trials. These participants were randomised and administered with 4 subcutaneous priming immunisations into upper arm with 15 μg or 75 μg of PD01A and were followed up till 91 weeks comprising of 52 weeks of initial follow up and then subsequent 39 weeks follow up. All patients were given 2 booster doses with 1st dose of 15 μg, or 75 μg post re-randomisation and then subsequent 2nd dose of 75 μg. All patients except one displayed transient local injection site reactions as TEAE (Alfaidi et al., 2025).

5.2.2 Passive immunization

A number of passive immunisation-based immunotherapies involving use of monoclonal antibodies have been developed against alpha-synuclein pathological form for treatment of PD and a few of them have reached different clinical trial phases yet none of them have been approved as of now. A Humanised IgG1 mAb, Prasinizumab developed by Prothena and Roche from mouse 9E4 mAb, which recognises amino acids 118–126 of human alpha synuclein. It has displayed decrease in neurotoxicity and neuropathology by reducing truncated form of alpha syn and preventing them from spreading across neurons (Xiao & Tan, 2025; Alfaidi et al., 2025). However, Certain post translational modifications such as nitration of Y125 of alpha synuclein and truncated forms of alpha synuclein such as C-terminal truncated alpha synuclein (α-SynΔC) are not recognised by Prasinezumab and thus can evade antibody binding, rendering it ineffective in degrading such pathological forms of alpha synuclein (Xiao & Tan, 2025). Another anti-alpha synuclein mAb, namely, Cinpanemab progressed up to clinical trials phase II (NCT03318523) (clinicaltrials.gov/ct2/show/NCT03318523) in PD but its subsequent development was halted post failure of SPARK trial in demonstrating clinical efficacy and failure to meet primary and secondary endpoints (Hutchison et al., 2024).

6. Preclinical and clinical evaluation

The misfolding and aggregation of α-syn can spread from cell-to-cell to different brain regions, as demonstrated by intrastriatal injection of synthetic α-syn PFF in WT mice. Similar injections of mouse α-syn PFF into rats also showed an increase in the accumulation of misfolded protein and further degeneration. This robust neurodegenerative pathology was seen 60–90 days post injection in different regions of the brain interconnected to each other. The spread of α-syn occurs in the form of phosphorylated α-synuclein (pS129), towards the SNpc. MPTP (1-methyl-4-phenyl-1,2,3,6-tetrahydropyri dine) is a mitochondrial toxin which is able to generate parkinson-like features in different animal models like mice, monkeys, and humans. It can cross the BBB due to its lipophilic nature and its active metabolite, 1-methyl-4-phenylpiridinium (MPP^+) made with the help of the enzyme monoamine oxidase B, can enter DA neurons using dopamine transporter (DAT). The mitochondrial respiratory chain is blocked due to the inhibition of complex I by MPP^+ and this leads to the generation of ROS and thus oxidative stress. The MPTP induction shows reduction in dopamine transporter (DAT) in the striatum, accompanied by the death of DA cell bodies in the SNpc. Several studies explore the MPTP dose-dependent activation of microglia (Merghani et al., 2021; Fornai et al., 2005). AFFITOPE (AFF) peptide vaccines, PD01A and PD03A, given in two different tg mouse models, were able to produce high titers of antibodies against α-Syn. The mouse models were overexpressing α-Syn under the PDGF promoter and the thymus cell antigen 1 (Thy1) promoter. AFF® PD01A immunization was able to reduce motor dysfunction, impaired memory, and α-Syn deposition. In the MSA mouse model, PD01A was able to provide protection against α-Syn aggregation (Mandler et al., 2014; Mandler et al., 2015). Two phase I trials evaluated the safety and tolerability of the vaccine in patients with MSA or PD. Similarly, AFF® PD03A was assessed in a separate clinical trial (NCT02267434) for its safety. It produces a sustained IgG antibody response against the PD03 peptide (Poewe et al., 2021). Another active immunization vaccine, UB-312 was proven to be well tolerated, safe, and produced anti-β-Syn antibodies in serum and CSF of all patients in a phase I study with 300/300/300 μg dose regimen (Yu et al., 2022).

The compound AFFITOPE® (AFF 1) was tested in the α-Syn transgenic mice, MBP, and it showed a reduction in the aggregation and an increase in the anti-inflammatory response in MBP (Mandler et al., 2015). The use of human-derived antibody BIIB054 in transgenic α-Syn A53T (M83) and BAC A53 mice targeted the N-terminus of α-Syn aggregates and showed improvement in motor symptoms (Weihofen et al., 2019). Similarly, PRX002 administration in the mThy1-α-Syn (line 61) caused a reduction in intracellular α-Syn and activation of astroglia and microglia(Games et al., 2014). The active immunotherapies, PD01A and PD03A, mimic α-syn C-terminal and cause reduction of α-Syn oligomers in CSF and IgG antibody response to α-syn epitope, with the completion of the safety and tolerability trial (Volc et al., 2020; Poewe et al., 2021). The monoclonal antibody PRX002/RG7935 (PRX002) has demonstrated good safety and tolerability with reduced free serum α-syn (Jankovic et al., 2018). Another passive immunotherapeutic antibody, BIIB054 (Cinpanemab) targeted aggregated α-syn but could not meet the primary and secondary outcomes of the Phase I trial (Brys et al., 2019).

7. Challenges and future scope

Although our understanding of neuroimmune processes in Parkinson's disease has improved, one major challenge that still remains is identifying the molecular link between α-synuclein aggregation and activation of the immune system. It is known that α-Synuclein aggregates activate microglia through mechanisms involving Toll-like receptors and the NLRP3 inflammasome, but the exact process that links protein misfolding to chronic inflammation is still unclear (Stefanova, 2022; Harms et al., 2021). Another challenge is the complexity of peripheral–central immune crosstalk. Peripheral immune cells, including monocytes and T lymphocytes, have been shown to enter the CNS and participate in neurodegeneration. Yet, the factors regulating this interaction and its timing during disease progression are not fully understood (Greenland et al., 2025; Brochard et al., 2009; Zhu et al., 2022). Therapeutic development in PD also remains challenging as many anti-inflammatory drugs suppress the immune system, which in turn increases susceptibility to multiple infections. In addition, many drugs cannot easily cross the blood–brain barrier, which reduces treatment effectiveness. Although α-synuclein vaccines and monoclonal antibodies appear safe, several have not shown clear benefits in clinical trials, highlighting the need for more precise therapeutic strategies and a deeper understanding of PD immunopathology studies (Volc et al., 2020; Hutchison et al., 2024). Future studies should aim to explain how α-synuclein aggregation triggers immune responses, particularly through pathways like Toll-like receptors, NF-κB, and inflammasomes (Stefanova, 2022; Harms et al., 2021). A clearer understanding of how the peripheral immune system (monocytes, T-cell activity, cytokines, and the gut microbiome) is involved in PD may provide important insights into how systemic inflammation contributes to disease progression (Greenland et al., 2025; Brochard et al., 2009). Another promising direction is the development of reliable biomarkers that link peripheral immune activation with neurodegeneration. Biomarkers in blood and cerebrospinal fluid, such as inflammatory cytokines, alpha-synuclein, and immune cell markers, may help in early detection improved monitoring of the progression of PD (Zhu et al., 2022). Improving vaccines and antibody therapies that target alpha-synuclein, along with personalized treatment approaches based on one's immune responses, may help develop better therapies that can slow or modify the progression of Parkinson's disease (Volc et al., 2020; Alfaidi et al., 2025).

8. Conclusion

Parkinson's disease is increasingly recognised as a multifaceted neurodegenerative disorder wherein immune dysfunction and persistent neuroinflammation play a crucial role in the progression of the disease. The aggregation of misfolded α-synuclein acts as a significant catalyst for immune activation, prompting microglia and astrocytes to release inflammatory cytokines like TNF-α, IL-1β, and IL-6, which lead to oxidative stress, mitochondrial impairment, and the loss of dopaminergic neurons. Furthermore, research suggests that neuroinflammation extends beyond the central nervous system and involves considerable communication between the peripheral and central immune systems. When the blood-brain barrier is weakened, immune cells such as monocytes, T cells, and B cells can enter the brain which further worsens inflammation. Growing research into the gut–brain axis suggests that inflammation in the gut and changes in the gut microbiome may promote the progression of α-synuclein pathology via the vagus nerve. Therapeutic approaches targeting immune mechanisms, especially α-synuclein–focused immunotherapies like peptide vaccines and monoclonal antibodies, have demonstrated promising outcomes in both preclinical and early clinical trials. Collectively, these observations highlight the importance of immune-related mechanisms in shaping the progression of Parkinson's disease and the development of targeted therapeutics.

References

Alahmari, A. (2021). Blood-brain barrier overview: Structural and functional correlation. *Neural Plasticity, 2021*. https://doi.org/10.1155/2021/6564585.

Alfaidi, M., Barker, R. A., & Kuan, W. L. (2025). An update on immune-based alpha-synuclein trials in Parkinson's disease. *Journal of Neurology, 272*(1), https://doi.org/10.1007/s00415-024-12770-x.

Anderson, J. P., Walker, D. E., Goldstein, J. M., De Laat, R., Banducci, K., Caccavello, R. J., ... Chilcote, T. J. (2006). Phosphorylation of Ser-129 is the dominant pathological modification of α-synuclein in familial and sporadic lewy body disease. *Journal of Biological Chemistry, 281*(40), https://doi.org/10.1074/jbc.M600933200.

Aggarwal, B. B., & Harikumar, K. B. (2009). Potential therapeutic effects of curcumin, the anti-inflammatory agent, against neurodegenerative, cardiovascular, pulmonary, metabolic, autoimmune and neoplastic diseases. *International Journal of Biochemistry & Cell Biology, 41*(1), 40–59. https://doi.org/10.1016/j.biocel.2008.06.010.

Beal, M. F. (2003). Bioenergetic approaches for neuroprotection in Parkinson's disease. *Annals of Neurology, 53*(S3), S39–S48. https://doi.org/10.1002/ana.10488.

Baxter, D. (2007). Active and passive immunity, vaccine types, excipients and licensing. *Occupational Medicine, 57*(Number 8), https://doi.org/10.1093/occmed/kqm110.

Bower, J. H., Maraganore, D. M., Peterson, B. J., Ahlskog, J. E., & Rocca, W. A. (2006). Immunologic diseases, anti-inflammatory drugs, and Parkinson disease: A case-control study. *Neurology, 67*(3), https://doi.org/10.1212/01.wnl.0000227906.99570.cc.

Boza-Serrano, A., Reyes, J. F., Rey, N. L., Leffler, H., Bousset, L., Nilsson, U., ... Deierborg, T. (2014). The role of Galectin-3 in α-synuclein-induced microglial activation. *Acta Neuropathologica Communications, 2*(Number 1), https://doi.org/10.1186/s40478-014-0156-0.

Braak, H., Del Tredici, K., Rüb, U., De Vos, R. A. I., Jansen Steur, E. N. H., & Braak, E. (2003). Staging of brain pathology related to sporadic Parkinson's disease. *Neurobiology of Aging, 24*(2), https://doi.org/10.1016/S0197-4580(02)00065-9.

Brochard, V., Combadière, B., Prigent, A., Laouar, Y., Perrin, A., Beray-Berthat, V., ... Hunot, S. (2009). Infiltration of CD4+ lymphocytes into the brain contributes to neurodegeneration in a mouse model of Parkinson disease. *Journal of Clinical Investigation, 119*(1), https://doi.org/10.1172/JCI36470.

Barnes, P. J. (2016). Glucocorticosteroids: Current and future directions. *British Journal of Pharmacology, 173*(1), 27–43. https://doi.org/10.1111/bph.13302.

Block, M. L., Zecca, L., & Hong, J. S. (2007). Microglia-mediated neurotoxicity: Uncovering the molecular mechanisms. *Nature Reviews. Neuroscience, 8*(1), 57–69. https://doi.org/10.1038/nrn2038.

Brys, M., Fanning, L., Hung, S., Ellenbogen, A., Penner, N., Yang, M., ... Cedarbaum, J. M. (2019). Randomized phase I clinical trial of anti–α-synuclein antibody BIIB054. *Movement Disorders, 34*(8), https://doi.org/10.1002/mds.27738.

Balasa, R., Barcutean, L., Mosora, O., & Manu, D. (2021). Reviewing the significance of blood–brain barrier disruption in multiple sclerosis pathogenesis and treatment. *International Journal of Molecular Sciences, 22*(16), 8370. https://doi.org/10.3390/ijms22168370.

Bennett, J., Basivireddy, J., Kollar, A., Biron, K. E., Reickmann, P., Jefferies, W. A., & McQuaid, S. (2010). Blood–brain barrier disruption and enhanced vascular permeability in the multiple sclerosis model EAE. *Journal of Neuroimmunology, 229*(1–2), 180–191. https://doi.org/10.1016/j.jneuroim.2010.07.011.

Cao, S., Theodore, S., & Standaert, D. G. (2010). Fcγ receptors are required for NF-kB signaling, microglial activation and dopaminergic neurodegeneration in an AAV-synuclein mouse model of Parkinson's disease. *Molecular Neurodegeneration, 5*(1), https://doi.org/10.1186/1750-1326-5-42.

Cote, S., Carmichael, P. H., Verreault, R., Lindsay, J., Lefebvre, J., & Laurin, D. (2015). Nonsteroidal anti-inflammatory drug use and the risk of Parkinson's disease: A systematic review and meta-analysis. *Neuroepidemiology, 44*(3), 178–187. https://doi.org/10.1159/000381106.

Cersosimo, M. G., & Benarroch, E. E. (2012). Pathological correlates of gastrointestinal dysfunction in Parkinson's disease. *Neurobiology of Disease, 46*(Number 3), https://doi.org/10.1016/j.nbd.2011.10.014.

Calder, P. C. (2015). Marine omega-3 fatty acids and inflammatory processes: Effects, mechanisms and clinical relevance. *Biochimica et Biophysica Acta (BBA) – Molecular and Cell Biology of Lipids, 1851*(4), 469–484. https://doi.org/10.1016/j.bbalip.2014.08.010.

Daneman, R., & Prat, A. (2015). The blood–brain barrier. *Cold Spring Harbor Perspectives in Biology,* 7(1), a020412. https://doi.org/10.1101/cshperspect.a020412.

Dias, V., Junn, E., & Mouradian, M. M. (2013). The role of oxidative stress in Parkinson's disease. *Journal of Parkinson's Disease, 3*(4), 461–491. https://doi.org/10.3233/JPD-130230.

Dinarello, C. A. (2011). Interleukin-1 in the pathogenesis and treatment of inflammatory diseases. *Blood, 117*(14), 3720–3732. https://doi.org/10.1182/blood-2010-07-273417.

Exner, N., Lutz, A. K., Haass, C., & Winklhofer, K. F. (2012). Mitochondrial dysfunction in Parkinson's disease: Molecular mechanisms and pathophysiological consequences. *EMBO Journal, 31*(14), 3038–3062. https://doi.org/10.1038/emboj.2012.170.

Eijsvogel, P., Misra, P., Concha-Marambio, L., Boyd, J. D., Ding, S., Fedor, L., ... Dodart, J. C. (2024). Target engagement and immunogenicity of an active immunotherapeutic targeting pathological α-synuclein: A phase 1 placebo-controlled trial. *Nature Medicine, 30*(9), https://doi.org/10.1038/s41591-024-03101-8.

Fornai, F., Schlüter, O. M., Lenzi, P., Gesi, M., Ruffoli, R., Ferrucci, M., ... Südhof, T. C. (2005). Parkinson-like syndrome induced by continuous MPTP infusion: Convergent roles of the ubiquitin-proteasome system and α-synuclein. *Proceedings of the National Academy of Sciences of the United States of America, 102*(9), https://doi.org/10.1073/pnas.0409713102.

Games, D., Valera, E., Spencer, B., Rockenstein, E., Mante, M., Adame, A., ... Masliah, E. (2014). Reducing C-terminal-truncated alpha-synuclein by immunotherapy attenuates neurodegeneration and propagation in Parkinson's disease-like models. *Journal of Neuroscience, 34*(28), https://doi.org/10.1523/JNEUROSCI.5314-13.2014.

Ghochikyan, A., Petrushina, I., Davtyan, H., Hovakimyan, A., Saing, T., Davtyan, A., ... Agadjanyan, M. G. (2014). Immunogenicity of epitope vaccines targeting different B cell antigenic determinants of human α-synuclein: Feasibility study. *Neuroscience Letters, 560*. https://doi.org/10.1016/j.neulet.2013.12.028.

Gomez-Isla, T., Irizarry, M. C., Mariash, A., Cheung, B., Soto, O., Schrump, S., ... Ashe, K. H. (2003). Motor dysfunction and gliosis with preserved dopaminergic markers in human α-synuclein A30P transgenic mice. *Neurobiology of Aging, 24*(2), https://doi.org/10.1016/S0197-4580(02)00091-X.

Greenland, J. C., Holbrook, J., Kahanawita, L., Camacho, M., Fryer, T. D., Hong, Y. T., & Williams-Gray, C. H. (2025). Peripheral-central immune crosstalk in Parkinson's disease and its association with clinical severity. *Brain, Behavior, and Immunity, 128*. https://doi.org/10.1016/j.bbi.2025.04.028.

Glass, C. K., Saijo, K., Winner, B., Marchetto, M. C., & Gage, F. H. (2010). Mechanisms underlying inflammation in neurodegeneration. *Cell, 140*(6), 918–934. https://doi.org/10.1016/j.cell.2010.02.016.

Grozdanov, V., Bliederhaeuser, C., Ruf, W. P., Roth, V., Fundel-Clemens, K., Zondler, L., ... Ludolph, A. C. (2014). Inflammatory dysregulation of blood monocytes in Parkinson's disease patients. *Acta Neuropathologica, 128*(5), 651–663. https://doi.org/10.1007/s00401-014-1345-4.

Gendelman, H. E., Appel, S. H., Mosley, R. L., & LaVoie, M. J. (2017). The role of regulatory T cells in Parkinson's disease. *Nature Reviews Neurology, 13*(11), 653–664. https://doi.org/10.1038/nrneurol.2017.120.

Hansson, O., Janelidze, S., Hall, S., Magdalinou, N., Lees, A. J., Andreasson, U., ... Blennow, K. (2017). Blood-based NfL: A biomarker for differential diagnosis of parkinsonian disorder. *Neurology, 88*(10), 930–937. https://doi.org/10.1212/WNL.0000000000003680.

Harms, A. S., Barnum, C. J., Ruhn, K. A., Varghese, S., Trevĩo, I., Blesch, A., & Tansey, M. G. (2011). Delayed dominant-negative TNF gene therapy halts progressive loss of nigral dopaminergic neurons in a rat model of parkinson's disease. *Molecular Therapy, 19*(1), https://doi.org/10.1038/mt.2010.217.

Harms, A. S., Ferreira, S. A., & Romero-Ramos, M. (2021). Periphery and brain, innate and adaptive immunity in Parkinson's disease. *Acta Neuropathologica, 141*(Number 4), https://doi.org/10.1007/s00401-021-02268-5.

Hirsch, E. C., & Hunot, S. (2009). Neuroinflammation in Parkinson's disease: A target for neuroprotection? *Lancet Neurology, 8*(4), 382–397. https://doi.org/10.1016/S1474-4422(09)70062-6.

Hutchison, R. M., Fraser, K., Yang, M., Fox, T., Hirschhorn, E., Njingti, E., ... Beaver, J. (2024). Cinpanemab in early Parkinson disease. *Neurology, 102*(5), https://doi.org/10.1212/wnl.0000000000209137.

Jang, H., Boltz, D., Sturm-Ramirez, K., Shepherd, K. R., Jiao, Y., Webster, R., & Smeyne, R. J. (2009). Highly pathogenic H5N1 influenza virus can enter the central nervous system and induce neuroinflammation and neurodegeneration. *Proceedings of the National Academy of Sciences of the United States of America, 106*(33), https://doi.org/10.1073/pnas.0900096106.

Jankovic, J., Goodman, I., Safirstein, B., Marmon, T. K., Schenk, D. B., Koller, M., ... Kinney, G. G. (2018). Safety and tolerability of multiple ascending doses of PRX002/RG7935, an anti-synuclein monoclonal antibody, in patients with Parkinson disease: A randomized clinical trial. *JAMA Neurology, 75*(10), https://doi.org/10.1001/jamaneurol.2018.1487.

Krashia, P., Cordella, A., Nobili, A., La Barbera, L., Federici, M., Leuti, A., ... Mercuri, N. B. (2019). Blunting neuroinflammation with resolvin D1 prevents early pathology in a rat model of Parkinson's disease. *Nature Communications, 10*(1), https://doi.org/10.1038/s41467-019-11928-w.

Krüger, R., Kuhn, W., Müller, T., Woitalla, D., Graeber, M., Kösel, S., ... Riess, O. (1998). Ala30Pro mutation in the gene encoding α-synuclein in Parkinson's disease. *Nature Genetics, 18*(2), https://doi.org/10.1038/ng0298-106.

Kalia, L. V., & Lang, A. E. (2015). Parkinson's disease. *The Lancet, 386*(9996), 896–912. https://doi.org/10.1016/S0140-6736(14)61393-3.

Korn, T., Bettelli, E., Oukka, M., & Kuchroo, V. K. (2009). IL-17 and Th17 cells. *Annual Review of Immunology, 27*, 485–517. https://doi.org/10.1146/annurev.immunol.021908.132710.

Lema Tomé, C. M., Tyson, T., Rey, N. L., Grathwohl, S., Britschgi, M., & Brundin, P. (2013). Inflammation and α-synuclein's prion-like behavior in Parkinson's disease–is there a link? *Molecular Neurobiology, 47*(Number 2), https://doi.org/10.1007/s12035-012-8267-8.

Loseva, E., Yuan, T. F., & Karnup, S. (2009). Neurogliogenesis in the mature olfactory system: A possible protective role against infection and toxic dust. *Brain Research Reviews, 59*(Number 2), https://doi.org/10.1016/j.brainresrev.2008.10.004.

Lindestam Arlehamn, C. S., Dhanwani, R., Pham, J., Kuan, R., Frazier, A., Rezende Dutra, J., ... Sette, A. (2020). α-Synuclein-specific T cell reactivity is associated with preclinical and early Parkinson's disease. *Nature Communications, 11*, 1875. https://doi.org/10.1038/s41467-020-15626-w.

Madsen, L., Labrecque, N., Engberg, J., Dierich, A., Svejgaard, A., Benoist, C., ... Fugger, L. (1999). Mice lacking all conventional MHC class II genes. *Proceedings of the National Academy of Sciences of the United States of America, 96*(18), https://doi.org/10.1073/pnas.96.18.10338.

Mahlknecht, P., Seppi, K., & Poewe, W. (2015). The concept of prodromal Parkinson's disease. *Journal of Parkinson's Disease, 5*(Number 4), https://doi.org/10.3233/JPD-150685.

Mandler, M., Valera, E., Rockenstein, E., Mante, M., Weninger, H., Patrick, C., ... Masliah, E. (2015). Active immunization against alpha-synuclein ameliorates the degenerative pathology and prevents demyelination in a model of multiple system atrophy. *Molecular Neurodegeneration, 10*(1), https://doi.org/10.1186/s13024-015-0008-9.

Mandler, M., Valera, E., Rockenstein, E., Weninger, H., Patrick, C., Adame, A., ... Masliah, E. (2014). Next-generation active immunization approach for synucleinopathies: Implications for Parkinson's disease clinical trials. *Acta Neuropathologica, 127*(6), https://doi.org/10.1007/s00401-014-1256-4.

Maroteaux, L., Campanelli, J. T., & Scheller, R. H. (1988). Synuclein: A neuron-specific protein localized to the nucleus and presynaptic nerve terminal. *Journal of Neuroscience, 8*(8), https://doi.org/10.1523/jneurosci.08-08-02804.1988.

McCoy, M. K., & Tansey, M. G. (2008). TNF signaling inhibition in the CNS: Implications for normal brain function and neurodegenerative disease. *Journal of Neuroinflammation, 5*, 45. https://doi.org/10.1186/1742-2094-5-45.

McGeer, P. L., Itagaki, S., Boyes, B. E., & McGeer, E. G. (1988). Reactive microglia are positive for HLA-DR in the: Substantia nigra of Parkinson's and Alzheimer's disease brains. *Neurology, 38*(8), https://doi.org/10.1212/wnl.38.8.1285.

Merghani, M. M., Ardah, M. T., Al Shamsi, M., Kitada, T., & Haque, M. E. (2021). Dose-related biphasic effect of the Parkinson's disease neurotoxin MPTP, on the spread, accumulation, and toxicity of α-synuclein. *Neurotoxicology, 84*. https://doi.org/10.1016/j.neuro.2021.02.001.

Mor, D. E., Ugras, S. E., Daniels, M. J., & Ischiropoulos, H. (2016). Dynamic structural flexibility of α-synuclein. *Neurobiology of Disease, 88*. https://doi.org/10.1016/j.nbd.2015.12.018.

Moustafa, A. A., Chakravarthy, S., Phillips, J. R., Gupta, A., Keri, S., Polner, B., ... Jahanshahi, M. (2016). Motor symptoms in Parkinson's disease: A unified framework. *Neuroscience and Biobehavioral Reviews, 68*. https://doi.org/10.1016/j.neubiorev.2016.07.010.

Nimmo, J. T., Smith, H., Wang, C. Y., Teeling, J. L., Nicoll, J. A. R., Verma, A., ... Carare, R. O. (2022). Immunisation with UB-312 in the Thy1SNCA mouse prevents motor performance deficits and oligomeric α-synuclein accumulation in the brain and gut. *Acta Neuropathologica, 143*(1), https://doi.org/10.1007/s00401-021-02381-5.

Nuytemans, K., Theuns, J., Cruts, M., & Van Broeckhoven, C. (2010). Genetic etiology of Parkinson disease associated with mutations in the SNCA, PARK2, PINK1, PARK7, and LRRK2 genes: A mutation update. *Human Mutation, 31*(Number 7), https://doi.org/10.1002/humu.21277.

Orihuela, R., McPherson, C. A., & Harry, G. J. (2016). Microglial M1/M2 polarization and metabolic states. *British Journal of Pharmacology, 173*(Number 4), https://doi.org/10.1111/bph.13139.

Pankratz, N., & Foroud, T. (2007). Genetics of Parkinson disease. *Genetics in Medicine, 9*(Number 12), https://doi.org/10.1097/GIM.0b013e31815bf97c.

Park, J. Y., Kim, K. S., Lee, S. B., Ryu, J. S., Chung, K. C., Choo, Y. K., ... Park, S. M. (2009). On the mechanism of internalization of α-synuclein into microglia: Roles of ganglioside GM1 and lipid raft. *Journal of Neurochemistry, 110*(1), https://doi.org/10.1111/j.1471-4159.2009.06150.x.

Perry, V. H., Cunningham, C., & Holmes, C. (2010). Systemic infections and inflammation affect chronic neurodegeneration. *Nature Reviews. Immunology, 10*(3), 217–226. https://doi.org/10.1038/nri2728.

Poewe, W., Seppi, K., Tanner, C., Halliday, G. M., Brundin, P., Volkmann, J., ... Lang, A. E. (2017). Parkinson disease. Nature reviews disease primers. *Nature Reviews Disease Primers, 3*(17014).

Poewe, W., Volc, Di, Seppi, K., Medori, R., Lührs, P., Kutzelnigg, A., ... Galabova, G. (2021). Safety and tolerability of active immunotherapy targeting α-synuclein with PD03A in patients with early Parkinson's disease: A randomized, placebo-controlled, phase 1 study. *Journal of Parkinson's Disease, 11*(3), https://doi.org/10.3233/JPD-212594.

Polymeropoulos, M. H., Lavedan, C., Leroy, E., Ide, S. E., Dehejia, A., Dutra, A., ... Nussbaum, R. L. (1997). Mutation in the α-synuclein gene identified in families with Parkinson's disease. *Science (New York, N. Y.), 276*(5321), https://doi.org/10.1126/science.276.5321.2045.

Pringsheim, T., Jette, N., Frolkis, A., & Steeves, T. D. L. (2014). The prevalence of Parkinson's disease: A systematic review and meta-analysis. *Movement Disorders, 29*(Number 13), https://doi.org/10.1002/mds.25945.

Pulendran, B., & Davis, M. M. (2020). The science and medicine of human immunology. *Science, 369*(Number 6511), https://doi.org/10.1126/science.aay4014.

Qin, X. Y., Zhang, S. P., Cao, C., Loh, Y. P., & Cheng, Y. (2016). Aberrations in peripheral inflammatory cytokine levels in Parkinson disease. *JAMA Neurology, 73*(11), 1316–1324. https://doi.org/10.1001/jamaneurol.2016.2742.

Ray Dorsey, E., Elbaz, A., Nichols, E., Abd-Allah, F., Abdelalim, A., Adsuar, J. C., ... Murray, C. J. L. (2018). Global, regional, and national burden of Parkinson's disease, 1990–2016: A systematic analysis for the Global Burden of Disease Study 2016. *The Lancet Neurology, 17*(11), https://doi.org/10.1016/S1474-4422(18)30295-3.

Rohn, T. T., & Catlin, L. W. (2011). Immunolocalization of influenza a virus and markers of inflammation in the human Parkinson's disease brain. *PLoS One, 6*(5), https://doi.org/10.1371/journal.pone.0020495.

Romero-Ramos, M., Chelpin, M. V. E., & Sanchez-Guajardo, V. (2014). Vaccination strategies for Parkinson disease: Induction of a swift attack or raising tolerance? *Human Vaccines and Immunotherapeutics, 10*(Number 4), https://doi.org/10.4161/hv.28578.

Ransohoff, R. M. (2016). How neuroinflammation contributes to neurodegeneration. *Science (New York, N. Y.), 353*(6301), 777–783. https://doi.org/10.1126/science.aag2590.

Schapira, A. H. V., Chaudhuri, K. R., & Jenner, P. (2017). Non-motor features of Parkinson disease. *Nature Reviews Neuroscience, 18*(Number 7), https://doi.org/10.1038/nrn.2017.62.

Scheiblich, H., Dansokho, C., Mercan, D., Schmidt, S. V., Bousset, L., Wischhof, L., ... Heneka, M. T. (2021). Microglia jointly degrade fibrillar alpha-synuclein cargo by distribution through tunneling nanotubes. *Cell, 184*(20), https://doi.org/10.1016/j.cell.2021.09.007.

Sonar, S. A., & Lal, G. (2017). Differentiation and transmigration of CD4 T cells in neuroinflammation and autoimmunity. *Frontiers in Immunology, 8.* https://doi.org/10.3389/fimmu.2017.01695 (Number NOV).

Sporici, R., & Issekutz, T. B. (2010). CXCR3 blockade inhibits T-cell migration into the CNS during EAE and prevents development of adoptively transferred, but not actively induced, disease. *European Journal of Immunology, 40*(10), https://doi.org/10.1002/eji.200939975.

Stefanova, N. (2022). Microglia in Parkinson's disease. *Journal of Parkinson's Disease, 12.* https://doi.org/10.3233/JPD-223237.

Su, R., & Zhou, T. (2021). Alpha-synuclein induced immune cells activation and associated therapy in Parkinson's disease. *Frontiers in Aging Neuroscience, 13.* https://doi.org/10.3389/fnagi.2021.769506.

Su, Y., Shi, C., Wang, T., Liu, C., Yang, J., Zhang, S., ... Xu, Y. (2022). Dysregulation of peripheral monocytes and pro-inflammation of alpha-synuclein in Parkinson's disease. *Journal of Neurology, 269*(12), https://doi.org/10.1007/s00415-022-11258-w.

Surmeier, D. J. (2018). Determinants of dopaminergic neuron loss in Parkinson's disease. *FEBS Journal, 285*(Number 19), https://doi.org/10.1111/febs.14607.

Sweeney, M. D., Sagare, A. P., & Zlokovic, B. V. (2018). Blood–brain barrier breakdown in neurodegenerative disorders. *Nature Reviews Neurology, 14*, 133–150.

Sommer, A., Marxreiter, F., Krach, F., Fadler, T., Grosch, J., Maroni, M., ... Winner, B. (2018). Th17 lymphocytes induce neuronal cell death in a human iPSC-based model of Parkinson's disease. *Cell Stem Cell, 23*(1), 123–131. https://doi.org/10.1016/j.stem.2018.06.015.

Storelli, E., Cassina, N., Rasini, E., Marino, F., & Cosentino, M. (2019). Do Th17 lymphocytes and IL-17 contribute to Parkinson's disease? *Journal of Neuroimmune Pharmacology, 14*, 23–31. https://doi.org/10.1007/s11481-018-9829-0.

Sulzer, D., Alcalay, R. N., Garretti, F., Cote, L., Kanter, E., Agin-Liebes, J., ... Sette, A. (2017). T cells from patients with Parkinson's disease recognize α-synuclein peptides. *Nature, 546*(7660), 656–661. https://doi.org/10.1038/nature22815.

Tansey, M. G., & Romero-Ramos, M. (2019). Immune system responses in Parkinson's disease: Early and dynamic. *European Journal of Neuroscience, 49*(3), 364–383. https://doi.org/10.1111/ejn.14290.

Tanaka, T., Narazaki, M., & Kishimoto, T. (2014). Interleukin-6 in inflammation, immunity, and disease. *Cold Spring Harbor Perspectives in Biology, 6*(10), a016295. https://doi.org/10.1101/cshperspect.a016295.

Tang, Y., & Le, W. (2016). Differential roles of microglia in neurodegenerative diseases. *Molecular Neurobiology, 53*(2), 1181–1194. https://doi.org/10.1007/s12035-014-9070-5.

Volc, D., Poewe, W., Kutzelnigg, A., Lührs, P., Thun-Hohenstein, C., Schneeberger, A., ... Medori, R. (2020). Safety and immunogenicity of the α-synuclein active immunotherapeutic PD01A in patients with Parkinson's disease: A randomised, single-blinded, phase 1 trial. *The Lancet Neurology, 19*(7), https://doi.org/10.1016/S1474-4422(20)30136-8.

Varatharaj, A., & Galea, I. (2017). The blood–brain barrier in systemic inflammation. *Brain, Behavior, and Immunity, 60*, 1–12. https://doi.org/10.1016/j.bbi.2016.03.010.

Vauzour, D., Vafeiadou, K., Rodriguez-Mateos, A., Rendeiro, C., & Spencer, J. P. (2010). The neuroprotective potential of flavonoids: A multiplicity of effects. *Genes & Nutrition, 5*(2), 115–126. https://doi.org/10.1007/s12263-010-0156-6.

Watson, M. B., Richter, F., Lee, S. K., Gabby, L., Wu, J., Masliah, E., ... Chesselet, M. F. (2012). Regionally-specific microglial activation in young mice over-expressing human wildtype alpha-synuclein. *Experimental Neurology, 237*(2), https://doi.org/10.1016/j.expneurol.2012.06.025.

Weihofen, A., Liu, Y. T., Arndt, J. W., Huy, C., Quan, C., Smith, B. A., ... Weinreb, P. H. (2019). Development of an aggregate-selective, human-derived α-synuclein antibody BIIB054 that ameliorates disease phenotypes in Parkinson's disease models. *Neurobiology of Disease, 124*. https://doi.org/10.1016/j.nbd.2018.10.016.

Wahner, A. D., Sinsheimer, J. S., Bronstein, J. M., & Ritz, B. (2007). Inflammatory cytokine gene polymorphisms and the risk of Parkinson's disease. *Neurogenetics, 8*, 181–188. https://doi.org/10.1007/s10048-007-0082-8.

Xiao, B., & Tan, E. K. (2025). Prasinezumab slows motor progression in Parkinsons disease: beyond the clinical data. *Npj Parkinson's Disease, 11*(1), https://doi.org/10.1038/s41531-025-00886-4.

Yu, E., Ambati, A., Andersen, M. S., Krohn, L., Estiar, M. A., Saini, P., ... Gan-Or, Z. (2021). Fine mapping of the HLA locus in Parkinson's disease in Europeans. *Npj Parkinson's Disease,* 7(1), https://doi.org/10.1038/s41531-021-00231-5.

Yu, H. J., Thijssen, E., van Brummelen, E., van der Plas, J. L., Radanovic, I., Moerland, M., ... Dodart, J. C. (2022). A randomized first-in-human study with UB-312, a UBITh® α-synuclein peptide vaccine. *Movement Disorders, 37*(7), https://doi.org/10.1002/mds.29016.

Zarranz, J. J., Alegre, J., Gómez-Esteban, J. C., Lezcano, E., Ros, R., Ampuero, I., ... De Yebenes, J. G. (2004). The new mutation, E46K, of α-synuclein causes Parkinson and lewy body dementia. *Annals of Neurology, 55*(2), https://doi.org/10.1002/ana.10795.

Zhang, W., Dallas, S., Zhang, D., Guo, J. P., Pang, H., Wilson, B., ... Zhang, J. (2007). Microglial PHOX and Mac-1 are essential to the enhanced dopaminergic neurodegeneration elicited by A30P and A53T mutant alpha-synuclein. *Glia, 55*(11), https://doi.org/10.1002/glia.20532.

Zhu, B., Yin, D., Zhao, H., & Zhang, L. (2022). The immunology of Parkinson's disease. *Seminars in Immunopathology, 44*(Number 5), https://doi.org/10.1007/s00281-022-00947-3.

Zierfuss, B., Larochelle, C., & Prat, A. (2024). Blood–brain barrier dysfunction in multiple sclerosis: Causes, consequences, and therapeutic implications. *The Lancet Neurology, 23*(1), 95–109. https://doi.org/10.1016/S1474-4422(23)00371-4.

CHAPTER FIFTEEN

Microglia-centered cellular crosstalk in neurodegeneration

Hao Huang[a,*] and Elvira Mass[b,*]

[a]Department of Medicine, University Medical Center Hamburg-Eppendorf (UKE), Hamburg, Germany; Institute of Neuroimmunology and Multiple Sclerosis, University Medical Center Hamburg-Eppendorf (UKE), Hamburg, Germany

[b]Developmental Biology of the Immune System, Life and Medical Sciences (LIMES) Institute, University of Bonn, Bonn, Germany

*Corresponding authors. e-mail address: h.huang@uke.de; elvira.mass@uni-bonn.de

Contents

Abstracts

Neuroinflammation shaped by aberrant cellular interactions represents a hallmark of neurodegenerative diseases of the central nervous system (CNS). Microglia are specialized tissue-resident macrophages that reside in the CNS parenchyma and have emerged as central regulators of this aberrant cellular crosstalk. They integrate local signals and orchestrate the cellular interaction networks that underlie disease progression. Recent advances in single-cell and single-nucleus omics, in combination with spatially resolved approaches, have substantially advanced our understanding of microglial dynamics in neurodegeneration. These technological and conceptual advances have revealed an unexpected diversity of disease-associated microglial states and highlighted microglia as central organizers of multicellular interaction networks within diseased CNS tissue. In this chapter, we discuss how these advances have reshaped our understanding of microglia-centered cellular crosstalk in neurodegeneration. We focus on the diversification of neurodegenerative CNS microglial states, the interaction of microglia with neurons,

Advances in Immunology, Volume 171
ISSN 0065-2776, https://doi.org/10.1016/bs.ai.2026.06.001

glial cells, adaptive immune cells, and the vasculature. We further discuss how this framework provides a basis for therapeutic strategies aimed at modulating, replacing, or reprogramming microglia in neurodegenerative disease.

1. Introduction

Microglia play essential roles in maintaining CNS homeostasis across the lifespan (Prinz et al., 2019). During development, microglia help ensure CNS integrity (Lawrence et al., 2024) and actively sculpt emerging neuronal circuits by regulating neuronal fates (Cunningham et al., 2013) and refining synaptic connections (Paolicelli et al., 2011). In the healthy adult CNS, microglia support tissue homeostasis through continuous surveillance of the parenchyma (Nimmerjahn et al., 2005) and engaging in dynamic interactions with neurons, glial cells, and vascular-associated elements to support tissue integrity (Prinz et al., 2019). In neurodegenerative disease, these homeostatic functions of microglia are progressively reprogrammed by chronic tissue stress, neuronal injury, myelin disruption, protein aggregation, metabolic imbalance and immune cell infiltration (Gao et al., 2023; Sadeghdoust et al., 2024; Shi & Yong, 2025; Wilson et al., 2023). How microglial functional states diversify across various neurodegenerative diseases and how these states influence communication with CNS cell populations are among the central questions in the field. In this chapter, we discuss how recent conceptual and technological advances have reshaped our understanding of microglial state diversification and microglia-centered cellular crosstalk in neurodegeneration, with particular emphasis on their interactions with neurons and adaptive immune cells.

2. Microglia in neurodegeneration – contributing to or causing diseases?

Neurodegeneration is characterized by progressive neuronal loss and encompasses remarkably diverse disorders (McKinney et al., 2026). In many of these diseases, the initiating etiology remains incompletely defined. Microglia, as the resident immune sentinels and highly plastic immune cells in the CNS, respond to insults across essentially all neurodegenerative conditions. Early in disease, they can support tissue integrity through debris clearance, synaptic surveillance, and local trophic functions. However, with chronic exposure to protein aggregates, neuronal and axonal injury, lipid disequilibrium, and inflammatory cues, these same programs can become ineffective or maladaptive, leading to loss of protective capacity or gain of pathogenic functions (McKinney et al., 2026; Wilson et al., 2023). Microglial contributions to distinct neurodegenerative diseases are not uniform, but instead emerge as distinct transcriptional states across different anatomical niches (Chhatbar et al., 2026; Fumagalli et al., 2025).

However, neurodegenerative disorders caused by intrinsic microglial dysfunction are collectively termed 'primary microgliopathies'. One such case is exemplified by a disease called polycystic lipomembranous osteodysplasia with sclerosing leukoencephalopathy (PLOSL) or Nasu-Hakola disease, a rare early-onset dementia. PLOSL is caused by microglial mutations in *TREM2* or its adaptor *TYROBP* (Paloneva et al., 2002; Xing et al., 2015). TREM2-DAP12/TYROBP signaling interacts with CSF1R and is critical for microglial sensing and homeostatic functions. Similarly, loss-of-function mutation in *CSF1R* causes a white matter degenerative disease called hereditary diffuse leukoencephalopathy with axonal spheroids (HDLS) or adult-onset leukoencephalopathy with axonal spheroids and pigmented glia (ALSP) (Rademakers et al., 2011; Wu et al., 2025). A further mechanistic example comes from the demonstration of a somatic *BRAF* mutation in erythro-myeloid progenitors, which give rise to mutant microglia that later drive neurodegeneration through chronic MAP kinase pathway activation and inflammatory reprogramming (Mass et al., 2017). Sandhoff disease provides another example of microglia as disease drivers. In this lysosomal storage disorder caused by *HEXB*-deficiency, microglia fail to provide neurons with β-hexosaminidase (HEXB) required for GM2 ganglioside turnover, thereby contributing directly to neuronal lipid storage and neurodegeneration (Frosch et al., 2025).

Together, these findings support the view that microglia can act not only as responders to neuronal disorders but also as primary drivers of CNS degeneration when their intrinsic homeostatic functions are disrupted.

3. Functional diversification of microglia in neurodegeneration

Microglial states in neurodegeneration are now understood to extend far beyond the classical concepts of "activation" or "microgliosis" (Depp et al., 2025; Paolicelli et al., 2022). Rather, neurodegenerative conditions include a broad diversification of microglial functional states that vary with disease context, stage, anatomical location, and local tissue environment. In this section, we outline how this conceptual shift emerged, from early histopathological descriptions to transcriptomic definitions such as disease-associated microglia, and then to the current view that microglial responses comprise heterogeneous, overlapping, and context-dependent programs across neurodegenerative diseases.

3.1 Early description of microglia states in neurodegeneration

As the dominant immune cells in the CNS, microglia execute essential functions to ensure CNS health across the lifespan. During development, microglia respond to changing demands of the developing CNS. They play essential roles in establishing tissue architecture and shaping neural circuits. These functions include ensuring structural integrity (Lawrence et al., 2024), the clearance of apoptotic cells (Anderson et al., 2022; Silva et al., 2026), regulation of the neuronal precursor pool (Cunningham et al., 2013), activity-dependent synaptic pruning (Paolicelli et al., 2011) and oligodendrogenesis (Wlodarczyk et al., 2017). In the mature CNS, the primary task of microglia is to maintain homeostasis. They continuously survey the parenchyma through highly motile processes (Davalos et al., 2012; Nimmerjahn et al., 2005) to maintain neuronal connectivity (Cserép et al., 2020), support the surrounding glial cell network (Du et al., 2022) and ensure vessel integrity (Bisht et al., 2021). These diverse developmental and homeostatic functions illustrate that microglia are not passive immune bystanders, but highly specialized regulators of CNS integrity, with their behavior being tightly tuned to the microenvironment. However, in neurodegenerative diseases, these same core functions are progressively reprogrammed by pathological protein aggregation, synaptic and neuronal network dysfunction, aberrant proteostasis, cytoskeletal abnormalities, altered energy homeostasis, DNA and RNA defects, inflammation, and neuronal cell death (Wilson et al., 2023). Microglial responses in neurodegeneration have been largely captured by the terms "microglia activation" or "microgliosis", which describe increased cell number and/or a marked morphological transition from highly ramified surveillant cells to less ramified or amoeboid forms (Gao et al., 2023). While useful as a histopathological description, this concept provides only a limited view of microglial biology (Depp et al., 2025; Paolicelli et al., 2022). It cannot resolve the molecular programs that govern microglial responses to neurodegeneration, nor can it distinguish disease-specific differences across neurodegenerative conditions.

3.2 The description of "disease-associated microglia"

The simplified view of microglia "activation" or "microgliosis" in neurodegeneration began to change with the emergence of high-throughput sequencing, especially single-cell and single-nucleus sequencing (scRNA-seq and snRNA-seq) technologies, which enabled microglial phenotypes to be resolved at much greater depth. An influential development in this field was the description of "disease-associated microglia (DAM)" in an Alzheimer's disease (AD) mouse model, with broader relevance proposed for mouse models of amyotrophic lateral sclerosis (ALS), and aging, as well as human neurodegenerative diseases (Keren-Shaul et al., 2017). In this study, DAM signatures were defined by the loss of homeostatic markers such as *P2ry12, Tmem119, Cx3cr1,* and *Sall1,* and acquisition of a transcriptional program enriched for *Apoe, Axl, B2m, Itgax, Trem2, Clec7a, Tyrobp, Lpl, Spp1, Cd9, Gpnmb,* and *Cst7.* DAM transition was proposed to occur in a stepwise manner, beginning with the downregulation of homeostatic microglial markers and followed by activation of a *Trem2*-dependent transcriptional program (Keren-Shaul et al., 2017). DAM represent only a fraction of microglia and are located in proximity to amyloid-β plaque in AD, suggesting that the DAM-state is dependent on the diseased microenvironment (Deczkowska et al., 2018; Keren-Shaul et al., 2017). At the same time as the description of DAM, another study also characterized microglia with similar signature genes in different CNS neurodegenerative mouse models with bulk RNA-seq, which were coined as "MGnD" – neurodegenerative microglia (Krasemann et al., 2017). Together, these studies established transcriptional frameworks for how neurodegenerative pathology reshapes microglial states. These frameworks had a major impact on the field. They moved microglial biology beyond the catch-all term of "activation" or "microgliosis" and provided tractable molecular signatures for studying microglial responses to neurodegeneration, and identified their spatial location in the diseased microenvironment. At the same time, however, the DAM concept was rapidly adopted as a standard term to describe microglial responses across neurodegenerative diseases. It has now become increasingly clear that this overgeneralization of DAM terminology is not sufficient to capture the full complexity of microglial responses in diverse neurodegenerative contexts (Depp et al., 2025; Paolicelli et al., 2022).

3.3 Heterogeneity of neurodegeneration-associated microglia

A recent review summarizes the current knowledge on microglial heterogeneity in development and across different neurodegenerative diseases uncovered by

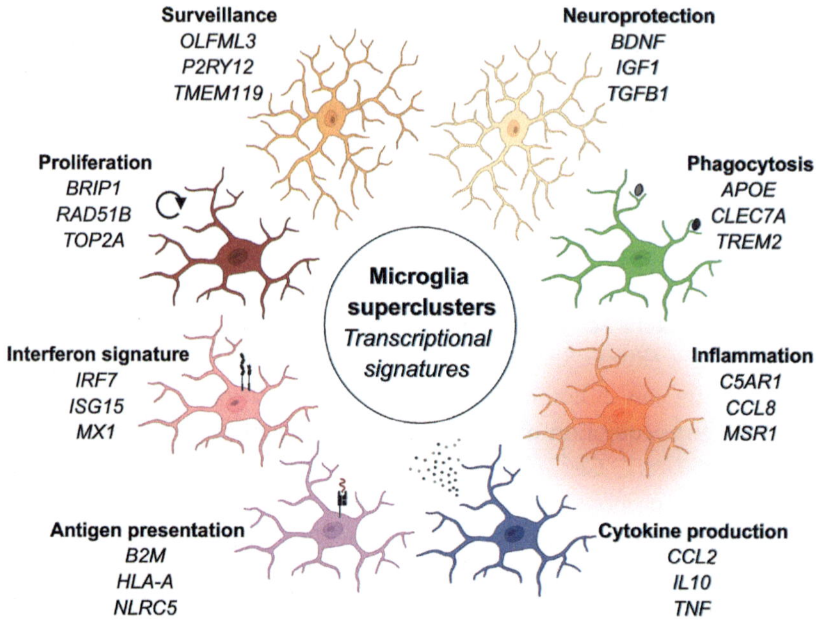

Fig. 1 Microglial state diversity in neurodegeneration. Schematic illustration of the heterogeneous microglial states in neurodegenerative disease. Based on (Chhatbar et al., 2026), microglial states across human neurodegenerative diseases can be classified into 8 transcriptionally distinct superclusters. These include surveillance microglia marked by *OLFML3*, *P2RY12*, and *TMEM119*; neuroprotective microglia expressing *BDNF*, *IGF1*, and *TGFB1*; phagocytic microglia marked by *APOE*, *CLEC7A*, and *TREM2*; inflammatory microglia expressing *C5AR1*, *CCL8*, and *MSR1*; cytokine-producing microglia marked by *CCL2*, *IL10*, and *TNF*; antigen-presenting microglia expressing *B2M*, *HLA-A*, and *NLRC5*; interferon-responsive microglia marked by *IRF7*, *ISG15*, and *MX1*; and proliferating microglia expressing *BRIP1*, *RAD51B*, and *TOP2A*. *Created in BioRender. Huang (2026) https://BioRender.com/jo3oggp.*

single-cell transcriptomics (Fumagalli et al., 2025). The review emphasizes that microglial heterogeneity emerges along multiple axes – including disease context, disease model, disease stage, anatomical regions, sex, and species. Despite varying nomenclature annotated by the original studies, five core transcriptional programs of microglia are summarized in this review that are consistent in different AD datasets: homeostatic, "DAM-like", antigen presentation clusters (enriched for HLA/MHC class II genes), cytokine-response microglia, and interferon-responsive microglia (IFM/IFN). Importantly, each of these broader programs still comprises heterogeneous microglial states with partially overlapping but variable signatures across studies (Fumagalli et al., 2025). In line with this review, a recent cross-disease snRNA-seq atlas and hierarchical taxonomy of

CNS myeloid cells suggest that microglial responses in neurodegeneration are best understood as overlapping and context-dependent programs rather than as a single disease-defining phenotype (Chhatbar et al., 2026). By analyzing over one million cells across more than 30 human and mouse conditions, the authors classified eight core microglial functional programs – surveillance, inflammation, proliferation, antigen presentation, phagocytosis, cytokine production, neuroprotection, and IFN signature (Fig. 1) – which resolve into 192 distinct clusters across various brain disorders. Spatial transcriptomic mapping revealed that these transcriptionally defined states occupy specific pathological niches, such as phagocytic clusters localizing near Aβ plaques in AD, supporting the view that microglial states are shaped by both intrinsic programs and immediate microenvironmental context. While core programs like phagocytosis and IFN signaling are largely conserved across species, human microglia display substantially greater transcriptional heterogeneity than mouse models, particularly regarding cytokine-producing states (Chhatbar et al., 2026). Similar conclusions of microglial heterogeneity have emerged from other recent studies, including a human microglia atlas using snRNA-seq across various human neurodegenerative diseases (Martins-Ferreira et al., 2025). Taken together, these studies demonstrate that microglial states are not a single universal disease-associated phenotype, but better viewed as heterogeneous, partially overlapping, and shaped by both local tissue environment and disease context.

4. Microglia-CNS cell interaction in neurodegenerative diseases

As outlined above, our understanding of heterogeneous microglial states in neurodegenerative diseases has advanced considerably with the widespread use of scRNA-seq and snRNA-seq, together with the emergence of spatial transcriptomic and proteomic technologies. This heterogeneity likely reflects functional diversification. These functions are executed through microglial interactions with neighboring CNS cells and are further shaped by local tissue context (Fig. 2). In this section, we discuss how the distinct microglial states identified in neurodegenerative settings may contribute to diseases within their respective cellular and spatial niches.

4.1 Microglia-neuron interaction

Neuronal viability and circuit connectivity are fundamental determinants of CNS function and are primary targets of injury in neurodegenerative disease

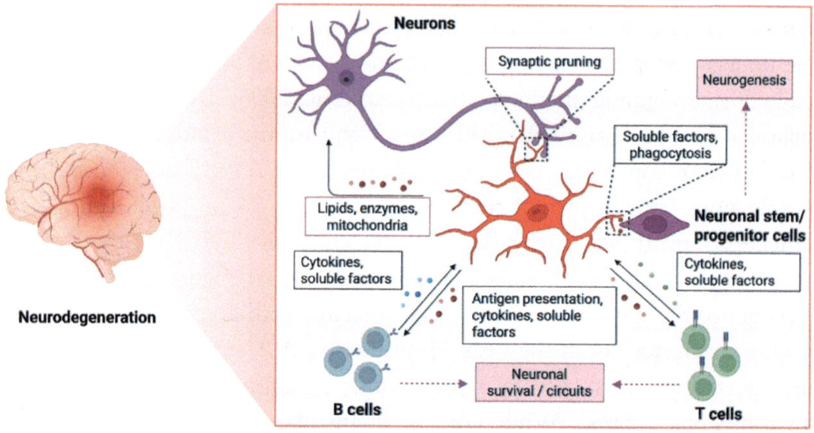

Fig. 2 Microglia-centered cellular interactions in neurodegeneration. Schematic illustration of microglial interactions with neurons, neural stem/progenitor cells, B cells, and T cells during neurodegeneration. Microglia communicate with neurons through synaptic pruning, phagocytosis, and the exchange of metabolites and cellular components, thereby contributing to synaptic and neuronal integrity. Microglia also regulate neural stem/progenitor cells through cytokines and soluble factors that influence neurogenesis. In parallel, microglia interact with adaptive immune cells through antigen presentation, cytokine production, and reciprocal inflammatory signaling with B and T cells. These cellular interactions collectively shape neuroinflammatory responses, neuronal survival, and circuit function in neurodegenerative disease. *Created in BioRender. Huang (2026) https://BioRender.com/ip94udg.*

(Balusu et al., 2023; Wilson et al., 2023). A large body of work has established that microglia are tightly integrated into this neuronal network, where they continuously sense and shape synaptic and neuronal integrity (Frosch et al., 2025; Lawrence et al., 2024; Paolicelli et al., 2011; Scheiblich et al., 2024; Sierra et al., 2010; Stevens et al., 2007). In the healthy CNS, microglia support neural circuit integrity through surveillance, synaptic remodeling, trophic support, and clearance of cellular debris (Nimmerjahn et al., 2005; Parkhurst et al., 2013; Petry et al., 2023; Zhao et al., 2024). In neurodegeneration, these same core functions are progressively reprogrammed by chronic tissue stress (Flury et al., 2025), protein aggregation (Wilson et al., 2023), disrupted lipid homeostasis (Li et al., 2024; Marschallinger et al., 2020), altered neuronal activity (Wilson et al., 2023), and persistent inflammatory signaling (Adamu et al., 2024). As a result, microglia no longer simply monitor the neuronal compartment, but actively shape synaptic vulnerability, neuronal survival, and the regenerative potential of adult neurogenic niches. This section summarizes how the mutual interaction between microglia and neurons is altered in neurodegeneration and how the alteration can influence disease progression.

4.1.1 Microglia and neurogenesis in neurodegenerative diseases

Microglia regulate neurogenesis across the lifespan through direct and dynamic interactions with neural stem and progenitor cells (NSCs/NPCs). During mouse development, microglia are present within the embryonic cortical precursor niches and influence precursor development (Antony et al., 2011). Microglia also colonize cortical proliferative zones and phagocytose NPCs as neurogenesis nears completion, directly controlling precursor number (Cunningham et al., 2013). More recently, this concept was extended to human development (Yu et al., 2025). In prenatal brain, microglia were shown to promote GABAergic neurogenesis in the medial ganglionic eminence through Insulin-like growth factor 1 (IGF1), directly linking a defined trophic factor to progenitor proliferation and neuroblast production (Yu et al., 2025). In adulthood, this regulatory role persists in canonical neurogenic niches. In adult mouse dentate gyrus, resident microglia rapidly engulf apoptotic newborn cells, establishing apoptosis-coupled phagocytosis as a physiological mechanism shaping baseline neurogenic output (Sierra et al., 2010). Adult mouse hippocampal neurogenesis is also regulated by fractalkine Cx3cl1-Cx3cr1 signaling, and disruption of this pathway alters microglial state and reduces neurogenesis (Bachstetter et al., 2011). In addition, phagocytic microglia release a distinct secretory program, such as neuropeptide VGF and growth factors VEGF and FGF2, that remodels adult mouse hippocampal neurogenesis (Diaz-Aparicio et al., 2020). Recent work links microglial control of neurogenesis to the PTEN–mTOR pathway: in the adult mouse hippocampus, inhibition of microglial TGF-β signaling increases neurogenesis, and this effect is reversed by rapamycin (Ware et al., 2026). Together, these studies provide direct evidence of microglial control over neuronal progenitors and newborn neurons in development and homeostasis. Mechanistically, microglia maintain the CNS neurogenic niche during development and adult homeostasis through apoptosis-coupled phagocytosis of excess newborn cells, secretion of neurotrophic mediators, and homeostatic signaling pathways such as Cx3cl1-Cx3cr1 (Früholz & Meyer-Luehmann, 2024).

In neurodegenerative disease, however, this microglia-NSC/NPC axis is likely progressively distorted. Indeed, adult hippocampal neurogenesis becomes progressively disrupted across multiple neurodegenerative disorders, such as ALS, Huntington's disease (HD), PD, dementia with Lewy bodies (DLB), and frontotemporal dementia (FTD) (Terreros-Roncal et al., 2021), as well as AD (Disouky et al., 2026). These studies suggest that defective NSC/NPC proliferation, neuronal differentiation, and niche support are not merely late consequences of tissue degeneration, but can emerge as early and disease-linked features of neurodegenerative pathology (Disouky et al., 2026; Hamilton et al., 2010; Scopa et al., 2020). Given the central role of microglia in regulating neurogenesis under physiological conditions, these findings implicate the involvement of microglia in regulating NSCs/NPCs in neurodegeneration (Früholz & Meyer-Luehmann, 2024). This microglia–neurogenesis relationship has been most extensively studied in AD. In APP/PS1 mice, Igf1 expression increases in parallel with microglial activation and reduced subgranular zone neurogenesis, linking altered microglial trophic signaling to impaired neurogenesis in AD (Myhre et al., 2019). Likewise, reduction of TGF-β signaling in another AD mouse model accelerates neurodegeneration and AD-like pathology (Tesseur et al., 2006). Conversely, in APP/PS1 mice, inhibition of microglial reactivity with minocycline increased the survival of newborn dentate granule cells and improved hippocampus-dependent learning, without altering brain Aβ levels or Aβ-associated morphological defects in the new neurons (Biscaro et al., 2012).

Taken together, current evidence supports a model in which neurodegenerative disease disrupts the microglia-NSC/NPC axis at multiple levels, including phagocytic niche maintenance and trophic support. This is mostly established in AD, where microglial state changes are linked to early deficits in adult neurogenesis and where partial restoration of neurogenesis can be achieved by modulating microglial activation. It remains to be established in the broader neurodegenerative contexts how defective microglia–NSC/NPC interactions may represent an impaired feature of diseased neurogenic niches.

4.1.2 Microglia-neuronal synapse interaction

Synapses form the core element of neuronal circuits in the CNS. It is well-appreciated that microglia sculpt synaptic connectivity (Paolicelli et al., 2011; Schafer et al., 2012; Stevens et al., 2007). These interactions are shaped by neuronal activity cues, metabolic states, and local extracellular composition. One of the best-characterized mechanisms of how microglia communicate with synapses is complement-mediated synaptic pruning during development and adult synapse surveillance (Schafer et al., 2012; Stevens et al., 2007). Microglia–synapse crosstalk can also be regulated by fractalkine

Cx3cl1–Cx3cr1 signaling, a major neuron-to-microglia communication axis that restrains excessive microglial activation and helps calibrate synaptic interactions (Paolicelli et al., 2011). In addition, IL-33–ST2 signaling has emerged as another instructive pathway for microglial synapse remodeling. In developmental and physiological settings, IL-33 promotes microglial engulfment of synaptic material, while downstream ST2–AKT signaling supports the metabolic adaptation and phagocytic capacity required for this process (He et al., 2022; Vainchtein et al., 2018). In the adult hippocampus, neuronal IL-33 further instructs microglial engulfment of the perisynaptic extracellular matrix, thereby promoting synapse plasticity and selective local remodeling responses (Nguyen et al., 2020). Together, these findings support the view that microglia shape synaptic structure and function through contact-dependent recognition, cytokine-mediated instruction, and remodeling of the local extracellular environment.

However, these mechanisms participating in synaptic refinement can be aberrantly engaged in disease and contribute to pathological synapse loss (Hong et al., 2016; Werneburg et al., 2020; Wilton et al., 2023). Central to this process is the complement cascade, particularly the C1q–C3–CR3 axis, which tags vulnerable synapses for microglial engulfment and has been strongly implicated in AD, MS and HD (Hong et al., 2016; Werneburg et al., 2020; Wilton et al., 2023). In addition, local exposure of phosphatidylserine and changes in neuronal activity state can further mark synapses for elimination in a C1q-dependent manner, linking molecular "eat-me" signals to structural circuit loss (Scott-Hewitt et al., 2020). On the contrary, Cx3cl1–Cx3cr1 signaling seems to safeguard synaptic connectivity, as perturbation of this pathway exacerbates synaptic loss in a *Cx3cr1*$^{-/-}$ 5xFAD AD model (Puntambekar et al., 2022). Collectively, current evidence supports the view that maladaptive microglial synapse elimination is a major pathway contributing to neuronal circuit dysfunction in neurodegenerative disease (Beiter et al., 2024; Hu & Tao, 2024).

4.1.3 Other modes of microglia-neuron interaction

Beyond neurogenesis and synapse-directed mechanisms, recent studies have shown that microglia–neuron interaction can influence neuronal fitness and survival (Chakraborty et al., 2026; Cserép et al., 2020; Frosch et al., 2025; Scheiblich et al., 2024).

Specialized somatic microglia–neuron junctions have been identified in mouse and human brain, showing that microglia interact with neurons not only at synapses but also at defined sites on the neuronal cell body. These contacts are organized for P2Y12-dependent purinergic signaling and link neuronal mitochondrial activity and activation state to microglial surveillance, thereby enabling microglia to monitor neuronal homeostasis in a highly localized manner (Cserép et al., 2020). In parallel, recent work has identified a stress-associated microglial state in which autonomous activation of the integrated stress response (ISR) drives microglia toward a dark microglia-like phenotype and induces secretion of neurotoxic lipids. These stressed microglia release lipid species that directly compromise neuronal homeostasis and survival. In AD models, microglial ISR activation aggravated synaptic loss and neurodegenerative pathology, whereas pharmacological inhibition of either the ISR or lipid synthesis mitigated the resulting neuronal and synaptic injury. These findings link chronic microglial stress to a metabolically maladaptive secretory program that converts tissue stress into neuronal damage (Flury et al., 2025).

Recent work has also identified tunneling nanotubes (TNTs) as a direct route of microglia–neuron communication in proteinopathy settings. In models of α-synucleinopathy (PD pathology) and tauopathy (AD pathology), microglia form TNTs with aggregate-burdened neurons, extract α-synuclein or tau aggregates, and donate healthy mitochondria, thereby reducing oxidative stress and restoring neuronal function (Scheiblich et al., 2024). Complementing this, impaired neuronal α-synuclein aggregate clearance was shown to enhance neuron-to-microglia TNT-mediated transfer of aggregates, which are subsequently degraded by microglia through increased autophagic flux (Chakraborty et al., 2026). Together, these studies suggest that TNTs support a bidirectional rescue pathway in which neurons offload proteotoxic material to microglia, while microglia reciprocally buffer neuronal stress through metabolic support.

Another recent study has described a microglia–neuron metabolic signaling axis in which microglia provide neurons with β-hexosaminidase (HexB), a lysosomal enzyme that degrades GM2 gangliosides, a class of neuronal membrane lipids. Through this pathway, together with neuronal MGL2, microglia help preserve neuronal lipid homeostasis, revealing a direct metabolic mode of microglia–neuron crosstalk in the healthy brain. Genetic disruption of this microglia-derived HexB pathway caused neuronal GM2 accumulation and disturbed neuronal membrane composition and function. Importantly, the study further linked this pathway to Sandhoff disease, showing that loss of HexB drives neuronal GM2 accumulation and downstream maladaptive microglial responses that contribute to neurodegeneration (Frosch et al., 2025).

Taken together, these studies show that microglia influence neuronal viability through multiple mechanisms beyond synapse pruning alone. Depending on context, microglia can monitor neuronal status, provide metabolic support, clear proteotoxic material, or, conversely, adopt stress-associated states that directly injure neurons. This broader view is important for neurodegenerative disease, where microglia-neuron interactions are likely to shape not only synaptic vulnerability but also the survival and functional resilience of neurons themselves.

4.2 Microglia–immune cell interaction

The classical idea of the CNS as an immune-privileged organ has undergone substantial revision (Smyth & Kipnis, 2025). CNS interfaces, including meninges, perivascular spaces, choroid plexus and CSF-associated compartments, are now understood as immunologically active sites that support surveillance, trafficking and communication (Van Hoecke et al., 2026). In addition, the skull bone marrow (sBM) has emerged as a local immune reservoir that can supply the dura with immune cells through direct vascular channels and thereby establishes a local periphery–brain axis of neuroimmune communication (Cugurra et al., 2021; Van Hoecke et al., 2026). During neurodegeneration, this axis can also directly contribute immune cells to the pathological CNS, further shaping the local inflammatory milieu (Mazzitelli et al., 2022; Soliman et al., 2025). Within this expanded neuroimmune framework, microglia are best viewed not as insulated parenchymal innate cells, but as integral components of a broader immune communication network that includes lymphocytes, CNS border-associated macrophages (CAMs), dendritic cells, and infiltrating monocyte-derived cells (Smyth & Kipnis, 2025; Van Hoecke et al., 2026). How microglia interact with these infiltrated immune cells in neurodegenerative diseases is therefore of considerable interest for understanding and modulating neuroinflammation in neurodegeneration.

4.2.1 Microglia–T cell interaction

T cell accumulation in the diseased CNS had long been viewed mainly as a secondary consequence of barrier dysfunction or peripheral immune activation (Pachter et al., 2003). Accumulating evidence has shown T cell infiltration into the CNS across several neurodegenerative diseases (Brochard et al., 2008; Chen et al., 2023; Frolov et al., 2025; Garofalo et al., 2022; Hartnell et al., 2024; Williams et al., 2021). Microglia and T cell crosstalk is increasingly recognized as an important component of neurodegenerative pathology.

A landmark study in tauopathy has shown that microglia promote T cell infiltration and establish an immune hub linked to neuronal loss (Chen et al., 2023). Depletion of either microglia or T cells attenuated neurodegeneration, indicating that pathogenicity arises not from either population alone, but from their coordinated interaction. Similarly, in an aging-associated white matter degeneration, maladaptive microglial states recruited cytotoxic CD8 T cells through Cxcl10 signaling and thereby drove axonal injury (Groh et al., 2025). Extending this concept to HD, another study used single-nucleus and spatial transcriptomics in an engineered pig model and identified an interferon-responsive microglial state associated with recruitment of cytotoxic CD8 T cells into the striatum (Li et al., 2026). Mechanistically, the authors implicated Cxcl8-mediated T-cell infiltration in accelerating neuronal loss, and showed that its neutralization mitigated neurodegeneration. These studies support the idea that microglia can function as local amplifiers of lymphocyte-engaging inflammatory niches.

Microglia not only recruit T cells, but can also shape their functional state within the CNS. Using an experimental autoimmune encephalomyelitis (EAE) mouse model, a study has shown that cognate interactions between microglia and CD4 T cells influence the regulatory T cell compartment, with microglial IFN-γ receptor signaling and MHC-II-dependent mechanisms contributing to this process. Thus, microglia are not merely recipients of lymphocyte-derived signals, but active regulators of T-cell differentiation and function in inflamed CNS tissue (Haimon et al., 2022). Our recent work in a murine model of spastic paraplegia 15 further supports this concept. Disease-associated microglial changes and CD8 T cell activation preceded overt neuronal loss, and single-cell analysis identified coordinated microglia–T cell interactive signaling (Frolov et al., 2025). Notably, microglia–T cell interaction may arise early in disease progression rather than simply appearing as a late consequence of tissue damage (Frolov et al., 2025).

At the same time, the microglia-T cell axis is not uniformly pathogenic. Recent work in tauopathy has shown that Granzyme K^+ CD8 T cells can slow disease progression by targeting microglia, indicating that T cells may, in some settings, constrain maladaptive microglial responses rather than amplify them. Together, these studies indicate that microglia-T cell interaction is bidirectional and context-dependent. It can promote immune recruitment, shape effector state, or even provide a layer of immune control over pathological microglial programs (Mason et al., 2025).

Taken together, current evidence indicates that microglia-T cell interactions are bidirectional, context-dependent, and increasingly relevant to neurodegenerative disease. Microglia can recruit and shape T cells, while T cells can either amplify or restrain maladaptive microglial responses.

4.2.2 Microglia–B cell interaction

Compared with the extensive body of work on T cells in neurodegeneration and their interactions with microglia, the role of B cells in neurodegenerative disorders and their crosstalk with CNS-resident microglia has remained much less well defined. Recent evidence, however, suggests that B cells can modulate microglial functional states in CNS disease through both indirect and direct mechanisms. These include peripheral production of immunoglobulins that accumulate within the CNS parenchyma, as well as CNS infiltration of B cells that subsequently engage local niche cells, including microglia (Kim et al., 2021; Sabatino et al., 2019; Zhang et al., 2025).

This concept is best established in MS and EAE. One study showed that secreted products from MS-implicated pro-inflammatory B cells can shift human brain-derived microglia toward an inflammatory phenotype, characterized by increased IL-12, IL-6, and TNFα, reduced IL-10 and quiescence-associated molecules, and impaired myelin phagocytosis. By contrast, secreted products from IL-10-expressing B cells promoted a more quiescent and phagocytically competent microglial state. The study further showed that factors released by pro-inflammatory microglia enhance B-cell activation, supporting the idea of a reciprocal and potentially self-reinforcing B cell-microglia inflammatory circuit in progressive MS. However, these conclusions are based mainly on human in-vitro assays, and the in-vivo organization and full molecular basis of this interaction remain incompletely resolved (Touil et al., 2023). A more direct in-vivo link comes from a recent EAE model showing that autoreactive B cells can trigger MS-like lesions when rescued from activation-induced cell death by Epstein-Barr Virus-like survival signaling (Kim et al., 2026). In this setting, lesion formation was associated with microglial activation and complement deposition, placing microglia downstream of pathogenic CNS B-cell activity rather than merely as bystanders of tissue injury. These findings support a model in which persistent autoreactive B cells initiate a local inflammatory circuit that includes activated microglia and demyelinating damage, although the precise molecular mediators of this crosstalk remain to be defined (Kim et al., 2026). Together, these findings suggest that in

MS, B cells provide antigen-directed inflammatory input, whereas microglia convert this signal into lesion-associated innate effector activity and simultaneously reinforce pathogenic B-cell responses within the CNS compartment.

Evidence for a related axis is also emerging in AD models. One study has reported activated B cells in the brain parenchyma together with immunoglobulin deposition around amyloid-β plaques. B cell depletion reduced disease-associated microglial changes and slowed cognitive decline, indicating that B cells can shape microglial state in amyloid-driven neurodegeneration (Kim et al., 2021). More recently, bone marrow-derived age-associated B cells (ABCs) have been shown to infiltrate the brain parenchyma during early amyloid pathology in both 5xFAD and APP/PS1 mice. Mechanistically, the study linked this process to sustained bone marrow B lymphopoiesis and showed that IL-6R blockade reduced ABCs, delayed cerebral amyloid-β pathology, and improved cognition (Zhang et al., 2025). These findings further support the idea that B cells can enter the CNS and participate in local inflammatory niches in AD, although the precise molecular basis of their interaction with microglia remains incompletely defined.

In addition, altered B-cell phenotypes have been reported in PD (Li et al., 2022; Scott, 2022) and ALS (Yildiz et al., 2023), but a clearly resolved mechanistic B cell-microglia circuit remains lacking. Overall, current evidence suggests that B cells can contribute to neurodegeneration, at least in part through reciprocal interactions with microglia. This concept is most strongly supported in MS/EAE and is increasingly emerging in AD, although the underlying mechanisms remain incompletely defined. In other neurodegenerative disorders, evidence for a functionally resolved B cell-microglia axis is still limited.

Taken together, the functional diversification of microglia in neurodegeneration is likely to have direct consequences for their interactions with T and B cells. Distinct microglial states differ in their capacities for chemokine production, antigen presentation, cytokine release, phagocytosis, and complement-associated responses (Chhatbar et al., 2026; Fumagalli et al., 2025), and are therefore likely to differentially control lymphocyte recruitment, activation, and retention within diseased CNS tissue. In this framework, interferon-responsive, antigen-presenting, and inflammatory microglial states may preferentially support T-cell recruitment and functional polarization (Groh et al., 2025; Haimon et al., 2022; Li et al., 2026), whereas lesion-associated and inflammatory microglial states may be particularly relevant for translating B cell-derived inflammatory, antibody, or complement-related signals into local innate effector activity (Kim et al. 2021, 2026; Touil et al., 2023; Zhang et al., 2025). Microglia-adaptive immune cell crosstalk should therefore be viewed not as a property of a single disease-associated phenotype, but as a state-dependent and context-dependent component of neurodegenerative pathology.

5. Targeting microglia–CNS interaction in neurodegeneration

Although our understanding of microglia-centered cellular crosstalk in neurodegenerative disease has expanded considerably, translating this knowledge into effective microglia-targeted therapies remains challenging. Recently, replacement of defective microglia by hematopoietic stem cell (HSC) or their progeny has been attempted in preclinical models of microgliopathies (Chen et al., 2025; Frosch et al., 2025; Mader et al., 2025; Tsourmas et al., 2025; Wu et al., 2025), MS (Mader et al., 2024) and AD (Chen et al., 2025; Yoo et al., 2023), as well as in human microgliopathy, ALSP (Wu et al., 2025). Microglia-replacement strategies have shown promise in preclinical models of neurodegenerative disease.

In Sandhoff disease, several recent studies support the view that defective microglia–CNS interactions are amenable to therapeutic intervention. Replacement of *HexB*-deficient microglia with donor-derived myeloid cells restored enzyme HexB activity, reduced substrate accumulation, improved neuronal phenotypes, and ameliorated behavioral deficits in mouse models (Frosch et al., 2025; Tsourmas et al., 2025). These disease-focused studies were further supported by recent methodological advances. Brain-wide microglia replacement using a non-conditioning strategy (Chen et al., 2025) or CNS-restricted, high-efficiency microglia replacement without conventional myeloablative preconditioning (Mader et al., 2025) showed therapeutic benefit in Sandhoff disease or AD. Related approaches have also been explored in AD, where replacement of dysfunctional microglia was used to restore protective microglial programs in the context of impaired TREM2 signaling (Yoo et al., 2023). In chronic EAE, myeloid cell replacement promoted neuroprotective and immunoregulatory states associated with improved pathology (Mader et al., 2024). This therapeutic concept has also received initial translational support in human microgliopathy. In *CSF1R*-deficient microgliopathy,

ALSP, replacement of defective microglia with *CSF1R*-normal cells attenuated pathology in mouse models and halted disease progression in treated patients during 24 months of follow-up (Wu et al., 2025).

However, as microglia remain mainly embryonically derived and receive minimal input from HSC-derived cells in most neurodegenerative conditions, the safety and long-term consequences of adoptive transfer require careful consideration. Recent work shows that monocytes can replace multiple brain macrophage compartments when niche access is created experimentally, but this does not necessarily result in full microglial identity. Adult monocytes retain durable ontogeny-associated features, whereas fetal liver progenitors more readily generate *bona fide* microglia-like cells (Bastos et al., 2025). Consistently, brain-engrafted monocyte-derived macrophages arising from blood or skull bone marrow acquire CNS-adapted states yet remain transcriptionally, epigenetically, and functionally distinct from endogenous microglia (Du et al., 2026). These observations suggest that successful engraftment and compartmental repopulation cannot be assumed as full restoration of resident microglial identity and function. Moreover, the therapeutic implications of microglia-centered cellular crosstalk are likely too complex to be fully addressed by global depletion or replacement strategies alone. Microglia exist in heterogeneous and dynamic states and engage in distinct interactions with neurons, infiltrating immune cells, and other CNS cell populations, as outlined above. However, tools to selectively target the microglial subsets that drive specific pathogenic interactions, while preserving subsets involved in tissue support and repair, remain limited. One challenge will therefore be to develop strategies that modulate defined microglial states and their disease-relevant cellular interactions with greater spatial, temporal, and functional precision.

6. Concluding remarks

Recent technological and conceptual advances have fundamentally changed how microglia are viewed in neurodegenerative disease. Rather than a uniform manifestation of "activation", microglial responses are now understood as heterogeneous, context-dependent, and spatially organized functional states. These states are closely linked to distinct interaction networks within the CNS, placing microglia at the center of multicellular crosstalk in the degenerating CNS. This framework provides an important basis for therapy, but also highlights the limits of current approaches.

A major challenge now is to move from increasingly rich descriptive maps to causal understanding. It will be important to determine which microglia-centered interactions are primary drivers of degeneration, which represent secondary adaptations to ongoing tissue injury, and which are compensatory responses that remain ultimately insufficient to preserve tissue integrity. Equally important will be to define which microglial states remain reversible and which reflect points of no return in disease progression. Addressing these questions will be essential for identifying which aspects of microglia-centered cellular crosstalk should be targeted therapeutically, and at which stage of disease. In this regard, an important next step for the field will be to develop tools that move beyond broad depletion or replacement and instead allow defined microglial states and their disease-relevant cellular interactions to be modulated with greater spatial, temporal, and functional precision.

Declaration of generative AI and AI-assisted technologies in the writing process

Generative AI and AI-assisted technologies were used exclusively for language refinement and editorial support during manuscript preparation, while all summaries, interpretation and conclusions were generated and critically evaluated by the authors.

References

Adamu, A., Li, S., Gao, F., & Xue, G. (2024). The role of neuroinflammation in neurodegenerative diseases: Current understanding and future therapeutic targets. *Frontiers in Aging Neuroscience, 16*. https://doi.org/10.3389/fnagi.2024.1347987.

Anderson, S. R., Roberts, J. M., Ghena, N., Irvin, E. A., Schwakopf, J., Cooperstein, I. B., ... Vetter, M. L. (2022). Neuronal apoptosis drives remodeling states of microglia and shifts in survival pathway dependence. *ELife, 11*. https://doi.org/10.7554/eLife.76564.

Antony, J. M., Paquin, A., Nutt, S. L., Kaplan, D. R., & Miller, F. D. (2011). Endogenous microglia regulate development of embryonic cortical precursor cells. *Journal of Neuroscience Research, 89*(3), 286–298. https://doi.org/10.1002/jnr.22533.

Bachstetter, A. D., Morganti, J. M., Jernberg, J., Schlunk, A., Mitchell, S. H., Brewster, K. W., ... Gemma, C. (2011). Fractalkine and CX3CR1 regulate hippocampal neurogenesis in adult and aged rats. *Neurobiology of Aging, 32*(11), 2030–2044. https://doi.org/10.1016/j.neurobiolaging.2009.11.022.

Balusu, S., Praschberger, R., Lauwers, E., De Strooper, B., & Verstreken, P. (2023). Neurodegeneration cell per cell. *Neuron, 111*(6), 767–786. https://doi.org/10.1016/j.neuron.2023.01.016.

Bastos, J., O'Brien, C., Vara-Pérez, M., Mampay, M., van Olst, L., Barry-Carroll, L., ... Movahedi, K. (2025). Monocytes can efficiently replace all brain macrophages and fetal liver monocytes can generate bona fide SALL1+ microglia. *Immunity, 58*(5), 1269–1288.e12. https://doi.org/10.1016/j.immuni.2025.04.006.

Beiter, R. M., Sheehan, P. W., & Schafer, D. P. (2024). Microglia phagocytic mechanisms: Development informing disease. *Current Opinion in Neurobiology, 86*, 102877. https://doi.org/10.1016/j.conb.2024.102877.

Biscaro, B., Lindvall, O., Tesco, G., Ekdahl, C. T., & Nitsch, R. M. (2012). Inhibition of microglial activation protects hippocampal neurogenesis and improves cognitive deficits in a transgenic mouse model for Alzheimer's disease. *Neurodegenerative Diseases, 9*(4), 187–198. https://doi.org/10.1159/000330363.

Bisht, K., Okojie, K. A., Sharma, K., Lentferink, D. H., Sun, Y.-Y., Chen, H.-R., ... Eyo, U. B. (2021). Capillary-associated microglia regulate vascular structure and function through PANX1-P2RY12 coupling in mice. *Nature Communications, 12*(1), 5289. https://doi.org/10.1038/s41467-021-25590-8.

Brochard, V., Combadière, B., Prigent, A., Laouar, Y., Perrin, A., Beray-Berthat, V., ... Hunot, S. (2008). Infiltration of CD4+ lymphocytes into the brain contributes to neurodegeneration in a mouse model of Parkinson disease. *Journal of Clinical Investigation*. https://doi.org/10.1172/JCI36470.

Chakraborty, R., Palese, F., Samella, P., Testa, V., Montero-Muñoz, J., Syan, S., ... Zurzolo, C. (2026). Impaired > \alpha > -synuclein aggregate clearance in neuronal cells drive their spread to microglia through tunneling nanotubes. *Nature Communications*. https://doi.org/10.1038/s41467-026-69930-y.

Chen, D., Wang, C., Chen, X., Li, J., Chen, S., Li, Y., ... Zhong, L. (2025). Brain-wide microglia replacement using a nonconditioning strategy ameliorates pathology in mouse models of neurological disorders. *Science Translational Medicine, 17*(796), https://doi.org/10.1126/scitranslmed.ads6111.

Chen, X., Firulyova, M., Manis, M., Herz, J., Smirnov, I., Aladyeva, E., ... Holtzman, D. M. (2023). Microglia-mediated T cell infiltration drives neurodegeneration in tauopathy. *Nature, 615*(7953), 668–677. https://doi.org/10.1038/s41586-023-05788-0.

Chhatbar, C., Sankowski, R., Schulz, M., Shimizu, T., Schwabenland, M., Staszewski, O., ... Prinz, M. (2026). A transcriptomic microglia taxonomy across mouse and human pathologies. *Nature Immunology*. https://doi.org/10.1038/s41590-026-02472-z.

Cserép, C., Pósfai, B., Lénárt, N., Fekete, R., László, Z. I., Lele, Z., ... Dénes, Á. (2020). Microglia monitor and protect neuronal function through specialized somatic purinergic junctions. *Science (New York, N. Y.), 367*(6477), 528–537. https://doi.org/10.1126/science.aax6752.

Cugurra, A., Mamuladze, T., Rustenhoven, J., Dykstra, T., Beroshvili, G., Greenberg, Z. J., ... Kipnis, J. (2021). Skull and vertebral bone marrow are myeloid cell reservoirs for the meninges and CNS parenchyma. *Science (New York, N. Y.), 373*(6553), https://doi.org/10.1126/science.abf7844.

Cunningham, C. L., Martínez-Cerdeño, V., & Noctor, S. C. (2013). Microglia regulate the number of neural precursor cells in the developing cerebral cortex. *The Journal of Neuroscience: The Official Journal of the Society for Neuroscience, 33*(10), 4216–4233. https://doi.org/10.1523/JNEUROSCI.3441-12.2013.

Davalos, D., Ryu, J. K., Merlini, M., Baeten, K. M., Le Moan, N., Petersen, M. A., ... Akassoglou, K. (2012). Fibrinogen-induced perivascular microglial clustering is required for the development of axonal damage in neuroinflammation. *Nature Communications, 3*, 1227. https://doi.org/10.1038/ncomms2230.

Deczkowska, A., Keren-Shaul, H., Weiner, A., Colonna, M., Schwartz, M., & Amit, I. (2018). Disease-associated microglia: A universal immune sensor of neurodegeneration. *Cell, 173*(5), 1073–1081. https://doi.org/10.1016/j.cell.2018.05.003.

Depp, C., Doman, J. L., Hingerl, M., Xia, J., & Stevens, B. (2025). Microglia transcriptional states and their functional significance: Context drives diversity. *Immunity, 58*(5), 1052–1067. https://doi.org/10.1016/j.immuni.2025.04.009.

Diaz-Aparicio, I., Paris, I., Sierra-Torre, V., Plaza-Zabala, A., Rodríguez-Iglesias, N., Márquez-Ropero, M., ... Sierra, A. (2020). Microglia actively remodel adult hippocampal neurogenesis through the phagocytosis secretome. *The Journal of Neuroscience, 40*(7), 1453–1482. https://doi.org/10.1523/JNEUROSCI.0993-19.2019.

Disouky, A., Sanborn, M. A., Sabitha, K. R., Mostafa, M. M., Ayala, I. A., Bennett, D. A., ... Lazarov, O. (2026). Human hippocampal neurogenesis in adulthood, ageing and Alzheimer's disease. *Nature*. https://doi.org/10.1038/s41586-026-10169-4.

Du, S., Ou, F., Drieu, A., Xu, E. Z., Cheng, Y., Storck, S. E., ... Kipnis, J. (2026). Brain-engrafted monocyte-derived macrophages from blood and skull-bone marrow exhibit distinct properties. *Neuron*. https://doi.org/10.1016/j.neuron.2026.01.032.

Du, Y., Brennan, F. H., Popovich, P. G., & Zhou, M. (2022). Microglia maintain the normal structure and function of the hippocampal astrocyte network. *Glia, 70*(7), 1359–1379. https://doi.org/10.1002/glia.24179.

Flury, A., Aljayousi, L., Park, H.-J., Khakpour, M., Mechler, J., Aziz, S., ... Ayata, P. (2025). A neurodegenerative cellular stress response linked to dark microglia and toxic lipid secretion. *Neuron, 113*(4), 554–571.e14. https://doi.org/10.1016/j.neuron.2024.11.018.

Frolov, A., Huang, H., Schütz, D., Köhne, M., Blank-Stein, N., Osei-Sarpong, C., ... Beyer, M. D. (2025). Microglia and CD8+ T cell activation precede neuronal loss in a murine model of spastic paraplegia 15. *Journal of Experimental Medicine, 222*(7), https://doi.org/10.1084/jem.20232357.

Frosch, M., Shimizu, T., Wogram, E., Amann, L., Gruber, L., Groisman, A. I., ... Prinz, M. (2025). Microglia-neuron crosstalk through Hex-GM2-MGL2 maintains brain homeostasis. *Nature, 646*(8086), 913–924. https://doi.org/10.1038/s41586-025-09477-y.

Frühholz, I., & Meyer-Luehmann, M. (2024). The intricate interplay between microglia and adult neurogenesis in Alzheimer's disease. *Frontiers in Cellular Neuroscience, 18*. https://doi.org/10.3389/fncel.2024.1456253.

Fumagalli, L., Nazlie Mohebiany, A., Premereur, J., Polanco Miquel, P., Bijnens, B., Van de Walle, P., ... Mancuso, R. (2025). Microglia heterogeneity, modeling and cell-state annotation in development and neurodegeneration. *Nature Neuroscience, 28*(7), 1381–1392. https://doi.org/10.1038/s41593-025-01931-4.

Gao, C., Jiang, J., Tan, Y., & Chen, S. (2023). Microglia in neurodegenerative diseases: Mechanism and potential therapeutic targets. *Signal Transduction and Targeted Therapy, 8*(1), 359. https://doi.org/10.1038/s41392-023-01588-0.

Garofalo, S., Cocozza, G., Bernardini, G., Savage, J., Raspa, M., Aronica, E., ... Limatola, C. (2022). Blocking immune cell infiltration of the central nervous system to tame Neuroinflammation in Amyotrophic lateral sclerosis. *Brain, Behavior, and Immunity, 105*, 1–14. https://doi.org/10.1016/j.bbi.2022.06.004.

Groh, J., Feng, R., Yuan, X., Liu, L., Klein, D., Hutahaean, G., ... Simons, M. (2025). Microglia activation orchestrates CXCL10-mediated CD8+ T cell recruitment to promote aging-related white matter degeneration. *Nature Neuroscience, 28*(6), 1160–1173. https://doi.org/10.1038/s41593-025-01955-w.

Haimon, Z., Frumer, G. R., Kim, J.-S., Trzebanski, S., Haffner-Krausz, R., Ben-Dor, S., ... Jung, S. (2022). Cognate microglia–T cell interactions shape the functional regulatory T cell pool in experimental autoimmune encephalomyelitis pathology. *Nature Immunology, 23*(12), 1749–1762. https://doi.org/10.1038/s41590-022-01360-6.

Hamilton, L. K., Aumont, A., Julien, C., Vadnais, A., Calon, F., & Fernandes, K. J. L. (2010). Widespread deficits in adult neurogenesis precede plaque and tangle formation in the 3xTg mouse model of Alzheimer's disease. *European Journal of Neuroscience, 32*(6), 905–920. https://doi.org/10.1111/j.1460-9568.2010.07379.x.

Hartnell, I. J., Woodhouse, D., Jasper, W., Mason, L., Marwaha, P., Graffeuil, M., ... Boche, D. (2024). Glial reactivity and T cell infiltration in frontotemporal lobar degeneration with tau pathology. *Brain, 147*(2), 590–606. https://doi.org/10.1093/brain/awad309.

He, D., Xu, H., Zhang, H., Tang, R., Lan, Y., Xing, R., ... Kuchroo, V. K. (2022). Disruption of the IL-33-ST2-AKT signaling axis impairs neurodevelopment by inhibiting microglial metabolic adaptation and phagocytic function. *Immunity, 55*(1), 159–173.e9. https://doi.org/10.1016/j.immuni.2021.12.001.

Hong, S., Beja-Glasser, V. F., Nfonoyim, B. M., Frouin, A., Li, S., Ramakrishnan, S., ... Stevens, B. (2016). Complement and microglia mediate early synapse loss in Alzheimer mouse models. *Science (New York, N. Y.), 352*(6286), 712–716. https://doi.org/10.1126/science.aad8373.

Hu, Y., & Tao, W. (2024). Current perspectives on microglia-neuron communication in the central nervous system: Direct and indirect modes of interaction. *Journal of Advanced Research, 66*, 251–265. https://doi.org/10.1016/j.jare.2024.01.006.

Keren-Shaul, H., Spinrad, A., Weiner, A., Matcovitch-Natan, O., Dvir-Szternfeld, R., Ulland, T. K., ... Amit, I. (2017). A unique microglia type associated with restricting development of Alzheimer's disease. *Cell, 169*(7), 1276–1290.e17. https://doi.org/10.1016/j.cell.2017.05.018.

Kim, H., Schneider, M., Raach, Y., Karypidis, P., Roux, J., Perdikaris, G., ... Derfuss, T. (2026). Myelin antigen capture in the CNS by B cells expressing EBV latent membrane protein 1 leads to demyelinating lesion formation. *Cell, 189*(2), 603–619.e25. https://doi.org/10.1016/j.cell.2025.12.031.

Kim, K., Wang, X., Ragonnaud, E., Bodogai, M., Illouz, T., DeLuca, M., ... Biragyn, A. (2021). Therapeutic B-cell depletion reverses progression of Alzheimer's disease. *Nature Communications, 12*(1), 2185. https://doi.org/10.1038/s41467-021-22479-4.

Krasemann, S., Madore, C., Cialic, R., Baufeld, C., Calcagno, N., El Fatimy, R., ... Butovsky, O. (2017). The TREM2-APOE pathway drives the transcriptional phenotype of dysfunctional microglia in neurodegenerative diseases. *Immunity, 47*(3), 566–581.e9. https://doi.org/10.1016/j.immuni.2017.08.008.

Lawrence, A. R., Canzi, A., Bridlance, C., Olivié, N., Lansonneur, C., Catale, C., ... Garel, S. (2024). Microglia maintain structural integrity during fetal brain morphogenesis. *Cell, 187*(4), 962–980.e19. https://doi.org/10.1016/j.cell.2024.01.012.

Li, J., Lin, Y., Gao, J., Yang, F., Li, C., Chen, Y., ... Yan, S. (2026). Single-nucleus transcriptomics of an engineered pig model reveals microglia–T cell interactions driving Huntington's disease neurodegeneration. *Nature Biomedical Engineering*. https://doi.org/10.1038/s41551-026-01621-x.

Li, R., Tropea, T. F., Baratta, L. R., Zuroff, L., Diaz-Ortiz, M. E., Zhang, B., ... Bar-Or, A. (2022). Abnormal B-cell and Tfh-cell profiles in patients with Parkinson disease. *Neurology Neuroimmunology & Neuroinflammation, 9*(2), https://doi.org/10.1212/NXI.0000000000001125.

Li, Y., Munoz-Mayorga, D., Nie, Y., Kang, N., Tao, Y., Lagerwall, J., ... Chen, X. (2024). Microglial lipid droplet accumulation in tauopathy brain is regulated by neuronal AMPK. *Cell Metabolism, 36*(6), 1351–1370.e8. https://doi.org/10.1016/j.cmet.2024.03.014.

Mader, M. M.-D., Napole, A., Wu, D., Atkins, M., Scavetti, A., Shibuya, Y., ... Wernig, M. (2024). Myeloid cell replacement is neuroprotective in chronic experimental autoimmune encephalomyelitis. *Nature Neuroscience, 27*(5), 901–912. https://doi.org/10.1038/s41593-024-01609-3.

Mader, M. M.-D., Scavetti, A., Yoo, Y., Chai, A. T., Uenaka, T., & Wernig, M. (2025). Therapeutic genetic restoration through allogeneic brain microglia replacement. *Nature, 646*(8086), 903–912. https://doi.org/10.1038/s41586-025-09461-6.

Marschallinger, J., Iram, T., Zardeneta, M., Lee, S. E., Lehallier, B., Haney, M. S., ... Wyss-Coray, T. (2020). Lipid-droplet-accumulating microglia represent a dysfunctional and proinflammatory state in the aging brain. *Nature Neuroscience, 23*(2), 194–208. https://doi.org/10.1038/s41593-019-0566-1.

Martins-Ferreira, R., Calafell-Segura, J., Leal, B., Rodríguez-Ubreva, J., Martínez-Saez, E., Mereu, E., ... Ballestar, E. (2025). The human microglia atlas (HuMicA) unravels changes in disease-associated microglia subsets across neurodegenerative conditions. *Nature Communications, 16*(1), 739. https://doi.org/10.1038/s41467-025-56124-1.

Mason, H. D., Latour, Y. L., Boughter, C. T., Johnson, K. R., Maric, D., Dorrier, C. E., ... McGavern, D. B. (2025). Granzyme K+ CD8 T cells slow tauopathy progression by targeting microglia. *Nature Immunology, 26*(7), 1152–1167. https://doi.org/10.1038/s41590-025-02198-4.

Mass, E., Jacome-Galarza, C. E., Blank, T., Lazarov, T., Durham, B. H., Ozkaya, N., ... Geissmann, F. (2017). A somatic mutation in erythro-myeloid progenitors causes neurodegenerative disease. *Nature, 549*(7672), 389–393. https://doi.org/10.1038/nature23672.

Mazzitelli, J. A., Smyth, L. C. D., Cross, K. A., Dykstra, T., Sun, J., Du, S., ... Kipnis, J. (2022). Cerebrospinal fluid regulates skull bone marrow niches via direct access through dural channels. *Nature Neuroscience, 25*(5), 555–560. https://doi.org/10.1038/s41593-022-01029-1.

McKinney, J. E., Bennett, M. L., & Bennett, F. C. (2026). Basic microglial functions and how they go awry in neurodegenerative disease. *Annual Review of Pathology: Mechanisms of Disease, 21*(1), 59–80. https://doi.org/10.1146/annurev-pathmechdis-042624-114332.

Myhre, C. L., Thygesen, C., Villadsen, B., Vollerup, J., Ilkjær, L., Krohn, K. T., ... Finsen, B. (2019). Microglia express insulin-like growth factor-1 in the hippocampus of aged APPswe/PS1ΔE9 transgenic mice. *Frontiers in Cellular Neuroscience, 13*. https://doi.org/10.3389/fncel.2019.00308.

Nguyen, P. T., Dorman, L. C., Pan, S., Vainchtein, I. D., Han, R. T., Nakao-Inoue, H., ... Molofsky, A. V. (2020). Microglial remodeling of the extracellular matrix promotes synapse plasticity. *Cell, 182*(2), 388–403.e15. https://doi.org/10.1016/j.cell.2020.05.050.

Nimmerjahn, A., Kirchhoff, F., & Helmchen, F. (2005). Resting microglial cells are highly dynamic surveillants of brain parenchyma in vivo. *Science (New York, N. Y.), 308*(5726), 1314–1318. https://doi.org/10.1126/science.1110647.

Pachter, J. S., de Vries, H. E., & Fabry, Z. (2003). The blood-brain barrier and its role in immune privilege in the central nervous system. *Journal of Neuropathology & Experimental Neurology, 62*(6), 593–604. https://doi.org/10.1093/jnen/62.6.593.

Paloneva, J., Manninen, T., Christman, G., Hovanes, K., Mandelin, J., Adolfsson, R., ... Peltonen, L. (2002). Mutations in two genes encoding different subunits of a receptor signaling complex result in an identical disease phenotype. *American Journal of Human Genetics, 71*(3), 656–662. https://doi.org/10.1086/342259.

Paolicelli, R. C., Bolasco, G., Pagani, F., Maggi, L., Scianni, M., Panzanelli, P., ... Gross, C. T. (2011). Synaptic pruning by microglia is necessary for normal brain development. *Science (New York, N. Y.), 333*(6048), 1456–1458. https://doi.org/10.1126/science.1202529.

Paolicelli, R. C., Sierra, A., Stevens, B., Tremblay, M.-E., Aguzzi, A., Ajami, B., ... Wyss-Coray, T. (2022). Microglia states and nomenclature: A field at its crossroads. *Neuron, 110*(21), 3458–3483. https://doi.org/10.1016/j.neuron.2022.10.020.

Parkhurst, C. N., Yang, G., Ninan, I., Savas, J. N., Yates, J. R., Lafaille, J. J., ... Gan, W.-B. (2013). Microglia promote learning-dependent synapse formation through brain-derived neurotrophic factor. *Cell, 155*(7), 1596–1609. https://doi.org/10.1016/j.cell.2013.11.030.

Petry, P., Oschwald, A., & Kierdorf, K. (2023). Microglial tissue surveillance: The never-resting gardener in the developing and adult CNS. *European Journal of Immunology, 53*(7), https://doi.org/10.1002/eji.202250232.

Prinz, M., Jung, S., & Priller, J. (2019). Microglia biology: One century of evolving concepts. *Cell, 179*(2), 292–311. https://doi.org/10.1016/j.cell.2019.08.053.

Puntambekar, S. S., Moutinho, M., Lin, P. B.-C., Jadhav, V., Tumbleson-Brink, D., Balaji, A., ... Lamb, B. T. (2022). CX3CR1 deficiency aggravates amyloid driven neuronal pathology and cognitive decline in Alzheimer's disease. *Molecular Neurodegeneration, 17*(1), 47. https://doi.org/10.1186/s13024-022-00545-9.

Rademakers, R., Baker, M., Nicholson, A. M., Rutherford, N. J., Finch, N., Soto-Ortolaza, A., ... Wszolek, Z. K. (2011). Mutations in the colony stimulating factor 1 receptor (CSF1R) gene cause hereditary diffuse leukoencephalopathy with spheroids. *Nature Genetics, 44*(2), 200–205. https://doi.org/10.1038/ng.1027.

Sabatino, J. J., Pröbstel, A.-K., & Zamvil, S. S. (2019). B cells in autoimmune and neurodegenerative central nervous system diseases. *Nature Reviews. Neuroscience, 20*(12), 728–745. https://doi.org/10.1038/s41583-019-0233-2.

Sadeghdoust, M., Das, A., & Kaushik, D. K. (2024). Fueling neurodegeneration: Metabolic insights into microglia functions. *Journal of Neuroinflammation, 21*(1), 300. https://doi.org/10.1186/s12974-024-03296-0.

Schafer, D. P., Lehrman, E. K., Kautzman, A. G., Koyama, R., Mardinly, A. R., Yamasaki, R., ... Stevens, B. (2012). Microglia sculpt postnatal neural circuits in an activity and complement-dependent manner. *Neuron, 74*(4), 691–705. https://doi.org/10.1016/j.neuron.2012.03.026.

Scheiblich, H., Eikens, F., Wischhof, L., Opitz, S., Jüngling, K., Cserép, C., ... Heneka, M. T. (2024). Microglia rescue neurons from aggregate-induced neuronal dysfunction and death through tunneling nanotubes. *Neuron, 112*(18), 3106–3125.e8. https://doi.org/10.1016/j.neuron.2024.06.029.

Scopa, C., Marrocco, F., Latina, V., Ruggeri, F., Corvaglia, V., La Regina, F., ... Cattaneo, A. (2020). Impaired adult neurogenesis is an early event in Alzheimer's disease neurodegeneration, mediated by intracellular Aβ oligomers. *Cell Death & Differentiation, 27*(3), 934–948. https://doi.org/10.1038/s41418-019-0409-3.

Scott, K. M. (2022). B Lymphocytes in Parkinson's disease. *Journal of Parkinson's Disease, 12*(s1), S75–S81. https://doi.org/10.3233/JPD-223418.

Scott-Hewitt, N., Perrucci, F., Morini, R., Erreni, M., Mahoney, M., Witkowska, A., ... Matteoli, M. (2020). Local externalization of phosphatidylserine mediates developmental synaptic pruning by microglia. *The EMBO Journal, 39*(16), https://doi.org/10.15252/embj.2020105380.

Shi, F.-D., & Yong, V. W. (2025). Neuroinflammation across neurological diseases. *Science (New York, N. Y.), 388*(6753), https://doi.org/10.1126/science.adx0043.

Sierra, A., Encinas, J. M., Deudero, J. J. P., Chancey, J. H., Enikolopov, G., Overstreet-Wadiche, L. S., ... Maletic-Savatic, M. (2010). Microglia shape adult hippocampal neurogenesis through apoptosis-coupled phagocytosis. *Cell Stem Cell,* 7(4), 483–495. https://doi.org/10.1016/j.stem.2010.08.014.

Silva, N. J., Anderson, S. R., Mula, S. A., Escoubas, C. C., Nakajo, H., & Molofsky, A. V. (2026). Microglial cathepsin B is necessary for neuronal efferocytosis in zebrafish and mice during brain development. *Nature Communications.* https://doi.org/10.1038/s41467-026-70350-1.

Smyth, L. C. D., & Kipnis, J. (2025). Redefining CNS immune privilege. *Nature Reviews. Immunology, 25*(10), 766–775. https://doi.org/10.1038/s41577-025-01175-0.

Soliman, E., Gudenschwager Basso, E. K., Ju, J., Willison, A., & Theus, M. H. (2025). Skull bone marrow-derived immune cells infiltrate the injured cerebral cortex and exhibit anti-inflammatory properties. *Brain, Behavior, and Immunity, 123*, 244–253. https://doi.org/10.1016/j.bbi.2024.09.023.

Stevens, B., Allen, N. J., Vazquez, L. E., Howell, G. R., Christopherson, K. S., Nouri, N., ... Barres, B. A. (2007). The classical complement cascade mediates CNS synapse elimination. *Cell, 131*(6), 1164–1178. https://doi.org/10.1016/j.cell.2007.10.036.

Terreros-Roncal, J., Moreno-Jiménez, E. P., Flor-García, M., Rodríguez-Moreno, C. B., Trinchero, M. F., Cafini, F., ... Llorens-Martín, M. (2021). Impact of neurodegenerative diseases on human adult hippocampal neurogenesis. *Science (New York, N. Y.), 374*(6571), 1106–1113. https://doi.org/10.1126/science.abl5163.

Tesseur, I., Zou, K., Esposito, L., Bard, F., Berber, E., Can, J. V., ... Wyss-Coray, T. (2006). Deficiency in neuronal TGF-β signaling promotes neurodegeneration and Alzheimer's pathology. *Journal of Clinical Investigation, 116*(11), 3060–3069. https://doi.org/10.1172/JCI27341.

Touil, H., Li, R., Zuroff, L., Moore, C. S., Healy, L., Cignarella, F., ... Bar-Or, A. (2023). Cross-talk between B cells, microglia and macrophages, and implications to central nervous system compartmentalized inflammation and progressive multiple sclerosis. *EBioMedicine, 96*, 104789. https://doi.org/10.1016/j.ebiom.2023.104789.

Tsourmas, K. I., Butler, C. A., Kwang, N. E., Sloane, Z. R., Dykman, K. J. G., Maloof, G. O., ... Green, K. N. (2025). Microglial replacement in a Sandhoff disease mouse model reveals myeloid-derived β-hexosaminidase is necessary for neuronal health. *Nature Communications, 16*(1), 7994. https://doi.org/10.1038/s41467-025-63237-0.

Vainchtein, I. D., Chin, G., Cho, F. S., Kelley, K. W., Miller, J. G., Chien, E. C., ... Molofsky, A. V. (2018). Astrocyte-derived interleukin-33 promotes microglial synapse engulfment and neural circuit development. *Science (New York, N. Y.), 359*(6381), 1269–1273. https://doi.org/10.1126/science.aal3589.

Van Hoecke, L., Van Acker, L., & Vandenbroucke, R. E. (2026). Decoding brain border immunity to enable future therapeutic avenues. *Trends in Immunology, 47*(4), 320–336. https://doi.org/10.1016/j.it.2025.12.007.

Ware, K., Peter, J., Yazell, J., Thapa, C., Taranov, A., Bedolla, A., ... Luo, Y. (2026). Inhibition of TGF-β signaling in microglia stimulates hippocampal adult neurogenesis and reduces anxiety-like behavior in adult mice. *Nature Communications, 17*(1), 1440. https://doi.org/10.1038/s41467-026-68885-4.

Werneburg, S., Jung, J., Kunjamma, R. B., Ha, S.-K., Luciano, N. J., Willis, C. M., ... Schafer, D. P. (2020). Targeted complement inhibition at synapses prevents microglial synaptic engulfment and synapse loss in demyelinating disease. *Immunity, 52*(1), 167–182.e7. https://doi.org/10.1016/j.immuni.2019.12.004.

Williams, G. P., Schonhoff, A. M., Jurkuvenaite, A., Gallups, N. J., Standaert, D. G., & Harms, A. S. (2021). CD4 T cells mediate brain inflammation and neurodegeneration in a mouse model of Parkinson's disease. *Brain, 144*(7), 2047–2059. https://doi.org/10.1093/brain/awab103.

Wilson, D. M., Cookson, M. R., Van Den Bosch, L., Zetterberg, H., Holtzman, D. M., & Dewachter, I. (2023). Hallmarks of neurodegenerative diseases. *Cell, 186*(4), 693–714. https://doi.org/10.1016/j.cell.2022.12.032.

Wilton, D. K., Mastro, K., Heller, M. D., Gergits, F. W., Willing, C. R., Fahey, J. B., ... Stevens, B. (2023). Microglia and complement mediate early corticostriatal synapse loss and cognitive dysfunction in Huntington's disease. *Nature Medicine, 29*(11), 2866–2884. https://doi.org/10.1038/s41591-023-02566-3.

Wlodarczyk, A., Holtman, I. R., Krueger, M., Yogev, N., Bruttger, J., Khorooshi, R., ... Owens, T. (2017). A novel microglial subset plays a key role in myelinogenesis in developing brain. *The EMBO Journal, 36*(22), 3292–3308. https://doi.org/10.15252/embj.201696056.

Wu, J., Wang, Y., Li, X., Ouyang, P., Cai, Y., He, Y., ... Peng, B. (2025). Microglia replacement halts the progression of microgliopathy in mice and humans. *Science (New York, N. Y.), 389*(6756), https://doi.org/10.1126/science.adr1015.

Xing, J., Titus, A. R., & Humphrey, M. B. (2015). The TREM2-DAP12 signaling pathway in Nasu-Hakola disease: A molecular genetics perspective. *Research and Reports in Biochemistry, 5*, 89–100. https://doi.org/10.2147/RRBC.S58057.

Yildiz, O., Schroth, J., Tree, T., Turner, M. R., Shaw, P. J., Henson, S. M., & Malaspina, A. (2023). Senescent-like blood lymphocytes and disease progression in amyotrophic lateral sclerosis. *Neurology Neuroimmunology & Neuroinflammation, 10*(1), https://doi.org/10.1212/NXI.0000000000200042.

Yoo, Y., Neumayer, G., Shibuya, Y., Mader, M. M.-D., & Wernig, M. (2023). A cell therapy approach to restore microglial Trem2 function in a mouse model of Alzheimer's disease. *Cell Stem Cell, 30*(8), 1043–1053.e6. https://doi.org/10.1016/j.stem.2023.07.006.

Yu, D., Jain, S., Wangzhou, A., Zhu, B., Shao, W., Coley-O'Rourke, E. J., ... Piao, X. (2025). Microglia regulate GABAergic neurogenesis in prenatal human brain through IGF1. *Nature, 646*(8085), 676–686. https://doi.org/10.1038/s41586-025-09362-8.

Zhang, J., Fang, W., Liu, H., Li, R., Zhu, Z., Wu, X., ... Chen, X. (2025). Bone marrow B lymphopoiesis accelerates early cerebral amyloid pathology. *Signal Transduction and Targeted Therapy, 10*(1), 312. https://doi.org/10.1038/s41392-025-02419-0.

Zhao, S., Umpierre, A. D., & Wu, L.-J. (2024). Tuning neural circuits and behaviors by microglia in the adult brain. *Trends in Neurosciences, 47*(3), 181–194. https://doi.org/10.1016/j.tins.2023.12.003.

9780443470547